# Praise for
# THE DEVELOPING MIND

"A tour de force of synthesis and integration. Siegel has woven a rich tapestry that provides a compelling account of how our interpersonal worlds and neural systems form two important pillars of the mind. The second edition brings the latest neuroscientific evidence to the fore; it is a 'must read' for any student or professional interested in mental health, child development, and the brain."
—RICHARD J. DAVIDSON, PhD, William James and Vilas Professor of Psychology and Psychiatry; Founder and Chair, Center for Investigating Healthy Minds, University of Wisconsin–Madison

"With the original publication of *The Developing Mind*, the field of interpersonal neurobiology was born. Siegel's genius for synthesizing and humanizing neuroscience, attachment, and developmental theory made the book a bestseller and attracted thousands to this new field. The second edition benefits from over a decade's worth of additional findings, reflections, ideas, and insights. I encourage you to take Siegel up on his offer to share this fascinating journey, whether for the first time or for a return trip. You won't be disappointed."
—LOUIS COZOLINO, PhD, Department of Psychology, Pepperdine University

"When *The Developing Mind* was first published, Siegel's proposal that mind, brain, and relationships represented 'three aspects of one reality' essential to human well-being still seemed closer to inspired speculation than teachable scientific knowledge. Just over a decade later, the neurobiology of interpersonal experience has grown into one of the hottest areas of psychological research. Over two thousand new references surveyed for the second edition testify to just how far neuroscientists, developmental psychologists, and clinicians have brought the field as they begin to more fully chart the interplay of mind, body, and relationships. This splendid second edition—at once accessibly written and meticulously documented—provides a comprehensive guide to this emerging science."—SARAH BLAFFER HRDY, PhD, Professor Emerita of Anthropology, University of California, Davis

"Siegel describes his book as 'a journey into the developing mind,' and no one is better equipped to invite psychotherapists and other students of human impulses to share this remarkable adventure. In clear and inspired prose, he reviews facts and theories about the human brain that can be difficult to grasp. He explains how the brain differentiates and enables the creative and passionate mind of a child to share meaningful intentions, experiences, imaginative beliefs, relationships, community, culture, and language. He puts this understanding in the service of a humane and respectful psychotherapy that can give integrity to young lives that have become anxious, chaotic, and rigid."
—COLWYN TREVARTHEN, PhD, FRSE, Professor Emeritus of Child Psychology and Psychobiology, University of Edinburgh, United Kingdom

"Fulfilled my wildest expectations. Instead of laboriously struggling to learn about neurobiology, I found myself fairly effortlessly assimilating information because 1) the author is able to present his material in the context of interpersonal relationships in general and the treatment dyad in particular, and 2) the author is a master of lucidity, avoids pedantry, and succeeds in making his data clinically useful."—*American Journal of Psychiatry*

"Readable, thoughtful, and informative."—*Educational Leadership*

"I knew that this book was one I should keep handy when I wanted to improve my understanding of information on which the future science of psychiatry will be based."—*Journal of Clinical Psychiatry*

"A remarkable book. . . . *The Developing Mind* boldly transcends the reductionism that characterizes so much of contemporary psychiatry."—*Psychiatric Times*

"Current, thorough, closely argued. . . . One of Siegel's major gifts is for presenting anatomical, neurological, research, and clinical information while still pointing out what remains unknown. He explores infant–parent relationships, emotions, states of mind, and how knowing about them can help one improve one's relationships and capabilities for developing successfully."—*Booklist*

"Why can't we remember what we did at age three? Why are some children unusually shy? What is the biochemistry of humiliation, and how can it be 'toxic to the developing child's brain'? New and plausible answers to these questions emerge from Siegel's synthesis of neurobiology, research psychology and cognitive science. . . . His subject—how we become the people we are— deserves to hold many readers spellbound."—*Publishers Weekly*

"The story Siegel tells is indeed fascinating, essentially describing the transactional processes that happen at the interface between developmental neurobiology and the environment of an individual. He links every level of the system from cell chemistry to brain architecture, to caregiver–infant attachments, to interpersonal relationships in adulthood. . . . This is a book to stimulate, illuminate, and drive our understanding of human developmental processes forwards and I suspect that *The Developing Mind* will be seen as a milestone work in the future."—*Journal of Child Psychology and Psychiatry*

"Brilliant. . . . It should probably not be read at one sitting, but sifted slowly as you would a 20 year old port. . . . This is not just a book for bright psychiatric residents or child fellows, but child psychiatrists young and old, overworked or underpaid. It offers a glimpse of new horizons in the profession."—*Canadian Child Psychiatry Review*

# THE DEVELOPING MIND

# The Developing Mind

## How Relationships and the Brain Interact to Shape Who We Are

### SECOND EDITION

## Daniel J. Siegel

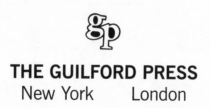

**THE GUILFORD PRESS**
New York    London

Published by The Guilford Press
A Division of Guilford Publications, Inc.
72 Spring Street, New York, NY 10012
www.guilford.com

Printed in the United States of America

This book is printed on acid-free paper.

Last digit is print number:   9   8   7   6   5   4   3   2   1

The author has checked with sources believed to be reliable in his efforts to
provide information that is complete and generally in accord with the standards
of practice that are accepted at the time of publication. However, in view of the
possibility of human error or changes in behavioral, mental health, or medical
sciences, neither the author, nor the editor and publisher, nor any other party
who has been involved in the preparation or publication of this work warrants
that the information contained herein is in every respect accurate or complete,
and they are not responsible for any errors or omissions or the results obtained
from the use of such information. Readers are encouraged to confirm the
information contained in this book with other sources.

**Library of Congress Cataloging-in-Publication Data**

Siegel, Daniel J., 1957–
    The developing mind : how relationships and the brain interact to shape who
we are / Daniel J. Siegel. — 2nd ed.
        p. cm.
    Includes bibliographical references and index.
    ISBN 978-1-4625-0390-2 (hardcover: alk. paper)
    1. Developmental psychology.    2. Interpersonal relations.    3. Intellect.
4. Brain—Physiological aspects.    I. Title.
    BF713.S525 2012
    155—dc23
                                                                2011052460

*For Maddi*

# About the Author

**Daniel J. Siegel, MD,** is an internationally acclaimed author, award-winning educator, and renowned child psychiatrist. He is Clinical Professor of Psychiatry at the School of Medicine of the University of California, Los Angeles, where he serves as Co-Investigator at the Center for Culture, Brain, and Development, and Co-Director of the Mindful Awareness Research Center. He is also the Executive Director of the Mindsight Institute, an educational center devoted to promoting insight, compassion, and empathy in individuals, families, institutions, and communities. Dr. Siegel's books include *Mindsight, Pocket Guide to Interpersonal Neurobiology, The Mindful Therapist, The Mindful Brain, Parenting from the Inside Out*, and *The Whole-Brain Child*.

# Preface to the Second Edition

Welcome to the fascinating world of interdisciplinary thinking. I invite you to join me on this journey to explore the intricate intertwining of mind, brain, and relationships. Since the publication of the first edition of *The Developing Mind* over a dozen years ago, much has emerged from the objective study of science and the subjective knowledge of internal reflection. This book honors these distinct but equally important realms of knowledge that will inform our travels.

In this second edition, I have had the deep honor to incorporate what I've learned from scientists, psychotherapists, educators, philosophers, contemplative practitioners, and community leaders. The field that the first edition of this book introduced—"interpersonal neurobiology," or simply "IPNB"—has grown in wonderful ways since then. It now has its own organizations (see the Global Association for Interpersonal Neurobiology Studies, or GAINS), in-depth educational programs (see *www.mindsightinstitute.com*), and a professional library of over two dozen textbooks.

My goal in thoroughly updating the references and revising the text for this edition is to make the ideas of IPNB and its scientific foundations as clear and concise as possible. I have had the good fortune of having 15 dedicated and bright research interns work by my side during the initial phases of this revision process. Their assignment was twofold: to "prove the first edition of this book and the ideas behind IPNB to be wrong" so that we could discard any proposals that were outdated or unfounded in the literature, and to offer any new research that presented alternative views. In this effort, over two thousand new scientific papers were reviewed; each paragraph of the book (projected on the wall at the Mindsight Institute) was collectively examined; and any necessary changes were made. In this process, we had the advantage of fresh minds exploring the foundations of IPNB to see whether any of the hypotheses set forth over a dozen years ago had since been proven with new studies and emerging technology. When we found that the majority of propositions were in fact supported by new findings, the shared experience was exhilarating.

We also had the opportunity to interview several readers of the first edition—many of them teachers of the book for over a decade now—and to ask them, "What should be changed in the second edition?" Their virtually uniform response was "Nothing, except to update the scientific references." So to stay true to the positive reception of the first edition, here in the second edition you'll find that the text has been thoroughly updated to reflect the research advances in various fields. I have also added special discussions of culture, gender, temperament, genetics, and the role of consciousness and its neural correlates in various mental and social processes. Most of the proposals have been supported by research findings enabled by recent technological advances, and for those that remain hypotheses, the text still reflects their status as educated guesses. Keeping the distinction between implications and data-supported findings clear was an important feature of the original text and remains a goal for this edition, and for the field of IPNB as a whole.

This new edition also has an epilogue reflecting on various practical and scientific aspects of this approach, as well as a glossary of terms to improve access to some of the intricate ideas and their vocabulary. In addition, there are new figures and frequent "pullout" quotations to support those who enjoy and benefit from these visual aids to learning. In discussing examples throughout the book, I alternate between the third-person singular pronouns "she" and "he" to avoid sexist usage. Naturally, all examples of individuals are presented without identifying features.

*The Developing Mind* has become a favorite book in a variety of programs; I hope that this second edition continues to be as well received. I love writing books, and returning to this first work to create a second edition has been a labor of love. This edition may have roughly the same sequence of chapters, but it is filled with fresh material and the integration of many new ideas and applications. I am grateful for all of the input we have received from readers from around the globe, and also to the many authors and conference co-faculty members who share in the passion for creating a consilient approach to this work. Marion Solomon and Bonnie Goldstein have been a wonderful team in bringing IPNB to the professional audience at our annual UCLA gatherings, and I thank them for their leadership in our professional community. Kitty Moore, the initial editor at The Guilford Press who brought this work into the world, is a joy to work with, and I am thankful for all of her support and wisdom over the years. Barbara Watkins worked with me on the day-to-day, line-by-line editing, and I cannot say enough in gratitude for her superb skills and for the way she kept the whole in mind while also paying such careful attention to detail and continuity. We had the exciting challenge of taking something people loved, updating it completely, and maintaining the essence of its heart and soul, while also refining the message with clear and integrated prose. It has been a pleasure to pore over these pages with her to get the book ready to go to press. Marie Sprayberry again magnificently copyedited the manuscript, and Martin Coleman served as production editor.

I would also like to thank the wonderful individuals who are a part of the Mindsight Institute, which serves as an intellectual home for IPNB. Our global online course participants' international perspective on the field and its application is invaluable for seeing the many ways in which this work can be applied across cultures. Input from students, both local and at a distance, has been a driving force for this work and motivates all of us to keep the field current. The members of our staff, including Stephanie Hamilton and Whitney Stambler, have made working here a pleasure. Whitney was devoted to making the extensive references and notes well integrated throughout the book, and I thank her for those efforts. I am also grateful for the assistance of Eric Bergemann and Aubrey Siegel in helping to do some of the final copyediting of the manuscript. Caroline Welch, our CEO, has been both an inspiration and a powerful presence in helping us to organize our work and create a vision for the many possible applications of IPNB in the world. I thank her for her leadership, which is at the heart of this second edition's message.

To dive into over a dozen disciplines of science and explore the consilient findings that emerge is naturally quite a challenge. For the first edition, the library was my second home, where I'd spend long hours wading into the stacks of periodicals. Since then, there has been an exponential increase in the number of journals and research articles accessible through our interconnected digital library via the Internet. Taking on this goal of updating the book was a joy with the fabulous group of interns who joined in on the intellectual adventure. Working together, we could explore research data, cross-reference a wide range of studies, integrate ideas, and weave all of these together in creating the second edition. I am deeply grateful for the companionship of this "mindful bunch": Lisa Baldini, Kimberly Clark, Hannah Farber, Julien Fyhrie, Victoria Goldfarb, Riley Kessler, Cyrus Nahai, Benjamin Nelson, Karen Olivares, Suzanne Parker, Francesca Reinisch, Gregory Sewitz, Katey Solzberg, Lucy Walsh, and Anabel Young. We went on a creative journey of discovery together, and I am thankful for their dedication to this project. It is my sincerest wish that this book you hold in your hands will maintain its usefulness as a solid resource, helping us to support the development of healthy and resilient minds throughout our lives.

# Preface to the First Edition

What is the mind? How does the mind develop? This book synthesizes information from a range of scientific disciplines to explore the idea that the mind emerges at the interface of interpersonal experience and the structure and function of the brain.

Like many adolescents, as a teenager I became filled with a particular intellectual passion: I was fascinated with people and the nature of the mind. Through a series of journeys, I eventually became a psychiatrist, specializing in the care of children and families. Along the way have been encounters with a wide variety of people and the stories of their lives. Trained in science and immersed in human struggles, I found myself naturally trying to understand the process of human development—of how people become who they are—by investigating what was known from research and getting as close as possible to the subjective experience at the core of people's lives. This book presents the integration of this effort to gain insights into the mind and human development.

From mountaintops and quiet conversations to lecture halls and the bustling discussions of a weekend conference, this exploration of the nature of the developing mind has come to involve people from many walks of life. At recent seminars, I have met with a range of professionals—in child development, education, medicine, neuroscience, psychology, public administration, and social work—to discuss basic questions regarding the mind and the ways experience shapes development. These experiences as an educator have motivated me to synthesize this work into a framework that provides an integrated scientific foundation regarding the interpersonal and neurobiological basis of the developing mind.

This book may be useful for those working in a variety of disciplines. Understanding these processes can enable clinicians to help patients heal. Academicians may find such an interdisciplinary effort useful in gaining insight into how their own work relates to independent fields of research.

Educators can benefit from insights into how emotion and interpersonal relationships are fundamental motivational aspects of learning and memory. For child development specialists and others who care for children, knowing how forms of communication directly shape a child's developing brain can be essential in creating programs that are scientifically based and that can optimize the care of children. For many other people, learning about how the mind emerges from the substance of the brain and the processes of interpersonal relationships can provide useful insights that can improve their professional as well as personal lives. Interpersonal experience shapes the mind as it continues to develop throughout the lifespan. This book is about *how* these interpersonal processes occur and how we can utilize ideas about neurobiology to help others, and ourselves, to grow and develop.

In my own field of psychiatry, the tremendous expansion of neuroscientific research seems to have been interpreted in the extreme by some as a call to "biological determinism"—that is, to a view of psychiatric disorders as a result of biochemical processes, most of which are genetically determined and little influenced by experience. This impression may sound reductionistic, but I wish that the sense of demoralization expressed by many educators and students in psychiatry didn't support the notion that the field has been losing its mind in favor of the brain. What is ironic, and what up until now has not been well known, is that recent findings of neural science in fact point to just the opposite: Interactions with the environment, especially relationships with other people, directly shape the development of the brain's structure and function. There is no need to choose between brain or mind, biology or experience, nature or nurture. These rigidly applied divisions are unhelpful and inhibit clear thinking about an important and complex subject: the developing human mind.

As I was finishing up the last chapter revisions for this book, an article by a renowned neuroscientist who is also trained as a psychiatrist appeared in the *American Journal of Psychiatry*. Eric Kandel's paper "A New Intellectual Framework for Psychiatry"[1] suggests that the field of psychiatry in recent times has suffered from a series of damaging divisions within its ranks. These divisions have blocked the ability to integrate a wide range of information about human experience, mind, and brain. It is my hope that presenting a scientifically grounded synthesis focusing on these domains will enable such professional divisions to give way to a new conceptual foundation that will be useful for clinicians and others who help people develop.

Although it is important to be aware of the significant and very real contributions of genetic and constitutional factors to the outcome of development, it is equally crucial that we examine what in fact is known about how experience shapes development. Such a balanced view enables us as parents, for example, to have a sense of responsibility for the experiences we provide without the unnecessary burden of guilt generated by the belief that our actions are solely responsible for the outcome of our children's development.

One factor turning some mental health care providers' attention away from the role of experience in human development may be our attempt to avoid some of the devastating errors of the past. Not so long ago, the mothers of children with autism were accused of being "refrigerators"; the families of patients with schizophrenia were said to be giving "double binds"; individuals with bipolar disorder were given thousands of hours of therapy, in search of the "psychological cause" of their mood swings; and people with obsessive–compulsive disorder were thought to be repressing some early trauma that may have produced their worries. In each of these painful examples, we as professionals looked toward experience to explain the causes of our patients' anguish and dysfunction. Despite the goodness of our intentions, these views were misguided and not helpful to our patients. They produced accusations of blame and a sense of guilt that were unfounded. They did not lead to growth or healing in our patients or their families.

Many people have been spared devastating amounts of pain and suffering because of our modern understanding of psychiatric illness and the appropriate use of pharmacological agents. Psychiatry has had to embrace the notion that the brain contributes to mental dysfunction, in order to pursue these extremely important avenues of medical care. But losing sight of the important role of experience, especially social experience, in shaping the mind does not help us to understand development or to help our patients.

If social factors—that is, human relationships—shape the development of the brain and the mind, *how* does this occur? The purpose of this book is to explore this question by examining some ways in which interpersonal experience shapes the developing mind and fosters emotional well-being.

An exciting challenge in writing this book has been to attempt to deepen an understanding of subjective everyday life, of the mind and human relationships, by drawing on the objective views of science. The benefit of this approach is that we can learn much more about what creates human experience than is possible with only everyday logic or self-reflection. For example, by learning how the circuits in the brain develop during the first years of life, we can gain insights into why older children or adults generally cannot consciously recall their experiences before the preschool years. By learning about the nature of how the brain creates an awareness of other minds, we can begin to understand the biological basis for emotional communication and what may be occurring when empathy is not a part of human relationships. In addition, understanding how trauma affects the developing brain can yield insights into the subsequent impairments in memory processing and the ability to cope with stress. Using science to understand the mind has provided a powerful tool for deepening our comprehension of subjective mental life and interpersonal relationships. These insights have proven tremendously useful in helping others grow and develop.

To see how these neurobiological ideas help others develop and heal not only has fueled my enthusiasm, but has generated the energy required for the completion of this book. This task would not have been possible without the loving support of my family. How many times they heard the excited call "It's finished!", only to find me working on the next draft a few weeks later. Their continuing encouragement is of immeasurable importance to me.

When The Guilford Press initially asked me to write this book, its focus was to be on memory and psychotherapy. Since that time, the topic of the book has broadened; it has come to include, with the helpful assistance of my patient editor, Kitty Moore, the much wider topic of these fundamental questions about the mind, the brain, and human relationships. I thank her for her belief in the work and her skillful help with the process of bringing it to completion. I would also like to express my appreciation to the efficient and responsive publication staff at Guilford, and especially to Anna Brackett and Marie Sprayberry, for their thoughtful attention to the text.

In my professional life, it can't be overstated that my patients have had the largest impact on my clinical education. In ways both professional and personal, they have taught me more than I ever dreamed I'd learn in a lifetime. I have also had the good fortune of having had several clinical teachers who have been especially supportive and helpful in my development as a psychotherapist, including Jim Grotstein, MD, Chris Heinicke, PhD, Regina Pally, MD, Arnold Scheibel, MD, and Don Schwartz, MD. Also along the journey have been many students—especially those in the Infant and Preschool Service, which I directed with Mary O'Connor, PhD, at UCLA, and at the Mindsight Institute and around the globe in our online class—whose questions keep an investigating and conceptualizing mind reflective and excited about trying both to understand and to communicate complex ideas. One of the most moving teaching experiences has come from the opportunity to work with many teams of psychotherapists from over a dozen nations in Eastern Europe who have been struggling to deal with the ravages of political wars and childhood abuse. The Children's Mental Health Alliance Foundation, directed by Pamela Sicher, MD, and Owen Lewis, MD, has developed a novel educational program to teach these devoted and sacrificing therapists the basic elements of evaluating, treating, and (we all hope) preventing child abuse in their developing nations. It is inspiring to see their dedication, and exhilarating to hear that the ideas of this book have been accessible and useful across cultures.

These issues about how experiences shape the brain and organize the mind were topics of passionate discussion for a local study group called, affectionately, the ID-CNS (Institute for Developmental and Clinical Neural Science). My thanks to its members—Lou Cozolino, PhD, Allan Schore, PhD, Judith Schore, PhD, and John Schumann, PhD—for our intellectual companionship on this journey into mind and brain. My childhood friend and longtime conversation partner in matters of the mind, Jonathan Fried, has offered valuable comments on the text and has been especially helpful in pointing out the abundance of "thuses" in the original manuscript; thus I thank him. Others who have read this work at various stages in its evolution and have provided immensely useful comments and questions include Daniel Attias, the late Lisa Capps, PhD, Leston Havens, MD, Erik Hesse, PhD, Althea Horner, PhD, Mary Main, PhD, Eleanor Ochs, PhD, Sarah Steinberg, Caroline Welch, and several anonymous reviewers through the editing process at The Guilford Press.

Several other people also need to be acknowledged. In medical school, Tom Whitfield III, MD, was my pediatric mentor and friend who taught me early on that "the way to care for patients is to care about them." The initial version of what was to become this book was begun on a trip to visit Tom and his wife, Peg, in the Berkshires before his death in 1996. The lessons I have learned from trying to make sense of the process of losing such an important attachment figure in my life are contained within these pages. Another person in those years who "saved my life" in medical school is Leston Havens, MD, who gave me the strength to hold on to my own experience in the confusing Boston psychiatric climate at the time. During my years of adult and child psychiatric residency, Joel Yager, MD, and Gordon Strauss, MD, and the late Dennis Cantwell, MD, supported my explorations of different directions and my efforts to organize my professional passions. In my National Institute of Mental Health research training years at UCLA, Marian Sigman, PhD, and Robert Bjork, PhD, were extremely supportive in guiding me through the wonderful interdisciplinary learning that the research fellowship allowed.

During many of those years as a trainee in psychiatry, I had the honor of being supervised by Robert Stoller, MD, who devoted much of his professional life to exploring the ways in which early life experiences shape development. We would spend hours discussing patients, the mind, and our own experiences as therapists. One of our topics was about human communication. As Bob wrote in one of his last books before his tragic accidental death:

> Still, yearning for clarity contains a pleasure of which I am only now fully aware. Sometimes, on paring a sentence down to its barest minimum, I find it transforms into a question, paradox, or joke (all three being different states of the same thing, like ice, water and steam). That is a relief: clarity asks; it does

not answer. Maybe then, in a hundred years, sitting on my haunches like a
Zen master, I shall finally write a clear sentence. But it will have no words.[2]

I have tried my best to use simple language, to avoid unnecessary jar-
gon, and to make sentences concise and clear. Though words are limited in
their ability to convey exactly what we mean, they are one of our only ways
of sharing information about complex ideas, as well as about simple truths.
Words enable us to communicate across the boundaries of time and space
that separate one mind from another. Words allow us to tell the stories of our
lives and relate the scientific explorations that reflect our drive to understand
ourselves and the world in which we live. I hope that the stories and science
in the book will help people to understand the social brain more fully and
to focus our attention on the many intriguing and important unanswered
questions about interpersonal experience and the developing mind across the
lifespan.

# Contents

# CHAPTER 1

# Mind, Brain, and Relationships
## *The Interpersonal Neurobiology Perspective*

The "mind" is rarely defined in fields that focus on mental experience. This avoidance may be due to any of several well-considered reasons. There is the understandable philosophical stance that definitions may restrict a full understanding, or the notion that the mystery of the mind makes us unable to characterize its defining features. Sometimes the word "mind" is used as a placeholder for the unknown, a marker of this mysterious source of our subjective inner life. In this book, I honor these positions while taking the risky step of exploring a working definition of the mind that has been of great value in understanding how our lives develop and what a healthy mind may actually be. After all, if we do not attempt to define at least a core aspect of the mind itself, how can we state what might constitute a healthy mind?

This book explores how recent findings from a range of sciences can bring us to a new understanding of the developing mind. The sciences give us many views of how the mind functions, providing in-depth but distinct perspectives on human experience. For example, neuroscience can inform us about how the brain gives rise to mental processes such as memory and perception. Developmental psychology offers us a view of how children's minds grow within families across time. Anthropology gives us insights into how relational experiences and communication patterns within different cultures directly shape the development of the mind. Psychiatry gives us a clinical view of how individuals may suffer from emotional and behavioral disturbances that profoundly alter the course of their lives. Often these disciplines function in isolation from one another. Yet when one attempts to synthesize their recent findings, an incredible convergence of many independent fields of study is revealed. This convergence can be called "consilience"—the discovery of common findings from independent disciplines.[1] These findings shed light on how the mind emerges from the substance of the brain and is

1

shaped by our communication within interpersonal relationships. My aim is to provide an overview and integration of some of these scientific perspectives, which serve as a foundation for a neurobiology of interpersonal experience.

More specifically, to help you to understand the developing mind, I provide an integration of mental processes (such as memory and emotion) with both neurobiology (such as neural activity in specific circuits) and interpersonal relationships (such as patterns of communication). This integration is indeed the challenge of the book, both in the writing and in the reading. My concern is with those who, like many of my past students, are new to neurobiology; the unfamiliar ideas and vocabulary may initially feel too overwhelming to continue. Numerous teaching experiences, however, have demonstrated that the outcome is worth the effort. I have tried to include enough of a background as the chapters evolve that each topic can be understood by those who may be totally unfamiliar with a given area. No prior expertise is required. New concepts and vocabulary are inevitable, but I have tried to incorporate information throughout the book in a "user-friendly" manner, summarizing the significance of certain findings and including reminders of certain trends as they recur in the book. Whatever your personal, scholarly, or professional pursuits, you will have a better understanding of unpredictable experiences after having studied this material. Learning this approach will support the scientific view that "chance favors the prepared mind," in that your own mind will be prepared with this integrative perspective to understand and respond to what arises in life. There are many readily accessible concepts and much useful information just below the surface of these sometimes new names and ideas. A shared understanding from the beginning will help you in making sense of the intricate and exciting findings about interpersonal relationships and the developing mind. For those who are charting new waters, I welcome you to the exciting world of interdisciplinary study!

## DEFINING THE MIND

Here is a definition of the mind that enabled dozens of scientists to communicate with one another about the mind: *"A core aspect of the mind is an embodied and relational process that regulates the flow of energy and information."* In the beginning of the Decade of the Brain, the 1990s, I offered this working definition to a group of over forty scientists in order to find a common starting place for us to address the connection between the mind and the brain. With this view, all of the researchers—from anthropologists to neuroscientists—could find a common way of describing each discipline's way of exploring the nature of reality. Energy and information flow is what is shared among people within a culture, and this flow is what is measured in subjects within a brain scanner. In this working definition, we also found a way

> The mind is an embodied and relational process that regulates the flow of energy and information.

to meet for over four years, sharing our various perspectives on the nature of what it means to be human. It was in the fertile soil of this gathering that the seeds of the interdisciplinary field that ultimately became interpersonal neurobiology (IPNB) were first sown. IPNB embraces everything from our deepest relational connections with one another to the synaptic connections we have within our extended nervous systems. It encompasses the interpersonal power of cultures and families, as well as insights into molecular mechanisms; each contributes to the reality of our subjective mental lives. IPNB is not a branch of neuroscience, but a broad field drawing on the findings from a wide range of disciplines that explore the nature of what it means to be human. Based on science, IPNB seeks to create an understanding of the interconnections among the brain, the mind, and our interpersonal relationships. IPNB can also be used to understand our relatedness beyond the interpersonal, to other living creatures and to our whole planet. With this approach, new strategies for both understanding and promoting well-being are possible. We can both define the mind and outline practical steps for how to cultivate a healthy mind as it develops across the lifespan.

The ideas of this framework are organized around three fundamental principles:

1. A core aspect of the human mind is an embodied and relational process that regulates the flow of energy and information within the brain and between brains.
2. The mind as an emergent property of the body and relationships is created within internal neurophysiological processes and relational experiences. In other words, the mind is a process that emerges from the distributed nervous system extending throughout the entire body, and also from the communication patterns that occur within relationships.
3. The structure and function of the developing brain are determined by how experiences, especially within interpersonal relationships, shape the genetically programmed maturation of the nervous system.

To put it simply, human connections shape neural connections, and each contributes to mind. Relationships and neural linkages together shape the mind. It is more than the sum of its parts; this is the essence of emergence.

One view of the mind parallels a dictionary definition of the psyche: "1. the human soul; 2. the intellect; 3. psychiatry—the mind considered as a subjectively perceived, functional entity, based ultimately upon physical processes but with complex processes of its own: it governs the total organism and its interaction with the environment."[2]

This book extends this notion of the mind's being more than "simply brain activity." It offers an IPNB perspective that draws on the full range of scientific disciplines to integrate everything from the societal to the synaptic. On the brain side of mental life, current neuroscience reveals the connection between brain structure and function, and provides us with new insights into how experience shapes mental processes.[3] By altering both the activity and the structure of the connections between neurons, experience directly shapes the circuits responsible for such processes as memory, emotion, and self-awareness. We now know, too, that experience and the firing of neurons can alter the regulatory molecules that control gene expression—a process called "epigenesis."[4] These epigenetic changes reveal the powerful ways in which experience modifies how the brain develops, sometimes across the lifespan. In fact, recent studies in neuroplasticity reveal how the brain continues to modify its structural connections with experience throughout life.[5] Moreover, studies of evolution suggest that our mammalian brains are profoundly social, and that relationships have a huge impact on neuronal function from the earliest days of our lives. On the relational side of our view of mind, we can draw upon a wide range of studies from development and family function to demonstrate the importance of patterns of communication between people to shape how the mind functions. We can use an understanding of the impact of experience on the mind to deepen our grasp of how the past continues to shape present experience and influence future actions. Insights into the mind, brain, relationships, and experience can provide a window into these connections across time, allowing us to see human development in a four-dimensional way.

This book synthesizes concepts and findings from a range of scientific disciplines, including those studying attachment, child development, communication, complex systems, cultural anthropology, emotion, evolution, information processing, memory, narrative, and neurobiology. I have attempted to provide enough of an introduction so that those totally unfamiliar with these domains can understand the material and apply the relevant findings in their professional work and personal lives. When we examine what is known about how the mind develops, we can gain important insights into the ways in which people can continue to grow throughout life. *The mind does not stop developing, even as we grow past childhood and adolescence.* Through understanding the connections between mental processes and brain functioning, we can build a neurobiological foundation for the ways in which interpersonal relationships—both early in life and throughout adulthood—continue to play a central role in shaping the emerging mind.

> The mind does not stop developing, even as we grow past childhood and adolescence.

## Energy and Information Flow

The mind—the regulatory process that creates patterns in the flow of energy and information—can be described as emanating in part from the activity of the neurons of the distributed nervous system.[6] Keep in mind that the "single-skull" view of mind as merely a product of the brain may be too limited. We have evolved to be social, and mental processes are a product of our inner neural connections as well as our interpersonal communicative connections with others. Without this reminder, it may be too easy to slip into the linear thinking that "mind is simply the brain's activity." The scientifically grounded view proposed in this text is that the mind arises from beyond the functioning of an isolated nervous system. Both our internal neural functions and our shared communicative processes give rise to the process defined here as mind.

It is important to underscore this issue right from the start. Sometimes neuroscience researchers or the popular media imply that the mind is simply the output of the brain. In this often-expressed view, mental life is equated with brain activity—an outcome of the firing of neurons within the brain. But in this book I take a broader view that perceives mental processes as emerging from neural functions throughout the whole body (not only the brain in the skull) *and* from relational processes (not only from one bodily self or nervous system). The mind is embodied, not just enskulled. And the mind is also relational, not a product created in isolation. These relationships include the communication an individual has with other entities in the world, especially other people. This book focuses especially on the important ways in which interpersonal relationships shape how the mind emerges in our human lives. But we also have a relationship with nature, with this planet, with the Earth upon which we live, that shapes our mental (and physical) lives as well. This is a vital form of relationship that sustains us in the air we breathe and the water we drink. But this book is focused primarily on the person-to-person aspect of our relationships. This is the social nature of the "embodied and relational process that regulates the flow of energy and information."

The implications of this definition are significant, as I hope you'll see in the journey through these pages. One implication is that we don't "own" our minds—that we, our individual "selves," are interdependent on others for the functioning of our minds. This relational part of the definition makes some people uncomfortable. Yet if you are in a family, or in a one-to-one relationship, you know that your subjective, inner mental life is profoundly influenced by others. On the scientific side, any anthrolopologist or sociologist knows from research how real this relational component of our mental lives truly is. And so what we need is a link that connects the social with the synaptic. To achieve the essential ability to move readily between these two levels of human reality, we will have to define the common ground that links them.

When one of us speaks to another, the voice box stimulates the movement of air molecules manifested as kinetic energy. The eardrum responds to this energy flow by creating electrochemical energy movement within the acoustic nerve and downstream neural circuits of the brain. Ions flow in and out of the neural membranes, and the release of chemical transmitters activates downstream neurons. When these patterns of neural firing match with prior learning, then this "energy flow" has informational value, and the listener can understand what the speaker has said.

Here we can see how "communication" is based on the *sharing* of energy and information. But what are these shared elements of mental life? Several different measures of *energy* can be used to study the different forms that energy flow takes. Brain imaging studies examine the metabolic, energy-consuming processes in specific neural regions, or the blood flow to certain areas that are thought to be a clustering of localized neuronal activity. Electroencephalograms (EEGs) assess the electrical activity across the surface of the brain as measured by electrodes on the head. These assessments of "energy flow" are not popularized, unscientific views of the flow of some mysterious substance through the universe. Neuroscience studies the way in which the brain functions through the energy-consuming activation of neurons. The degree and localization of this arousal and activation within the brain—this flow of energy—directly shape our mental processes.

But the mind is involved in more than the regulation of the flow of energy. The mind is also about regulating the flow of *information*.[7]

What is information? At the most basic level, "information" consists of swirls of energy that have symbolic meaning. If I say the term "glicanera," and you do not understand Greek, you will not derive information from that sound. Yes, the letters themselves have information; a "g" is pronounced "gee," and when it is combined with all the other letters, you can say the word "glicanera." In that way, the letters are bits of information—squiggles that stand for certain sounds. But the whole word may have no symbolic reference. If you speak Greek, you will "know" that this word means "sweet water," and that it is also the name of a magnificent beach

> "Information" consists of swirls of energy that have symbolic meaning.

on Crete. Now you know that the word "glicanera" stands for something more than the sounds of the letters. This information comes from the way the symbolic meanings are embedded in that set of sounds—the pattern of energy flow in "glee-kah-nehr-ah."

Within IPNB, we view mind, brain, and relationships as three aspects of energy and information flow. Brain is the embodied neural *mechanism* shaping that flow; relationships are the *sharing* of the flow; mind is the embodied and relational process that *regulates* the flow of energy and information. If we ask, "Where is the mind?", we can say that its regulatory functions are embodied in the nervous system and embedded in our interpersonal relationships. This emergent process of both the neural and the interpersonal locates the mind within both the physiological and relational frame of reality. The mind develops in the interaction of at least these two facets of our human lives.

Mind, brain, and relationships are not three separate elements. Instead, we are proposing that they are "three aspects of one reality"—that is, energy and information flow. Just as we have heads and tails of one coin, we can have many facets of one entity. This aspect of mind *regulates* the flow of energy and information as it is *shared* within relationships and moves through the physical *mechanisms* of the brain, the embodied neural connections within the extended nervous system distributed throughout the whole body. This "embodied brain" is simply referred to hereafter as the "brain," for ease of reference, reading, and writing. Please note, too, that a self-organizing process like the mind is an emergent property of a system. This process both *arises from* the interaction of the system's elements (energy and information flow within the body and are shared between people) and also *regulates* in a recursive way the very elements from which it arose. This recursive, reentry property of mind, typical of self-organizing emergent processes, means that relationships and brain shape mind and mind shapes relationships and brain. Mind, brain, and relationships are three aspects of one system: regulation, embodied mechanism, and sharing of energy and information flow. We'll be exploring these intricate and fascinating aspects of the mind throughout the pages of our journey together. Figure 1.1 shows this triangle of human experience, with mind, brain, and relationships representing aspects of energy and information flow.

This may be a new way for you to think, but embracing mental, neural, and relational processes as involving energy and information flow patterns is a powerful way to blend science with the subjective nature of our human lives. Naturally, our mental experience is far more than a regulatory process; it involves the subjective quality of our consciousness and the inner ways of knowing that enrich our sense of feeling, meaning, purpose, love, connection, and wholeness. However, learning about the regulatory aspect of mind

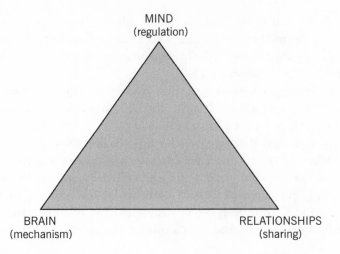

**FIGURE 1.1.** Three aspects of energy and information flow. Adapted from *The Mindful Therapist: A Clinician's Guide to Mindsight and Neural Integration* by Daniel J. Siegel. Copyright © 2010 by Mind Your Brain, Inc. Used by permission of W. W. Norton & Company, Inc.

empowers us to see more deeply into the ways the mind develops as the brain changes and as relationships evolve over time. As you'll see, certain patterns of this flow involve a flexible and adaptive outcome; mind, brain, and relationships can be intentionally moved toward health. This pattern of healthy living involves the *integration of energy and information within the nervous system and between people.* Integration is the organizing principle that links the ways energy and information flow is shared (relationships), is shaped (the mechanisms of the embodied nervous system or, termed simply, the brain), and is regulated (the mind).

## Integration

The mind has distinct modes of processing information. For example, our sensory systems can respond to stimuli from the outside world, such as sights or sounds, and can "represent" this information as patterns of neural firing that serve as mental symbols. The activity of the brain creates "representations" of various types of information about the outer and inner worlds. For example, we have representations of sensations in the body, of perceptions from our five senses, of ideas and concepts, and of words. Each of these forms of representation is thought to be created in different circuits of the brain. These information-processing modes can act independently, and they also have important interactions with one another that directly affect their processing. We can have complex representations of sensations, perceptions, ideas, and linguistic symbols as we think, for example, of some time in the past. The weaving together of these distinct modes

> Linking differentiated parts into a functional whole is called "integration."

of information processing into a coherent whole may be a central goal for the developing mind across the lifespan. *This process of linking differentiated parts into a functional whole is called "integration."* As we'll see, integration is a unifying principle that will help us to understand the linkage of mind, brain, and relationships throughout our discussions. Furthermore, in IPNB, we propose that integration is the heart of health.

Interpersonal relationships may facilitate or inhibit this drive to integrate a coherent experience. Relationships early in life may shape the very neural structures that create representations of experience and allow a coherent view of the world: Interpersonal experiences directly influence how we mentally construct reality. This shaping process occurs throughout life, but is most crucial during the early years of childhood. Patterns of relationships and emotional communication directly affect the development of the brain. Studies in animals, for example, have demonstrated that even short episodes of maternal deprivation have powerful neuroendocrine and epigenetic effects on the ability to cope with future stressful events. Studies of human subjects reveal that different patterns of child–parent attachment are associated with differing physiological responses, ways of seeing the world, and interpersonal relationship patterns.[8] The communication of emotion may be the primary means by which these attachment experiences shape the developing mind. Research suggests that emotion serves as a central organizing process within the brain. In this way, an individual's abilities to organize emotions—a product, in part, of earlier attachment relationships—directly shapes the ability of the mind to integrate experience and to adapt to future stressors.

## Differentiation and Linkage

To understand integration, we must unpack its two fundamental components: "differentiation" and "linkage." Differentiation is how parts of a system can become specialized, unique in their growth, individualized in their development. Linkage involves the connection of separate areas to each other, often involving the sharing of energy and information flow. When differentiated areas become linked, they retain some of their essential qualities while also becoming a part of a functional whole. Here we see how integration makes the whole greater than the sum of its parts. In mathematics, we use terms such as "complexity" and "coherence" to describe such linkage of differentiated parts. In biological terms, we can see how individuals develop, growing ever more differentiated and interconnected over a lifetime and across the generations. In day-to-day terms, vitality and harmony emerge from integration. From simple, less integrated stages of development, differentiation and linkage can create more sophisticated and intricate functions. Such integration gives rise to flexible and adaptive functions. This is the essence of health.

There are important scientific implications for systems that link differentiated parts to one another. Like a choir, they move toward harmony in an integrated state. Yet if such integration is impaired, the result is chaos, rigidity, or both. Chaos and rigidity can then be seen as the "red flags" of blocked integration and impaired development of a mind. Taking note of this pattern has profoundly useful implications for understanding impediments to health and for promoting health through integrative development. For example, attachment can be understood as how parents have come to integrate their own inner self-awareness with their relationship with their children—honoring differences, cultivating compassionate linkages. An integrated relationship is a healthy relationship.

Here is a fabulous finding verified by studies in neuroplasticity: How we learn to focus the mind can change the brain. If we learn the basic approach of linking differentiated parts of our lives—our nervous systems and our social connections with others—we can move internally and interpersonally toward integration and health. Lack of integration can help explain otherwise mysterious patterns underlying how some individuals become stuck in their growth and development.[9] Given that the focus of the mind can change brain activity and structure, knowing something about brain anatomy and function can empower us to transform our lives and intentionally move our development toward health. This book creates a view of the developing mind by examining the interdependent mental, relational, and neural processes that are the foundational aspects of energy and information flow within and among people.

## THE ORGANIZATION OF THE BOOK

This book is composed of two general forms of information. First, scientific findings from a range of disciplines are summarized and synthesized to construct a conceptual foundation for an "interpersonal neurobiology" of the developing mind. This scientific foundation creates a new, interdisciplinary view of established knowledge. Second, conceptual implications and new proposals derived from data, clinical experience, and synthetic reasoning across disciplines can then be drawn from this framework. Here we are "moving beyond the data" with caution and intention, but doing so out of necessity. Much as in the old Indian fable of the blind men and the elephant, we need to fill in the gaps in our knowledge to create a "whole-elephant" view of reality. I have tried my best to clarify where we are synthesizing established views from science and where we are making hypotheses from this existing data.

Each chapter explores a major aspect of human experience: awareness, memory, attachment, emotion, states of mind, representations, self-regulation, interpersonal connection, and integration.

## Brain Anatomy and Awareness

In the remainder of this first chapter, we will dive into the basics of brain anatomy and function so that we start with a common understanding of this point on our triangle. Much remains unknown about neural processes, but having a basic scaffold of shared knowledge will be of great benefit. We will also begin to explore the wonderful and mysterious world of consciousness, examining some aspects of its subjective nature and its neural correlates. The fact is, we don't really know how the physical property of neural firing and the subjective experience of being aware of something create each other. I raise this issue from the start because it is a fundamental unanswered question. Conscious awareness is a useful modality for examining this fascinating question, and we will explore the science of how neural function may be correlated with the subjective experience of being aware.

> We don't really know how the physical property of neural firing and the subjective experience of being aware of something create each other.

## Memory

In Chapter 2, I summarize research on various forms of memory to help us understand how our earliest experiences shape not only what we remember, but also how we remember and how we shape the narrative of our lives. Memory can be seen as the way the mind encodes elements of experience into various forms of representation. As a child develops, the mind begins to create a sense of continuity across time, linking past experiences with present perceptions and anticipations of the future. Within these representational processes, generalizations or mental models of the self and the self with others are created; these form an essential scaffold for the growing mind's interactions with the world.

The narrative process is one way that the mind attempts to integrate these varied representations and mental models. Autobiographical narratives are reviewed to explore how the mind creates coherence within its own processes and how this central integrative function influences the nature of interpersonal relationships.

## Attachment

Awareness, memory, and autobiographical narrative set the stage for Chapter 3, which examines attachment in children and adults. Repeated patterns of children's interactions with their caregivers become "remembered" in the various modalities of memory and directly shape not just what children recall, but how the representational processes develop. Behavior, emotion, perceptions, sensations, and models of others are engrained by experiences that occur before children have autobiographical memory processes available to them.

A profound finding from attachment research is that the most robust predictor of a child's attachment to parents is the way parents narrate their own recollections of childhood during the Adult Attachment Interview. This implies that the structure of an adult's narrative process—not merely *what* the adult recalls, but *how* it is recalled—is the most powerful feature in predicting how an adult will relate to a child. These attachment studies provide a framework for understanding how communication within relationships facilitates the development of the mind.

## Emotion

The primary ingredient of secure attachment experiences is the pattern of "emotional communication" between child and caregiver. This finding raises the fundamental question of why emotion is so important for the evolving identity and functioning of a child, as well as in the establishment of adult relationships. It also raises the question as to what exactly is "emotion." Why does a child require emotional communication and the alignment of emotional states for healthy development? To attempt to answer these questions fully, we need to synthesize a number of independent perspectives. The way the mind establishes meaning is closely linked to social interactions and both meaning making and relationships appear to be mediated via the same neural circuits responsible for initiating emotional processes. Emotion can thus be seen as an integrating process that links the internal and interpersonal worlds of the human mind.

## States of Mind

Chapter 5 examines how different mental processes are organized within a state of mind. These states allow disparate activities of the brain to become linked at a given moment in time. A single brain functions as a system that can be understood by examining the "theory of nonlinear dynamics of complex systems," or, more briefly, "complexity theory." Chapter 5 proposes how the laws of complex systems that deal with emergent processes and self-organization can be applied not only to the single mind, but also to the functioning of two or more minds acting as a single system. This new application allows us to deepen our discussion of states of mind and their fundamental importance in creating internal subjective experience and shaping the nature of human relationships.

## Representations

Chapter 6 reviews in detail how the mind creates representations—mental symbols—of experience. Our internal experiences are constructive processes. That is, our emotions, states of mind, and interpersonal relationships help shape the ways in which these representational processes develop.

This chapter also looks at how differences in the hemispheres of the brain shape the creation of representations. The brain has an asymmetry in its circuitry, which leads to the specialization of func-

> Our internal experiences are constructive processes.

tions on each side of the brain. The capacities to sense another person's emotions, to understand others' minds, and even to express one's own emotions via facial expressions and tone of voice are all mediated predominantly by the right side of the brain. In certain insecure attachment patterns, communication between parent and child may lack these aspects of emotions and mental experience. In contrast, secure attachments seem to involve the sharing of a wide range of representational processes from both sides of the brain. In essence, balanced interpersonal communication allows the activity of one mind to sense and respond to the activity of another. The ways we connect with each other directly shape how we "regulate" our emotions and alter our states of mind. In other words, dyadic regulation directly shapes "self-regulation," the topic of the next chapter.

## Self-Regulation

Chapter 7 explores self-regulation—the way the mind organizes its own functioning. Self-regulation is fundamentally related to the modulation of emotion and self-organization. As we'll see, this process involves the regulation of energy and information flow via the modulation of arousal and the appraisal of meaning. Emotion regulation is initially developed from within interpersonal experiences in a process that establishes self-organizational abilities.

## Interpersonal Connection

Chapter 8 examines the nature of the connections between minds. Interpersonal relationships shape the mind by allowing new states to emerge within interactions with others. Early in development, patterns of communication between parent and child help determine the ways in which self-regulation emerges. Self-organization thus emerges out of self–other interactions. These patterns can help us to understand how relationships throughout life may facilitate emotional well-being. Examples from families and individual patients in psychotherapy are offered to illustrate these ideas.

## Integration

How the self creates a sense of coherence across time is reflected in the concept of integration, the central topic of Chapter 9. As noted earlier, "integration" refers to the way the mind links differentiated parts. The mind establishes a sense of coherence by linking states of mind across time.

By organizing the self across past, present, and future, the integrating mind creates a sense of coherence and continuity. Integration can be assessed by examining the structure of autobiographical narratives. Narrative coherence is reflected in the way a life story is told and the manner in which life is lived. In this way, an attachment history revealed in an adult attachment narrative reflects the individual's capacity to integrate a coherent sense of self. Various forms of mental dysfunction may signal that integration is impaired, leading to a sense of paralysis or chaos. From the perspective of interpersonal neurobiology, the signs, symptoms, and syndromes described in the *Diagnostic and Statistical Manual of Mental Disorders* (the DSM-IV-TR)[10] can be interpreted as actually describing chaos, rigidity, or both. However, human relationships can foster resilience and emotional well-being by facilitating an integrative capacity.

Throughout our journey together, we'll be exploring new ways to understand established findings that move us further in understanding human development. My overall goal is to create a scientifically grounded, interdisciplinary view that deepens our grasp of the developing mind and helps create stronger minds, healthier relationships, and more integrated brains for the generations ahead.

Let us now turn to look at the "brain" aspect of energy and information flow—but please keep in mind the complete triangle of mind, brain, and relationships as it reveals the interdependent nature of these three aspects of one reality. What are the mechanisms by which human relationships shape brain structure and function? How is it possible for the interactions between people to affect something so inherently different as the activity of neurons?

Exploring insights from neurobiology—the study of the way neurons work and how the brain functions—will greatly enhance our ability to address these basic questions. We'll then turn to some basic ideas about how we can use awareness, the mental experience of consciousness, to intentionally alter the structure of the brain. The very focus of our attention can create neural firing patterns that can change the brain's physical connections. Given that interpersonal relationships guide how we focus our attention and therefore how our neural firing patterns emerge, our social

> Our social experiences can directly shape our neural architecture.

experiences can directly shape our neural architecture. Put simply, our relational connections shape our neural connections. This interactive process occurs throughout the lifespan.

## THE EMBODIED BRAIN

### The Organization of the Brain

The brain is a complex system of interconnected parts. At its most basic level, the skull-based portion of the nervous system consists of over one hundred billion "neurons" and trillions of supportive "glia" cells. Collectively, these neurons are over two million miles long. Each neuron has an average of ten thousand connections that directly link it to other neurons.[11] Thus there are thought to be about one million billion of these connections, making it "the most complex structure, natural or artificial, on earth."[12] A neuron is one of the basic types of cells in the nervous system; it consists of a cell body, receiving ends called "dendrites," and a long axonal length that reaches out to other neurons. The neuron sends an electrical impulse, called an "action potential," down its long axons; this releases a neurotransmitter at the space at the end, called a "synapse," which then excites or inhibits the downstream neuron. This is an example of electrochemical energy flow. A synapse is the connection that functionally links neurons to one another. These synaptic connections help form the linkages that are the foundation for the intricate architecture of the brain. Because of the spider-web-like interconnections, activation of one neuron can influence an average of ten thousand other neurons. The resulting set of neurons that are firing together is called a "neural net profile," which signifies a pattern of neural activity clustered into a functional whole. Such a neural net profile, for example, can be a neural representation activated when we think of the Golden Gate Bridge or the Eiffel Tower. Each time we think of that particular structure, a similar neural net profile will become activated. The vast numbers of neural connections are not static; the brain continually changes its synaptic interconnections in response to experience.[13] This means that the number of firing patterns possible across a lifespan is virtually infinite. The number of possible "on–off" patterns of neuronal firing even in a given moment of time is immense, estimated as a staggering ten times ten one million times (ten to the millionth power). The brain is obviously capable of an imponderably huge variety of activity; the fact that it is often organized and functional is quite an accomplishment!

Neurons and glia are organized in various levels of complexity, from small clusters called "nuclei" to larger assemblies called "circuits," "regions," and "hemispheres." These various groupings have internal interconnections that enable neural firing to cluster into specialized patterns limited to that specific area; the output of these differentiated areas then links with the output of other regions by way of intergroup fibers that enable cross-group communication to occur. These neural clusters can be classified in a number of ways, including their anatomical placement in the lower, central, and upper areas of the brain. Figure 1.2 is a schematic drawing of the basic structure of the brain.

## Lower Brain Structures

The "lower structures" include those circuits of the brainstem deep within the skull that mediate basic elements of energy flow, such as states of arousal

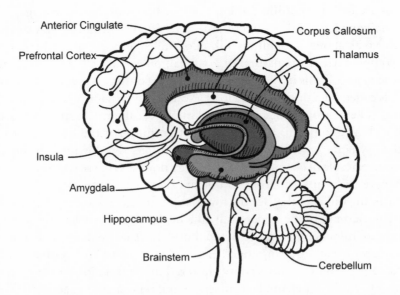

**FIGURE 1.2.** Diagram of the right hemisphere of the human brain. The lower areas include the cerebellum and the brainstem; the central areas include the limbic regions (amygdala, hippocampus) and thalamus; the upper areas include the cortical regions. Copyright 2012 by Mind Your Brain, Inc.

and alertness and the physiological state of the body (temperature, respiration, heart rate). Clusters of neurons in this region are also responsible for the survival reactions of fight–flight–freeze and are fundamental to the "polyvagal theory" of self-regulation.[14] This theory suggests that our interactions with others directly shape how these deep structures in the brain respond with a sense of safety and receptivity or with a sense of danger or life threat. At the top of the brainstem is the thalamus, an area that serves as a gateway for incoming sensory information. It has extensive connections to other regions of the brain, including the neocortex, just above it. As we shall see, one theory of awareness considers the activity of a thalamocortical circuit to be a central process for the mediation of conscious experience.[15] Other proposals suggest that various regions contribute to different elements of consciousness, and to a wide range of senses of a self.[16]

The lower regions of the brain also house the hypothalamus and the pituitary, which are responsible for "physiological homeostasis," or bodily equilibrium, established by way of neuroendocrine activity (neuronal firing and hormonal release). The body proper is intimately integrated with skull-based neural tissue by way of these hormonal and other regulatory processes, such as the immune and musculoskeletal systems. When we use the term "brain," we can now see that it makes no sense in our conceptualizations to separate this skull-based structure from the body as a whole. Stress is often responded to by the "hypothalamic–pituitary–adrenocortical (HPA) axis," and this system can be adversely affected by trauma. Studies reveal that early childhood stress can even negatively affect the ways in which gene expression is regulated in these important areas of the brain's stress response system. Such gene regulation alterations in response to experience are a part of a process called "epigenesis."[17] This HPA neuroendocrine axis, along with the autonomic nervous system (regulating such things as heart rate and respiration) and the neuroimmune system (regulating the body's immunological defense system), are ways in which the function of the brain and body are intricately intertwined. When we see that social interactions directly shape the ways in which these integrative processes function, we can see how relationships and the embodied brain are really part of one larger system.

> Relationships and the embodied brain are really part of one larger system.

## Central Brain Structures

The more centrally located "limbic regions"—including the clusters of neurons called the "hippocampus" and "amygdala"—play a central role in coordinating the activity of various regions. The limbic regions are thought to play an important role in mediating emotion, motivation, and goal-directed behavior, as well as in the integration of memory and the engagement of an attachment system that enables mammalian young to depend upon their parents for safety and security. Limbic structures permit the integration of a wide range of basic mental processes, such as the appraisal of meaning, the processing of social signals, and the activation of emotion. This region houses the medial temporal lobe (toward the middle of the brain, just to the sides of the temples), including the hippocampus, which is thought to play a central role in flexible forms of memory (e.g., in the recall of facts and auto-biographical details) and identifying the context of an ongoing experience.

## Upper Brain Structures

The "upper structures" toward the top of the brain, such as the cerebral cortex (sometimes called the "neocortex"), mediate more complex information-processing functions such as perception, thinking, and reasoning. This "outer bark" of the brain consists of highly folded layers, usually about six cells deep, that are filled with "cortical columns" of highly linked neuronal clusters. The grouped columns process information, and their communication with other columnar areas allows increasingly complex functions to emerge. In general, the cortex matures from back to front, with the frontal regions continuing active growth well into young adulthood. These frontal neocortical areas are considered to be the most evolutionarily "advanced" in humans; they mediate the complex perceptual and abstract representations that constitute our associational thought processes.

The frontmost part of the frontal neocortical region—the "prefrontal cortex"—has two important aspects: the ventral and medial zones, and the lateral prefrontal cortex (also known as the dorsolateral prefrontal cortex). The dorsolateral prefrontal cortex rests to the sides (thus "lateral"). It is thought to play a major role in working memory—placing something in the chalkboard of the mind to dial a phone number, for example—and the focusing of conscious attention. The middle prefrontal area includes the orbitofrontal cortex (just behind and above the orbits of the eyes), the dorsal and ventral aspects of the medial prefrontal cortex, the ventrolateral prefrontal cortex, and the anterior cingulate cortex. Some authors consider the anterior cingulate and the orbitofrontal regions as part of the limbic area, while others recognize the interface role these regions play between the lower limbic and the higher cortical areas and refer to them at times as "par-alimbic cortex." In this manner, the middle prefrontal region can be seen, in fact, as the uppermost part of the limbic system as well as a part of the frontal lobes of the neocortex. These bridging areas are part of a "team" of middle prefrontal regions that work together as a functional whole to link widely separated areas to one another. They have important integrative functions that help coordinate and balance cortical activity of thought and feeling with the lower limbic, brainstem, and bodily areas' functions. As we'll soon see, this region also links the perception of communication signals from other people to these internally mediated neural firing patterns, creating a wide spectrum of integration ranging from the somatic to the social.

## Neural Integration

The brain as a whole functions as an interconnected and integrating system of subsystems. "Interconnected" means that the long axonal fibers link widely separated clusters of neurons to each other in a spider-web-like configuration. "Integrated," as we've seen, means that these separate, differentiated areas maintain their unique features while also becoming linked. It's crucial to keep in mind that integration is not becoming blended or "all one," but rather involves the maintenance of differences while facilitating connection. This is truly how the whole is greater than the sum of the parts. The linkage of differentiated parts of a system is the definition of integration, and when it occurs in the brain, we call this "neural integration." The outcome of neural integration is optimal self-regulation with the balancing and coordination of disparate regions into a functional whole. Although each element of such a system contributes to the functioning of the whole, certain regions play an important role in integrating brain activity. These include the limbic areas (especially the hippocampus), the prefrontal regions, the corpus callosum (which links the left and right sides of the brain to each other), and the cerebellum (which plays a role in linking bodily motion, mental states, and cognitive processing). All of these areas have unique and extensive input and output pathways linking widely distributed areas in the brain. When we look to understand how the mind develops, we need to examine how the brain comes to regulate its own processes. Such self-regulation appears to be carried out in large part by the process of integration that may depend on these and other integrative circuits.

To summarize this point succinctly, self-regulation appears to depend upon neural integration. As we'll see, optimal relationships are likely to stimulate the growth of integrative fibers in the brain,

> Self-regulation appears to depend upon neural integration.

whereas neglectful and abusive relationships specifically inhibit the healthy growth of neural integration in the young child.[18] Even impairments to health that are not experientially derived, such as autism, bipolar disorder, and schizophrenia, have now been shown to reveal impairments to neural integration.[19]

To gain a visual grasp of some of this brain structure, it may be help-ful to use a readily available, three-dimensional model. It will enable you to have neuroanatomy in the palm of your hand, so to speak. (See Figure 1.3.) If you make a fist with your thumb bent toward the center of your palm, and your fingers curled around it and resting on the lower part of your hand, you'll have a model of the brain. Your lower arm represents the loca-tion of the spinal cord inside the backbone, and your wrist is at the base of the skull. The various parts of your hand represent the three major regions discussed above—brainstem, limbic (central), and neocortical (upper) areas. If you look directly at your fist from the palmar side, the orbits of the eyes emerge around the areas of the fingernails of your third and fourth fingers. The ears extend from either side of your fist. Your fingers represent the neo-cortex. Facing you are its frontal lobes; at the top are the neocortical areas that mediate motor control and somatosensory representations; to the sides and back of your hand are the posterior parts that generally mediate percep-tual processing of the outside world but also play important roles in social perception, such as the temporal lobe of the cortex. The lower parts of the brain are represented by the midline portion of your lower palm. Just below your knuckles, deep inside your fist where the end of your thumb rests, is the limbic region. Most of the brain is split into the left and right hemispheres, which are connected with bands of tissue called the corpus callosum and

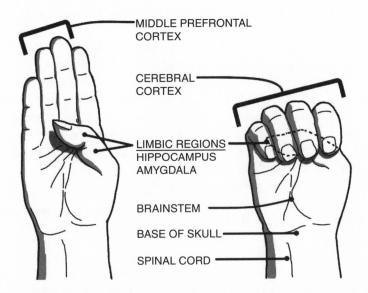

**FIGURE 1.3.** Hand model of the brain. Adapted from Siegel (2010a, p. 15). Adapted with permission from Bantam Books. Copyright 2012 by Mind Your Brain, Inc.

the anterior commissures, thought to serve as direct sources of information transfer between the two sides of the brain. The cerebellum, located at the back of your hand near its connection to your wrist, may also indirectly transfer information across the division that separates the two halves of the brain. The cerebellum itself may carry out a number of informational and integrating processes.

The areas of your fist jutting out from the front of your palm are the frontal lobes, beginning from your second knuckles forward to your fingernail areas. The very front of this anterior region, in front of the last knuckles, is the prefrontal cortex—an area we will be exploring throughout the book. The lateral prefrontal cortex rests to the sides and is represented by your index finger on one side and your fifth finger on the other. On your fist model, the more centrally located orbitofrontal area lies, as you may have guessed, just behind and above the orbits of the eyes, especially where your last knuckles bend and the tips of your fingers push inward toward your palm. These middle two fingernail areas in your hand model also symbolically represent the related ventral and medial zones of this prefrontal region, and so let us refer to this cluster of horizontally and vertically "middle" regions simply by the term "middle prefrontal" cortex. Notice on your hand model that these middle two fingernail areas representing the position of the middle prefrontal region are adjacent to a number of areas from which they receive and to which they send information: the deeper structures of the brain that process sensory and bodily data, the limbic areas, and the neocortex just above it. This three-dimensional hand model thus gives you a direct experiential/visual example of neural interconnections and the relevance of anatomy for coordinated function.

The brain is highly interconnected, and controversy exists in academic circles about how distinct these regions actually are in anatomy and function.[20] The notion of a limbic "system," for example, has been challenged, because defining its limits (where it starts and where it ends) has been scientifically difficult to accomplish. Nevertheless, the limbic and paralimbic regions appear to utilize specific neurotransmitters, to have highly interconnected circuitry, to carry out complementary functions, and to have similarities in their evolutionary history. For example, the middle prefrontal regions, sitting at the top of the limbic area and anatomically connected to a wide array of circuits in the neocortex and the deeper structures of the brain, carry out a vital role in the coordination of the activity from all three regions.[21] As we shall see, recent studies from neuroscience suggest that this middle prefrontal region may play a major role in many of the integrating processes we will be examining, such as self-awareness, empathy, memory, emotion regulation, and attachment.

## Brain Development

The activation of neural pathways directly influences how connections are made within the brain and how the regulation of genes is altered. Though experience shapes the activity of the brain and the strength of neuronal connections throughout life, experience early in life may be especially crucial in organizing the way the basic regulatory structures of the brain develop. These include, as suggested earlier, the integrative fibers of the brain. For example, traumatic experiences at the beginning of life may have profound effects on the integrative structures of the brain, which are responsible for basic regulatory capacities and enable the mind to respond later to stress.[22] Thus we see that abused children have abnormal responses of their stress hormone levels, which are in part due to changes in the regulation of the genes in these areas of the brain responsible for reacting to stress.[23] Cortisol in sustained and elevated levels can become toxic to the brain.[24]

The essential take-home message here is that early experience shapes the regulation of synaptic growth and survival, the regulation of response to stress, and even the regulation of gene expression. Experience directly shapes regulation.

More common, everyday experiences also shape brain structure. The brain's development is in part an "experience-dependent" process, in which experience activates certain pathways in the brain, strengthening existing connections and creating new ones. Development is also in part "experience-expectant," in that genes instruct specific circuits to be

> Early experience shapes the regulation of synaptic growth and survival.

created, such as the visual system, but that maintenance of those synaptic linkages requires stimulation from species general experiences, such as receiving light to the retina of the eyes. Lack of experience for these circuits can lead to cell death in a process called "apoptosis," or to the diminution of synaptic connections in a process called "parcellation" or "pruning." This is sometimes called a "use-it-or-lose-it" principle of brain development. Whether experience-expectant or experience-dependent development is occurring, synaptic connections are maintained by ongoing neural firing that is created with experience.

An infant is born with a genetically programmed excess of neurons, and the postnatal establishment of synaptic connections is determined by both genes and experience. Genes contain the information for the general organization of the brain's structure, but experience plays an important role in determining which genes become expressed, how they will be activated, and the timing of that activation. The expression of genes leads to the production of proteins that enable neuronal growth and the formation of new synapses.

Experience—the activation of specific neural pathways—therefore directly shapes gene expression (i.e., "epigenesis"), and leads to the maintenance, creation, and strengthening of the connections that form the neural substrate of the mind. In epigenesis, the sequence of DNA in a chromosome does not change, but the molecules that control gene expression do. Early in life, interpersonal relationships are a primary source of the experience that shapes how genes express themselves within the brain. Changes in epigenetic regulation of gene expression induced by experience can be long-lasting and may even be passed on to the next generation by way of the alterations of epigenetic regulatory molecules in the sperm or egg.[25]

At birth, the cortex of the infant's brain is the most undifferentiated part of the body. Genes and early experience shape the way neurons connect to one another and thus form the specialized circuits that give rise to mental processes. The early years are when basic architecture in the brain is laid down. The differentiation of circuits within the brain involves a number of processes, including these:

1. The growth of axons into local areas, and the development of axonal connections among widely distributed regions.
2. The growth of new neurons and the establishment of new and more extensive synaptic connections between neurons in certain regions, such as the hippocampus.
3. The growth of myelin along the lengths of neurons, which increases the speed of nerve conduction by one hundred times and reduces the refractory period during which a just-fired neuron must rest before firing again by thirty times. Thus myelin functionally enhances the linkage among synaptically connected nerve cells by three thousand times.
4. The modification of receptor density and sensitivity at the postsynaptic "receiving" cells, making connections more efficient.
5. The balance of all these factors with the dying away or pruning of neurons and synapses resulting from disuse or toxic conditions such as chronic stress.

In experimental animals, enriched environments and exercise have been shown to lead to increased density of synaptic connections, and especially to an increased number of neurons and actual volume of the hippocampus, a region important for learning and memory.[26] Experiences also lead to increased activity of neurons, which enhances the creation of new neurons and the growth of new synaptic connections or the strengthening of existing synapses. This experience-dependent brain growth and differentiation is thus referred to as an "activity-dependent" process.

Studies suggest, too, how gene expression is altered following experiences. The fundamental mechanism of epigenesis is that neural firing can lead to the "turning on" or "expression" of genes that enable protein production. Protein production in turn creates structural changes, allowing neurons, for example, to form new synaptic linkages or to strengthen existing ones. Experience can also induce changes in the molecules on the chromosome that do not code for protein synthesis, but instead function to regulate the expression of the adjacent gene. Epigenetic changes induced by experience alter how and when genes are expressed, and thus have a powerful impact on neural connections. Studies are now beginning to reveal the important ways in which we may have embedded in our own nuclear material the ways in which our parents and even our grandparents experienced stress, had alterations in their epigenetic control mechanisms, and then passed these changes on to us via the gametes from which we were formed.[27] There are profound implications of these new findings for our understanding of development and the emergence of patterns of growth, temperament and other inborn qualities of nervous system functioning, and the intergenerational transmission of stress and trauma.

Interpersonal experiences continue to influence how our minds function throughout life, but the major structures—especially those that are responsible for self-regulation—are initially formed in the early years. As proposed earlier, regulation emerges from integration. And for this reason, it will be helpful to keep a close eye on unfolding research that may continue to reveal how interpersonal experience shapes the growth of the integrative regulatory circuits of the brain. The essential proposal is that the integrative communication stimulates the healthy growth of integrative fibers in the brain. Given the proposal that integration enables regulation, we will look closely at the early years of life to understand the ways in which the mind develops and comes to regulate its own processes through interactions with important caregivers. New findings on the study of neuroplasticity reveal that the brain is open to further development throughout the lifespan.[28] From studies of early interpersonal experience, we can try to understand how relationships may continue to foster the development of the mind throughout life.

> Interpersonal experiences continue to influence how our minds function throughout life.

## Information Processing and Neurobiology

From an information-processing perspective, brain anatomy and neural circuit functioning can be understood as follows. Signals consisting of electrochemical energy flow patterns from the brain's deep structures represent physiological data from the body. They are received and processed by the centrally located limbic structures. More elaborately processed data from the activities of the limbic region itself are integrated by the adjacent paralimbic areas, including the orbitofrontal cortex and anterior cingulate. Another middle prefrontal area, the "insula" (which is a portion of the ventrolateral prefrontal cortex), receives direct input from the body as well. These areas send emotional and somatosensory input to the neocortex, which also processes perceptual representations via the thalamus and the sensory cortices, conceptual representations from the associational cortices, and linguistic representations from the language-processing centers. In one view, information-processing links input from various regions by way of integrative circuits, such as the associational cortices and middle prefrontal cortex, which take in the different neural "codes," coordinate the information contained within these signals, and "translate" them into transformed neural activity. The transformed information is then sent as output to the various regions. Such neural translation of the various forms of representations allows for information to be both processed and then communicated in different codes to the relevant regions. This translation process allows for a type of neural integration of complex information within the brain and yields highly complex neural output and mental capacities.[29]

An analogy is this: We can transmit information in an electronic mail message containing the twenty-six letters of the alphabet, spacing, and a handful of punctuation marks. This email is transmitted as energy flow through cables or the air. The energy flow is then translated back into information—its symbolic value as letters, spacing, and punctuation marks. Through the same wires, we can send an entire photograph or even a video. Though the message contains different information (note, photo, video), the fundamental medium in which the data are transmitted is identical—electrical impulses flowing as patterns of energy through a wire of a cable, or through the air for WiFi. The information contained within the different messages varies in its patterns and its complexity. Without the proper receiving device to translate these electrical impulses into words, pictures, or video, the complex representation has no meaning. This will happen if you open a .pdf file with a word-processing program. You will find symbols that make no sense. Energy will abound on your computer screen, but the pattern of that energy will be indecipherable. It will have no informational value; it will not be symbolic of something other than being a mess of squiggles on a screen. If I spoke to you in Greek and you did not know that language, you would receive the energy, but it would not have informational value for you. Information is in the eye and ear of the beholder.

The same principle is true with the brain. Neural activity is the fundamental form in which energy flows and then information can be transmitted.

This electrochemical energy flow consists of action potentials with ions moving in and out of the membrane, release of the chemical neurotransmitters, and chemical activation of the downstream receptors. The sending area is capable of transmitting a certain kind of information as neural codes. The receiving circuits or systems must be capable of processing such signals for them to have any meaning; in other words, they need to stand for something that is useful beyond just the neural firing itself. The brain is genetically programmed to be able to differentiate its regions, which carry different forms of sending and receiving information—swirls of energy flow that stand for something other than merely neural firing patterns. These forms vary in pattern and complexity from the most "simple" signals of the deeper structures (such as heart rate) to the more complex ones of the neocortex (such as ideas about freedom or about the mind itself).

Experience not only serves to activate the energy flow to these regions; it is necessary for the proper development of the brain itself. Experience-expectant and experience-dependent maturation are a part of even the basic sensory systems of our brains. The brain must "use it or lose it" in many cases of brain specialization. For example, studies in animals reveal that the lack of exposure to certain types of visual information, such as vertical lines, during a critical period early in life leads to loss of the capacity for perceiving such lines later in life. Specific forms of experience are necessary for the normal development of information-processing circuits in the visual cortex.[30] As discussed earlier, this has been called "activity-expectant" development, in that genetically created circuits "expect" exposure to minimal inputs (light or sound) to maintain those pathways. The same process may occur for other systems in the brain, such as the attachment system. Children who have had no experience with an attachment figure (not merely suboptimal attachment, but a lack of attachment) for the first several years of life may suffer a significant loss of the capacity to establish intimate interpersonal relationships later on.[31] Even the ability to perceive the mental side of life may require interactions with caregivers in order to develop properly.[32]

In this way, we can reexamine one of our initial questions: How does experience shape the mind? A general principle can be proposed here: *Experiences can shape not only what energy and information enters the mind, but also how the mind processes that information.* To "process" here means to make meaning out of energy flow patterns, to create symbolic value out of swirls of neural firing patterns. How this occurs can be seen as the modification of the actual circuits of the brain responsible for processing that particular type of information. If you don't speak Greek, you won't know what "glicanera" means. Experience

> Experiences can shape not only what energy and information enters the mind, but also how the mind processes that information.

creates representations, as well as stimulating the capacity for specific forms of information processing. This is how learning occurs.

## The Brain as a System and as Part of a Larger System

The brain can be considered as a living system that is open and dynamic. It is also a part of a larger system. Its integrated, component subsystems interact in a patterned and changing way to create an irreducible quality of the system as a whole.[33] Furthermore, the brain is a complex system, meaning that there are multiple layers of component parts capable of chaotic behavior.[34] These parts can be conceptualized at various levels of analysis, and include the single neuron and its sending and receiving functions; neuronal groups; circuits; systems; regions; hemispheres; and the whole brain within the skull. This skull-based neural collection is also intricately interconnected with an array of neural, immune, endocrine, metabolic, cardiovascular, and musculoskeletal processes in the rest of the body. When we add to this that the brain is a "social organ" and takes in the neural signals from other brains, we can see that viewing the "brain" as limited to the skull makes no biological sense. It is "bio-illogical" to view component elements of a whole as isolated from one another.

Examining the brain in context, we can temporarily tease apart its many layers of input and output to get a glimpse of how the parts make up the whole. The basic components, the neurons, are the simplest. As we move up the levels, the units become more and more elaborate. Some authors use the terms "lower-order" to refer to the basic level of organizational unit and "higher-order" to refer to the more intricate level of organization. For the most part, each subsystem can be considered to have both lower and higher orders of systems with which it relates. For example, the activity of the visual cortex is made up of the lower-level input from the eyes, but itself contributes to the higher-level processing of the entire perceptual system.[35]

A living system must be open to the influences of the environment in order to survive, and the brain is no exception. The system of the brain becomes functionally linked to other systems, especially to other brains. The brain is also dynamic, meaning that it is forever in a state of change. An open, dynamic system is one that is in continual emergence with a changing environment and the changing state of its own activity. From the point of view of the brain as an open system, each region may take in unique input from outside itself. Certainly we have input from outside our bodies as we receive signals from other people and engage in interactions with the world. Within the body, the nervous system receives input from the many physiological processes mentioned above. Yet the embryonic origins of the nervous system itself as coming from what initially was ectodermal cells—the layer destined to become our skin, which encases the body and forms the boundary of inner and outer—reveals that our neural tissue is always about linking this inner bodily world with the outer world.

It is quite natural, from this developmental perspective, to see the brain as both embodied and relational. The deeper structures of the skull-based brain receive sensory input from the body and from the external world; the limbic region receives input from the deeper structures and from the neocortex; and the neocortex receives data from the limbic area, the brainstem, and the body itself. Neuroanatomic studies reveal that the neocortical regions are also intricately interwoven with the "lower" levels of the system, and thus that our "higher thinking" is actually directly dependent upon activity of the entire brain, and indeed the entire body. The regions balancing and coordinating the state of activation of the brain's subcomponents play an important role in the regulation of the body and emotions. It is an important and fascinating finding that those regions, such as the middle prefrontal cortex, that serve to regulate internal states are integrative in their functions and in their structural connections. As stated earlier, this integrative linkage of differentiated areas of the nervous system may be the fundamental mechanism underlying regulation. Integration is how the nervous system becomes coordinated and balanced. This is the outcome of the integrative circuits of the brain that perform such a regulatory function.

The field of complex systems theory derives from the probability field of mathematics.[36] From this perspective, a complex system is said to have a "self-organizing" property that emerges in the interaction of elements of the system. *I am proposing in this book that the emergent process of energy and information flow within bodies and within relationships is one important aspect of "the mind."* This embodied and relationally embedded process is regulatory, in that it self-organizes the movement of energy and information flow within bodies and among people interacting with one another.

Does the self-organizing emergent property that derives from complexity theory overlap with "self-regulation," a primary focus in the field of psychopathology? If so, this may be a conceptual bridge linking two independent fields. One implication of this possible overlap is that "impairments to self-regulation" suggested by the field of developmental psychopathology as central to mental dysfunction may be fundamentally "impairments to self-organization." And if self-organization moves the system to the most flexible, adaptive, and harmonious states with integration, then perhaps self-regulation, too, is dependent on integration. This is the basis of the proposal being made here that regulation comes from integration. And now we can state the

> The emergent process of energy and information flow within bodies and within relationships is one important aspect of "the mind."

notion that dysregulation comes from nonintegrated functioning. Given that integration produces harmonious and flexible functioning and that impairments to integration yield chaos, rigidity, or both, we can predict that dysregulation will result in this pattern of dysfunction. Indeed, DSM-IV-TR's entire listing of psychiatric disorders can be reframed within this perspective as revealing chaos and/or rigidity, and so as reflecting impaired integration. Recent studies in trauma[37] and in neural functioning in the non-task-performing default mode or "resting state"[38] support this proposal that impaired integration is the common mechanism among disorders of health, whether they have primarily experiential or non-experiential (e.g., genetic, toxic, infectious, or random) origins.

Another implication is that the basic process we call "emotion" is actually an aspect of this self-organizing emergent property reflecting changes in states of integration. If this is true, it makes our emotional lives fundamental to our minds. For example, some suggest that emotions, generated and regulated by the activity of the subcortical areas—those beneath the cortex—are integral parts of our neocortically derived "rational thoughts" as well as the overall functioning of our minds.[39] Furthermore, the "regulation of emotion" may be dependent on large-scale integrative processes—ones that emerge from prefrontal coordination and balance, as well as from interpersonal experiences within one-on-one relationships, families, communities, and even the larger culture in which we live. Relationships that are attuned—ones that honor differences and cultivate compassionate connections—are integrative relationships that promote health. These issues also suggest that specific circuits within the brain may function as somewhat distinct "subsystems" that create their own predominant states of processing. For example, the left and right sides of the brain have distinct circuits that become predominant early in life, even in the embryo. Each of these pathways has its dominant neurotransmitters and involves distinct evaluative components that serve to direct each hemisphere to process information in distinct manners. How each hemisphere is activated will directly shape our subjective sensations and the ways in which we communicate with others. Naturally, we need to be skeptical about oversimplifying reality and also to remain cautious of overgeneralizations, but (as we'll see) distinct patterns that have emerged through millions of years of evolution support the notion that the two sides of the brain are specialized in their neural functions.[40] Again, integrating the two differentiated sides of the nervous system appears to support healthy growth and development.

The broader "system" view is of energy and information flow; we can detect its integrative quality with harmony or its impediments with chaos and rigidity. Integration, in relationships and in the brain, is the substrate for well-being from this perspective. Integration can be seen as a deep mechanism that enables us to gain insight into both synaptic and societal connections and how they impede or promote the development of a healthy mind. The principles of integration become our guiding framework, whatever level of micro- or macroanalysis we examine.

## Genes, Epigenetic Regulation, and Experience

In an era when science is enabling us to understand human experience in new ways, it is important to examine the common debate about how much of development and personality can be attributed to "nature" or genetics, as opposed to "nurture" or experience. Misinterpretations of genetic studies have led to beliefs such as "What parents do has no effect on their children's development." It is certainly true that temperament and other constitutional variables play a huge, and perhaps previously underrecognized, role in child development.[41] However, riding the pendulum swing of "What shapes development?" to either the genetics end or the experience end can lead to erroneous conclusions.[42]

A wide range of studies[43] has in fact clarified that development is a product of the effects of experience on the unfolding of genetic potential. Genes encode the information for how neurons are to grow, make connections with each other, and die back as the brain attains differentiation of its circuitry. These processes are genetically preprogrammed *and* experience-dependent. Genes have two major functions.[44] First, they act as "templates" for information that is to be passed on to the next generation; second, they have a "transcription" function based on the information encoded within their DNA, which determines which proteins will be synthesized. Molecules on the chromosome directly affect when, which, and how genes are expressed. Transcription is directly influenced by experience. Experience alters the molecular mechanisms that regulate gene expression, (i.e., the process of epigenesis) and determines when genes express themselves via the process of protein synthesis. For the brain, this means that experience directly influences how neurons will connect to one another—creating new synaptic connections, altering their strengths, and allowing others to die away.[45]

In other words, genes do not act in isolation from experience. Experience has a long-lasting impact on how we learn, and it directly involves gene expression. In turn, the nature of our genes and of their regulation directly affects how we respond to experience. Genes and experience interact in such a way that certain biological tendencies can create characteristic experiences. For example, certain temperaments may produce characteristic parental responses and may shape how each child responds to parents.[46] These responses in turn shape the way in which neuronal growth, interconnections, and pruning (dying back) occur.

   The development of the mind has been described as having "recursive" features.[47] That is, what an individual's mind presents to the world can reinforce the very things that are presented. A typical environmental/parental response to a child's behavioral output may reinforce that behavior. Therefore, the child plays a part in shaping the experiences to which the child's mind must adapt. In this way, behavior itself alters genetic expression and regulation, which then shapes neural connections and their firing patterns, ultimately influencing behavior. In the end, changes in the organization of brain function, emotional regulation, and long-term memory are mediated by alterations in neural structure. These structural changes are due to the activation or deactivation of genes encoding information for protein synthesis. Experience, gene expression and gene regulation, mental activity, behavior, and continued interactions with the environment (experience) are tightly linked in a transactional set of processes.[48] Such is the recursive nature of development and the way in which nature and nurture, genes and experience, are inextricably part of the same process. Embracing this approach to the nature–nurture issue allows us to stand on scientifically solid ground as we try to understand human development and the growth of the mind. The question isn't "Is it heredity *or* experience?" but "How do heredity, epigenetic changes, *and* experience interact in the development of an individual?"

   Genetic studies of behavior commonly note that fifty percent of each of the personality features measured is attributable to heredity. The majority of the other half of the variability is thought to be due to "nonshared" aspects of the environment, such as school experiences and peer relationships.[49] But siblings—even identical twins, who are raised by the same parents at the same time—actually have a "nonshared" environment, in that parental behavior is not identical for each child.[50] The recursive quality of mental development magnifies initial individual differences and creates a challenge to the sometimes held opinion that growing up in the same family is a shared (statistically identical) experience. This reminds us that each individual's history reflects an inseparable blend of how the environment, random events, gender, and temperament all contribute to the creation of experiences in which adaptation and learning recursively shape the development of the mind.

   Gender-based differences in brain development, in conjunction with cultural expectations, may be a factor in moving development in a certain direction that reinforces itself across the lifespan.[51] However, it is important to avoid conclusions drawn from adult differences that may be due to cultural factors experienced throughout childhood and adolescence. I do not want to overstate the innate neural differences between individuals of either gender. (For various studies of how culture shapes neural development, please see the wide range of research projects described at our Foundation for Psychocultural

Research–UCLA Center for Culture, Brain, and Development website, *cbd. ucla.edu.*) Excessive judgments about these gender differences can cause an observer to miss the reality that there is far more in common across the genders than there are neurally determined distinctions.

The complicated interaction of genes, experience, and epigenetic regulation is also revealed in the inheritance patterns of certain psychiatric disorders, such as schizophrenia.[52] In identical twins, who share all of their genetic information, there is slightly less than fifty percent concordance in the behavioral expression of the illness. This implies that many factors determine how a "genotype" (genetic template or information) becomes expressed as a "phenotype" (genetic transcription function leading to protein synthesis and external manifestation as physical or behavioral features). *In utero* factors such as infections and exposure to toxins can influence the early development of the nervous system in ways that are not dependent upon the genes themselves. Genetic variables may influence vulnerability to a condition such as schizophrenia, but they may require exposure to such an agent for disease to be induced. Studies of individuals with certain atypical neurotransmitter variants, called "alleles," reveal observable differences in those individuals only when they are exposed to a severe developmental challenge such as abuse early in life.[53] Those with the atypical variants do extremely poorly in their lives, whereas those with the typical variants are less severely affected. Without the experience of the abuse, the individuals may have no phenotypic difference discernible to an observer.

The epigenetic regulation of gene expression may vary even in individuals who share the same genes. Adolescence is a period of intense pruning of the nervous system, and vulnerable brains may be especially at risk following this period of development. This parcellation, also called pruning or "apoptosis," can unmask latent vulnerabilities. The timing of this parcellation process can help us explain the unfolding of serious psychiatric disturbances during and immediately following adolescence. For these reasons, too, how the child's environment offers support or intensifies stress can directly influence the occurrence and progression of psychiatric illness. Children who are exposed to significant trauma early in life, for example, have epigenetic changes that make the HPA axis less adaptive in ways that appear to last a lifetime.[54] Future studies will need to investigate whether clinical interventions with such individuals may be able to reverse these structural and epigenetic impacts of trauma on the developing brain.

For the growing brain of a young child, the social world supplies the most important experiences influencing the expression and regulation of genes. This in turn determines how neurons connect to one another in creating the neuronal pathways that give rise to mental activity. The function of these pathways is determined by their structure; thus alteration in genetic expression changes brain structure and shapes the developing mind. The functioning of the mind—derived from neural activity—in turn alters the physiological environment of the brain, and thus itself can produce changes in gene expression. These interdependent processes are all a part of the complex systems of our mental lives.[55] This is clearly seen in the production of corticosteroids as a response to stress, which directly influences gene function.[56] In children with shy temperaments, for example, there is a huge physiological response to even mild environmental changes. Such individuals create their own internal world of stress responses that heighten their brains' reactivity to novelty.[57] Likewise, a child traumatized early in life will have an alteration in physiological response, such that small stressors lead to large hormonal responses.[58] Thus both constitutional and experientially "acquired" reactivity can lead to further physiological features that maintain the hypervigilant response over time. Jerome Kagan and his colleagues have demonstrated that parenting behavior makes a large difference for the trajectory of development.[59] In their research, those parents who supportively encouraged their shy children to explore new situations enabled the children to develop more outgoing behaviors than those parents who did not help their children with their fears. These and other studies clearly demonstrate that parenting has a direct effect on developmental outcome, even in the face of significant inherited features of physiological reactivity.[60] Throughout this book, we will return to discussions of shy and traumatized children as examples of the interactions between constitutional and experiential variables in development.

## Relationships and the Brain

I am proposing in this book that the mind develops as relationships and the brain change across time, and that the regulatory function of the mind emerges within the interactions of neurophysiological processes and interpersonal relationships. In other words, the mind is an emergent property that regulates the flow of energy and information within bodies and between people. Relationship experiences have a dominant influence on the brain because the circuits responsible for social perception are the same as or tightly linked to those that integrate the important functions controlling the creation of meaning, the regulation of bodily states, the modulation of emotion, the organization of memory, and the capacity for interpersonal communication. Interpersonal experience plays a special organizing role in determining the development of brain structure early in life and the ongoing emergence of brain function throughout the lifespan.

One fundamental finding relevant for this IPNB view of the mind comes from numerous studies on attachment across a wide variety of cultures.

Attachment is based on collaborative communication. Secure attachment involves contingent communication, in which the signals of one person are directly responded to by the other. Ultimately this is "integrative communication," in which the distinction between two people is honored and compassionate, caring communication linking the two people is created. It sounds simple. But why is this type of reciprocal communication so important? Why do people even with a common cold have improved immune function and recover one day sooner when they see a physician who is empathic?[61] Why doesn't such integrative communication happen in all patient–clinician relationships? And why doesn't this contingent compassionate communication happen in all families?

During early development, a parent and child "tune in" to each other's feelings and intentions in a dance of connection that establishes the earliest form of communication. Mary Ainsworth's early studies suggest that healthy, secure attachment requires a caregiver to have the capacity to perceive and respond to the child's mental state.[62] This way of reflecting on the child's mental life—of seeing the mind beneath behavior and respecting the existence of an internal subjective world—has been identified as a possible core mechanism underlying secure attachment.[63] These studies propose that a "reflective function" enabling the parent to carry out "mentalization" may be at the heart of Mary Ainsworth's original notion that parental sensitivity is at the heart of attachment security.[64] This is essentially the extent to which a parent is "mind-minded" and has a "theory of mind"—that is, the extent to which the parent is able to conceptualize the real entity called "mind" both in the self and in others.[65] We'll see that this reflective function enables a parent to be sensitive to the child's signals and respond to the child's inner experience, not merely to the manifest behavior.

In Chapter 3, I review findings from neuroscience that can help us to understand what mechanisms underlie these early reciprocal communication experiences; how they are remembered; and how they allow a child's brain to develop a balanced capacity to regulate emotions, to feel connected to other people, to establish an autobiographical story, and to move out into the world with a sense of vitality. The capacity to reflect on mental states, both of the self and of others, emerges from within attachment relationships that foster such processes.[66] I call this capacity "mindsight"—the ability to see the internal world of self and others. It may be essential in healthy relationships of many kinds. *Mindsight permits integrative communication in which individuals are honored for their differences and compassionate connections are cultivated that link one mind to another.* My proposal is that *interpersonal integration promotes the growth of integrative fibers in the brain.* These neural circuits linking differentiated areas to one another are the regulatory and social circuits of the brain. In this way, the concept of mindsight builds on the illuminating work of mentalization and extends the exploration further by embedding notions of neural integration and interpersonal relation-

> "Mindsight"—the ability to see the internal world of self and others.

ships as interdependent aspects of the flow of energy and information. Mindsight can thus be conceptualized as the way we perceive energy and information flow within the neural and the relational systems from which the mind emerges. When we see the flow of energy and information clearly, mindsight enables us to then intentionally move this flow toward integration and thus toward health.

These patterns of respectful, compassionate interpersonal communication literally shape the structure of the child's developing brain toward integration. These important early interpersonal experiences are encoded within various forms of memory and shape the architecture of the brain. The integrative function of the brain is what permits flexible and adaptive neural regulation, and so interpersonal relationships that are integrative promote healthy self-regulation. It is important to keep in mind that development does not only occur during childhood or adolescence. The brain continues to change in response to experience throughout the lifespan. We are in lifelong development, as reflected in the ever-changing structure of the brain throughout our lives. The need for integrative communication and connection does not end with childhood. As adults, we need not only to be understood and cared about, but to have other individuals simultaneously experience a state of mind similar to our own. We need to be a part of a whole larger than our bodily defined selves. We are continually emerging within our connections with others. It is for this reason that healthy relationships are an important part of health as we age.[67] With shared, collaborative experiences, life can be filled with an integrating sense of connection and meaning.

So far, the emphasis in this chapter has been on the embodied brain aspect of energy and information flow. In the next section, emphasis shifts more directly to mind and how it emerges from the interface of relationships and neural function.

## MIND: REGULATION AND CONSCIOUSNESS

We do not know how the physical property of neurons firing and the subjective experience of our inner mental lives mutually create each other. No one knows how the scent of a rose is "created" when chemicals from the flower stimulate our olfactory nerves. And so with this humbling reality, we can propose that, for now, we can see the subjective side of mental life and the objective (measureable) side of neural life as representing two primes, or irreducible aspects, of our human existence.[68] Just as we do not struggle to resolve the primes of two sides of one coin, we can also consider that mental and neural are two aspects of one reality of energy and information flow.

That said, we can describe at least three dimensions of the mind. One is the mind's regulatory function that governs the flow of energy and information, as described earlier. If we define this first core feature, we can be in a scientifically grounded position to offer new and (let us hope) helpful ways of making our minds stronger, our mental lives healthier, our sense of well-being more robust. The second core aspect of mind is the phenomenon of being aware, of having an internal sense of knowing that is part of what we call "consciousness." A third aspect of mind is our subjective internal life, which shapes our sense of self and our connections to others in the world. Ultimately, this subjective aspect of mind is a wondrous mystery. What are these aspects of mind, truly—this sense of knowing within awareness and the subjective texture of that which is known? Although we may never truly "explain" awareness and this subjective side of mind, we can actually come to practical insights that are quite useful. In teasing apart these three core dimensions of mind—regulation, awareness, and subjective experience— I am not attempting to eliminate the magnificence and mystery of mind, but rather to illuminate its core and differentiable features so that we can improve our mental lives.

## Regulating Energy and Information Flow

When we regulate anything, we need to monitor and then modify that which is being regulated. These are two fundamental aspects of regulation. When you are driving a car, you must have your eyes open to perceive where you are going and then to alter the direction and speed of the vehicle. When we regulate our emotions, we monitor our internal states and then modify our degrees of arousal and excitation to bring more balance into our lives. The outcome of healthy regulation is to coordinate and balance our functions so that we are adapting to our ever-changing environment.

The fascinating view that emerges from IPNB's consilient approach to the developing mind is that *regulation results from integration*. When our relationships are integrated, they are the most flexible and adaptive—and the most rewarding and meaningful. When the brain links its differentiated circuits to each other, the nervous system achieves homeostasis and develops new levels of

> Regulation results from integration.

intricacy in its functions. In this way, defining this aspect of the mind as a regulatory process can purposefully lead to the growth of a healthy brain and relationships. This is an empowering and practical definition of a core feature of mind that can improve the way we raise our children, teach, conduct therapy, and live our day-to-day lives.[69] The underlying possibility is that the power of awareness can be used intentionally to cultivate integration in our relational and neural lives. If being aware in this way can transform lives, what do we know about the process of consciousness? What does it mean to be consciously aware?

## Consciousness: Knowing and Subjective Experience

Any exploration of the mind will be strengthened if we acknowledge that our mental lives cannot be fully measured in a quantitative or objective way. Even if we develop ways of measuring integration and the regulatory aspect of mind, we still have the inner subjective experience of being aware, which is not measureable. Even self-report measures, reliable as they may or may not be, are not the same as inner subjective awareness. *Your* internal mental experience—your sense of knowing and being aware, and the subjective nature of what is known in your conscious experience—cannot be fully known by me or anyone else. Our internal sea is a private world we can share only in communications that approximate our internal world; we can never fully reveal to others its true nature. In science, for example, we can explore the "neural correlates" of consciousness, but these and other measurements only describe physical changes at the time of the study participants' subjective experience. Even more, it is important to keep in mind that these correlations are not necessarily revealing a linear causal influence. Systems often function in nonlinear ways, and we need to be scientifically cautious about drawing premature conclusions about the directionality of causation. Awareness may also influence the state of neural firing as much as neural firing influences awareness: Causality may be bidirectional, as often happens in emergent self-organizing processes.[70]

These important and fascinating studies of neural correlations do not solve the "hard problem" of how the physical property of neurons' firing in the many complex ways they do "gives rise" to the subjective experience of being aware.[71] And they leave us with the important issue of how subjective awareness may shape the firing of neurons. Studies have also revealed that a wide array of specific brain regions and their interactions appear to play an important role in the emergence of conscious experience.[72] Physically interconnected circuits of the brain, from the brainstem up through the thalamus and connecting with the cortex, may weave a neural pattern that gives rise to consciousness.[73] But it is important to keep in mind that these proposals, even if true, do not answer the basic question. Even if the physical and the mental occur simultaneously in time, we just don't have a clear model for how the way you see the color red in your subjective life and the firing of the areas of your brain responsible for vision work together. How a person is aware of vision relies on a complex array of neural firing patterns linking widely separated areas to one another.[74] Recent studies of imagery and its impact on how the brain changes raise important questions about how conscious mental experience (imagery) can alter the brain's physical structure (synaptic connections). These studies of neuroplasticity reveal that focusing internal awareness on a self-generated image can alter the activity and the neural connections in specific regions of the brain. Imagining the playing of scales on a piano is associated with expansion in the motor areas of the brain responsible for the fingers and is similar to the change that occurs with actually playing the scales.[75] Although we certainly can propose that the neural firing is what creates the imagery in the first place, how does the person *initiate* this imagery-based neural change? What does it mean to have intention and will to carry out an action?[76]

These are important and challenging questions—and the point of this brief discussion is to invite us to embrace the possibility that the mind is more than simply the "output" of the brain.[77] At a minimum, energy and information flow between and among people in one-to-one relationships, families, communities, and societies. This flow directly activates our mental experience in ways that are beyond our own private neural firing pattern proclivities. Anyone in a close, intimate relationship knows how our mental lives are shaped directly by our interactions with others. Let's try to keep an open mind for the possibility that the arrows of causality of the triangle of human experience point in all directions: Brain influences mind and relationships; relationships influence mind and brain; mind influences brain and relationships. If the mind is an emergent property of the system of energy and information flow that is fundamental to our neural nature and our relational connections with others, then viewing the causal processes as "emergent" and not merely linear (as in "Brain creates mind alone") will be a useful starting place.[78] Being aware in our mental lives permits conscious choice. An aware mind can choose with intention how to shape neural and relational functioning. This empowering point of view has deep implications, as we shall see.

Some neuroscientists may propose that mind is "simply an outcome" of the activity of the brain. Brain is primary, and mind is an outcome of neural firing, a "secondary effect" of the nervous system's function. Others suggest just the opposite, stating that our mental lives are in a different domain of reality that has little correlation with the physical

> Being aware in our mental lives permits conscious choice.

world.[79] Our position in IPNB is to embrace the view that there are at least three "primes" of one reality—mind, brain, and relationships, as mentioned earlier. Each is a unique and irreducible aspect of energy and information flow. Our mental lives—awareness, subjectivity, and the regulatory facet of the mind—are emergent processes that arise from both neural and relational processes and their interface with each other. Let us consider the subjective side of this mental experience a prime, an irreducible aspect of the emergent property we are calling "mind." This stance will become clearer as we move forward through the ensuing chapters, with research-based data supporting this interdisciplinary perspective.

As a reminder, we are defining "mind" as an emergent process, part of which involves the regulation of energy and information flow, the "brain" as an embodied mechanism of that flow, and "relationships" as the sharing of that flow. These are not three separate elements, three different worlds, or three items to check off on a biopsychosocial model of the world. Instead, these are elements of "one reality" that is energy and information flow; mind, brain, and relationships are three aspects of the one reality of patterns in the flow of energy and information.

Much of what occurs within our neural, relational, and mental lives is not within the experience of awareness. And so I am not equating mind with consciousness. Mental life includes consciousness but is not limited to it; the regulation aspect of the mind can be with or without our being aware. Sigmund Freud made a major contribution to our understanding of mental life by pointing out that the processes outside our awareness have a significant influence on the quality of our lives.[80] In this text, however, I use the term "nonconscious" rather than "unconscious" to refer to the processes of which we are not aware, in order to avoid the many historical and sometimes limiting nonconscious associations that arise with the "unconscious" term. I hope Freud would approve.

Information that enters consciousness is important because it permits choice and change. Items within consciousness become temporarily more stable and thus available for mental and neural manipulation. "Consciousness" is not the same as "attention."[81] Some forms of attention are within conscious awareness, and some forms are not. Attention itself can be defined as a process that directs the flow of energy and information—and that can proceed with or without awareness. "Nonfocal attention" is the term for the focus of energy and information that does not involve the experience of being aware. "Focal attention" is that form of guiding the flow of energy and information in the mind that involves our conscious awareness of that flow. Within our everyday lives—and within the developmental processes of parenting, education, and psychotherapy—using the conscious focus of attention, harnessing focal attention, can enable significant changes to occur within our scaffold of knowledge. Awareness stabilizes that which we are aware of. As we'll see in Chapter 2, focal attention enables a form of flexible memory called "explicit processing" to be created in the brain. With conscious awareness, we also create purpose and can plan and engage our lives intentionally as we deepen an understanding of ourselves and the world in which we live.

### Subjective Experience

One aspect of consciousness is the quality of our internal subjective experience. This is sometimes called "phenomenal consciousness." The quality of your internal subjective experience of seeing red and my experience of seeing the same red may not be exactly the same. No one's unique subjective world is quantifiable, and comparing one's own subjective mental life to another's is limited by its internal nature. For this reason, the contemporary scientific field of psychology may have understandably moved away from introspective reports as a source of reliable data, seeking instead a more "objective" and often quantifiable way of measurement that can be statistically analyzed as self-reports, as observable behaviors, and as measureable scans of brain activations. Yet the subjective world is real, even if science cannot "prove it" with controlled forms of measurement. I was once in a debate with a fellow psychiatry trainee who took the position that psychiatrists should not learn psychotherapy, because there was no evidence from science that feelings were "real." The only natural response I could muster was to suggest that I wasn't certain how we could proceed with our conversation, because we didn't have the scientific evidence that he was "real."

One thing we do know is that when parents attune themselves to the internal subjective experience of a child, the child thrives. In fact, this is true with all close personal relationships. When a child is interested in a bug, for example, and has a caregiver who shares her interest and excitement, focusing their shared attention together on the insect, the child feels seen and enriched. That child will thrive in the moment. Repeated experiences in which caregivers attune themselves to children's internal worlds and join with the children at this subjective sharing level result in scientifically demonstrable positive outcomes for the children. In other words, although we cannot quantify a child's excitement or disappointment, we can in fact observe such joining experiences and then measure the various healthy ways in which such respect leads to positive developmental outcomes. As noted earlier, patients with a common cold who see an empathic physician have been shown to recover one day faster and to have better immune function than patients who see a nonempathic physician.[82] Again we see measureable scientific findings that the nonmeasureable subjective world is

> Our relationships directly influence our internal experience of being aware.

of vital importance. Researchers have viewed this intersubjective aspect of consciousness as a primary influence in how the experience of awareness develops.[83] Our relationships directly influence our internal experience of being aware.

Conscious awareness can also involve a relationship with our own internal subjective lives; it can be a way of taking "time-in" to focus on our internal subjective states. As children develop, their interactions with caregivers can influence how they become aware of their own internal worlds. How we pay conscious attention to our own bodily experiences can profoundly influence how consciousness arises.[84] This overlap between the bodily sense of self in the physical world and the relational sense of self within our interpersonal connections is exemplified by the finding that the same middle prefrontal area (the anterior cingulate) is responsive both to physical pain and to social rejection.[85] Again and again, we'll be able to illuminate the ways the neural, relational, and mental aspects of our lives are intimately intertwined.

As Helen Keller, who became blind and deaf at the age of nineteen months, stated in her autobiography,[86] her "mind was born" at the moment she knew what her teacher *meant* by the sign for "water." Shared experience within interpersonal relationships, as Lev Vygotsky proposed,[87] is an important source of our mental lives and directly develops our thought processes and internal states. The mind is both embodied and relational. In other words, mental life is not just affected by synaptic connections in the brain, but extends beyond the skull; it is both embodied and relational. The sharing of energy and information (relationship) occurs as you read this book. You remember the experience by altering the brain mechanism of that flow as synaptic connection. You can change the way you regulate energy and information flow (mind) within awareness and choose to move this flow with intention.

## Knowing and the Awareness of Content

A second aspect of consciousness is the sense of knowing its content, or the "known." If conscious awareness is holding something "in the front of your mind," making it more stable for a brief period of time, what exactly does this mean? Knowing—the *access* dimension of awareness, also known as "cognizance"—is how we subjectively sense knowledge or clarity about something. We can "pay attention" to the path in front of us as we walk, knowing that we are taking one step at a time. In this example, focal or conscious attention enables us to have a clear view of where we are walking. We have the phenomenal or qualitative aspect of our subjective experience within consciousness, and we have an access aspect of knowing the path ahead of us. With the knowing of such focal attention, we can choose to walk along a different path and change our direction with intention and awareness. With focal attention, with something known within awareness, the mind has the ability to choose and change its course of functioning with intention and purpose. With this "attentional flashlight,"[88] we can choose which part of our experience to illuminate and bring into cognizance. In this way, consciousness plays an important role in what are called "executive functions"; these include attentional control, cognitive flexibility, goal setting, impulse regulation, and complex information processing, and planning.[89] The unfolding of conscious awareness over children's lives is influenced by a range of experiences from infancy onward that also shape the executive functions, which play an important role in how their lives unfold.[90] As the example of Helen Keller illustrates, our sense of awareness even of who we are is directly shaped by the relational experiences we have of sharing our sense of knowing, our mutually created sense of meaning and connection.

I use "*consciousness*" to signify the experience of being aware, the internal state of knowing that something is happening in the present moment. The term "cognition" can be used to signify the broad way in which energy flow patterns with symbolic value—what I have defined as "information"—move across time. This flow involves alterations in representation, the clustering of it with related representations, and the performing of designated informational transformations (such as comparing and contrasting, finding meaning, recalling similar elements, rhyming, and various other ways of shifting and recombining the symbolic representations of information). "Cognition," as the broad term referring to information processing in general, does not need awareness and exists across a wide array of other species.

> *Consciousness* is the experience of being aware, the internal state of knowing that something is happening in the present moment.

"Sentience" is a term that sometimes is used to refer to the "ability to perceive or to feel things" or a "state of elementary or undifferentiated consciousness."[91] We have our sentient experience as the essence of our inner subjective lives. The feelings of sentience may be more akin to being aware of energy flow patterns that have no symbolic value, such as the smell of a rose, the exhilaration of an astonishing sunset, or the glorious feeling of the harmony of a choir in full voice. The awareness of these inner states is a direct feeling and knowing beyond information; they are as close to the sense of "the thing itself" as we can get within our conscious experience.

The ability to perceive and to understand other people's minds, a form of "metacognition" sometimes called "mentalization," begins within the first year of life[92] and is proposed to play a role in the unfolding of consciousness.[93] Other terms for this capacity are "theory of mind," "mind-mindedness," "mind perception," and the IPNB term "mindsight." While seeing the mind of another seems to catalyze the development of self-awareness, what more broadly do we understand about how consciousness develops? Some propose that intersubjective consciousness emerges during the first year of life,[94] whereas more internally based senses of awareness emerge during the second year of life.[95] Is the moment we share meaning via language use with another person, as Helen Keller experienced, a special form of the "mind [being] born"? When does this inner sense of being alive and being aware of that sense actually occur? And how would we even know? There are clearly many aspects of "self" that appear to emerge within our interpersonal worlds.[96] Some people remember clearly recognizing a sense of "self-awareness" as it emerged at a particular time in their lives, but these retrospective reports are constrained by the nature of recollection. In other words, we may be aware long before we can remember that we were aware. Clinically, some people have reported recollections of a kind of psychological birth of consciousness, in which such clear "beginnings" happened during their adolescence or beyond. Others recall a sense of self much earlier, during the earliest days of elementary school or earlier. Innate neural features and their interaction with family communication patterns may each contribute to the timing and nature of how awareness of the self develops across childhood and beyond.

What indeed is this awareness of the "self"? When do you first realize that you are a person and occupy space and can think? Is it when you first realize that you are in the present moment remembering something from the past? How does awareness differ from self-awareness? And does the "self" need to be limited to the boundaries of the body? In other words, can a "sense of self" include a sense of "me" and "you" and perhaps even a membership in a "we"? With all the ways in which life and the brain change over time, perhaps the self can be viewed as more of a verb than a noun—as a process that evolves as we grow and change. These are all intriguing questions that remain to be illuminated with future explorations.[97] The important point here is to consider these open questions so that we can imagine how mind, brain, and relationships co-influence their own development across the lifespan.

## Mindful Awareness

One form of awareness is the recently researched but ancient practice called "mindfulness" or "mindful awareness." Though the specific scientific definitions of mindfulness vary, we can state here the general perspective that being mindful involves a way of paying attention, on purpose, to present experience as it emerges moment by moment without being swept up by judgments.[98] This is the opposite of being on "automatic pilot" or being "mindless" in our actions. When we speak of "awakening the mind," this often refers to the way in which we can become alive and attend to the details of ordinary experience as if it were extraordinary.[99] Mindful awareness can enable our inner sense of knowing and subjective experience of being alive to attain a new sense of vitality, detail, and clarity. Being present in this way has been scientifically demonstrated to support mental, physical, and social well-being.[100]

The study of mindfulness explores both inherent traits and intentionally created states. Mindful traits include being aware of what is happening as it is happening, being nonjudgmental (not being taken over by prior expectations) and nonreactive (coming back to emotional baseline readily), being able to label and describe the internal world, and having self-observation.[101] These traits may be related to some combination of temperament and a relationship history that has fostered this way of being grounded in the present moment-to-moment unfolding of experience.

With intention, it is also possible to engage in a training of the mind that can be called "mindful awareness practice," in that it creates a state of being alert and open to the novel way of experiencing in that moment. This form of awareness has the qualities described above, but also can be thought of as having the features of self-compassion and other-directed compassion. In other words, some consider that mindful awareness is a way of being aware of one's own inner life and the surrounding world with kindness, a form of positive regard for self and others. When we "take time-in" with positive regard for ourselves and others, we cultivate mindfulness as a trait in our lives.

Mindful awareness practices may have origins in ancient or modern times, and may come from the East or West. They include mindfulness meditation, yoga, tai'chi, qigong, and centering prayer. I myself also do mindful dishwashing at home. Each dish, the sensations of the water, the movement of sponge over plate, the sound of the stream flowing from the faucet, the feel of the towel, and the circular motion of the towel as each dish is dried and put away—these all become the focus of moment-to-moment attention. The beauty of mindful awareness is that it can be applied to everyday life in a secular fashion. Research has clearly demonstrated that it can improve the health of the mind with increased flexibility, concentration, and sense of well-being. Improved empathy and compassion enhance relationships, and a shift in the baseline activity of the brain occurs, which is associated with approaching rather than withdrawing from challenging situations.[102] This can be seen as a sign of "neural resilience." Primary care physicians who are taught mindful awareness, for example, have less burnout and enhanced empathy for their patients.[103] A study of intensive meditation training reveals that the cultivation of mindful awareness leads to increased telomerase, the enzyme that maintains the integrity of chromosomes by supporting the telomeres at their ends, and thus increasing cell life.[104] Patients listening to a mindfulness recording during the light treatment for psoriasis heal four times more quickly than other patients.[105] The overall idea is that the intentional creation of a mindful state is healthy for the body in that moment. With repeated practice, it can become a mindful trait—a way of being that shapes the ongoing health of the individual's life.

A recent study suggests that parents who have mindful traits may also have a state of mind called "secure with respect to attachment." This enables them to have children who themselves are securely attached to their parents and develop well.[106] As we'll see, this connection between mindfulness as a way of being and the open, receptive way of participating in healthy relationships may rest within the process of integration. In other words, when we are loving of others, we are in an interpersonally integrated and mindful state, and when we are loving of ourselves with self-compassion and kindness, we are in an internally integrated and mindful state.

Mindful awareness is a profoundly integrative internal process.[107] The observing self is open and receptive to the experiencing self, moment by moment. Research has demonstrated that being present with mindful awareness promotes health across the entire triangle of well-being, involving mind, brain, and relationships. Attachment relationships that promote well-being involve interpersonal communication that honors the unique, differentiated qualities of each person, while also promoting the partners' linkages through compassionate and empathic communication. Having a mindful state enables a parent to take in the child's nature and attune to it without distorting perceptions or expectations. This secure relationship is based on the integration of the caregiver's and child's states of mind; the internal world of each person is encouraged to be differentiated and linked—to become integrated.

We return to the topic of attachment and how it influences the developing mind in Chapter 3. In the next chapter, we explore the nature of memory, the ways in which experiences shape its development, its neural basis, and its crucial role in the mind's creation of a coherent sense of self.

# CHAPTER 2

# Memory

## A GENERAL DEFINITION OF MEMORY

We often think of "memory" as what we can consciously recall about what happened in the past. If you think about what you did last weekend or last year, for example, you may begin to visualize some event or interaction with other people. How are those experiences remembered? How does recollection actually happen? In this chapter, we explore answers to these questions by looking at what is known about the mechanisms of memory. Although people have been fascinated with memory for thousands of years, it is only recently that we have been able to understand in a scientific way what some of the basic elements of memory actually are.[1]

As we explore the remembering mind, try to keep an eye on your everyday basic assumptions about memory. You may be surprised to find that many of them are helpful, but that some of them may be in need of revision. Common misconceptions about memory include the following: that we are always aware of what we have experienced; that when we remember something, we have the feeling of recollection; and that the mind is somehow able to make a sort of photograph of experiences, which is stored without further modification. Recollection is thus often seen as the presentation of information, independent of the time of recall or of bias by prior experiences. As we'll see, the structure of memory is quite complex: It constructs the past, the present, and the anticipated future, and it's sensitive to both external and internal factors.[2]

Memory is more than what we can consciously recall about events from the past. A broader definition is that *memory is the way past events affect future function.* In this view, the brain experiences the world and encodes this interaction in a manner that alters future ways of responding. What we shall soon

46

see is that this definition of memory allows us to understand how past events can directly shape how and what we learn, even though we may have no conscious recollection of those events. Our earliest experiences shape our ways of behaving, including patterns of relating to others, without our ability to recall consciously when these first learning experiences occurred.

As discussed in Chapter 1, the brain is composed of spider-web-like neural networks capable of firing in a myriad of patterns, called "neural net profiles."[3] Scientists studying the behavior of such networks have found that the structure of a neural net allows it to learn through an encoding process that initially activates a specific set of associated neuronal firing patterns distributed throughout the brain.[4] Writers who explore this phenomenon describe it in terms of "connectionist theory" and "parallel distributed processing." The essential feature of these studies is that the connection of neurons in an intricate network (i.e., the structure of the brain) allows learning to occur.[5] Abnormalities in this interconnectivity may underlie significant disorders of how the brain processes information, such as autism.[6] Another perspective is reflected in the term "grandmother cells." This refers to the finding that some forms of information (e.g., face recognition of your grandmother) are contained within single neurons. This localized view of information processing actually has robust support from a range of biological studies. This cellular way of representing information is distinct from but not incompatible with parallel distributed/neural information processing, and studies suggest that both forms of neural representations may occur in the brain.[7] It is thought that the firing of single or collective components of a neural network alters the probabilities of patterns of firing in the future. If a certain pattern has been stimulated in the past, the probability of activating a similar profile in the future is enhanced. If the pattern is fired repeatedly, the probability of future activation is further increased. The increased probability is created by changes in the synaptic connections within the network of neurons. Changes at the level of the cell membrane thus alter the firing probability of specific combinations of neurons.[8] The process of "long-term potentiation" has been described as one way in which such alteration of connection strengths among neurons occurs.[9] The specific pattern of firing (i.e., the energy flow within a certain neural net profile) contains within it "information." Thus the network learns from its past experiences. *The increased probability of firing a similar pattern is how the network "remembers."* Information is encoded and retrieved through the synaptic changes that direct the flow of energy through the neural system, the brain.

In a direct way, experience shapes the structure of the brain. As we've seen in Chapter 1, this general process is called "experience-dependent" brain development; the term refers to the general processes by which neuronal connections are maintained, strengthened, or created during experience. As we continue to learn and remember throughout life, our brains and our minds can be seen as having ongoing development across the lifespan. The infant brain has an overabundance of neurons with relatively few synaptic connections at birth, compared to the highly differentiated and interwoven set of connections that will be established in the first few years of life. Experience, genetic information, and epigenetic regulatory factors will determine to a large extent how those connections are established. Memory utilizes the processes by which chemical alterations strengthen associations among neurons for short-term encoding. For long-term memory storage, neural firing actually activates the genetic machinery for protein production necessary for the establishment of new synaptic connections.

As Milner, Squire, and Kandel have noted, "recent work on plasticity in the sensory cortices has introduced the idea that the structure of the brain, even in sensory cortex, is unique to each individual and dependent on each individual's experiential history."[10] Thus the structure and function of the brain are shaped by experience. Developmental and memory processes may actually be based on similar neural and molecular mechanisms underlying synapse formation.[11] These changes in synaptic connection alter the ways in which the brain functions. What we usually think of as "memory" refers to the way in which events can influence the brain and alter its future activity in a specific manner. As we'll see, the brain has a wide array of direct mechanisms by which it "remembers" experience.

How we recall the past will be determined by which components of the massive network of the brain are activated in the future. For example, if you see the Eiffel Tower on a trip to Paris, your visual system (and other parts of your brain) will activate its circuitry, creating a representation or image of the Tower within your mind. This is called "encoding" a memory. The next stage is the "storage" of memory. This is the increased probability that a similar neural net profile will be activated again in the future. Note that there is no "storage closet" in the brain in which something is placed and then taken out when needed. *Memory storage is the change in probability of activating a particular neural network pattern in the future.* Your brain will have the potential to reactivate the visual circuitry (i.e., the neural net profile), similar to the initial encoding. Memory, then, is a process that is based on altering the probabilities of neuronal firing. "Retrieval" is the activation of that potential neural net profile, which resembles—but is not identical with—the profile activated in the past. Thus, when you intentionally try to recall the Eiffel Tower, you may experience an internal visual image of the structure, as well as other aspects of your Paris journey.

The neural net of the brain can activate a set of anatomically and chronologically associated firings in response to the environment. This profile is encoded, stored, and retrieved on the basis of a simple axiom defined

in 1949 by Donald Hebb: Neurons that
fire together at one time will tend to
fire together in the future.[12] Or, in Carla
Shatz's paraphrase: Cells that fire together

> Neurons that fire together wire
> together.

wire together. As Hebb pointed out, "The general idea is an old one, that
any two cells or systems of cells that are repeatedly active at the same time
will tend to become 'associated,' so that activity in one facilitates activity in
the other."[13] In fact, Sigmund Freud postulated a "Law of Association" in
1888, which proposed just this phenomenon.[14] This neural association that
functionally links the activity of neurons is now understood to involve transient metabolic changes for short-term memory and more stable structural
changes for long-term memory storage. The principle of linkage involves
both anatomic and temporal association of neuronal activity. As we'll see,
because of this temporospatial integration of function at the neural level, it
is fundamentally through memory that the complex neural network creates
anatomically distributed and functionally clustered assemblies of activation
across time. The alteration of synaptic connections or "synaptic strengths,"
either by the creation of new connections or the modification of existing
ones (e.g., by way of changes in neurotransmitter release or receptor sensitivity), directly changes the probabilities of neuronal firing. This is the essence
of how the neural net remembers.

Let's continue with the example of the Eiffel Tower. You may be able—
if you've actually seen the Tower or a picture of it—to "see" an image of the
Tower in your mind's eye. What does this actually mean? Recent brain studies suggest that, given the task to visualize an object, the parts of your brain
responsible for visual processing will become active.[15] What is believed to be
occurring is that a neural net profile similar to the one activated at the time
you actually saw the object is now being reactivated in the same parts of the
brain. This is called a "visual representation." Thus the mind is able to generate a pattern of neural firing at the time of seeing with your eyes, as well
as to generate an image independently in the process of imagining with your
mind. Representations come in many forms, including perceptual ones (like
visualizing the Eiffel Tower), semantic ones (like seeing the words "Eiffel
Tower" and knowing their meaning), and multiple sensory ones (such as
having a feeling of hunger because when you were at the Tower you had to
wait for a picnic, and now your mind is bringing up the associated sensation
of hunger).[16]

Our memories are based on the binding together of various aspects of
these neuronal activation patterns. These "associational linkages" make it
more likely that items will be activated simultaneously during the retrieval
process. Representations are linked together via a wide range of internal
neural processes unique to each individual. Brain imaging studies suggest

that the representation of an experience may be stored in the particular regions of the brain that initially were activated in response to the experience, such as the perceptual areas in the posterior part of the neocortex at the back of the head. Encoding and retrieval processes may be mediated via regions distinct from those involved in storage (such as the orbitofrontal part of the prefrontal cortex, just in back of and above the eyes).[17] Thus specific regions may actively mediate a process whereby neural patterns (representations) are activated and then bound together in the act of encoding or during recollection.[18] What are stored are the probabilities of neurons firing in a specific pattern—not actual "things." Your recollection of the Eiffel Tower will differ from mine for many reasons, encompassing the unique aspects of several factors: the nature of our experiences, the ways in which our brains create representations, and the manner in which the encoding and retrieval process may function. For example, if you were bitten by a dog during that Parisian picnic, you may begin to feel a sense of fear or even pain (emotional and bodily representations, respectively) when you think of the Tower. If you loved France, your sensory representations may be quite different than they would be if you disliked France when you first visited. How you feel at the time you are remembering will also profoundly influence which elements become associated with this complexly bound representation during retrieval.

In memory research, the initial impact of an experience on the brain has been called an "engram."[19] If you visited the Eiffel Tower with a friend and were talking about existential philosophy and Impressionist paintings as you were having your picnic, your engram might include the various levels of experience: semantic (factual—something about philosophy or art or knowledge about the Tower), autobiographical (your sense of yourself at that time in your life), somatic (what your body felt like at the time), perceptual (what things looked like, how they smelled), emotional (your mood at the time), and behavioral (what you were doing with your body). Your original Eiffel Tower engram would include linkages connecting each of these forms of representations.

Scientists have used different terminology to identify these distinct aspects of memory. Some researchers use the term "explicit semantic" memory for how we recall facts, whereas "explicit episodic" or "autobiographical" memory are terms used for recollections of the self in time. If we are remembering one episode of life, the term "episodic" is used. But if we are recalling many events of a similar kind, such as all the experiences we've had at the Eiffel Tower, then we use the term "autobiographical" memory.[20] Some studies suggest that the distinctions between semantic and episodic memory are not as sharply defined as the terms imply.[21] A similar notion to the broad category of explicit memory is the idea of "declarative" memory, in which we can use words to declare the nature of such a recall. The other layers of memory are at a different level of integration from explicit or declarative forms of memory and are grouped together as "implicit" or "nondeclarative" memory.[22] For the purposes of this book, the terms "implicit" and "explicit" are used to identify these functionally distinct forms of memory described further below.

Some authors use the notion of "trace theory" to describe the encoding, storage, and retrieval processes of memory. In this view, your engram or memory trace has both a "gist" (the general notion that you were in France at the Tower) and specific details.[23] With time, the details of an experience may begin to fade away and become less tightly bound together. The gist, however, may remain easily accessible for retrieval and quite accurate. When we try to retrieve an "original memory," in fact, we may be calling up the gist at first ("I was at the Eiffel Tower when I was in my early twenties") and then later trying to reconstruct the details. This reconstruction process may be profoundly influenced by the present environment, the questioning context itself, and other factors, such as current emotions and our perception of the expectations of those listening to the response.[24] Memory is not a static thing, but an active set of processes. Even the most "concrete" experiences, such as recalling an architectural structure, are actually dynamic representational processes. Remembering is not merely the reactivation of an old engram; it is the construction of a new neural net profile with features of the old engram and elements of memory from other experiences, as well as influences from the present state of mind.

> Memory is not a static thing, but an active set of processes.

## IMPLICIT MEMORY:
## MENTAL MODELS, BEHAVIORS, IMAGES, AND EMOTIONS

From the first days of life, infants perceive the environment around them. Research has shown that infants are able to demonstrate recall for experiences in the form of behavioral, perceptual, somatosensory, and emotional learning.[25] Examples of these forms of memory are numerous and demonstrate how active infants are in perceiving and learning about their environment. Babies can turn their heads to a learned stimulus. They can perceive visual patterns and can even relate these to other perceptual modalities, such as touch or sound. If they become frightened by a loud noise associated with a particular toy, they will get upset when shown that toy in the future. These forms of memory are called "implicit." They are available early in life and, when retrieved, are not thought to carry with them the internal sensation that something is being recalled. An infant who sees that toy just gets upset;

the infant probably does not sense, "Oh, yes, I remember that toy. It made a loud noise before. Perhaps it will make one again. Oh, no!" Instead, the neural net/Hebbian associations automatically link the visual input of the toy with an internal emotional response of fear.

Implicit memory involves parts of the brain that do not require conscious processing during encoding or retrieval.[26] When implicit memory is retrieved, the neural net profiles that are reactivated involve circuits in the brain that are a fundamental part of our everyday experience of life: behaviors, emotions, bodily sensations, and images. These implicit elements form part of the foundation for our subjective sense of ourselves that filter our experience in the moment: We act, feel, and imagine without recognition of the influence of past experience on our present reality.

Implicit memory relies on brain structures that are intact at birth, mature throughout development, and remain available to us throughout life. These structures include the amygdala and other limbic regions for emotional memory, the basal ganglia and motor cortex for behavioral memory, and the perceptual cortices for perceptual memory. Somatosensory (bodily) memory is also a part of implicit processes, and is probably mediated by the somatosensory cortex, the orbitofrontal cortex, the anterior insula, and the anterior cingulate (regions responsible for bodily representations), especially on the right side of the brain.[27]

## Mental Models

With repeated experiences, the infant's brain—functioning with its rapidly developing neural net/parallel processor—is able to detect similarities and differences across experiences. From these comparative processes, the infant's mind is able to make "summations" or generalized representations from repeated experiences as encoded in these areas of the brain. This is a fundamental aspect of learning. These generalizations form the basis of "mental models" or "schemata," which help the infant (in fact, each of us) to interpret present experiences as well as to anticipate future ones. *Mental models are basic components of implicit memory.* Our minds use mental models of the world in order to assess a situation more rapidly and to determine what the next moment in time is most likely to offer.

The brain uses many perceptual channels to create neural representations of the outside world. These images of reality cross modalities such as touch and sight to create multimodal models—models that span perceptual modalities. For example, if infants are allowed to feel the shape of a nipple with their mouths in a darkened room, they later will be able to pick out the familiar nipple from a visual display.[28] Their minds have created a mental image from touch, which then can be used to sense a familiar pattern by sight. The brain can also average across different experiences. Infants can be shown an array of facial images and then later pick out the ones that are summations of those seen earlier. From the first days of life, the infant's brain is capable of creating a multimodal model of the world. These capacities further suggest that the mind is capable from the very beginning of creating generalizations from experience.

These mental models are derived from encounters with the world. Mental models in turn help the mind to seek out familiar objects or experiences and to know what to expect from the environment. Deviations from the usual can be ascertained, and the world becomes a familiar and negotiable place to live. Studies of children and adults suggest that here-and-now perceptual biases are based on these nonconscious mental models.[29] For example, if you've seen numerous city streets before, you may be more likely to see the next one from a similar viewpoint, without examining subtle differences in detail. On the other hand, if you have never been to a city before, you will see each street as unique "for what it is" rather than making automatic perceptual presumptions. *The brain can be called an "anticipation machine," constantly scanning the environment and trying to determine what will come next.*[30] Mental models of the world are what allow our minds to carry out this vital function, which has enabled us as a species to survive. Prior experiences shape our anticipatory models, and thus the term "prospective memory" has been used to describe how the mind attempts to "remember the future," based on what has occurred in the past.[31] Each moment, the brain automatically tries to determine what is going on; it does this by activating a mental model and classifying experience. This helps to bias present perceptions, and thus to allow for more rapid processing of the immediate environment. Readiness for response is enhanced by anticipating the next moment in time—what the world may offer next and what behavior to initiate in response.

Let's look at an example. If prior encounters with animals with large teeth have shown that they present a danger, then within the memory of such an animal will be the association of fear. The next time we encounter such a beast, we will be motivated by fear to run for safety. If we did not have the capacity to create a mental model that establishes the generalization "Large-toothed animals are dangerous," then encounters with a slightly different type of beast might not prompt us to run. We would have to learn anew with every experience. Mental models, the generalizations from past experiences, are the essence of learning. These models, derived from the past, shape our perceptual experience of the present and help us to anticipate and act in the future. As we'll see, *anticipating* the future may be a fundamental component of implicit memory, distinct from the capacity to *plan* for the future. The more complex and deliberate aspect of planning may depend upon the explicit memory processes discussed in later sections.

Parenthetically, the procedure of asking how a mental process was used adaptively in our evolutionary past is sometimes called "reverse-engineering the mind."[32] The brain, after all, is constructed by genetics, by aspects of the physiological internal environment (such as nutrients, hormones, toxins, drugs, or lack of oxygen), and by experience. The genetic contribution to brain functions and mental processes can be seen through the eyes of the evolutionary biologist: Those functions enhancing the probability that the genes would be replicated (passed on through creating offspring) were also most likely to be passed on through the generations. In this way, the genetic determination of mental processes may reflect adaptations to past environments, not necessarily to our current ones. Recent findings from the study of the regulation of gene expression—the field of "epigenetics"—reveal, too, that experience shapes the molecular control of how genetic information shapes brain growth. Studies now suggest that these regulatory changes can be directly passed through the egg or sperm to future generations. For the mind, what this means is that processes such as memory, attention, perception, and emotional responses may be understood (at least in part) by their past function in the evolutionary history of our species, as well as by present conditions, the earlier experiences of individuals, and perhaps even our immediate ancestors' experiences as well.[33]

## Developmental Implications of Implicit Memory

The following examples illustrate the ubiquitous role of implicit memory throughout the lifespan. They also introduce some ideas about attachment, which are explored in greater detail in Chapter 3.[34] An infant who has a healthy, secure attachment has had the repeated experience of nurturing, perceptive, sensitive, and predictable caregiving responses from her mother, which have been encoded implicitly in her brain. She has developed a generalized representation of that relationship with her caregiver—a mental model of attachment—which helps her know what to expect from her mother. Given that these repeated experiences have been predictable, and that when there have been disruptions in mother–infant communication the mother has been relatively quick and effective at repairing the ruptures, this fortunate infant has been able to develop a secure, organized mental model of their emotional relationship. Her implicit memory anticipates that the future will continue to provide such contingent communication. When the child's mind has been seen clearly and responded to with affection and compassion, the implicit self of the child develops well.

An infant with an insecure attachment may have experienced his parents as less predictable, emotionally distant, or perhaps even frightening.

These experiences, too, become encoded implicitly, and the infant's mind has a generalized representation of this relationship that can be filled with uncertainty, distance, or fear. Being alone with a parent

> These implicit memory encodings . . . shape the growing child's architecture of the self.

who has been the source of confusion and terror can reactivate these implicit representations and create a very unpleasant, disorganizing, and frightening internal world for the infant. This state of mind, a part of his emotional memory, is implicitly learned during the first year of his life. These implicit memory encodings are more than simply recollections; they shape the growing child's architecture of the self. This is the heart of implicit memory.

By a child's first birthday, these repeated patterns of implicit learning are deeply encoded in the brain. Indeed, attachment studies at this time yield striking differences in infants' behavior when they are with each parent. An infant's states of mind when she is with the mother can affect her differently from those that are activated when she is with her father. As we'll see in Chapter 3, this is the origin of the differences that can be seen in the infant's attachment to the two parents. By eighteen months, the maturation of various parts of the child's brain has allowed for the blossoming of her comprehension and expression of language. At about this time, frontal parts of the brain are developing rapidly and enable her to have evocative memory, in which it is believed she is able to bring forward in her mind a sensory image of a parent in order to help soothe herself and regulate her emotional state.[35] Infants are likely to be calmed by the image of a parent with whom they have a secure attachment, and to be anxious, distant, or fearful with a parent with whom they have an insecure attachment.

The patterns of particular states of mind in an infant can be seen as an implicit form of memory. Repeated experiences of terror and fear can be engrained within the circuits of the brain as states of mind. With chronic occurrence, these states can become more readily activated (retrieved) in the future, so that they become characteristic traits of the individual.[36] In this way, our lives can become shaped by reactivations of implicit memory, which lack a sense that something is being recalled. We simply enter these engrained states and experience them as the reality of our present experience.

Insights into the ways in which early experiences have shaped the implicit memory system can aid in the understanding of various aspects of human relationships. Being with a particular person can activate distinct mental models that affect our perceptions, emotions, behaviors, and beliefs in response to this other person. The notion of implicit memory's influencing our experiences with others is one way of understanding the complex feelings and perceptions arising within interpersonal relationships. Each of us filters our interactions with others through the lenses of mental models created from patterns of experiences in the past. These models can shift rapidly outside of awareness, sometimes creating abrupt transitions in states of mind and interactions with others. In this way, "transference"—the activation of old mental models and states of mind from our relationships with important figures in the past—happens all the time, both inside and outside the psychotherapy suite. Knowing about implicit memory allows us the opportunity to free ourselves from the possibly repetitive behaviors and automatic reactions derived from the past.

## EXPLICIT MEMORY: FACTS, EVENTS, AND AUTOBIOGRAPHICAL CONSCIOUSNESS

By the second birthday, toddlers have developed new capacities: to talk about their recollections of the day's events, and to remember more distant experiences from the past. These abilities probably reflect the maturation of the brain's medial temporal lobe (which includes a part called the hippocampus), parietal, and orbitofrontal cortex; this maturation process allows them to have "explicit" memory.[37] Explicit memory is what most people mean when they refer to the generic idea of memory. When explicit recollections are retrieved, they have the internal sensation of "I am remembering." Two forms of explicit memory are "semantic" (factual) and "episodic" (autobiographical or oneself in an episode in time). Table 2.1 provides an overview of the types and characteristics of memory.

The development of the unique aspects of explicit memory involves a number of domains in a child's experiencing. A sense of sequencing, thought to be a function of the hippocampus as a "cognitive mapper," develops during the child's second year of life.[38] Recalling the order in which events in the world occur allows the child to develop a sense of time and sequence. Children come to expect what typically comes first and what comes next in a given situation, with at times intense and passionate reactions to deviations. Associated with this hippocampal ability is the establishment of a spatial representational map of the locations of things in the world. Loss of hippocampal functioning in animals, for example, leads to loss of memory for running a maze.[39] What is interesting in this finding is the notion that this cognitive mapper is thus able to identify context and to create a four-dimensional sense of the self in the world across time. The brain's ability to create such a temporal and spatial representation is clearly of great survival value. Explicit memory plays the important role of providing a sense of space and time, allowing people to remember where things are and when they were there.

## TABLE 2.1. Implicit and Explicit Memory

Implicit memory

Early form of memory—present before birth.
Devoid of the subjective internal experience of "recalling," of self, or of time.
Involves mental models and "priming."
Includes behavioral, emotional, perceptual, and somatosensory memory.
Focal attention *not* required for encoding.
Mediated via brain circuits involved in the initial encoding and independent of the
    medial temporal lobe/hippocampus.

Explicit memory

Late memory—present beginning in first year of life:
    Semantic (factual) memory: Initial development by one to two years of age.
    Autobiographical (collections of episodic memory): Progressive development with
        onset after second year of life.
Requires conscious awareness for encoding and having the subjective sense of
    recollection (and, if autobiographical, of self and time).
Focal attention required for encoding.
Hippocampal processing required for storage and initial retrieval.
Cortical consolidation makes selected events a part of permanent memory and
    independent of hippocampal involvement for retrieval.

Paller, Voss, and Westerberger have stated:

> Models of declarative memory generally posit that these distinct features or fragments must become linked together for enduring memory storage to be successful. Retrieval, rehearsal, and consolidation would thus entail synchronous activation across dispersed cortical networks, and this synchronous cross-cortical activity may be of the same type necessary for conscious experience more generally.[40]

In this way, we can see how the emergence of consciousness as development progresses may be intimately related to the development of memory. Both memory and consciousness depend upon integrative processes in the brain for their creation. This linkage of differentiated elements can also be seen in how energy and information is shared within relationships with caregivers and in the larger communities of interconnected relationships in which we live.[41] Memory has been shown, for example, to be influenced by the use of language within the communication patterns of both the microculture of a family and the macroculture of our larger

> The emergence of consciousness may be intimately related to the development of memory.

society.[42] In these ways, the conscious experience we have of a "self" is formed in part by how our synapses are shaped by our social experiences within the family and broader society.

As children grow into their second year, they begin to develop a more complex image of themselves in the world. This sense of self has been identified by studies examining how children respond to seeing themselves in the mirror with a red mark placed on their faces. They notice something different in their reflection, suggesting that they have a mental image in their minds of what they usually look like. By eighteen months, they are able to touch themselves rather than the mirror in exploring the red mark. Taken together, these studies on the developmental phase of the second year suggest that a child is developing a sense of the physical world, of time and sequence, and of the self, all of which form the foundation of explicit autobiographical memory.[43] Before this time, events in the child's life may have been remembered ("event memory"), but it is thought that these are semantic recollections of experiences without an enriched sense of self across time, which is the hallmark of autobiographical (episodic) recollection.[44]

Wheeler and other researchers have summarized a range of neuroimaging studies revealing that memory for facts (semantic memory), including events, is functionally quite distinct from memory of the self across time (episodic memory).[45] Semantic memory allows for propositional representations—symbols of external or internal facts that can be declared with words or in graphic form and can be assessed as "true" or "false." Such semantic knowledge has been called "noesis" and allows us to know about facts in the world. In contrast, autobiographical or episodic memory requires a capacity termed "autonoesis" (self-knowing) and appears to be dependent upon the development of frontal cortical regions of the brain. These regions undergo rapid experience-dependent development during the first few years of life (continuing possibly into adulthood) and are postulated to mediate autonoetic consciousness. The ability of the human mind to carry out what Tulving and colleagues have termed "mental time travel"—that is, to have a sense of recollection of the self at a particular time in the past, awareness of the self in the lived present, and projections of the self into the imagined future—is the unique contribution of autonoetic consciousness.[46] By the middle of the third year of life, a child has already begun to join caregivers in mutually constructed tales woven from their real-life events and imagining.[47] The richness of self-knowledge and autobiographical narratives appears to be mediated by the interpersonal dialogues in which caregivers co-construct narratives about external events and the internal, subjective experiences of the characters.

Nelson describes the process this way:

The major developmental transition in the preschool years can be viewed as a move toward a social–cultural–linguistic self in society. This transition to a new level of social-cognitive consciousness is apparent in major shifts between the 2- and 5-year-old levels of functioning in myriads of situations, experimental and everyday, that are now well documented in the developmental literature.[48]

She then goes on to illuminate the implications of this growth:

The changes observed are not caused by some single factor, but are dependent on the achievements of many related skills unique to human development. Nor are they the product of a sudden shift in cognitive level, but of a continuous, overlapping process of developing functions. Among the achievements of this period of development, the most powerful and profound is that of an advanced level of social and cultural language functions. The transition to a "cultural self" depends on the experiences of language in social use, thus on social practices, but its effects are also profoundly personal, involving the child's social and cognitive awareness and capacity for new levels of mental representation and reflective thought. This process is slow and massively interactive, eventuating in a culturally saturated concept of self, an autobiographical memory self with a specific self-history and imagined self-future that reflects the values, expectations, and forms of the embedding culture.[49]

Interventions to increase parental reflection on shared experiences has been shown to improve the child's growing autobiographical sense of self.[50] As Fivush and Nelson reveal, "Parent-guided reminiscing about past events that includes discussion, comparison, and negotiation of internal states of self and other, and places these internal states in explanatory narratives of behavior, allows children to construct a psychologically imbued representation of relations between past and present, and self and other."[51] In this way, we can hypothesize that attachment experiences—that is, communication with parents and other caregivers—directly enhance a child's capacity for autonoetic consciousness. This may be one reason why shared communication about remembered events enhances recollection. In other words, our relationships not only shape what we remember, but how we remember and the very sense of self that remembers.[52] An example of empirical support for this view comes from Jack and colleagues' study:

Conversations about past events between 17 mother–child dyads were recorded on multiple occasions between the children's 2nd and 4th birthdays. When these children were aged 12–13 years, they were interviewed about their early memories. Adolescents whose mothers used a greater ratio of elaborations to repetitions during the early childhood conversations had earlier memories than adolescents whose mothers used a smaller ratio of elaborations to repetitions. This finding is consistent with the hypothesis that past-event conversations during early childhood have long-lasting effects on autobiographical memory.[53]

How parents engage with children in focusing attention and encouraging elaboration on their shared reflections appears to have a direct impact on the autobiographical development of the self.

Our autobiographical sense of self emerges within our interpersonal experiences. Fivush summarizes this process succinctly:

> Autobiographical memory is a uniquely human system that integrates memories of past experiences into an overarching life narrative. . . . (a) autobiographical memory is a gradually developing system across childhood and adolescence that depends on the development of a sense of subjective self as continuous in time; (b) autobiographical memory develops within specific social and cultural contexts that relate to individual, gendered, and cultural differences in adults' autobiographical memories, and, more specifically, (c) mothers who reminisce with their young children in elaborated and evaluative ways have children who develop more detailed, coherent, and evaluative autobiographical memories.[54]

The encoding process for both forms of explicit memory (semantic and episodic) appears to require focal, conscious, directed attention to activate the hippocampus.[55] As encoding occurs, stimuli are placed initially in "sensory" memory, which lasts for about a quarter to half a second. This sensory "buffer" contains the initial neural activations of the perceptual system. Only selected items from this huge immediate sensory process are then placed in "working" memory, which lasts up to half a minute if there is no further rehearsal. If the mind rehearses or refreshes the activity of these activated circuits of working memory, then the items can be either maintained for longer periods of time in this process (such as practicing a phone number long enough to dial it repeatedly if the line is busy) or placed into longer-term storage.

Working memory has been called the "chalkboard of the mind." It is the mental process involved when we say that we are "thinking about something"; it allows us to reflect upon items perceived in the present and recalled from the past.[56] When we consciously think of a problem or an event, working memory allows us to link together various representations and manipulate them in our minds. The product of such cognitive processing can then enter a more stable component, "long-term" memory. In some individuals with disorders of attention, working memory appears to be unable to handle as many items for as long as the working memory of nondisordered individuals can. Imaging studies have supported this clinical finding by identifying abnormalities in the lateral prefrontal cortex, the site thought to be a primary mediator of working memory.[57]

Although this prefrontal region may play an important role in working memory, research suggests that this function is not limited to one area, but rather is a distributed process arising from the interaction of many neural components. Buchsbaum and D`Esposito state:

> One conclusion that arises from this research is that working memory can be viewed as neither a unitary nor a dedicated system. A network of brain regions, including the prefrontal cortex (PFC), is critical for the active maintenance of internal representations that are necessary for goal-directed behavior. Thus, working memory is not localized to a single brain region but probably is an emergent property of the functional interactions between the PFC and the rest of the brain.[58]

Long-term explicit memory is thought to be the process by which items are stored for extended periods of time beyond working memory.[59] For example, recalling a close friend's phone number requires it to be placed in long-term storage. Remembering the phone number of a shop we need to call only once requires working memory to hold on to those digits just long enough to dial the number. After the call, the shop's number vanishes from any form of permanent storage. If working memory persisted, we would be bombarded by irrelevant information from the past. Placing a needed item into long-term memory allows us to recall important data. When we ask others to recall their experiences from the last month, we are in effect requesting them to activate a representational process that has been "stored" as an increased probability of firing within a neural net. This is mediated by genetically activated structural alterations in synaptic connections within the network. In contrast, working memory is thought to be independent of gene-activated protein synthesis. It involves functional (not structural) alterations in synaptic strengths, such as increases in synaptic excitability that temporarily enhance the probability of specific neuronal firing. Recollection can be viewed as the actual activation of a potential or latent representation. The hippocampus is essential for both encoding items into and retrieving them from long-term explicit memory. The linkage of this process to the circuits of the lateral prefrontal cortex is one view of the mechanism for having working memory activate the structurally embedded elements of long-term memory, where they can be consciously examined, manipulated, and reported to others. Controversy exists, however, in regard to how distinct "working" and "long-term" memory are from one another.[60]

> Recollection can be viewed as the actual activation of a potential or latent representation.

Long-term memory does not last forever. For these items to become a part of permanent explicit memory, a process called "cortical consolidation" is thought to occur.[61] Though the mechanism has not been elucidated thus far, some views suggest that cortical consolidation requires a nonconscious activation or rehearsal process that allows representations to be stored in the "associational cortex."[62] This region of the cerebral cortex appears to integrate representations from various parts of the brain. Consolidation appears to involve the reorganization of existing memory traces, not the laying down of new engrams. In this manner, consolidation may make new associational linkages, condense elements of memory into new clusters of representations, and incorporate previously unintegrated elements into a functional whole. In cortical consolidation, information is finally free of the need for the hippocampus for retrieval. This consolidation process may depend on the rapid-eye-movement (REM) sleep stage, which is thought to be attempting to make sense of the day's activities.[63] Though filled with a combination of seemingly random activations, aspects of the day's experiences, and elements from the more distant past, dreams may be a fundamental way in which the mind consolidates the myriad of explicit recollections into a coherent set of representations for permanent, consolidated memory. Other studies suggest that REM and dreaming are not necessary for memory consolidation and learning.[64] Although sleep itself is essential for optimal health, it remains unclear exactly how either REM or slow-wave sleep contributes directly to the long-term processing of memory.

Research is still in its infancy regarding the details of the consolidation process.[65] Interestingly, cortical consolidation may take weeks, months, or perhaps years to occur. For example, if a man sustains a head injury in a motorcycle accident on the first of January, he may lose recollection of events from November and December of the prior year, but may be able to recall those from October and earlier without difficulty. This is called "retrograde" amnesia and involves impairment in the ability of the hippocampus to retrieve not-yet-consolidated memories. He may also experience severe difficulty recalling events after the accident, called "anterograde" amnesia. This involves damage to the hippocampus's ability to encode new items into long-term explicit memory. Working memory may remain unimpaired. Also, the man's ability to encode or retrieve items from implicit memory will be intact. He can learn new skills and have emotional associations to recent events, but he will be unable to recall when he acquired the new knowledge or to have any sense of time or self connected with the recollections.

Many forms of amnesia involve the impairment of explicit processing in the setting of intact implicit memory. Explicit recollections, as we've seen, require focal, conscious attention, and are processed through the initial phases of encoding in working memory and then in long-term memory on their way toward cortical consolidation. There are certain situations, however, in which there is a dis-association between implicit and explicit memory. "Infantile" or "childhood" amnesia is one such example (to be discussed below), in which normal infants' and young children's implicit memory is intact, but their explicit recall, especially episodic memory, is impaired. Other examples include hypnotic amnesia; the effects of certain medications, such as the benzodiazepines (minor tranquilizers); surgical anesthesia; some neurological conditions, such as brain injury and Korsakoff's syndrome; and divided-attention phenomena, such as an experiment in dichotic listening. In this last case, a participant is asked to pay attention to only one ear while listening to two auditory lists on a set of headphones. For example, in the left ear is played a list of zoo animals, in the right a list of flowers. When asked to repeat what was heard in the focally attended ear (say, the left), most participants have excellent recall of the animals. When asked what was heard in the right ear, participants usually state that they don't know. When asked to fill in the blank spaces on partially spelled words, such as "r ___ ___ e," they are much more likely than participants exposed to a different list to fill in the word "rose." This is an example of indirect recall, a measure of implicit memory. A participant's brain has encoded the flowers implicitly, so that the brain is "primed" (i.e., made more likely) to bring up a flower when given a cue. Participants have no conscious recall of

> Without focal attention, items are not encoded explicitly.

what they heard, or even a sense that what they are writing is a reflection of something they experienced. *Without focal attention, items are not encoded explicitly.* Implicit memory may be more fully intact, but explicit memory is impaired for that stimulus or event.[66]

## THE SUBJECTIVE EXPERIENCE
## OF EXPLICIT AND IMPLICIT MEMORY

When either semantic or episodic explicit memory is retrieved, there is an internal sensation of "I am recalling something." This distinguishes explicit recollections from implicit ones, in which there is no such subjective sense of remembrance. Explicit memories take a number of forms. Semantic memory is a type in which we can recall factual information, such as the capitals of the major countries of Europe. If we recall that we were once in those cities but cannot summon the sensation of the self in time on the trip, then this reflects a semantic memory for a personally experienced event. In the past, this form of memory may have been considered by academicians as a part of autobiographical recall, but recent neuroscientific studies support

the notion that semantic recall lacking a sense of self is in fact quite different from but highly interactive with episodic recall.[67] Noetic consciousness
(knowing the fact that we were once in Europe) is thought to be distinct
from autonoetic consciousness (recalling our experience of the trip), both
in subjective experience and in the involvement of the prefrontal cortices in
the latter process. Episodic recall activates autobiographical memory representations and evokes a process of mental time travel—the sense of the self
in time—which differentiates it from semantic recollections. The content of
autobiographical recollection will also influence the neural regions recruited
during such activations. As Svoboda, McKinnon, and Levine state regarding autobiographical memory (which they abbreviate as AM): "Our findings support a neural distinction between episodic and semantic memory
in AM. . . . Emotional events produced a shift in lateralization (toward the
right) of the AM network with activation observed in emotion-centered
regions and deactivation (or lack of activation) observed in regions associated
with cognitive processes.[68]

The distinct experiential aspects of memory are thought to involve different centers of activation and patterns of electrical (EEG) waves within
the brain.[69] For example, although there may be significant overlap in the
neural areas involved, semantic recall appears to generally involve a dominance of left over right hippocampal activation. Autobiographical recall, in
contrast, involves more of the right hippocampus and right orbitofrontal
cortex.[70] Here we see that structure and function within the brain correlate
with our day-to-day encounters with subjective experience. This distinction
may reveal itself when we know a fact without any feeling that it is a part
of our experienced life. Though semantic and episodic memory have much
in common—they are flexibly accessible, have virtually unlimited capacities for representing "data," are encoded with contextual features, and can
be retrieved in a declarative manner via language or drawing—they in fact
appear to be mediated by somewhat distinct mechanisms.[71]

For episodic memory, there appears to be a much larger process involved
than merely the autobiographical content of representations of personally
experienced events: Autonoetic awareness involves the experience of mental
time travel and is directly linked to the processes of the prefrontal regions
of the brain. Autonoetic consciousness is created within the various layers of prefrontal function.[72] These include an integrating capacity, in which
more posteriorly stored information can be organized and sequenced into
a meaningful set of representations; executive functions, which provide a
more global control of widely distributed brain processes; and the mediation
of self-reflection and social cognition.[73] We can see that mental time travel is
more than a subjective sense of feeling oneself in the past, present, or future:
It is an actively constructive mental process that creates the self within a

social world. It turns out that several independent lines of research point to the midline prefrontal regions—especially the orbitofrontal cortex in the right hemisphere—as a crucial area for integrating memory,[74] attachment,[75] emotion,[76] bodily representation and regulation,[77] and social cognition.[78]

Within explicit autobiographical memory, we can find a number of variations on these elements of self in time. For example, you may recall a general sense of yourself from your senior year in high school. This generic episodic recollection can be thought of as a general descriptor summating across your perceptions of a year of specific episodes. In a sense this is a self-concept, or a self-schema made conscious, about yourself during that year. In contrast, you may be able to recall a specific event during that time, such as your last day of high school. In retrieving this memory, you may recall it as an event you observed from a distance, as if you were taking an outsider's perspective. This is an "observer" recollection, which some might consider a distanced form of episodic retrieval, but which others would label an event memory within semantic recall.[79] In contrast, you may recall the event as if you were actually there; this is a "participant" or "field" recollection. In this case, you would be able to see things from your actual perspective. Observer recollections appear to involve less emotional intensity than field recollections do. Autonoesis thus evokes elements of the self's lived experience, rather than merely the propositional (factual) representations of noetic consciousness.

The process of reactivating representations from explicit memory is often dependent on the context, that is, the features of the internal and external environment. When there is a match between retrieval cue and memory representation, the process is called "ecphory."[80] Ecphory depends upon the features of the eliciting stimulus and the form in which the representation has been stored in memory. Retrieval is enhanced when conditions at the time of recall are similar to those of the initial encoding. The similarities may be in the physical world (sights, sounds, smells) or in one's state of mind (emotions, mental models, states of general arousal). In this way, explicit memory is said to be "context-dependent." The hippocampus is able to encode its cognitive mapping on experiences, giving them a context in which they are both registered and stored. The actual representations of such experiences are thought to be stored in more posterior portions of the brain. The prefrontal regions are thought to carry out the process of creating an episodic "retrieval state" in which a match between retrieval cue and stored representation (ecphory) can occur.[81]

Individuals may have recollections and lack an understanding of how the context cued the specific event being recalled. They may explore these memories by searching for a match between the features present at the time of retrieval and at the time of the original event. Such a search can sometimes reveal the underlying emotional meaning or gist of a particular recollection. However, the sense of mental time travel by itself does not mean that the recollection is accurate. It merely implies that the prefrontally mediated autonoetic awareness circuits are involved in the activation, not that ecphory has occurred. In this manner, the prefrontal region may attempt to create accurate assemblies of representations—but, accurate or not, they may contain a sense of the self recalling the past. This can be viewed as what we can call an "ecphoric sensation," which has a sense of conviction that the recalled memory is indeed accurate. We can have a clear sense that something happened when in fact it did not. Such subjective sensations may be a part of imagination, dreaming, or inaccurate as well as accurate recollection.

> We can have a clear sense that something happened when in fact it did not.

The richness we may feel in reflecting on past experiences is shaped in part by internal or external context cues, which can then initiate a cascade of further related recollections. Initial ecphory (the retrieval cue's matching the stored memory representation) is followed by a series of sometimes unpredictable associative linkages influenced by both memory and present experience. These associated recollections and retrieval cues can be woven into the process of remembering and can become a part of the "reconstructed" memory. Representations resembling those of the past are reassembled anew during the process of recollection. Retrieval is thus, as Robert Bjork and colleagues have suggested, a "memory modifier": The act of reactivating a representation can allow it to be stored again in a modified form.[82] The frontal lobes, in carrying out the integrative, executive, and socially constructive remembering of the self, can directly shape the nature of autobiographical recollections and life stories. These processes explain one way in which our memories—things we may regard as facts—can actually change over time and evolve over the lifespan.

Often cues will activate both explicit and implicit elements of memory. The initial subjective experience of this frequent process can often be a wave of internal, nonverbal sensations and images or behavioral impulses (implicit recollections), that may not feel as if something is being recalled. As explicit memory retrieval becomes linked to these implicit counterparts, we may begin to get a sense of some factual elements or images that begin to have the sensation of "I am remembering something now." On a daily basis, we actively reconstruct neural net profiles that have encoded both implicit and explicit circuits. The internal, subjective sensations of these distinct forms of memory parallel their anatomic distinction within the brain.[83]

Explicit memory is often communicated to ourselves and to others in the form of descriptive words or pictures as a story or sequence of events. If these involve the sense of self at some time in the past, then they are a part of explicit autobiographical memory. We listen to the words and receive a linguistic message, or see the pictures and have a conscious sense of the story being told. But recollections usually involve the association of these explicit elements with their implicit counterparts. To sense these, it is important to recall (explicitly) that implicit memory does not have a sense of "something being remembered." We sense, perceive, or filter our explicit memory through the mental models of implicit memory. We can watch for the shadows that such implicit "recollections" cast on the stories we tell, as well as on nonverbal aspects of behavior and communication.

For example, a thirty-five-year-old woman began to recount her experiences of being raised by a violent, alcoholic father. When she began to tell her story, her eyes became filled with tears, her hands began to tremble, and she turned away from her therapist. She stopped speaking and seemed to become frozen, with a look of terror on her face. For the therapist, the feeling in the room was intense and consuming. The patient began to speak again, but this time spoke of her father's "positive attributes." Though she wiped away her tears, and tried to "compose" herself and not "worry so much about the past," her nonverbal communication remained. In this case, the patient was being flooded by the implicit elements of her early experiences, evoked in part by her recounting the story of her father's rages. As she began to divert the narrative she was relating, only parts of the implicit memories were able to be diffused. Despite this diversion, for the remainder of the session she continued to feel frightened and humiliated.

The challenge in cases like this one is not only to listen to the words, but also to observe the nonverbal elements of communication that let us know what others are experiencing and remembering. We must keep in mind that only a part of memory can be translated into the language-based packets of information people use to tell their life stories to others. Learning to be open to many layers of communication is a fundamental part of getting to know another person's life.

## CHILDHOOD AMNESIA

For over a century, clinicians have been aware of an impairment in the ability of older children or adults to recall the first years of their lives. Initial impressions suggested that this "memory barrier" is for the period before the ages of five to seven years. Psychoanalytic writings from the past suggested that infantile amnesia was due to some traumatic, overwhelming experiences that were being blocked, and that one focus of treatment should be to uncover this "repression barrier."[84] Modern analytic thinking does not support this notion, however. Developmental psychologists also view childhood amnesia differently. They suggest that immaturities in the sense of self, in the sense of time, in verbal ability, and in narrative capacity may be the factors limiting recall for the period before the age of about two to three years.[85] Neurobiologists investigating this form of amnesia have looked at the development of the hippocampus/medial temporal lobe and the orbitofrontal region during the first years of life as a possible mediator of the phenomenon of childhood amnesia.[86] This view supports the developmental psychologists' observations in providing the likely neurobiological underpinnings to this typical developmental form of amnesia. In this way, explicit memory may require the neural maturation of the hippocampus to allow for the full expression of first semantic and then later episodic memory.

Let's explore the development of explicit memory by examining the experiences of a young girl. A one-year-old is able to have implicit recollection of all sorts of experiences: becoming excited when she hears the car pull into the garage, knowing emotionally on some level that her mother is coming home; learning to walk; or generating mental models for repeated experiences. She has already developed the capacity for generalized recollections, called "general event knowledge."[87] Before the age of eighteen months, she has begun to develop the ability to recall the sequence of events in her world.[88] She thus can encode and retrieve facts from specific experiences. This can be considered a form of semantic memory, in which knowledge of specific events can be recalled after a long delay.[89]

After about eighteen months, the child develops self-referential behaviors that reveal a sense of continuity of the self through time. By her second birthday, she can now begin to talk about events that have happened to her. As she continues to mature, her sense of self develops more fully and may allow for the gradual emergence of episodic memory and the capacity for mental time travel—for remembering herself in specific experiences in the past. As her prefrontal regions develop, this capacity becomes increasingly complex and sophisticated. These regions may continue to develop into adulthood and may explain the deepening capacity for self-awareness and autonoetic consciousness throughout the lifespan. At the early age of two, the child can say that she saw a dog that morning, or that she went to visit her grandfather at the park. She can narrate her ongoing experience and can verbalize her anticipation of future events. Though now she can talk about her recent recollections, she cannot episodically remember when she was an infant. Some facts that she has learned during her second year of life, however, may be quite available to her within semantic memory, such as the names of objects and what things do. Though controversy exists over the nature and timing of the onset of declarative or semantic explicit memory,[90] some investigators suggest that even preverbal infants can recall the facts of experiences at this early age.[91] The work of Patricia Bauer and her colleagues suggests that even experiences that occurred after a child's first birthday but before the advent of spoken language may be recalled verbally with considerable accuracy after many months. These recollections are likely to be part of explicit semantic memory and not derived from the yet-to-be-accessible autobiographical process.[92]

Some authors argue that childhood amnesia is not an impairment in general explicit recall, but rather is very specifically due to the developmental lag in the onset of episodic memory within explicit processing.[93] Support for this view comes from findings that children even in their second year of life have a remarkable ability to retain facts about novel experiences with great accuracy.[94] Thus these studies suggest that semantic explicit memory is intact from a very early age.

How does episodic memory develop? A few findings that explore the impact of experience on autobiographical memory may be useful in examining this question. Children who have more experiences of talking about their memories with their parents are able to recall more details about their lives later on.[95] "Memory talk" is a common process in which parents focus their attention on the contents of a child's memories. A similar observation is that parents who participate in an "elaborative" form of communication have children with a richer sense of autobiographical recall. Elaborative parents talk with their children about what they, the children, think about the stories they read together. In contrast, "factual" parents—the classification designating parents who are found to talk only about the facts of stories, not a child's imagination or response—have children with a less developed ability for recall of shared experiences. Similarly, "emotion knowledge" is higher in children whose parents elaborate on the nature and the emotional meaning of an experience in their discussions with their children.[96] There is probably a range of communication styles between the extremes of these two research categories. Nevertheless, these findings support the general principle that interpersonal experiences appear to have a direct effect on the development of explicit memory, as well as on the understanding of the mind's inner nature. As Bauer and colleagues have stated, "The talk in which children and parents engage prior to, during, and/or after an event works to organize, integrate, and, thereby, facilitate children's memory for it."[97]

> Interpersonal experiences appear to have a direct effect on the development of explicit memory.

Are these merely genetic findings revealing that parents give rise to offspring who naturally, genetically, will have their same traits? To be sure, we must await further studies, such as those that might examine the narratives of identical twins raised apart, to clarify the origin of these differences in

narrative style.[98] There is clearly a difference in narrative experience, whatever the origin: Some families participate in frequent co-construction of
narrative and elaborative memory talk. In reinforcing this kind of experience, parents may facilitate their children's ability to describe their memories, as well as their imaginations. In a similar fashion, research has shown
that children raised in families that discussed people's emotional reactions
tended to be more interested in and able to understand others' emotions.[99]
Such children are also taught that what they have to say about the contents
of their minds is important.

Cross-cultural studies suggest that culturally mediated communication
patterns may directly impact the emergence of a sense of self in the growing child. One study found that Japanese-born individuals perceived a visual
image of an aquarium by noting its holistic features: how plants, rocks, and
fish all formed part of a larger whole marine scene. In contrast, American-
born Japanese presented with the same image noted the individual characteristics of a single fish, highlighting its colors and anatomy, rather than
perceiving the overall aquatic environment.[100] As we'll see in future chapters, such a finding of culturally influenced perceptual biasing may reflect
the preferential growth of the right versus the left hemisphere in individuals
within traditional Japanese culture, versus the more individually oriented
emphasis in mainstream U.S. society. Culture plays an important role in
mediating patterns of social relatedness, and hence the growth of the brain
and the mind.

As families shape the developing minds of children, culture also shapes
and continues to shape how minds develop across the lifespan. Memory processes and a sense of self and identity are all shaped by our social experiences.
Our most intimate sense of our individual lives—our autobiographical
memories and our identities—are actually shaped, in part, by our relational
worlds. Each of these experiences may enhance the capacity for emotional
regulation.[101] These effects may be mediated by the experience-dependent
growth of the orbitofrontal regions responsible for affect regulation and the
encoding and retrieval of episodic memory.[102]

The lack of explicit recall for the first years of life reveals a differential
development among several modalities of memory. The first year appears to
enable implicit but not explicit encoding and retrieval. The circuits mediating the various forms of implicit memory are fairly well developed at birth.
The second year has been shown to allow for a form of explicit recollection
that is most likely to be semantic in nature. Such a capacity is likely to be
mediated by the maturation of the medial temporal lobe, including areas of
the hippocampus. By eighteen months to two or three years of age, episodic
memory begins to emerge. The emergence of this process may be facilitated
by the development of the prefrontal regions of the brain, especially the

orbitofrontal cortex. As these regions develop actively during the preschool years, episodic memory undergoes significant maturation. The ongoing development of a sense of self during this time enables this form of autonoesis to grow rapidly and become more elaborate. As the sense of self continues to develop, the intricacies of self-experience evolve.

Nelson and Carver explain:

> What makes possible the changes in explicit memory through the preschool period is the development of various prefrontal functions that can come to the assistance of the medial temporal lobe (explicit) memory system. For example, it is generally not until the preschool period that children begin to routinely employ strategies to help them remember things; the use of strategies, of course, is a quintessential prefrontal function. . . . [They further state that] the neural circuitry involved in long-term memory develop slowly over the infancy and preschool period. The relevant structures that are thought to develop during this interval include the circuits that pass along information from the medial temporal lobe, where initial encoding and consolidation is performed, and the cortex, where memory is stored. It is neural maturation, then, that likely accounts for the gradual "recovery" from infantile amnesia."[103]

In general, childhood amnesia raises the larger issue about remembering and forgetting. Our internal sense of who we are is shaped both by what we can explicitly recall, and by the implicit recollections that create our mental models and internal subjective experience of images, sensations, emotions, and behavioral responses.

## EMOTION, REMEMBERING, AND FORGETTING

Is everything that is experienced remembered? No. Forgetting is an essential aspect of explicit memory; if we were to have easy access to every experience we have encoded, our working memory would be flooded with extraneous facts and images, and efficient functioning would become impaired.[104] Which events, then, are more likely to be remembered and which forgotten? It turns out that many studies of emotion and memory point to an inverted-U-shaped-curve effect.[105] Experiences that involve little emotional intensity seem to do little to arouse focal attention, and have a higher likelihood of being registered as "unimportant" and therefore of not being easily recalled later on. Events experienced with a moderate to high degree of emotional intensity seem to get labeled as "important" (probably by anatomic structures in the limbic region and closely aligned areas, such as the amygdala and orbitofrontal cortex, which are discussed in more detail later in the book) and are more easily remembered in the future. If events are overwhelming and filled with terror, a number of factors may inhibit the hippocampal processing of explicit memory, and therefore may block explicit encoding and subsequent retrieval. As Elzinga and colleagues report in a study of how the stress hormone cortisol influences subsequent recall, "These results suggest that stress-induced cortisol specifically affects long-term consolidation of declarative memories. These findings may have implications for understanding the effects of traumatic stress on memory functioning in patients with stress-related psychiatric disorders."[106] While cortisol may impede explicit processing by blocking the hippocampus functioning, other factors such as divided attention may also contribute to the blockage of explicit memory encoding.[107] At the same time, other elements occurring during an overwhelming event may actually increase the strength of implicit encoding. Such factors may include amygdala discharge and the release of noradrenaline in response to massive stress. Such conditions may allow and even reinforce implicit memory encoding, while divided attention and cortisol secretion may simultaneously impede explicit processing of the traumatizing event. This proposes that trauma may have a differential impact on implicit and explicit memory; however, the exact interactive mechanisms of these two layers of memory need to be clarified in future research.[108]

Although even one-time occurrences can alter synaptic strengths, repeated experiences and emotionally arousing experiences have the greatest impact on the connections within the brain. In other words, not all encounters with the world affect the mind equally. Studies have demonstrated that if the brain appraises an event as "meaningful," it will be more likely to be recalled in the future. Some of these studies suggest that the interaction of stress-related neuromodulatory chemicals, cortisol and adrenaline, may be directly involved in the activation of regions involved in memory encoding.[109] The brain appraises the significance of stimuli in numerous ways, including the activation of areas such as the amygdala. If the amygdala is activated, then the engram encoded at that particular time is thought to be marked as significant; this has been called a "value-laden"

> If the brain appraises an event as "meaningful," it will be more likely to be recalled in the future.

memory.[110] The neuronal mechanism for this labeling is the pronounced increase in synaptic strengths at the time of that specific experience. As we'll see in Chapter 4 on emotion, value systems in the brain may serve as neuromodulatory circuits with processes that (1) enhance neuronal excitability and activation; (2) enhance neuronal plasticity and the creation of new synaptic connections; and (3) have extensive innervation linking various brain regions. This emotionally charged value-laden memory is thus made more likely to be reactivated among the myriad of infinite engrams laid down throughout life.

The relationship between emotion and memory suggests that emotionally arousing experiences are more readily recalled later on. As James McGaugh has stated,

> the evidence suggests the possibility that the influences of several neuromodulatory systems on memory may be integrated by interactions occurring within the amygdala. . . . The evidence thus strongly supports the general hypothesis that endogenous neuromodulatory systems activated by experience play a role in regulating memory storage. [He goes on to suggest that] the strength of memories depends on the degree of emotional activation induced by learning. Highly emotional stimulation may well, as William James (1890) suggested, "almost . . . leave a scar on the cerebral tissue" in the form of lasting changes in synaptic connectivity.[111]

In other words, emotion involves a modulatory process that enhances the creation of new synaptic connections via increases in neuronal plasticity.

What are the mechanisms of this increased plasticity? The exact link between emotion and the activation of genes to initiate new synapse formation as a part of neuroplastic changes has not yet been fully clarified. However, some intriguing possibilities are suggested by studies done on the molecules of memory in invertebrate animals.[112] A protein called CREB-1 (for "cyclic AMP response element binding-1") appears to lead to the activation of genes that initiate the protein synthesis necessary to establish synaptic connections. The growth of new synapses is normally constrained by inhibitory memory-suppressing genes that appear to regulate the transfer of information from short-term storage, such as working memory, into long-term memory. This suppression may be mediated by a protein called CREB-2. If this process studied in "lower" animals is found to be utilized by human memory processes, then perhaps it is the human brain's way to ensure that irrelevant stimuli are not encoded into long-term memory: Some active process would need to be initiated to produce structurally based encoding of events into long-term memory. This overall process is part of "long-term potentiation." These are exciting findings with relevance to human memory—specifically, to the emotional mechanisms by which the amygdala and other structures enhance memory encoding, as well as to the overall process of neuroplasticity by which brain structure is changed by experience.[113]

The "emotion circuits of the brain" that are activated when we have an emotionally engaging experience also serve as evaluative centers that directly influence our focus of attention and our state of arousal. During an "emotionally meaningful experience," it may be that our attention is concentrated and our state of arousal heightened, so that certain regions of the brain, such as the nucleus basalis,[114] are activated and release acetylcholine; this enhances the likelihood of gene activation in those neurons that are firing together. Concentrated attention may also increase the localized release of brain-derived neurotropic factor, which increases gene expression.[115] In other words, this view proposes that "emotion" is a process that helps focus attention and creates the neurochemical conditions that heighten neuroplastic changes in the brain.

The relationships among memory, emotion, and the self are complex. Looking toward neurobiology for some insights into these processes can be enlightening. As Robert Post and colleagues have suggested:

> The amygdala is thought to be involved with imparting the emotional significance to an object and linking it to other memory systems initially imparted by the hippocampus but then subserved by other complex cerebral pathways potentially involving many hundreds of thousands if not millions of synapses. Just the way the properties of objects are synthesized convergently by different pathways, we can surmise that the historical and emotional significance of objects are likewise "synthesized," but also edited, updated, and revised based on new experiences. In this fashion, the more complex associative experiential properties and cues may be attached to critical objects in the environment, such as one's parents, siblings, and even the concept of oneself.[116]

By creating meaning, our emotional neuromodulatory systems help organize and integrate our memories. Our lives are filled with implicit influences, the origins and impact of which we may not be aware. *In the case of childhood amnesia, this intact implicit memory in the presence of an impairment in explicit recall is a typical finding, unrelated to trauma.* As children's lives unfold, they are able to recall more and more of the events in their lives as these are woven into a narrative picture of the self across time. This narrative emerges as value-laden memories are consolidated and become a part of the permanent explicit autobiographical memory system. Not every experience will be episodically recalled; this is a part of normal forgetting. Our minds must selectively inhibit the encoding, recollection, and consolidation of many events that have occurred. If we were to become bombarded by irrelevant explicit detail, we would become confused and overwhelmed.

## STRESS, TRAUMA, AND MEMORY

Stressful experiences may take the form of highly emotional events or, when the stress is overwhelming, overtly traumatizing experiences. The degree of stress will have a direct effect on memory: Small amounts have a neutral effect; moderate amounts facilitate memory; and large amounts impair memory. The effect of stress appears to be mediated by the characteristic neuroendocrine responses involving the immediate transient effects (lasting seconds to minutes) of noradrenaline release and the more sustained effects (lasting minutes to hours) of glucocorticoids such as cortisol, also known as "stress hormones." The mechanisms of and the interactions between these agents are complex. Studies suggest that the HPA axis involves the release of stress hormones that directly affect the hippocampus, a region with the highest density of receptors for these blood–borne agents.[117] Chronic stress may produce elevated baseline levels of stress hormones and abnormal daily rhythms of hormone release. The effects of high levels of stress hormones on the hippocampus may initially be reversible and involve the inhibition of neuronal growth and the atrophy of cellular receptive components called "dendrites."[118] Not only do high levels of stress transiently block hippocampal functioning, but excessive and chronic exposure to stress hormones may lead to neuronal death in this region—possibly producing decreased hippocampal volume, as found in patients with chronic posttraumatic stress disorder (PTSD).[119] Activation of the autonomic nervous system leads to the release of adrenaline and noradrenaline (known as the catecholamines), which are thought to affect the amygdala directly. The amygdala, as we've seen, plays an important role in establishing the value of an experience and integrating elements of encoding with the hippocampal processing of the event. As proposed earlier, excessive cortisol secretion may impair the hippocampal contribution to explicit memory processing, while noradrenaline secretion may enhance the implicit encoding facilitated by the amygdala.[120]

Highly emotional events may involve a certain degree of stress response. Particular cascades of physiological and cognitive reactions may reinforce the effects of stress on memory. Bower and Sivers have noted:

> Several factors working in concert promote better memory for highly emotional events. Prominent among these are the personal significance of the event, its distinctiveness or rarity and selective rehearsal. . . . When emotionally aroused, the brain triggers reactions from the autonomic nervous system and the endocrine system; the latter releases stress hormones into the blood stream, creating persistent arousal and reactivation of whatever thoughts are salient in the cognitive system. This arousal persists for several minutes and has an effect analogous to involuntary recycling of the stressful occurrence and the events leading up to it. Such rehearsal enhances the degree of learning of whatever aspects of the event were encoded. Beyond this physiological arousal that continues for several minutes, our minds have a tendency to return repeatedly over many hours or days to memories of emotionally upsetting events, perhaps triggered by external cues or ideational sequences that have been associated with the aversive event.[121]

In this manner, emotionally arousing experiences become better remembered by a combination of direct physiological effects (perhaps on the genetic activation leading to synapse formation, as discussed above) and complex cognitive effects on the encoding of memory via the retrieval, rehearsal, and reencoding process.

Under some conditions, explicit memory may be blocked from encoding at the actual time of an experience. Trauma may be such a situation. Various factors may contribute to the inhibition of hippocampal functioning needed for explicit memory at the time of a severe trauma.[122] During a trauma, the victim may focus his attention on a nontraumatic aspect of the environment or on his imagination as a means of at least partial escape. Divided-attention studies suggest that this situation will lead to the encoding of parts of the traumatic experience implicitly but not explicitly.[123] Furthermore, the release of large amounts of stress hormones in response to threat may impair hippocampal functioning. The outcome for a victim who dissociates explicit from implicit processing is an impairment in autobiographical memory for at least certain aspects of the trauma (explicit blockage may refer to "psychogenic" amnesia). Implicit memory of the event is intact and includes intrusive elements such as behavioral impulses to flee, emotional reactions, bodily sensations, and intrusive images related to the trauma.[124] Individuals who dissociate during and after a traumatic experience have been found in some studies but not in others to be the most vulnerable to developing PTSD.[125] As we've discussed, chronic stress may actually damage the hippocampus itself, as suggested by the finding of decreased hippocampal volume in patients suffering from chronic PTSD.[126] Under such conditions, future explicit processing and learning may be chronically impaired. Furthermore, in addition to damaging the hippocampus, early child maltreatment may directly affect the structure and epigenetic regulation of circuits that link bodily response to brain function: the autonomic nervous system, the HPA axis, and the neuroimmune process.[127] These ingrained ways in which adverse child experiences are "remembered" may explain the markedly increased risk for medical illness in adults with histories of childhood abuse and dysfunctional home environments.[128]

> Chronic stress may actually damage the hippocampus itself.

On the basis of this information, one can propose that psychological trauma involving the blockage of explicit processing also impairs the victim's ability to cortically consolidate the experience.[129] With dissociation or the prohibition of discussing with others what was experienced, as is so often the case in familial child abuse, there may be a profound blockage to the pathway toward consolidating memory. Unresolved traumatic experiences from this perspective may involve an impairment in the cortical consolidation process, which leaves the memories of these events out of permanent memory. But the person may be prone to experiencing continually intrusive implicit images of past horrors. Nightmares, occurring during the dream stage of sleep and involving active REM sleep disturbances, may reveal futile attempts of the brain to resolve and consolidate such blocked memory configurations. Both the dream and the slow-wave stages of sleep are thought to play a central role in reorganizing memory and in reinforcing the connections between memory and emotion.[130]

Although they are not linked within their independent domains of study, dream research, memory investigations, and the study of adaptation to trauma may help us understand some important processes in memory and trauma. Endel Tulving and coworkers have proposed a model of "hemispheric encoding–retrieval asymmetry,"[131] which has been generally supported and further elaborated by subsequent research,[132] though not by all studies.[133] In brief, this model draws on a range of investigations suggesting that the left prefrontal cortex plays a dominant role in the *encoding* of episodic memory, whereas the right prefrontal cortex is essential in episodic *retrieval*. The dreams of REM sleep involve markedly increased brain activity. Eye movements have been associated with the activation of the opposite side of the brain (i.e., movement to the left is associated with right-hemisphere activation).[134] (This finding explains why so many individuals look to the left during autobiographical recall—which, as we now know, activates right prefrontal regions.)

All of these findings taken together raise the following proposal, which remains to be substantiated by specific research. During the typical dreaming state, the left and right hemispheres are activated in an alternating, rhythmic, and synchronous fashion. Activation of the right orbitofrontal region of the prefrontal cortex mediates a "retrieval state" for the reactivation of episodic representations. Left orbitofrontal activation initiates an "encoding state" in which representations can be registered, linked together, and encoded into a reorganized or consolidated form. Slow-wave sleep may participate in the reassembly of various neural representations of memory, and REM sleep appears to function as a crucial process for memory consolidation that may facilitate long-term potentiation, allowing the strengthening of synaptic connections.[135] Thus memory may be "reorganized" during the various stages of sleep. The prefrontal regions have extensive innervation to various parts of the brain, including the neocortical associational cortex. The newly reorganized episodic memory becomes consolidated within the associational cortex, where it is now independent of the hippocampus and available for later retrieval. Future access of these newly reorganized memory representations can occur within autonoetic consciousness as mediated by the right orbitofrontal regions. The essential feature of such a process is the synchronous activation of right and left hemispheres to synthetically retrieve and encode episodic memory into a consolidated form. Dreaming thus permits episodic memory representations to become the engrams for consolidative encoding. Neural synchronization in both slow-wave and REM stages of sleep, as well as during daytime reflections, may play an important role in the consolidation process in general.[136] The result of such synchronization may be, literally, a "consolidation" of episodic memory into a coherent set of reprocessed and more fully integrated representations. The result of this integration and consolidation, we can propose, is the stuff of our life narratives.

We can further propose that autonoetic consciousness of traumatic events is disturbed in individuals who have experienced trauma that remains "unresolved." As we'll see in future chapters, this unresolved state of mind has important implications for the mind's functioning and for interpersonal relationships. Some individuals may become flooded by excessive implicit recollections, in which they lose the self-monitoring features of episodic recall and feel not as if they are intensely recalling a past event, but rather that they are in the event itself.[137] Others have knowledge of a traumatic event but no sense of self: They have noetic but not autonoetic awareness of the experience. The capacity of the left prefrontal region to encode episodic memory may have been impaired by blocked explicit encoding as proposed above, and/or by the flood of right-hemisphere representations of emotion and bodily sensations from the overwhelming event. Various studies of trauma patients reveal a significant asymmetry in hemispheric activity, with unresolved traumatic memories being associated with an excessively right-dominant activation pattern.[138] Traumatized children have also been found to have asymmetric brain abnormalities and altered development of the corpus callosum, the band of tissue that allows for interhemispheric transfer of information.[139] These findings, combined with the clinical observation of REM sleep disturbances in those with PTSD, support the proposal that bilateral cooperation of the hemispheres may be necessary for the consolidation of memory in general—and that failure to consolidate memories of traumatic events may be at the core of unresolved trauma. Such a view also points to the generalization that impairment in bilateral integration of information (the flow of energy and representations across the hemispheres) may be proposed as a marker of psychological impairment following traumatic experience.[140]

In individuals with chronic PTSD, the damage documented in hippocampal structure and function may reveal one aspect of their difficulties in resolving traumatic experiences.[141] Other studies suggest that childhood neglect and abuse lead to impairments in the growth of integrative fibers of the brain.[142] The resolution process can thus be proposed to involve the integration of the trauma into a larger associational matrix within the brain so that the mind can become "coherent," as we'll discuss in later chapters on regulation and neural integration. In essence, such proposed integration may result in a more coherent autobiographical narrative and a resolution of disturbances in REM sleep. These possibilities are explored in detail in the final two chapters.

As we shall also see in subsequent chapters, a lack of cortical consolidation may be seen clinically in the absence of a narrative version of a traumatic experience. An individual may find a way to "stick together" as a cohesive but constricted way of functioning—but more fluid, flexible, and adaptive "coherence" may be lacking. This impediment to coherent functioning may be at the heart of a range of compromises to mental and interpersonal well-being. Furthermore, there may also be an inability to establish a sense of coherence and continuity across various states of mind. Traumatic states may remain isolated from the typical integrative functioning of the individual and thus impair development. Implicit elements of major and perhaps even minor traumatic events may continue to shape the individual's life without conscious awareness of their origins. In other words, the implicit impact of trauma may influence a person's nonconscious and conscious experience, but without a sense of its origins from the past. In this view, negative influences on development may impair mental health by blocking the typically unrestricted flow of information within the mind.

This restricted flow may impair the creation of life stories that would otherwise allow for emotionally significant events to be placed in the larger associational network of permanent, consolidated memory. Schemata of the self and of others in the world help shape the structure of such a cognitive framework of memory. In other words, implicit mental models help shape the organization of explicit autobiographical memory. Traumatic memories that are unresolved do not reach this point of being consolidated into the larger framework of implicit–explicit consolidated narrative memory. They can be seen instead as remaining in an unstable state of potential implicit activations, which tend to intrude upon the survivor's internal experiences and interpersonal relationships.

## THE ACCURACY OF MEMORY AND THE IMPACT OF TRAUMA

Clinicians, educators, journalists, attorneys, and lawmakers all share questions concerning remembering and forgetting, especially in cases involving allegations of childhood abuse. As one reviews the research findings and wades through the controversies and politics, a few simple truths become clear. Individuals can experience traumatic events and be unable to recall them explicitly later on; a wide range of research over the last hundred years supports this view, with recent findings supporting the proposal that implicit memory for traumatic events may be greater in those with PTSD.[143] Research has also supplied a neuroscientific explanation for this old knowledge.[144] Years can go by before a contextual change in an individual's life occurs and the recollection of a traumatic event can become available to conscious recollection.[145] This has sometimes been referred to as "delayed recall." Although delayed recollection may be quite accurate, explicit memory is exquisitely sensitive to the conditions of recall. Recounting the elements of explicit autobiographical memory is a social experience that is profoundly influenced by social interaction. Thus what is recounted is not the same as what is initially remembered, and it is not necessarily completely accurate in detail.

The human mind is extremely suggestible throughout life, particularly in childhood.[146] This suggestibility allows us to attend schools and to permit our minds to become deeply influenced by the views of others. Often we maintain critical analyses of whether the information we are being supplied is trustworthy, and thus whether it should become a part of our memory systems. However, the determination by such "metamemory" processes of the accuracy of a memory can be distorted by a number of factors, including drug states, hypnosis, and intense and repeated questioning within certain forms of interrogation. Some individuals may be more susceptible to suggestive influences than others. Suggestibility studies indicate that it is possible for an individual to be firmly convinced of the veridicality of a "recollection" when in fact the event being recalled has never occurred. Thus a person's degree of conviction about the accuracy of a memory may not correspond to its accuracy.[147] The use of internal corroborations may be useful in understanding how past experiences have influenced a person's life. These can include the structure of memory systems and the relationship between implicit and explicit components of the memory of an event. External corroborations, such as the reported experiences of other family members, police reports, photo albums, and journals, may be useful in creating a fuller picture. Knowing that memory is social and suggestible, and that the act of retrieving a memory can actually alter its form for subsequent storage, is important for interviewer and interviewee alike.

To put it simply, actual events can be forgotten, and nonexperienced "recollections" can be deeply felt to be true memories. These findings leave us with several important principles. Patients are vulnerable to the suggestive conditions of psychotherapy. Clinicians must be careful to take a neutral stance with respect to the accuracy of patients' recollections. Conditions that enhance suggestibility and that suspend critical metamemory processes should either be avoided altogether or used only

> Actual events can be forgotten, and nonexperienced "recollections" can be deeply felt to be true memories.

with extreme caution and informed consent. These conditions include hypnosis, amytal interviews, and intense, repeated questioning by an examiner. Clinicians should make special efforts to be aware of professional and personal biases that may directly influence their views about trauma and psychopathology. These views may manifest themselves in both the verbal and nonverbal behavior of a therapist. Excessive interest in a patient's traumatic experience versus interest in the patient himself can lead to a nonconscious pressure within the patient to keep the therapist involved by elaborating stories of trauma.

On the other hand, those who deny or are unaware of the effects of trauma on the functioning and development of the mind (such as the adaptations of dissociation and amnesia) are also likely to inhibit the elaboration of others' actual life histories, both verbally and nonverbally. If a person's history includes trauma, then a relationship with a nonaware friend, spouse, or therapist will not provide the safe haven in which the traumatized individual can begin to explore the often fragmented and frightening aspects of memory. Traumatized individuals may be extremely cautious about revealing the humiliating and painful past experiences they may have had. They may have a deep sense of shame about these traumatic events, which can make them exquisitely sensitive to the attitudes of others and vulnerable to a sense of being misunderstood or discounted. Victims of childhood abuse may be especially susceptible to feeling that they are "not being believed" and will be wary of revealing their hidden pain to a nonsupportive listener. For example, a therapist who is not able to entertain the possibility that a given individual may indeed have an accurate, perhaps delayed recall of a traumatic event may inhibit proper therapy from occurring.

There is great societal concern, controversy, and confusion about the accuracy of memories and the effects of trauma. Memory researchers have focused their efforts on how best to study the effects of trauma on memory, and can help bring our attention to the impact of trauma on us as individuals, communities, and a society. A special issue of the journal *Development and Psychopathology* compiled a compendium of thinking about these issues.[148] The following reflections on the impact of trauma have been provided by some of our leading investigators in the study of memory.

The investigation of trauma and memory is challenging because the laboratory setting of experiments, as well as available naturalistic experiences of highly stressful events (e.g., visits to the doctor, invasive medical procedures, or even natural disasters), are in some ways inherently different from intrafamilial child maltreatment. Robyn Fivush has stated:

> The research on traumatic memories conducted thus far, however, has focused on public events, events which may be painful or stressful, but do not

involve secrecy or shame. But many traumas experienced by young children are silenced. The ability to discuss past events with others, and to verbally rehearse these events to oneself, may play an instrumental role in children's developing abilities to understand and interpret their experiences. Placing past events in the context of one's ongoing life history allows one to integrate past experiences into a cohesive sense of how the world works and who one is. Children experiencing traumatic experiences who are not given the opportunity to discuss these events with others may not be able to integrate these negative experiences, and thus may be left with recurring fragments of memory that are associated with highly negative affect that cannot be resolved.[149]

Other memory researchers share this compassionate view of the impact of trauma and urge us to work toward alleviating the suffering that trauma produces both in individuals and in our societies. Christianson and Lindholm suggest:

Although there are documentation of forgotten, as well as of remembered, childhood trauma, it seems that most often the memory processes associated with traumas experienced in early age are not simply a matter of either/or, such that we either remember or forget them. Instead, both forgetting and remembering can occur selectively, and individuals may represent these memories in very different ways. . . . Children lack the experiences and resources to handle trauma on their own and therefore they need a lot of support from parents to overcome these experiences. Children who have been involved for example in accidents or catastrophes, usually process the experience by talking about it with their parents who help them come to terms with the event. If a close relative, on the other hand, is responsible for inflicting the trauma, such as in incest cases or domestic violence, a child is not in the same position to deal with the experience. . . . Unprocessed and disintegrated memories of a childhood trauma may not only cause problems and suffering for the individual him/herself, but can also constitute a serious threat for other people. Perpetrators of serious crimes, such as murder or rape, have often experienced severe traumas in childhood for which they have never received any help.[150]

Violence in our society has multiple causes.[151] The impact of violence on children may be complicated by the fact that their inherent mental models of the world as a safe place are directly affected by their witnessing of violence in the community. According to Lynch and Cicchetti:

Children exposed to ongoing stress and trauma, such as that associated with exposure to community violence, may develop schemas of the world as a hostile place (Cicchetti and Lynch, 1993, Dodge, 1993) and experience changed attitudes about people, life, and the future (Terr, 1991). Significant figures such as children's caregivers may come to be viewed as incapable of keeping children safe from the dangers present in their environment. Likewise, children may feel that they are not worthy of being kept safe. If such beliefs persist, then they may contribute to the development of insecure relationships with caregivers among children who live in threatening and violent environments.[152]

These learning experiences in the community may thus have a direct effect on children's models of attachment to their caregivers. As we shall see in the next chapter, these experiences and their associated models directly influence a wide range of mental processes, from memory to emotion regulation.[153] Lynch and Cicchetti describe one aspect of the cascading effect of trauma on security of attachment by noting that

> secure children may attend to interpersonal information more flexibly, resulting in increased relationship success. If children who have been traumatized can develop and maintain representational models that are open and secure, then the likelihood that they will experience successful interpersonal relationships and more positive overall adaptation may be greater. Traumatized children with insecure representational models may be more likely to experience traumatic stress reactions, in part because they may be less able to engage in successful and supportive interpersonal relationships.[154]

In other words, attachment relationships that offer children experiences that provide them with emotional connection and safety, both in the home and in the community, may be able to confer resilience and more flexible modes of adaptation in the face of adversity.

The impact of trauma is also mediated by the direct toxic effects of chronic stress on the brain. As Bremner and Narayan have urged us to note:

> Findings of hippocampal atrophy and memory deficits in stress have broad implications for public policy. With recent data showing that 16% of women have a history of childhood sexual abuse, it is clear that childhood trauma is a major public health problem. If stress results in damage to the hippocampus, this could have far reaching effects on childhood development. Given the important role that the hippocampus plays in learning and memory, victimized children may suffer in terms of academic achievement. These deficits in academic achievement may plague them throughout the rest of their lives. An increased emphasis is needed to direct resources and attention to the prevention and treatment of childhood victimization as well as stress at other stages of development.[155]

Memory forms the foundation for both the implicit reality (behavioral responses, emotional reactions, perceptual categorizations, schemata of the self and others in the world, and possibly bodily memories) and explicit recollections of facts and of the self across time. In this way, we must understand the many layers of memory in order to comprehend other persons' present and past life experiences and the ways they anticipate and plan for the future. As we shall see, the disorganizing effects of trauma and its lack of resolution can be passed from generation to generation. The emotional suffering, the stress-induced damage to cognitive functioning, the internal chaos of intrusive implicit memories, and the potential interpersonal violence created as a result of trauma produce ripple effects of devastation across the boundaries of time and human lives. As we will explore in the chapters ahead, disruptive interpersonal relationships produce incoherent functioning of the individual mind. This connection between interpersonal and individual processes is clearly seen in an important aspect of memory: the narrative telling of our life stories.

## MEMORY AND NARRATIVE

The telling of stories has a central place in human cultures throughout the world and plays a crucial role in the interactions between adults and children.[156] From an early stage in development, children begin to narrate their lives—to tell the sequence of events and internal experiences of their daily existence.[157] What is so special about stories? Why are we as a species so consumed by the process of telling and listening to stories?

As fundamental creations of social experience, stories embody shared cultural rules and expectations, exploring the reasons for human behavior and the consequences of deviations from the cultural norm. Meaning embedded in culturally transmitted stories can directly influence how individuals interpret overwhelming events, as well as how those events are subsequently processed.[158] Stories also captivate our attention, in that they require us to participate in the active construction of the characters' mental lives and experiences. In this way, a story is created by both teller and listener.

By the second year of life, children begin to develop the "later" form of memory, called declarative or explicit, which includes both semantic (factual) and episodic (remembering oneself in an episode in time) memory.[159] "Narrative" memory is a term referring to the way in which we may store and then recall experienced events in story form. "Co-construction of narrative" is a fundamental process, studied across cultures by anthropologists, in which families join together in the telling of stories of daily life.[160] Children can be encouraged to see themselves as the locus of action; this "agentic self-focus" influences the way memory is encoded and retrieved. As Wang has noted in exploring the interplay of cultural and parental practices:

Regardless of culture, children who had a greater agentic self-focus showed more advanced in̶d̶e̶p̶e̶n̶d̶e̶n̶t̶ ̶m̶emory skills than those who were less oriented tow̶a̶r̶d̶ ̶w̶h̶e̶n̶ defining themselves. Children's cultural bac̶k̶g̶r̶o̶u̶n̶d̶ ̶w̶a̶s̶ ̶d̶i̶r̶e̶c̶tly related to their shared and independent ̶m̶e̶m̶o̶r̶y̶ ̶w̶h̶e̶n̶ controlling for other factors. Mediation ̶a̶n̶a̶l̶y̶s̶e̶s̶ ̶f̶o̶u̶n̶d̶ ̶t̶h̶a̶t̶ ̶m̶aternal elaborations and evaluations func̶t̶i̶o̶n̶e̶d̶ ̶i̶n̶ ̶e̶xplaining cultural differences in children's ̶m̶e̶m̶o̶r̶y̶,̶ ̶a̶n̶d̶ ̶m̶a̶t̶ernal evaluations and child agentic self-focus ̶p̶l̶a̶y̶e̶d̶ ̶r̶o̶l̶e̶s in children's independent memory reports. ̶T̶h̶e̶s̶e̶ ̶r̶e̶s̶u̶l̶t̶s̶ ̶l̶e̶n̶d̶ support to the social interactionist theories ̶o̶f̶ ̶m̶e̶m̶ory development as a result of collaborative ̶n̶a̶r̶r̶a̶t̶i̶v̶es of the past between children and signifi-

̶p̶s̶y̶c̶h̶o̶l̶o̶gist Lev Vygotsky said that a child's inter-̶a̶c̶t̶i̶o̶n̶s̶ ̶w̶i̶t̶h parents creates thought.[162] In this view, ̶c̶h̶i̶l̶d̶r̶e̶n̶ ̶w̶ith their parents will begin to narrate such ̶e̶v̶e̶n̶t̶s̶ ̶.̶.̶.̶ ̶b̶e̶ginings and the contents of their memories will become active parts of their internal and conscious worlds. This view also reveals the possibility that some of our most cherished personal processes, such as thought or even self-reflection, may have their origins as interpersonal communication. Our sense of self is shaped by our relational experiences with our parents, within the larger culture in which we live.[163] Conway and colleagues state:

> Children who narrate life events with their parents will begin to narrate such events to themselves.

> Self systems with an independent focus feature the early establishment of a coherent, elaborate, emotionally charged, and self-focused autobiographical history. In contrast, self systems with an interdependent focus show a later establishment of a brief, skeletal, emotionally unexpressive, relation-centered autobiographical history.[164]

Independent self-focus has been found to be characteristic of Western cultures, whereas interdependent self-focus has been found in many East Asian cultures.[165] Conway and colleagues further conclude from their research that

> the presence of similar periods of childhood amnesia [less than five years] and reminiscence bump [ten to thirty years of age] across cultures suggests that culturally independent processes may mediate the emergence of these periods in the life-span retrieval curve. These processes might be related to an alignment of cultures and/or they may be neurodevelopmental. In contrast, general differences in memory content across cultures point to society-

specific influences on the relation of memory to the self during development. Cultural (e.g., independent vs. interdependent self-focus) and individual (including neurological) factors thus exhibit a complex, dynamic, and interactive relation in shaping the content, accessibility, and life-span distribution of autobiographical memory and further creating cultural diversity and commonalities in individuals' life stories.[166]

The hippocampus and prefrontal (including orbitofrontal) regions mediate explicit autobiographical memory, and thus this form of memory is directly related to an integrated spatial and temporal map. As the millions of traces of perception within explicit encoding are laid down through working memory, only a selected portion will be brought into long-term memory. Of this selected set of memory traces, much fewer will survive the translation of these into permanent memory. This latter process of cortical consolidation, as discussed above, may be fundamentally related to dreams and to the "narrativization" of episodic memory. Dreaming is a multimodal narrative process containing various elements of our daily experience, past events, mental models, and present perceptual experience. The unit of a day, marked by the consolidation process of sleep, may thus be seen as a form of chapter in a life story. Each day is literally the opportunity to create a new episode of learning, in which recent experience will become integrated with the past and woven into the anticipated future.

Stories involve the perspective of the teller (first or third person, past or present), various characters' activities and mental states (emotions, perceptions, beliefs, memories, intentions), and the depiction of conflicts and their resolution.[167] Several genres of narrative are present from early life onward: fictional, schematic (general descriptors of events), and factual. These stories can be about others, or they can be autobiographical. Stories of each type may actually overlap to varying degrees with the other genres. For example, fictional stories often involve elements of the teller's own life story, even if this is unintentional on the part of the teller. Autobiographical accounts may often incorporate generalizations from repeated experiences or aspects of imagined events. Thus the emergence of a story may involve multiple layers of narrative genres.

Stories, in the form of bedtime routines, myths, films, plays, novels, diary entries, dinner conversations, or psychotherapy sessions, are present throughout our lives. Many forms of human interaction—from children's play and drawing to adults' joint attention to autobiographical reflections—involve the co-construction of narrative around the memory talk between individuals.[168]

Narrative can be seen as a fundamental process that reveals itself in various ways. It creates shareable stories (often called "narratives"), determines patterns of behavior (called "narrative enactments" or "performances"), and may influence our internal lives (in the form of dreams, imagery, sensations, and states of mind). As discussed in later chapters, we can also propose that the narrative process directly influences emotional modulation and self-organization.

The storytelling and story-listening process often involves the essential features of social interaction and discourse. The teller produces verbal and nonverbal signals that are received by the listener, and then similar forms of communication are sent back to the teller. This intricate dance requires that both persons have the complex capacity to read social signals, to share the concept of a subjective experience of mind, and to agree to participate in culturally accepted rules of discourse. Stories are thus socially co-constructed. One can argue that even writers working in "isolation" have an imagined audience with whom they are engaged in active discourse. It is no wonder that the story process requires an intact social system of the brain to mediate this exquisite circle of communication.[169]

The creation of narrative coherence can be facilitated by social experiences. It is by focusing on this narrative system that we can begin to see the relationship between narrative co-construction and the acquisition of more adaptive self-organization, leading to coherent functioning. In the next chapter, we explore the ways in which attachment relationships promote narrative processing, emotional communication, and the development of the mind.

The influence of narrative on internal experience is revealed most dramatically in dreams, guided imagery, and journal writing. The myriad of representations in each of these processes may often surprise the conscious mind. Dreams weave elaborate stories incorporating a wide array of images from various points in time. Guided imagery brings to the fore sets of vivid experiences that contain active reflections and themes about an individual's priorities and present life challenges. Journal writing can often reveal concerns and perspectives about life that have been unavailable to simple introspection. By defining the process of narrative as more than just the verbal creation of stories, we can identify how each of these internal experiences is shaped by the central narrative themes in our lives.

Narrative enactments can be seen in the patterns of behavior, of relating, and of decision making that steer the course of an individual's life.[170] Why call this "narrative" and not just "learned behavior"? Recognizing the central role of *themes* in bringing some sense of continuity to a person's life directions is helpful in understanding why the person does what he does—and how to help him change that behavior if necessary. Our nonconscious mental models may be revealed as narrative themes. The central, coherence-creating, narrative process has a unifying quality that links otherwise disparate aspects

> Our nonconscious mental models may be revealed as narrative themes.

of memory within the individual. Enactments, then, are the behavioral manifestations of this core narrative process that links past, present, and future. Awareness of the role of early life experiences in shaping both *what* is processed and *how* information about the mind itself is handled can help us to negotiate our way through the complexities of the mind and social relationships.

Narratives reveal how representations from one system can clearly intertwine with another. Thus the mental models of implicit memory help organize the themes around which the details of explicit autobiographical memory are expressed. Though we can never see mental models directly, their manifestation in narratives allows us at least to view the shadows they cast on other systems of the mind.

## THE REMEMBERED AND THE REMEMBERING SELF

Each of us has innumerable anecdotes that can serve to illustrate particular sentiments or sets of events from our pasts. The notion of a single narrative for a human life is too limited, as memory and the nature of our selves are forever changing. As our present state of mind reflects the social context in which our narrative is being told, we weave together a tapestry of selected recollections and imagined details to create a story driven by past events as well as by the need to engage our listeners. Thus the expectations of the audience play a major role in the tone of storytelling. This social nature of narrative means that the remembering self is perpetually in a process of creating itself within new social contexts.[171] Indeed, as we continue to change as individuals through time, our narratives will also evolve as a reflection of the dynamic nature of life and human relationships.

Edward Reed states that "perception is to self as memory is to selves,"[172] emphasizing the important point that in any given moment we perceive and interpret experience from a new view. As we accumulate lived moments across time, we are capable of recalling not as one self, but as the many types of selves that have existed in the past. Narrative recollection, then, is the opportunity for those varied states to be created anew in the present.

To extend this argument a bit further, we actually perceive in the present in various dimensions. The "self" at any given moment in time is filled with myriad layers of mental representations, only some of which are selected as a part of conscious experience. Thus the remembered self is multilayered. As time passes and we shift across various states, we can indeed recall various ways of being from the past. As our state in the present may also vary from one moment to the next, the state-dependent quality of retrieval suggests that we will also narrate our lives from the standpoints of multiple selves.

With all of this flexibility and change in response to the environment and to internal factors, what makes for any kind of continuity in the narrative process? Though states of mind, social context, and selective recollection certainly influence narrative telling, specific and consistent patterns in the structure of the narrative process do appear to emerge within an individual. One feature that may lend longitudinal continuity to the narrative process is the important role of mental models in shaping the themes of stories. These pervasive elements of implicit memory help create the "between-the-lines" messages of the stories we tell and the lives we live. Another element is the structure of the individual's narrating process itself. As we shall see in the next chapter, early attachment experiences are associated with specific patterns of how people narrate their lives.

## REFLECTIONS: SELF AND OTHER ACROSS TIME

From the beginning of life, the brain responds to experience with the establishment of connections among neurons. Those pathways activated simultaneously become associated with one another and are more likely to be activated together again in the future. As noted earlier in this chapter, this is Hebb's axiom. Before the development of the hippocampus in the medial temporal lobe, the brain is only able to have implicit memory. This form of memory is diverse and is thought to include behavioral, emotional, perceptual, and possibly somatosensory memory. When implicit memory is reactivated in the future ("retrieved"), it does *not* have a sense of self, of time, or of something being recalled. It merely creates the mental experience of behavior, emotion, or perception. Such experiences are generalized in the creation of schemata or mental models, which are fundamental to implicit memory.

During the second year of life, the hippocampus matures enough for a second form of memory to become available. Explicit memory requires focal attention for encoding and leads to the long-term and then permanent accessibility of elements of first factual and later autobiographical memory. The encoding of explicit memory, which is dependent upon the hippocampus, yields a form of retrieval that involves the sense of recollection—and, if autobiographical, of the self at some time in the past. A process called "cortical consolidation" appears to be essential for items in long-term explicit storage to be placed in permanent memory within the associational regions of the neocortex, where they become independent of the hippocampus for retrieval.

The autobiographical narrative process is directly influenced by both implicit and explicit memory. Autonoetic consciousness is the experience in which we are able to perform "mental time travel," creating representations of the self in the past, present, and future. As a child develops into the third year of life, the orbitofrontal cortex becomes capable of mediating episodic memory or autonoesis. In a fundamental manner, the narrative process allows individuals to shape the flow of information about the self and others.

When we attend a funeral and are surrounded by others who have also known and shared the life of someone we love who has now passed away, we can feel the deceased's "spirit" within us. And, indeed, the patterns of activation of those trillions of neuronal connections within each of us at the memorial service may have similarities because of our parallel experiences with the deceased. As survivors, we attempt to deal with the loss by creating a sense of coherence with the loved one within the narratives we construct of our lives together. At such a memorial service, stories often will be told to "capture the life and the essence" of the person who has just died. This sharing of stories reflects the central importance of narratives in creating coherence in human life and connecting our minds to each other. Stories are passed from generation to generation and help keep the human soul alive.

The psyches of those who have been an intimate part of our development live on within us in both the details and the structure of our lives' ongoing stories. Altering our life paths may require examination of these influences on our core narrative structures and themes. Through an elaborative form of contingent communication—the connection between two individuals' mental states, and their joint attention to each other's life stories— interpersonal relationships of many forms may facilitate turning points in individuals' lives, reflected in the changing architecture of their narrative processes. Enabling people to achieve a fuller coherence within their own minds and in their connections to others may help them meet the challenge of living, in which the self is continually emerging in ever-enriching and complex ways. In the next chapter, we explore the features of human relationships that facilitate the development of emotional resilience and a coherent narrative process.

# CHAPTER 3

# Attachment

## THE ATTACHMENT SYSTEM

"Attachment" is an inborn system in the brain that evolves in ways that influence and organize motivational, emotional, and memory processes with respect to significant caregiving figures. The attachment system motivates an infant to seek proximity to parents (and other primary caregivers) and to establish communication with them. At the most basic evolutionary level, this behavioral system improves the chances of the infant's survival.[1] At the level of the mind, attachment establishes an interpersonal relationship that helps the immature brain use the mature functions of the parent's brain to organize its own processes.[2] The emotional transactions of secure attachment involve a parent's emotionally sensitive responses to a child's signals,[3] which can serve to amplify the child's positive emotional states and to modulate negative states. In particular, the aid caregivers can give in reducing uncomfortable emotions, such as fear, anxiety, or sadness, enables children to be soothed and gives them a haven of safety when they are upset.[4] Repeated experiences become encoded in implicit memory as expectations and then as mental models or schemata of attachment, which serve to help a child feel an internal sense of what John Bowlby called a "secure base" in the world.[5]

Studies of attachment have revealed that the patterning or organization of attachment relationships during infancy is associated with characteristic processes of emotional regulation, social relatedness, access to autobiographical memory, and the development of self-reflection and narrative.[6] Mary Main has summarized the following principles:[7]

1. The earliest attachments are usually formed by the age of seven months.
2. Nearly all infants become attached.
3. Attachments are formed to only a few persons.
4. These "selective attachments" appear to be derived from social interactions with the attachment figures.
5. They lead to specific organizational changes in an infant's behavior and brain function.

The attachment system serves multiple functions. For an infant, activation of the attachment system involves the seeking of physical proximity. Proximity seeking allows the infant to be protected from harm, starvation, unfavorable temperature changes, disasters, attacks from others, and separation from the group. For these reasons, the attachment system is highly responsive to indications of danger. The internal experience of an activated attachment system is thus often associated with the sensation of anxiety or fear and can be triggered by frightening experiences of various kinds, as well as by a threat of separation from the attachment figure.[8]

Attachment relationships thus serve a vital function in providing the infant with protection from dangers of many kinds. Two broad qualitative terms are used to describe the nature of attachments: They are seen as "secure" or "insecure." Another important distinction is between "organized" and "disorganized" attachment patterns, as we shall see. Attachment relationships are crucial in organizing not only ongoing experience, but the neuronal growth of the developing brain. In other words, these salient emotional relationships have a direct effect on the development of the domains of mental functioning that serve as our conceptual anchor points: memory, narrative, emotion, representations, and states of mind.

Attachment relationships may serve to create the central foundation from which the mind develops. Disorganized forms of insecure attachment may serve as a significant risk factor in the development of psychopathology.[9] Secure attachment, in contrast, appears to confer a form of emotional resilience but by no means is a guarantee of mental health, as other factors play important roles in the development of well-being.[10] Many factors contribute to the overall development of the individual, including experiences, temperament, peers, chance, culture, and various genetic and epigenetic factors. Weinfield, Sroufe, Egeland, and Carlson state:

> Attachment relationships may serve to create the central foundation from which the mind develops.

Thus, although insecure attachment is considered a risk factor for pathology, not all, or even most, insecurely attached infants will develop psychopathology. Psychopathology is a developmental construction involving a myriad of influences interacting over time. Similarly, secure attachment is not a guarantee of mental health, but rather is viewed as a protective factor or buffer.[11]

Although attachment behavior is seen primarily in children, adults continue to manifest attachment-related behavior and mental processes throughout the lifespan. Especially under times of stress, many adults will internally or externally engage in proximity-seeking behavior[12]—for example, by monitoring the whereabouts of a few selected "attachment figures" and seeking them out as sources of comfort, advice, and strength. For adults, such attachment figures may be mentors, close friends, or romantic partners. There are, however, research and conceptual differences between the study of romantic adult attachment (i.e., adult–adult pair bonds) and the developmental form of attachment (i.e., the asymmetric parent–child relationship).[13] The differences between developmental attachment and romantic attachment are important to keep in mind when we are comparing research data from these two valid but distinct forms of attachment. Adults often can choose to whom they become attached, but for children, such options are not readily available. Furthermore, a child's immature and dependent state creates vital needs for connection to assure survival—needs that are often quite different from the external realities of adult life.

## HUMAN COMMUNICATION AND STATES OF MIND

A thirty-year-old woman sits quietly in the chair in my therapy office. She looks puzzled as I repeat my question: "How was your visit with your mother last weekend?" She bites her lip, looks away, and gazes down toward the floor, saying nothing. She reaches up and covers her eyes with her arm. Her breathing becomes more rapid and shallow. She taps her foot nervously on the floor. Silence. My heart begins to accelerate. I find myself looking down at the floor and notice my own foot tapping. My own state of mind is revealed in nonverbal signals: facial expression, eye gaze, bodily motion, tone of voice, and the timing of verbal signals (whether fast, slow, in response to other comments, or the like). My voice is low in volume, and I slowly say, "Oh . . . it was a hard weekend." My head feels as if it is about to burst. "HORRIBLE!" the woman suddenly exclaims. The pressure in my head dissipates with a sense of relief. The muscles in my face begin to relax from their drawn, tightened state as hers also relax. The patient's body becomes less tense. "Horrible . . . ," she moans, now with tears in her eyes.

As this story of my patient illustrates, engaging in direct communication is more than just understanding or even perceiving the signals—both verbal and nonverbal—sent between two people. For "full" emotional communication, one person needs to allow his state of mind to be influenced by that of the other.[14] In this example, my sensitivity to this patient's array of signals allows my own state to become aligned with that of the patient. The sense that my head is "about to burst," followed by the release of pressure, shows how the patient's shifts from bewilderment to rage to sadness are experienced by another person. The shifts in my own state may be a part of the internal process that makes me aware of the often subtle and rapid nonverbal signals sent in this direct form of emotional communication. The alignment of my own state allows me to have an experience as close as possible to the patient's subjective world at that moment. In being sensitive to my own internal response, I can become aware of my perceptions of the patient's experience. This yields important experiential information. Such an alignment also permits a nonverbal form of communication to the patient that she is being "understood" in the deepest sense. After feeling better at the conclusion of therapy, this patient tells me that what has helped her in our work together is that she "feels felt" by me. I will never forget that illuminating term. Her state directly influences mine, and she knows that she exists within my own mental world; she is "feeling felt" by another person. This attunement of states forms the nonverbal basis of collaborative, contingent communication.[15] The capacity to achieve this attuned form of communication, sometimes called "affect attunement,"[16] is dependent on an individual's sensitivity to signals. Parental sensitivity to signals is the essence of secure attachments and can inform us about how two people's "being" with each other permits emotional communication and a sense of connection to be established at any age.[17] In these transactions, the brain of one person and that of another are influencing each other in a form of "co-regulation."[18]

This chapter examines the developmental evidence from attachment research demonstrating the importance of this co-regulating contingent communication. The attunement of states of mind is the fundamental way in which the brain activity of one person directly influences that of the other. Collaborative communication allows minds to "connect" with each other. During childhood, such human connections allow for the creation of brain connections that are vital for the development of a child's capacity for self-regulation.[19] Studies reveal that such relationship experiences are grounded in *patterns of communication*. Let us review how the infant's mind develops within these emotional relationships, in order to understand the research-based views of what forms of interpersonal experience facilitate the development of psychological resilience and emotional well-being.

One essential message is that the developing mind uses an attachment figure's states of mind to help organize the functioning of its own states. As we shall see, "states" or "states of mind" involve various aspects of brain activity. The momentary alignment of states is dependent upon parental sensitivity to the child's signals; it allows the mind of the child both to regulate itself in the moment and to develop regulatory capacities that can be utilized in the future.[20] Attunement between child and parent, or between patient and therapist, involves the intermittent alignment of states of mind. As two individuals' states are brought into alignment, a form of what we can call "mental state resonance" can occur, in which each person's state both influences and is influenced by that of the other. There are moments in which people also need to be alone and not in alignment; an attuned other knows when to "back off" and stop the alignment process. Intimate relationships involve this circular dance of attuned communication, in which there are alternating moments of engaged alignment and distanced autonomy. At the root of such attunement is the capacity to read the signals (often nonverbal) that indicate the need for engagement or disengagement.[21]

Patterns in the flow of energy and of information within and between people comprise the fundamental components of a state of mind. In this way, *attuned communication involves the resonance of energy and information between two people.* For the nonverbal infant, this intimate, collaborative communication is mediated without words. This need for nonverbal attunement persists throughout life. Within adult relationships of all sorts, words can come to dominate the form of information being shared, and this can lead to a different form of representational resonance. Such a verbal exchange may feel quite empty if it is devoid of the more primary aspects of each person's internal states.[22] Infant attachment studies remind us of the crucial importance of attuned nonverbal communication in all forms of human relationships. It is a way of responding to more than merely external behaviors.

## ATTACHMENT THEORY

In the middle of the twentieth century, a British psychoanalyst and psychiatrist, John Bowlby, turned to animal behavior studies to enrich the traditional analytic views of child development.[23] Bowlby wrote about attachment, separation, and loss in ways that led to the establishment of primary caregivers in orphanages and in pediatric hospital wards. His idea was simple and powerful: The nature of an infant's attachment to the parent (or other primary caregiver) will become internalized as a working model of attachment. If this model represents security, the baby will be able to explore the world and to separate and mature in a healthy way. If the attachment relationship is "insecure," the internal working model of attachment will not give the infant a sense of a secure base, and the development of secure-base behaviors (such as play, exploration, and social interactions) may be impaired. Of course, if circumstances change, a securely attached infant or young child can become insecurely attached, and an insecure attachment can become secure.

An "internal working model of attachment" is a form of mental model or schema.[24] It is postulated that children can use a form of remembering called "evocative" memory by the age of eighteen months to bring an image of an attachment figure forward in their minds, which helps to comfort them.[25] Children carry those to whom they are attached inside of them, in the form of multisensory images (faces, voices, smell, taste, touch), mental representations of their relationships with them, and the sense that they can be with them if this is needed. As described in Chapter 2, the formation of mental models is a fundamental way in which implicit memory allows the mind to create generalizations and summaries of past experiences. One form of such a mental model is a "script" that serves as a blueprint for expected interpersonal patterns of behavior and communication.[26] These models are then used to bias present cognition for more rapid analysis of an ongoing perception, and also to help the mind anticipate what events are likely to happen next. In this way, forming mental models is the essential manner in which the brain learns from the past and then directly influences the present and shapes future actions.

> An "internal working model of attachment" is a form of mental model or schema.

Attachment studies examine the active nature of both children's and parents' mental models of attachment relationships. How can such learned, implicit models be assessed? Models exert their effects on an array of observable phenomena, including overt behavior, interpersonal communication, emotional regulation, autobiographical memory, and narrative processes. For example, these models directly influence how a parent interacts with a child. Parental expectations, perceptions, and behavior interact with the inborn temperamental features of the child in determining what the exact nature of the parent–child transaction will be like. Attachment research has shown that parents' expectations and patterns of relating are profoundly influenced by their own attachment history and attitudes in the present, as revealed in what Main has termed their "state of mind with respect to attachment."[27]

Attachment relationships also need to be seen through the lens of the cultural context in which they reside. Anthropologists and other researchers have importantly noted that the patterns of communication between a caregiver and an infant are powerfully shaped by culture and other aspects of a family's social world. For example, high degrees of physically controlling touch in one culture may support secure attachment, whereas similar active handling in another setting would be associated with insecurity.[28] Having a number of attachment figures in a village or other community setting may be the norm in one culture but unheard of in another. Children are capable of forming secure attachments to more than one caregiver.[29] Indeed, the unfortunate situation in many contemporary societies is to have a parent, isolated from others, caring for one or more young children. This may be in conflict with how we have biologically evolved to live within cooperative groups of caregiving individuals.[30] Children, though, do the best they can to respond to what they are given. The essential point is that it is imperative to view attachment patterns as adaptive, culturally sensitive ways in which children respond to their experiences with caregivers. The term "insecure attachment" for some social scientists may seem pejorative rather than descriptive. As we'll see, organized forms of insecure attachment are simply adaptations to particular patterns of caregiver communication and are less likely to result in compromises to mental health in later development than disorganized forms. Security does not guarantee anything, and organized insecurity is not synonymous with mental dysfunction, though it may have increased tendencies toward inflexible, chaotic, or other forms of non-optional self-regulation. Children do the best they can with the organized attachment experiences they are offered. In contrast, disorganized attachment appears to be incompatible with the attachment system's goals of proximity seeking, secure base, and safe haven. In this way, disorganized attachment confers high risk for compromised mental functioning and health, whereas insecure attachment by itself may be seen as an organized, adaptive strategy children have learned in order to survive.

## ASSESSING ATTACHMENT

### Infant Attachment Research: The Strange Situation

Mary Ainsworth, a research psychologist, collaborated with Bowlby, a psychoanalyst, at London's Tavistock Clinic in the 1950s.[31] As a psychologist, she was interested in developing a quantifiable research measure capable of assessing the security of attachment. Her idea was to study mother–infant interactions over the first year of life, and then to do something that would enable observers to access and classify the proposed internalized working model of attachment. Her Baltimore study[32] did just that and has been replicated hundreds of times since then by other researchers throughout the world. In this study, after a year of observations in the home, each mother–infant pair or dyad was brought to a laboratory setting. At various times in the twenty-minute procedure, the infant stayed with the mother, with the mother and a stranger, with only the stranger, and then alone for up to three minutes. The idea was (and still is) that separating a one-year-old from her attachment figure within a strange environment and at times with a stranger should activate the infant's attachment system. One should then be able to study the infant's responses at separation and at reunion. The most useful assessments came at the reunion episode of this paradigm.

What Ainsworth found in her initial landmark study was that infants' behavior at reunion fell into specific patterns of responding. Each of these patterns corresponded in a statistically significant way to the independently performed home observation ratings for the year prior to the laboratory assessment. This lab measure is called the Ainsworth or Infant Strange Situation.[33] The initial study classified three distinct attachment patterns. Now we also use a fourth, developed by Mary Main and Judith Solomon,[34] which helps further define the nature of some infants' behavior. Naturally, there are also some patterns that are "unclassifiable," in that they do not meet criteria for any of the prior four categories.[35] The right side of Table 3.1 lists the four categories of Infant Strange Situation behavior patterns.

At the time of reunion, the infant's response to the mother's return is coded for the way he seeks proximity to the mother, the ease with which he can be soothed, and the rapidity of his return to play. The idea is that an infant who has developed an internal working model of a secure attachment will be able to use the parent to soothe himself quickly and return to his childhood task of exploration and play. If the infant has an insecure attachment model, then the return of the parent will not facilitate such an emotional regulatory function or allow the child to use the parent to return to playing.

The Strange Situation classifications at one year of age have been associated with numerous findings as children grow into adolescence, such as emotional maturity, peer relationships, and academic performance.[36] These correlations suggest that patterns of relating between parent and child have significant influences later in life. Since most of these children have continued to have the same parents, these correlations by themselves only support, but do not prove, some views that the first year of life is a critical period of development.[37] Further studies of adoptive and foster parents also support the notion that parents who can make sense of the internal lives of their children have children who are securely attached.[38] Parents and other caregivers continue to influence us throughout childhood. Bowlby coined the term "internal working model of attachment" in order to emphasize the manipulable working nature of the attachment system.[39] In other words, changing conditions will change a child's, adolescent's, or adult's working model of attachment as development unfolds across the lifespan. Patterns established early in life have a major impact on functioning, but the individual's experiences

## TABLE 3.1. AAI Classifications and Corresponding Patterns of Infant Strange Situation Behavior

| Adult state of mind with respect to attachment | Infant Strange Situation behavior |
| --- | --- |
| Secure/autonomous (F) | Secure (B) |
| Coherent, collaborative discourse. Valuing of attachment, but seems objective regarding any particular event/relationship. Description and evaluation of attachment-related experiences is consistent, whether experiences are favorable or unfavorable. Discourse does not notably violate any of Grice's maxims. | Explores room and toys with interest in preseparation episodes. Shows signs of missing parent during separation, often crying by the second separation. Obvious preference for parent over stranger. Greets parent actively, usually initiating physical contact. Usually some contact maintaining by second reunion, but then settles and returns to play. |
| Dismissing (Ds) | Avoidant (A) |
| Not coherent. Dismissing of attachment-related experiences and relationships. Normalizing ("excellent, very normal mother"), with generalized representations of history unsupported or actively contradicted by episodes recounted, thus violating Grice's maxim of quality. Transcripts also tend to be excessively brief, violating the maxim of quantity. | Fails to cry on separation from parent. Actively avoids and ignores parent on reunion (i.e., by moving away, turning away, or leaning out of arms when picked up). Little or no proximity or contact seeking, no distress, and no anger. Response to parent appears unemotional. Focuses on toys or environment throughout procedure. |
| Preoccupied (E) | Resistant or ambivalent (C) |
| Not coherent. Preoccupied with or by past attachment relationships/experiences, speaker appears angry, passive, or fearful. Sentences often long, grammatically entangled, or filled with vague usages ("dadadada," "and that"), thus violating Grice's maxims of manner and relevance. Transcripts often excessively long, violating the maxim of quantity. | May be wary or distressed even prior to separation, with little exploration. Preoccupied with parent throughout procedure, may seem angry or passive. Fails to settle and take comfort in parent on reunion, and usually continues to focus on parent and cry. Fails to return to exploration after reunion. |
| Unresolved/disorganized (U/d) | Disorganized/disoriented (D) |
| During discussions of loss or abuse, individual shows striking lapse in the monitoring of reasoning or discourse. For example, individual may briefly indicate a belief that a dead person is still alive in the physical sense, or that this person was killed by a childhood thought. Individual may lapse into prolonged silence or eulogistic speech. The speaker will ordinarily otherwise fit Ds, E, or F categories. | The infant displays disorganized and/or disoriented behaviors in the parent's presence, suggesting a temporary collapse of behavioral strategies. For example, the infant may freeze with a trance-like expression, hands in air; may rise at parent's entrance, then fall prone and huddled on the floor; or may cling while crying hard and leaning away with gaze averted. Infant will ordinarily otherwise fit A, B, or C categories. |

*Note.* From Hesse (1999b, p. 399). Copyright 1999 by The Guilford Press. Reprinted by permission. Descriptions of the adult attachment classification system are summarized from Main, Kaplan, and Cassidy (1985) and from Main and Goldwyn (1984, 1998). Descriptions of infant A, B, and C categories are summarized from Ainsworth, Blehar, Waters, and Wall (1978), and the description of the infant D category is summarized from Main and Solomon (1990).

continue to influence the internal model of attachment. This suggests that new relationship experiences have the potential to move individuals toward a more secure state of mind with respect to attachment. Intervention studies support the idea that a relationship-based treatment focus can enable proper development to occur.[40]

It may at first seem artificial to reduce complex behavior into segmented, distinct categories. But research must often try to cluster participants into groups in order to find statistically meaningful patterns. These groupings are general patterns, and a given individual or relationship may reveal elements of several classifications. Nevertheless, this way of thinking scientifically about organizational forms can inform us greatly about global patterns of behavior. Longitudinal attachment studies, which follow parents and infants as they develop throughout the lifespan, require such classifications and have yielded some fascinating and powerful findings useful in understanding the nature of human experience.[41] As we review the specific attachment categories, keep in mind that a child may have a different pattern with each attachment figure. A given individual may then experience a number of elements from each classification as they mature from childhood to adulthood and coalesce a variety of attachment relational patterns into an internalized sense of self. The manner in which an individual has come to integrate a coherent model across numerous relationship patterns may in fact be at the heart of how attachment experiences shape a coherent mind.[42]

## A Brief Overview of Infant Attachment Classifications

### Secure Pattern

Parents who are emotionally available, perceptive, and responsive to their infants' needs and mental states—that is, those who are sensitive to their children's signals—have infants who are most often "securely" attached. Ainsworth initially postulated that it might be maternal warmth that predicted security, but she updated this view in her Baltimore study with the notion of maternal sensitivity. Sensitivity requires that the infant's internal world be perceived by the caregiver, made sense of, and then responded to in a timely and effective manner. This contingent communication emerges from the parent's capacity to see the mental life of the child, not merely to respond to external behaviors or even to be a warm presence. An infant who experiences this can be said to "feel felt" and to be "understood" by the parent. This important capacity to perceive the child's mind is at the heart of secure attachment relationships. The ability to understand behavior in mental terms is also a part of how parents make sense of their inner lives. This may explain why Mary Ainsworth initially found that a parent's ability to be a good informant—to be able to discuss in detail the nature of a child's unique

personality and emotional features—is
what also seemed to correlate with secure
attachment.[43] Securely attached children
seek proximity and quickly return to play
in the Strange Situation. The Strange

> Securely attached children seek proximity and quickly return to play in the Strange Situation.

Situation activates the attachment system; this leads a child to engage in
proximity-seeking behavior, which is then terminated after contact with the
figure to whom the child has a secure attachment.[44] In low-risk, nonclinical
populations, security of attachment to mothers is found in about fifty-five to
sixty-five percent of infants.[45]

### Avoidant Pattern

Parents who are emotionally unavailable, imperceptive, rejecting, and unre-
sponsive are associated with "avoidantly" attached infants. These babies seem
to ignore the return of their parents in the Strange Situation. Their attentional and representational state is a "deactivating" one, which leads to an
external behavior that minimizes proximity seeking when in the presence
of the parent with whom they have an avoidant attachment.[46] In low-risk
samples, about twenty to thirty percent of infants are found to be avoidantly
attached to their mothers.

### Resistant or Ambivalent Pattern

Those parents who are inconsistently available, perceptive, and responsive,
and who tend to intrude their own states of mind onto those of their children, tend to have children with "resistant" or "ambivalent" attachments.
These infants seem anxious, are not easily soothed, and do not readily return
to play in the Strange Situation at the time of reunion with the parent with
whom they are ambivalently attached. In this case, there is an "overactivation" of the attachment system, in which a child's attentional/representational
state leads to external proximity-seeking behavior that is *not* terminated by
contact with the parent. In other words, the relationship with the parent is
not able to turn the attachment behavior "off" after reunion, and the child
remains with an overactivating or maximizing strategy toward attachment
filled with a sense of anxiety.[47] In nonclinical, low-risk populations, five to
fifteen percent of infants display this type of attachment to their mothers.

### Disorganized/Disoriented Pattern

Finally, parents who show frightened, frightening, or disoriented communications during the first year of life tend to have infants Main and colleagues

have identified as "disorganized/disoriented" in their attachments.[48] During the Strange Situation, such an infant appears disorganized and disoriented during the return of the parent; for example, some have been observed turning in circles, approaching and then avoiding the parent, or entering a trance-like state of "freezing" or stillness.[49] Dyads falling into this attachment category are also given a best-fitting alternative primary classification of one of the prior three organized forms of attachment; for this reason, the sum of all of the percentages reported here is over one hundred. In nonclinical populations, disorganized attachments are found in twenty to forty percent of infants studied. In parentally maltreated infants, disorganized attachment is found in an average of seventy percent.[50]

Studies of genetics reveal that in general, attachment categories are independent of genes or related issues, such as temperament of the child.[51] Genes may confer a vulnerability to response in the setting of suboptimal attachment experiences. One study revealed that children with a certain "allele" or variant of the dopamine transport gene are differentially susceptible to unresolved loss and trauma.[52] Genetic variants do not produce attachment patterns, but their presence may make the adaptation to certain experience more difficult.

As we'll also see, the regulation of genes by "epigenetic" changes in the regulatory molecules controlling gene expression may also be influenced by attachment experience. For example, Michael Meaney's lab has revealed that "low-licking" rat mothers provide experiences that alter brain structure and lead to epigenetic alterations in the stress response. Meaney's research group has also revealed that children exposed to maltreatment early in life have epigenetic regulatory changes in the areas of the brain responsible for the HPA axis—changes that intensify the stress response.[53] These epigenetic changes not only influence the present experience of the individual, but also may be passed down through the sperm and eggs of the parents, and so may shape neural structure in the offspring.[54] Future research will need to illuminate the contributions of epigenetic and genetic variations that create increased vulnerability in adapting to stressful childhood environments. Although a child's particular attachment pattern appears to be developed in response to his or her caregiving environment, the response of that child may be exacerbated by possible genetic and epigenetic factors.[55]

In a review of this issue, Bokhorst and colleagues state:

> In a sample of 157 monozygotic and dizygotic twins, genetic and environmental influences on infant attachment and temperament were quantified. Only unique environmental or error components could explain the variance in disorganized versus organized attachment as assessed in the Ainsworth Strange Situation Procedure. For secure versus nonsecure attachment, 52%

of the variance in attachment security was explained by shared environment, and 48% of the variance was explained by unique environmental factors and measurement error. The role of genetic factors in attachment disorganization and attachment security was negligible. Genetic factors explained 77% of the variance in temperamental reactivity, and unique environmental factors and measurement error explained 23%. Differences in temperamental reactivity were not associated with attachment concordance.[56]

Environmental factors, such as stressful socioeconomic conditions, may increase the probability of disorganized attachment.[57]

Nevertheless, the routes of transmission for disorganized attachment remain to be fully elucidated, and further studies will need to pursue many (some as yet undiscovered) factors in a child's life that may help illuminate the origins of this form of attachment.[58]

Attachment theory suggests that a child's attachment system adapts to experiences with the attachment figure. Each of the classification categories in the Strange Situation is shaped by the pattern of communication between parent and child. In this way, the genetically preprogrammed, inborn attachment system is shaped by experience. This adaptation produces characteristic organizational changes in the way the child's mind develops. In other words, the mind as an embodied and relational process that regulates the flow of energy and information is directly shaped by the relational environment and the synaptic adaptations to that ongoing environmental experience. The caregiving adult's mind and patterns of communication directly shape the organization of the developing child's brain.

> The caregiving adult's mind and patterns of communication directly shape the organization of the developing child's brain.

In particular, the child's patterns of brain function—influencing the child's emerging state of mind—become activated within the context of a specific relationship. They are "context-dependent," as is much of brain function. This neuroscience principle can explain how one child can have distinct attachment strategies for each caregiver. In this manner, we can propose that the interpersonal relationship with each particular caregiver directly shapes the neurobiological state of the infant's brain activated within interactions. These states create an attentional and representational set of activations that are thought to minimize distress, regulate behavior, and help the child organize the self.[59] Ultimately, attachment interactions are all about how dyadic regulation shapes self-regulation. In other words, the child learns to regulate her own states of arousal and inner processing through interactions with another. The activation of a particular state in the presence of a particular caregiver is an adaptive process. This is how typical development unfolds within a relational setting. As we'll see below, both secure attachment and the "organized" forms of insecure attachment (avoidant and ambivalent) reveal effective modes of adaptation. In contrast, Main and Hesse have proposed that the nonorganized form of attachment (disorganized/disoriented) reveals that the infant has been presented with an unsolvable problem or "paradoxical injunction."[60] When the parent is the source of fear and disorientation, it is impossible for the child to achieve an organized, effective adaptive state.[61]

## Adult Attachment: Moving to the Level of Mental Representations

Mary Main pursued the question of why parents act in such distinctly different patterns with their children and she was able to move the field of attachment beyond the study of infant behavior and into the representational level of analysis.[62] As a graduate student, she had worked with Mary Ainsworth just after Ainsworth's original attachment studies in Baltimore. Presently a professor at the University of California at Berkeley, Main, with her students Carol George and Nancy Kaplan, developed a series of questions to ask the parents in her attachment studies to recollect their own childhood experiences.[63]

In the early 1980s, Mary Main and Ruth Goldwyn (then a visiting graduate student from London), later joined by Erik Hesse, created a way of analyzing the transcripts of this protocol—now called the Adult Attachment Interview (AAI).[64] What they found was that a parent's pattern of narrating the "story" of her early family life within a semistructured interview could be correlated with the Strange Situation classification of that parent's child. In this manner, Main began what is now a powerfully rewarding set of investigations. Studies using the AAI are being carried out throughout the world, with over ten thousand AAIs having been analyzed and over two hundred peer-reviewed studies published.[65] The AAI is a narrative assessment of an adult's "state of mind with respect to attachment," which reflects a particular organizational pattern or engrained state of mind of that individual at the time of the interview. As mentioned earlier, this developmental assessment of adult attachment is quite distinct from the romantic form of adult attachment as measured by self-report inventories.[66] The AAI's robust correlation with an adult's relationship with his offspring suggests that developmental attachment is in fact quite tenacious in the person's life.[67] Furthermore, attempts to correlate the AAI with features of an adult's personality as assessed by brief self-report measures have not revealed any significant associations.[68] This demonstrates that some of the measures of personality found in behavioral genetics to have a large degree of heritability are not associated with AAI findings; it therefore supports the notion that the AAI is measuring some feature of the adult derived primarily from the individual's experiences.[69]

Results from carefully performed longitudinal studies using Main and Gold-wyn's analysis of the AAI in fact have found that secure versus insecure childhood attachment status as observed in Ainsworth's Strange Situation can often predict later adult attachment findings, although this relation is not observed in all studies.[70]

All indications point to a primary role of experiential factors (includ-ing childhood attachment and more recent relationship experiences in cer-tain AAI results, as discussed later); however, the possible contributions of genetic factors will need to be further examined in future studies that utilize standard behavioral genetics approaches, such as twin and adoption studies. A few such studies have already been conducted.[71] Because of the research-supported way in which the AAI reveals how an adult's mind has been shaped by and has made sense of early attachment experiences, this instrument is a valuable tool in the basic assessment of individuals at the start of psychotherapy. I have used the AAI in clinical practice for over twenty years, and it is a profoundly useful instrument in both the assessment and the treatment-planning phases of clinical work.[72]

The strength of the correlations between parents' AAI results and their infants' Strange Situation results across socioeconomic and cultural groups has been reinforced by a number of findings suggesting that the AAI is measuring some feature of the adults that is robust, persists across time, and is independent of other variables. The psychometric properties of this instrument include that the AAI is stable over repeated assessments across a one-month to four-year period, as well as unrelated to most measures of intelligence.[73] It is also unrelated to long- and short-term memory, social desirability, or interviewer style.[74] The AAI is even more predictive of the Strange Situation results than it is predictive of direct research observations of parenting behavior available in prior studies. Marinus van IJzendoorn and his colleagues have termed this a "transmission gap"[75]—a finding that has yet to be fully understood. One preliminary suggestion is that parental "mind-mindedness" or "reflective function" may be a crucial feature that is present in the caregiver but not directly measureable in standard parental "sensitiv-ity" observations in many prior studies.[76] Essentially, "reflective function" is the capacity of the parent to perceive the internal mental world—to have mindsight or mentalization—so that the child is seen as having an internal center of subjective life worthy of being the focus of the parent's attention.[77] In fact, this aspect of a parent's sensitivity was initially a fundamental part of Mary Ainsworth's original formulation of the key factors involved in attach-ment security in which she postulated that a sensitive parent would be able to see things "from the baby's point of view."[78] The concept of the transmission gap reinforces the notion that the AAI is assessing some fundamental mental process of the parent that ultimately influences the parent's communication and interactions with the child. Many factors yet to be determined may also play a role in influencing this gap, including neurobiological factors (some related to genetics), in both the behavioral output of parents[79] and children's differential susceptibility to environmental influences.[80] All of these findings suggest that understanding the processes underlying the AAI, including memory, social communication, and some integrating process creating coherence of mind, will enable us to explore more fully the interpersonal nature of the mind's development.

The AAI is a semistructured autobiographical narrative in which an adult, or sometimes a teenager (usually a parent or parent-to-be), is asked a series of questions about her own childhood.[81] These questions include versions of the following: What were growing up and the person's early relationship with each parent like? What was the experience of being separated, upset, threatened, or fearful? Was there an experience of loss, and, if so, what was the impact on the individual and the whole family? How did the person's relationship with her parents change over time? How have all of these things shaped the development into adulthood of the individual's personality and parenting approach?

The AAI narrative is a subjective account of the individual's recollections. It does not claim to be an exact accounting of what occurred in the past. The method of interview analysis developed by Main and her colleagues begins with an examination of the elements of the recalled and inferred experiences with parents. Each of the speaker's parents is ultimately scored for the extent to which the rater concludes that the parent was loving, rejecting, involving/role-reversing, neglecting when present, and pressuring to achieve.[82] However, the most critical aspects of interview analysis rest upon the speaker's ways of presenting and evaluating his history. It is here that the AAI offers a unique perspective on the relationships among attachment, memory, and narrative.

The AAI rater also examines the transcript for the pattern of communication between the interviewer and the speaker.[83] In the discourse, and indeed in our daily conversations, how we talk with people reflects our internal processes and our response to the social situation of a conversation with another person. The analysis leads to ratings of what is called the current "state of mind with respect to attachment." Domains of this state of mind include the overall coherence of the transcript, idealization of parent, insistence on lack of recall, involved/involving (preoccupying) anger, passivity or vagueness of discourse, fear of loss, dismissing derogation, metacognitive monitoring, and overall coherence of mind. In some individuals, there is some disorganization or disorientation in reasoning or discourse when focusing on the topic of loss (of a family member by death) or abuse; this is assessed by scales for unresolved loss and/or trauma.[84]

The final classification, ascertained after several in-depth readings of the transcript, is based on examination of the numerically determined profiles across the domains of mental states with respect to attachment, together with directions for classifying the speaker's current state of mind (determined by the discourse analysis). This interview has a tremendous capacity to bring out subtle aspects of autobiographical narratives. Interviewees are often amazed at how this forty-five- to ninety-minute interview with a stranger can bring out such personally meaningful and often previously unrealized aspects of their early histories. As a parallel to the Strange Situation, the AAI also places a participant in an unusual setting in which "the unconscious is surprised" by the discussion of such intimate attachment issues, early memories, and reflections on how these experiences have shaped the adult's development and parenting behavior.[85]

As Erik Hesse has suggested, the AAI requires that the speaker perform the dual tasks of collaborative communication and searching for memories.[86] The search for memories of one's own childhood while maintaining typical discourse can lead to characteristic violations of Grice's four maxims of discourse that pertain to quality, quantity, relation, and manner. Violations are seen as types of incoherences in the narrative process.[87] These maxims form a core feature of the AAI assessment: "1) Quality—be truthful, and, have evidence for what you say; 2) quantity—be succinct, yet complete; 3) relation—be relevant or perspicacious, presenting what has to be said so that it is plainly understood;

> The AAI requires that the speaker perform the dual tasks of collaborative communication and searching for memories.

and 4) manner—be clear and orderly."[88] According to Main and Goldwyn, optimal discourse can be succinctly described as "truthful and collaborative," and they conceptualize violations of Grice's maxims as having to do with (internal) consistency (quality) versus collaboration with the interviewer or interview process (quantity, relation, and manner).[89] Assessment of the AAI examines how a speaker's state of mind at the time of the interview facilitates or impedes the ability to carry out a truthful/collaborative discourse while simultaneously conducting autobiographical reflections.

The ways in which the narrative reflects such a process is encoded in the scale assessing the overall coherence of the transcript. With the addition of the other elements that examine features of the narrative process, an overall "coherence-of-mind" rating is achieved, which assesses the global state of mind with respect to attachment. It is important to note that generally this adult stance represents an overarching state of mind toward attachment—not the attachment to each of the adult's parents. In contrast to a child's Strange Situation classification, an adult receives a single "state-of-mind" classification, not a relationship-specific category. Hesse has described an emerging "cannot classify" category—revealed in about five to ten percent of low-risk samples—which may reveal those individuals who are unable to attain such a unifying overall stance toward attachment.[90] As we'll explore in detail in Chapter 9 of this book, the capacity to integrate various elements of mental functioning, including autobiographical memory and social communication, can be viewed as a fundamental integrating process with which the mind creates coherence across its various states and mental processes.

The AAI results in an interviewee's being assigned a classification. The left side of Table 3.1 lists the four adult classifications. A parent's insecure–secure classification tends to correspond to the quality of her infant's attachment to her in sixty-five to eighty-five percent of cases.[91] These percentages are statistically quite meaningful, even without one hundred percent predictability.[92] Future research will need to examine the role of a parent's narrative functioning and other variables related to parental sensitivity, and how these may serve as mediating factors in the correlation of AAI results and the child's attachment classification at one year of age. As of this time, of all available measures—including intellectual functioning, personality assessments, and socioeconomic factors—the AAI remains the most robust predictor of how infants become attached to their parents,[93] probably because it reveals coherent autobiographical reflections and the capacity to reflect on the mind.

The AAI has been administered to parents at various stages of their children's lives: during pregnancy, at one year of age when the Strange Situation is performed, and at six years of age.[94] In each of these contexts, the AAI has a robust association with the specific classification of the infant–parent attachment. This means that the AAI findings are strong, seem to be stable across time, and have predictive power even before an infant is born. The prebirth research studies support the idea that the AAI is measuring some variable of a parent—not just some reaction of the parent to a feature of the child's inborn characteristics, such as temperament.[95]

An infant's attachment is specific to each parent and corresponds to each parent's AAI classification in a largely independent manner.[96] This parental specificity also suggests that the adult–infant correlations are not merely determined by genetic or other features of the child alone, but are a function of the history of parent–child interactions. Having differing attachment statuses dependent on the state of mind with respect to attachment of each parent (or other caregiver) is an important factor in understanding the development of these attachment patterns. Overall, these findings support the view of childhood attachment as relationship-based.[97]

Studies have also been done in which children who received Strange Situation classifications as infants were administered the AAI in late adolescence. In the majority of these studies, the Strange Situation results generally predict, about two decades later, the AAI classifications for the now grown children.[98] Some deviations from these predictions seem to be related to adverse life events, such as trauma and loss during the later years of childhood and adolescence.[99]

Temperament plays a role in eliciting particular reactions from parents, but it is not the major variable in determining attachment classifications within the child–parent relationship.[100] The temperament and genetically determined features of the parent certainly play a role in overt behavior. Some studies of parenting behavior suggest a strong genetic influence on particular patterns of emotional availability and parental discipline, for example.[101] As noted earlier, future studies of infant attachment and of the AAI will need to specifically examine the genetic contribution to these different patterns of attachment, and how such experiences might predispose individuals to various developmental pathways. Thus far, studies of identical twins compared to fraternal twins and research on foster children have been helpful in revealing the statistical finding of a minimal role of genetic factors in attachment.[102] At this point, the findings from attachment studies support the notion of child attachment as the result of a relationship, not of a feature of the child alone.

If a child has different attachment patterns with different caregivers,[103] how does this affect the child's future adult attachment status? The most dominant experiences—for example, those with a primary caregiver—may be those that tend to exert the most influence on the adult's narrative and attachment status.[104] Research correlations between Strange Situation status and later AAI classification are based on the infant's primary attachment relationship, most often with the mother. One notion is that different attachment patterns may be activated in the future, depending on the social situation. This might be revealed in the therapeutic setting, in which a clinician finds different "states of mind with respect to attachment" evoked within different moments of psychotherapy. The distinct findings of romantic attachment may reveal some elements of an overlap between the developmental attachment states of mind and how an individual may behave with different romantic partners in an adult-to-adult pair bond.[105]

The centrality of our attachment relationships was captured well by Mary Ainsworth:

> Many of the most intense emotions arise during the formation, the maintenance, the disruption, and the renewal of attachment relationships. The formation of a bond is described as falling in love, maintaining a bond as loving someone, and losing a partner as grieving over someone. Similarly, threat of loss arouses anxiety, and actual loss gives rise to sorrow; whilst each of these

situations is likely to arouse anger. The unchallenged maintenance of a bond is experienced as a source of security, and the renewal of a bond as a source of joy.[106]

Our various ways of engaging in close attachment relationships and maintaining these bonds as sources of security and joy may depend in part on our developmental histories as well as on our temperaments as we move into adulthood. The developmental influences on this capacity for intimate connections are the primary focus of attachment theory and research.

Different child–parent pairs may evoke different patterns of relating from the same parent, which may lead to different attachment classifications for different offspring of this parent. These variations may explain why the AAI does not have one hundred percent predictability to the Strange Situation.[107] It also raises the important issue of how the AAI may change with life experiences, such as the establishment of new forms of emotional relationships in parenting, romance, friendship, or psychotherapy.[108] In this way, different relationships may evoke different patterns of relating in each of us. The states of mind we experience, including the mental models activated in response to communication patterns with others, can in turn shape the manner in which we establish new relationships. We can find ourselves with a very different experience of the self and the self with others within different relationship contexts.

These social-context-dependent changes reflect the mind's capacity to adapt to new situations. However, attachment research and clinical experience suggest the existence of some tenacious process that maintains similar characteristics of the individual over time. Some of these traits can be seen as elements of implicit memory: mental models of the self and others, behavioral response patterns, and emotional reactions. As an individual reflects on the self across time, these characteristic traits can be seen in the autobiographical narrative process within the AAI. Main's term "state of mind with respect to attachment" refers to an engrained, temporally stable, self-organizing mental state.[109] This is not a transient, randomly activated state; rather, from repeated experiences with caregivers, it has become a characteristic self-defining state—or "trait"—of that individual. We will explore the notion of self-defining states of mind later in the book.

Let us now review in more detail the findings from attachment research with both children and adults, in order to explore these topics more fully. A complete review of this fascinating and important area of research is beyond the scope of this chapter, but such surveys are available in a number of helpful references.[110] Attachment research provides us with a set of rigorously collected data about human communication and mental coherence, which, as noted earlier, can teach us important principles about how the mind develops within interpersonal relationships. In the detailed discussions that follow, we explore the implications of this important work for understanding developmental processes, as well as the functioning of the human mind.

## ATTACHMENT, MIND, AND PSYCHOPATHOLOGY

Experiences throughout life shape the functioning of the mind. Those that occur in the early years mold our synaptic connections and so may set the stage for continued transactions with the world, which then reinforce those mental functions. Longitudinal research on attachment suggests that certain early relationship experiences promote emotional well-being, social competence, cognitive functioning, and resilience in the face of adversity.[111] However, because development is a process, older children, adolescents, and adults may be able to continue to grow and change despite suboptimal early life experiences.

Insecure attachment is not equivalent to mental disorder, but it creates a risk of psychological and social dysfunction.[112] For example, social competence in those with avoidant attachments may be compromised: Avoidantly attached children have been found to be controlling, aggressive, and disliked by their peers.[113] Ambivalently attached children may have a predisposition for social anxiety.[114] Disorganized/disoriented attachments are sometimes associated with dissociative symptomatology, and if such individuals are exposed to overwhelming experiences later in life, they may be prone to developing PTSD, as MacDonald and colleagues report:

> Disorganized attachment status at 12 months, compared with nondisorganized attachment status, significantly predicted both higher avoidance cluster PTSD symptoms and higher reexperiencing cluster PTSD symptoms. These findings suggest that the quality of early dyadic relationships may be linked to differences in children's later development of posttraumatic stress symptoms following a traumatic event.[115]

Persons in this attachment grouping, along with others who have experienced significant maltreatment in early childhood, also have deficits in attention and the regulation of emotion and behavioral impulses.[116] Intervention studies that offer young children the opportunity to develop secure attachments with their caregivers have yielded positive outcomes in the development of emotional, social, and cognitive competence.[117]

For example, if an infant does not receive predictable, warm, and emotionally available communication from caregivers, he may adapt by avoiding dependence on others in the future and deactivating the attachment system.[118] If his caregiver's behavior does not undergo a favorable change, or if other secure attachments do not predominate, this adaptation may make him withdraw from others' attempts to establish close, warm relationships with him. At five, ten, or twenty years of age, such an individual may be experienced by others as "aloof." Some might interpret such a trait as constitutional rather than as adaptive to the past environment. Of note is that studies of rats have found that maternal deprivation is associated with social behavioral problems. Rentesi and colleagues studied the impact on a nineday-old rat of a twenty-four-hour period of separation from its mother. They state: "The findings of this study showed that maternal deprivation results in long-term modifications in HPA axis and serotonergic activity indicating a clear relationship between early life stressful events and the development of anxiety-like disorders later in adulthood."[119] Of note, too, some studies suggest that these behavioral and social abnormalities can be ameliorated by serotonin medications.[120] These findings support the notion that early attachment experiences directly affect the development of the brain.[121] The fact that the behavioral problems return after cessation of the medications also supports the view that these brain changes are engrained within the neural pathways and possibly within the related epigenetic regulatory mechanisms that also shape basic functions, such as behavior, emotional regulation, and social relations.[122] Furthermore, such findings importantly remind us that an individual's favorable response to a medication does not deem the dysfunction as "due to genetics, not experience." Early experience shapes the structure, function, and epigenetic regulation of the brain. This reveals the fundamental way in which gene expression is determined by experience.[123]

As Brodsky and Lombroso have noted,

> The fact is that neither genetics nor environmental theories have led to a fundamental understanding of the etiologies of the vast majority of psychiatric disorders. If we have learned anything from recent studies, it is that a delicate interplay exists between nature and nurture. [They go on to address the consistent finding that even in studies of inherited disorders with identical twins, the concordance is rarely complete:] These results suggest that although genetic factors may provide [the] underlying diathesis or vulnerability for a disorder, environmental factors play a critical role in the ultimate expression of symptoms.[124]

Environmental factors play a crucial role in the establishment of synaptic connections after birth.[125] For the infant and young child, attachment relationships are the major environmental factors that shape brain development during its period of maximal growth. Therefore, caregivers are the architects of the way in which experience influences the unfolding of genetically preprogrammed but experience-dependent brain development. Genetic potential is expressed within the setting of social experiences, which directly influence how neurons connect to one another. Human connections create neuronal connections.

One example of risk for emotional disturbances is seen in the development of children who experience trauma at an early age.[126] As Glaser and colleagues suggest,

> For the infant and young child, attachment relationships are the major environmental factors that shape brain development during its period of maximal growth.

> [childhood trauma] may have long-lasting and enduring effects on adult psychological functioning, as exposed individuals continually react more strongly to small stressors occurring in the natural flow of everyday life. The finding that emotional stress reactivity is most pronounced for subjects who experienced trauma early in life confirms prior evidence suggesting that the effects of trauma are more detrimental when trauma occurs at a younger age.[127]

Allan Schore addresses a relevant aspect of the neurobiology of this situation:

> Although the critical period of overproduction of synapses is genetically driven, the pruning and maintenance of synaptic connections [are] environmentally driven. This clearly implies that the developmental overpruning of a corticolimbic system that contains a genetically encoded underproduction of synapses represents a scenario for high risk conditions.[128]

"Developmental overpruning" refers to a toxic effect of overwhelming stress on the young brain: The release of stress hormones leads to excessive death of neurons in the crucial pathways involving the neocortex and limbic system— the areas responsible for emotional regulation.[129] Children who may have a "genetically encoded underproduction of synapses," or who may have a genetic variant that dysregulates the production of related neurotransmitters such as dopamine, may be at especially high risk if exposed to overwhelming stress. In this way, we can see how experience and genetics interact in the development of risk for future disorder. Such risk is ultimately expressed within the neural connections of the brain.

An individual's personality is created from the continual interaction of genetically determined constitutional features and experiential exchanges with the environment, especially the social environment shaped by the family and by culture.[130] Vulnerability to dysfunction emerges from this interaction—not from genes and experience in isolation from each other. If the capacity of the mind to adapt remains into adulthood, then the emotional relationships we have throughout life may be seen as the medium in which further development can be fostered. These attachment relationships and other forms of close, emotionally involving interpersonal connections may serve to allow synaptic connections and possibly epigenetic alterations to continue to be molded, even into adulthood.

But how "plastic" is the brain? How open is the brain to further development beyond the early years of life? Which circuits remain capable of establishing new connections, and which are relatively "fixed" after certain early periods of development? Though these are open questions in neuroscience, we are discovering that the adult brain continues to change throughout the lifespan.[131] For some individuals who have experienced suboptimal attachment relationships, the brain may remain open to further growth and development. For others, early life histories that lack any attachment experience (as in severe neglect) or that include experience of overwhelming trauma (as in physical, sexual, or emotional abuse) may markedly alter the neurobiological structure of the brain in ways that are long-lasting and challenging to repair.[132] The questions that need to be asked are these: How can such experiences be prevented? And if they have already occurred, how can lasting improvement in these individuals possibly be achieved? A major theme of attachment research and effective treatment studies is that intervention via the medium of the attachment relationship is the most productive approach to creating lasting and meaningful results. Attachment research suggests a direction for how relationships can foster healthy brain function and growth: through contingent, collaborative communication that involves sensitivity to signals, reflection on the importance of mental states, and the nonverbal attunement of states of mind.[133]

Research into the relationship of attachment to psychopathology suggests a number of findings.[134] A meta-analysis of AAI studies conducted by van IJzendoorn and Bakermans-Kranenburg indicates that insecure attachment appears to be associated with a higher prevalence of mental disturbance, including anxiety (ambivalent attachment) and dissociative (disorganized attachment) disorders.[135] In general, ambivalent attachment predicts vulnerability for anxiety problems,[136] whereas avoidant attachment and disorganized attachment predispose an individual to develop conduct problems,[137] and disorganized attachment also predicts dissociation and personality disorder symptoms.[138] A study conducted by Carlo Schuengel and his colleagues suggests that the presence of an unresolved loss in a parent who has a primary insecure state of mind with respect to attachment leads to a less optimal outcome for children than does the presence of unresolved loss in a parent who has a primary secure status.[139] Adult security of attachment therefore appears to convey a form of resilience—at least for offspring—even in the face of trauma or loss. This finding is consistent with the general conclusion that attachment provides a framework for adaptation to life experiences:

Security conveys resilience, whereas insecurity conveys risk. Also, a genetic variant may make a child's response to suboptimal parenting related to unresolved loss or trauma in the parent more intense.[140] Van IJzendoorn's meta-analysis indicated that in psychiatric populations, insecurity in the AAI is far more prevalent and security ("secure/autonomous" status; see below) is far less prevalent than in the general population.[141]

> Adult security of attachment therefore appears to convey a form of resilience—at least for offspring—even in the face of trauma or loss.

The essential issue here is how the pattern of communication with attachment figures has allowed the mind to maintain proximity to them and establish self-organizing processes.[142] In this manner, Main suggests that the "maintenance of a 'minimizing' (avoidant) or 'maximizing' (resistant) behavioral strategy is therefore likely eventually not only to become dependent on the control or manipulation of attention but also to necessitate overriding or altering aspects of memory, emotion, and awareness of surrounding conditions."[143] Attachment history is correlated with a wide variety of mental processes central to the regulation of emotion and behavior. This finding may be understood in the context of neurobiological studies that implicate the same attachment-experience-dependent regions (prefrontal, especially the orbitofrontal cortex) in integrating these functions.[144] In this way, the link between insecurity of attachment and risk for psychopathology may be found within the brain regions that are dependent upon patterns of communication early in life for proper development, and also responsible for the regulation and integration of various processes (including memory, perception, and emotion). Dysregulation of this central integrating process will undermine successful self-organization, which may produce various forms of disturbances in emotional regulation and lead to mental suffering.

The rest of this chapter takes a closer look at each Infant Strange Situation classification and the corresponding parental state of mind regarding attachment from the AAI, in order to explore more fully the interactions between child and parent. These interactions—the patterns of the sharing of energy and information between caregiver and infant—are what influence neural growth and directly shape the developing mind of the child.

## SECURE ATTACHMENTS

In the Strange Situation, securely attached one-year-old infants (classified as "B") seek proximity after separation, are quickly soothed, and return rapidly to play. In Ainsworth and her colleagues' home observations of secure parent–child dyads during the first year of life, the parents were sensitive to the children's signals—emotionally available, perceptive, and effective at meeting the children's needs.[145] One could say that these parents were "tuned in" to the infants' emotional state of mind.[146] Peter Fonagy and Mary Target have described this ability as a product of the adults' "reflective function," in which parents are able to reflect (using words) on the role of states of mind in influencing feelings, perceptions, intentions, beliefs, and behaviors.[147] For this reason, reflective function has been proposed to be at the heart of many secure attachments, especially when the parent has had a difficult early life. The nonverbal component of this reflective ability can be seen in the capacity for affect attunement as seen in these dyads, in which the emotional expression of each member of a pair is contingent with that of the other.[148] Attunement involves the alignment of states of mind in moments of engagement, during which affect is communicated with facial expression, vocalizations, body gestures, and eye contact. This attunement does not occur for every interaction.[149] Rather, it is frequently present during intense moments of communication between infant and caregiver.[150]

Healthy attunement therefore involves the parent's sensitivity to the child's signals and the collaborative, contingent communication that evokes what has been described earlier as a "resonance" between two people's states of mind: the mutual influence of each person's state on that of the other. Such attunement involves disengagement at moments when alignment is not called for, and reengagement when both individuals are receptive to state-to-state connection. The states being aligned are indeed psychobiological states of brain activity.[151] Each individual becomes involved in a mutual co-regulation of resonating states.[152]

In emotional relationships of many sorts—including romance, close friendships, psychotherapy, and student–teacher relationships—there may be aspects of attachment present in which there are the basic elements of seeking proximity, using the other as a safe haven to help soothe oneself when upset, and internalizing the other person as a mental image providing a sense of a secure base.[153] These later forms of attachment can be established in the same manner that allows a secure attachment to develop in childhood. For the first two, "symmetrical" forms of relationship (friendship and romance), each member of the dyad demonstrates consistent, predictable, sensitive, perceptive, and effective communication. In therapist–patient and teacher–student relationships—which, like parent–child relationships, are "asymmetric"— the sensitivity to signals is the primary responsibility of the former individual, who serves as the sole "attachment figure" providing a safe haven and secure base for the other. The capacity of an individual to reflect upon the mental state of another person may be an essential ingredient in many forms of close, emotionally engaging relationships. This reflection on mental states is more than a conceptual ability; it permits the two individuals' minds to enter a form of resonance in which each is able to "feel felt" by the other. This intense and intimate form of connection is manifested both in words and in the nonverbal aspects of communication: facial expressions, eye contact, tone of voice, bodily movement, and timing of responses. This type of communication is what reveals attunement of states of mind.

The verbal component of communication can encompass many issues. Communication that is about the content of the other person's mind—such as "memory talk" or the elaborative style of discourse that focuses on the perceptions, memory, and imagination of another, as discussed in Chapter 2—enhances the mental processes of memory and self-reflection.[154] Intimate elaborative dialogues also focus on the other essential features of mental states: thoughts, feelings, intentions, beliefs, and perceptions. At the most basic level, therefore, secure attachments in both

> The matter of the mind matters for secure attachments.

childhood and adulthood are established by two individuals' sharing a nonverbal focus on the energy flow (emotional states) and a verbal focus on the information (representational processes of memory and narrative) of mental life. The matter of the mind matters for secure attachments.

## ADULT SECURE/AUTONOMOUS STATE OF MIND WITH RESPECT TO ATTACHMENT: FREEDOM TO REFLECT

Securely attached children tend to have parents who have an AAI classification of "secure/autonomous" present state of mind with respect to attachment (coded as "F"; think of "free").[155] A parent of a securely attached child stated:

> "My mother was a very caring person, and I remember feeling very close. My mother used to ask me what happened during the day after I came home from school. I remember one day when I was very upset. She was a very busy person. I came in the room, and I remember her putting her books down, and she went with me to my room so that we could talk in private. I don't remember exactly what she said, but I do remember how good she made me feel."

This portion of this adult's AAI narrative reveals a balanced perspective that is not overly idealizing. There is an ease of access to general autobiographical knowledge (e.g., the person's mother was caring and she felt close to her), and specific autobiographical details are provided to support these terms. This narrative segment reveals that there is general knowledge of what occurred and evidence for what is being said. The overall coherence of the narrative is very high and satisfies Grice's maxims of discourse. As Hesse has noted, such narratives reveal that an adult has the capacity to engage in collaborative and coherent discourse while simultaneously examining memories of attachment-related experiences.[156] Another aspect frequently found in these adults is the ability to reflect on mental processes within these narrative accounts.[157] Such a reflective function, in which the mind is able to represent other minds, reveals that the adult has what Fonagy and colleagues suggest is a "mentalizing" capacity.[158] This may be essential for a child's states of mind to be perceived and responded to by a parent.

Even though some narratives may contain descriptions of less-than-ideal parenting experiences, a coherence of mind is reflected in the flow of the narrative discourse; this coherence reveals an ease in talking objectively about the past and an ability to see parents as influential in the adult's development. The parent quoted above had this to say about her father:

"My father was very troubled by his being unemployed. For several years, I think that he was depressed. He wasn't very fun to be around. He'd go out looking for work, and when he didn't find any, he would yell at us. When I was young, I think that it was very upsetting to me. I didn't feel close to him. As I got much older, my mother helped me understand how painful his situation was for him, and for me. I had to deal with my anger with him before we could have the relationship we developed after my teen years. I think that my drive today is in part due to how difficult that period was for all of us."

These reflections on her relationships reveal an ability to balance positive and negative aspects of her experiences and to reflect on how they may have affected her during youth and then into adulthood.

Adults with a secure/autonomous state of mind may have a fluidity in their narratives, self-reflection, and access to memory. They may have a range of mental models of attachment relationships, which allows them to be flexible in their perceptions and plan of action. As Main has described, their attentional/representational state does not require a minimizing or maximizing strategy in addressing attachment-related issues.[159] Informal observations suggest that they can also be seen as having the ability both to enjoy and to modulate high levels of emotional intensity, and to experience rewarding emotional connections with others.

The narratives of secure/autonomous parents reveal that their internal working models of attachment are secure, that they acknowledge the importance of attachment relationships, and that they are free to live in the present. If their internal working models of attachment are secure, there is little "leftover business" that interferes with their narratives or, presumably, with their parenting approach to their children. There is a sense that secure/autonomous parents have life stories that allow them to live fully in the present, unimpaired by troubles from the past, denial in the present, or attachment-related worries about the future. The minds of such individuals can be described as having an organized and unimpaired flow of energy and information. We can propose that the coherence of narrative seen in this group of individuals may reflect a well-functioning ability to integrate aspects of the self over time—a subject we will explore in greater detail in Chapter 9.

An informal subset of secure/autonomous adults consists of those with an "earned" secure/autonomous status.[160] These are individuals whose described experiences of childhood would have been likely to produce some form of insecure attachment (avoidant, ambivalent, or disorganized). However, the coherence of their transcripts reveals a fluidity in their narratives and a flexibility in their reflective capacity, so that their present state of mind with respect to attachment is rated as secure/autonomous. From information contained within their AAI narratives, these individuals often appear to have had a significant emotional relationship with a close friend, romantic partner, or therapist, which has allowed them to develop out of an insecure status and into a secure/autonomous AAI status.[161] In studies comparing "earned" secure/autonomous, "continuous" secure/autonomous, and insecure parents, several findings emerge.

One overall finding is that the attachment of children to parents in the "earned" and "continuous" secure/autonomous categories appears to be indistinguishable.[162] When parent–child interactions were assessed, even under conditions of significant stress, these two groups were indistinguishable from one another. This may be a limitation of the present assessment measures, or an illumination of the ways in which one can significantly alter present functioning even in the face of difficult childhood experiences that resulted in earlier insecurity. Another general finding is that a subset group called "retrospective earned" secure/autonomous parents tends to report more depressive symptomatology than either a "prospective earned" or a "continuous secure/autonomous" group, and as much symptomatology as (or more than) the insecure group. How can this be explained? There are various ways of interpreting the notion of "earned security," and researchers will need to explore its retrospective and prospective nature in future assessments to clarify these important issues.[163]

In terms of our discussion, these findings with the "earned" secure/autonomous adults may reflect a flow of knowledge about the self across time. Implicit elements from early life experiences are quickly activated in intense emotional relationships, such as those with children and spouses. If the "prospective earned" category truly represents the emotional development of an individual from an insecure to a secure/autonomous state of mind with respect to attachment, then the narrative coherence within the AAI may reflect some important integrative process that enables parents to break the transgenerational passage of insecure attachment patterns.[164] Further studies of this population may be helpful in understanding the factors and mechanisms the mind can use to achieve a coherent integration in the face of suboptimal attachment history.

## AVOIDANT ATTACHMENTS

In the Strange Situation, avoidantly attached one-year-old infants (coded "A" in Table 3.1) demonstrate no overt response to the return of their parents, who are likely to have a "dismissing" stance toward attachment (see below).[165] They continue to play and behave as if the parents hadn't left or returned. Studies have revealed, however, a significant response by their nervous systems, as measured by heart rate changes.[166] Externally, to an observer, they appear avoidant of the parents' return.

Ainsworth and colleagues found that during the first year of life, these pairs were characterized by emotional distance and by neglectful and rejecting behavior on the part of the parents.[167] These parents appeared to be emotionally unavailable, relatively insensitive to their children's state of mind, imperceptive of their children's needs for help, and not effective at meeting those needs once perceived. Later studies would show that such parents demonstrated low degrees of affect attunement; language expression independent of facial emotions; and difficulty in relating to their children at the children's level of development in various situations, such as problem-solving tasks.[168]

The view of such a child's internal working model of attachment is that the parent has never been useful at meeting his emotional needs and is not attuned to his state of mind; therefore, behaviorally, it serves no purpose to seek the parent upon reunion. Connecting or emotionally joining in an avoidantly attached pair is limited, keeping parent and child relatively isolated compared to a securely attached dyad. In this manner, the organized adaptive strategy is to have an attentional/representational state that minimizes proximity seeking, reduces expectations, and shapes other attachment-related behaviors and mental processes accordingly.[169] The sense of self in this state is disconnected.

In an avoidantly attached dyad, the parent is significantly lacking in the enactment of the ability to conceptualize the mind of the child.[170] This lack may be evident in the decreased tendency of the parent, and then of the child, to reflect on the mental states of others or of the self. Some individuals may have a sense of disconnection of which they may be quite unaware. This sense of distance from others, and from the self, may dominate their experiences. It may also be apparent in how they describe their awareness of their own emotions. Informal observations suggest that they tend to engage in dry, logical, analytic thinking that lacks a sensory or intuitive component. As we'll see below in the discussion of adults classified as dismissing with the AAI, there is also a characteristic lack of richness and depth in the autobiographical narrative and self-reflections.[171]

As described at the beginning of this chapter, and as Bowlby proposed many years ago,[172] human infants have an inborn, genetically determined motivational system that drives them to become attached to their caregivers like other ground-living primate infants. Infants become attached to their caregivers whether or not those caregivers are sensitive and responsive. If primary caregivers do not offer the elements of secure attachment, the children must adapt to suboptimal interactions. In avoidantly attached children, such experiences seem to shape expectations and produce an organized adaptation involving a behavioral response that minimizes frustration: The children act as if the parents never left and show no outward signs of needing the parents. At the same time, however, the physiological studies of avoidantly attached children and their dismissing parents clearly demonstrate that the internal value placed on

> If primary caregivers do not offer the elements of secure attachment, the child must adapt to suboptimal interactions.

attachment has remained intact and intense.[173] The behavioral adaptations in infants, and the cognitive adaptations in older children and adults (paucity of autobiographical memory and narrative; beliefs in the unimportance of relationships in development and in life), are in contrast to the continued internal and nonconscious importance placed on attachment.

## ADULT DISMISSING STATE OF MIND WITH RESPECT TO ATTACHMENT: MEMORIES FROM AN EMOTIONAL DESERT

"My parents were very helpful to me growing up. They gave me excellent experiences with classes in school and outside of the regular curriculum. I was able to learn a foreign language and to play two instruments proficiently. [In response to a query about her relationship with her parents from early on, she stated:] My parents were very generous people. My father was very, very funny, and he taught me the importance of a good sense of humor. My mother was very neat, and she taught me the benefits of organization. Overall, my family was very good. [When asked for specific memories of her childhood, she stated:] I have very fond memories of my childhood. I don't remember specific experiences, but I do know that we had a very good family life. There were a lot of good times. [She also stated:] I believe in hard work and finding your own way in life. I am raising my children to achieve what I was able to: independence and stick-to-it-ness."

This excerpt from an AAI narrative shows the individual's lack of interpersonal connections from her childhood. Adults with this type of narrative often have the unique feature of insisting that they do not recall their childhoods. Their general descriptors are not supported by specific memories, and hence their transcripts have an incoherence defined by violations to Grice's maxim of quality (consistency) of discourse. Their responses are also generally excessively brief, violating Grice's maxim of quantity. For example, in response to a question about the mother–child *relationship*, they may state, "My mother was good. I cannot remember anything she did to support that word. I just think she was good, that's all." Often the implied sense in the interview is that there was not much emotional connection between parent and child. There are also reported examples of subjects' describing rejecting or neglecting behaviors on the part of the parents to support positive general statements offered about them. Overall, these narratives suggest that the mentalizing processes of the interviewees and their primary attachment figures may have been minimal.[174] The parent–child interaction appears to have had a suboptimal quality and quantity of mutual sharing of reflections on the mental states of others.

The internal working model of attachment in a "dismissing" (coded as "Ds") adult is thought to resemble that of an avoidantly attached child: "My parent is rejecting, and I cannot expect any emotional comfort or connection from this parent, so I will live on my own as an adaptation." This is a mental adaptation, not a conscious, deliberate choice on the part of the young infant. If a parent has shown little attunement to a child's internal state, the child will experience a world that remains emotionally isolated from the parent's world. The child's sense of self also remains fundamentally separate from that of the parent.

The narrative of past experiences quoted above has an underlying theme: "Life was good. I learned important things from my parents. I want my children to learn to be independent too." This person's account does not actually address the question about the quality of her relationship with her parents. Her past is summarized positively in terms of the products her parents gave her, not their connection to or communication with her. As noted earlier, another feature of the narrative is the person's insistence on her inability to recall details of her childhood. This amnesia seems to include a period far beyond five years of age (the time when most of us begin to have ease of access to explicit autobiographical memory). Her "blockage" of memory for her childhood experiences includes most of her adolescent years as well. We can view these findings as suggestive of the possibility that autonoetic consciousness may be quite underdeveloped in dismissing individuals, at least for childhood events.

Dismissing adults' insistence that they do not recall their childhood is often robust. Main and her colleagues are cautious, however, in their interpretation, since it could also serve to block discourse. This lack of recall should not be misinterpreted as a blocked memory of some trauma. Attachment studies suggest that this lack of recall is associated with the neglecting, rejecting, and emotionally disconnected pattern of relationships seen in avoidant attachments, rather than with some form of trauma-induced blockage as might be seen with physical or sexual abuse.[175] Studies also suggest that other aspects of personal knowledge, such as which television shows were popular or what major world events occurred at particular times in these adults' lives, are normally present.[176] In other words, noetic consciousness appears to have developed normally in these individuals.

The emotional distance and rejection that dominate avoidant relationships create a kind of low-affect environment. It is particularly interesting that preliminary findings from the prospective Minnesota Longitudinal Study of Parents and Children suggest that avoidantly attached children reveal dissociative symptoms throughout childhood, which seem to remit as adulthood approaches.[177] This project is an ongoing study examining adaptation in an "at-risk" sample of over 150 children and their families, who have been followed since the late 1970s (before the births of the children). These children were considered to be at high risk for poor adaptational outcome due to poverty and other factors, such as the youth of the mothers. In general, the findings from this study support the view that interpersonal relationships shape the way the mind develops. Specifically, the relationships that lead to avoidant attachments appear to foster a dis-association among, or disavowal of, elements of mental life.[178] For example, the need for emotional connection is repeatedly met with frustration within the interpersonal matrix of avoidantly attached dyads.

Why would such an emotional climate produce a lack of access to explicit autobiographical details of family life? Are these events encoded, but is access then blocked? Is there some different process of encoding in avoidantly attached children and in adults with dismissing states of mind with respect to attachment? Could it be that the lack of emotion does not allow the relationship experiences to be encoded as "value-laden" memories, which are then more likely to be recalled? Do these families not engage in the sorts of elaborative discussions that would develop the contents of the children's memories and imaginations more fully and enable them to express these more readily? The answers to these questions are open for investigation.

These questions suggest a number of possible routes to the lack of recall and lack of autobiographical narrative richness seen in dismissing and avoidant attachments. If future studies confirm their validity, then they may also point the way to what approaches might be useful to enable reflection to develop in these individuals' lives: emotionally involving, elaborative, and contingent communication with others. As noted briefly earlier, and as we'll explore in the chapters ahead, the region of the brain most central to attachment also appears to be the primary mediator of autonoetic consciousness. This right orbitofrontal region, along with other areas of the middle prefrontal cortex, serves the vital integrative function of coordinating social communication, empathic attunement, emotional regulation, registration of bodily state, stimulus appraisal (the establishment of value and meaning of representations), and autonoetic consciousness.[179] These exciting convergent findings suggest a preliminary view of how early emotional relationships shape self-knowledge and the capacity to integrate a coherent state of mind with respect to attachment.

The assessment of AAI narratives examines how specific explicit recollections correspond with generalized autobiographical themes and descriptions. In this way, the rater is able to uncover inconsistencies among the subjects' episodic recall, their semantic knowledge, and the themes of their life stories. Life narratives are not merely accumulations of autobiographical detail, but are driven by both explicit memory and implicit recollections of repeated experiences. We've discussed in Chapter 2 how the themes of life stories may be created by generalizations of the past (such as mental models),

> Life narratives are . . . driven by both explicit memory and implicit recollections of repeated experiences.

as well as by nonconscious wishes and by fantasies of what could have been a more desired past. This reconstructive aspect of memory can have strategically adaptive functions in creating a narrative sense of self that can serve to reduce anxiety about the actually lived past.[180] The "minimizing" strategy of the avoidant or dismissing stance may produce very specific adaptations of the access to and focus of autonoetic consciousness. As we'll see next, the "maximizing" strategy of the ambivalent or preoccupied stance may also produce characteristic patterns of autonoetic consciousness in which there is a blurring of past, present, and future representations during the AAI. Because autonoesis permits mental time travel, it can involve quite distinct dimensions of the experience of recollection during the challenging setting of the AAI.

We can think of autobiographical memory as organized into three categories of recollection: general periods, general knowledge, and specific events.[181] We can first think of our past in general periods, such as "when I was in high school." Next, we may have general autobiographical knowledge, such as the view that "I was good at basketball." Finally, we may recall specific events from our past, such as "when I was at that last basketball game during my junior year in high school." AAI narratives show that dismissing adults appear to lack recall for the details of specific relationship-related events in their lives.

This finding may be understood in terms of Wheeler, Stuss, and Tulving's notion of autonoetic consciousness as distinct from autobiographical memory.[182] Autonoesis is the mind's ability to perform mental time travel with a sense of the self in the personally experienced past, as described in Chapter 2. Memory for general periods or general knowledge of events in one's past can exist as a part of autobiographical memory, but may be experienced only within noetic consciousness. In other words, we may know that a past event occurred, but we do not have a sense of ourselves in the past. This factual knowledge of even personal past events is recalled as a semantic (factual) recollection, rather than as part of the episodic process of mental time travel. In episodic recall, the self as experienced is represented in memory. The finding that differing brain structures support autonoetic versus noetic recollection suggests that those with dismissing states of mind with respect to attachment may in fact be utilizing differing neurological mechanisms in their narrative recounting. Most individuals look to the left when recalling autobiographical memories, a process thought to activate right-hemisphere circuits predominantly.[183] Do those with dismissing states of mind look to the right side during the AAI—suggestive of the activation of the left hemisphere, where semantic recall is thought to be mediated? Main and Hesse, as well as others, have been examining the answer to this question both with respect to the AAI and with respect to a self-visualization task conducted at Berkeley.[184] An exploratory study by Behrens and colleagues supporting this hypothesis reveals the following findings:

> For the hemispheric activation analyses, the mother with Dismissing status had significantly stronger brain activation in her left hemisphere regardless of picture type, consistent with the idealization that characterizes a Dismissing status (Main, et al., 2002), and indicative of this mother's disconnect in perceiving even Negative pictures in a positive manner. The mother with Preoccupied status showed stronger activation in her right hemisphere for all but the Neutral pictures, consistent with the involving anger often present in the Preoccupied status (Main, et al., 2002).[185]

Further research will need to validate these initial supportive findings of an asymmetric bias across the patterns of insecure attachment.

Some of those with dismissing states of mind insist on complete lack of recall for personal events in their lives. Not only do they appear not to recall themselves in the past; they do not seem even to recall the facts of experiences. Beyond mere autonoetic impairments, there appears to be a blockage in recall or impaired encoding of facts about relationship-related experiences. To attempt to understand this insistence on lack of recall, we can look toward the general studies of memory and emotion, which suggest that emotionally charged experiences are more likely to be remembered.[186] The parts of the brain responsible for assigning priorities to incoming engrams, including the amygdala and orbitofrontal cortex, probably mediate this "red-flagging" of experiences as being value-laden, emotionally meaningful, and therefore memorable.[187] Emotional experiences are more likely to be remembered in the long term, suggesting that the cortical consolidation process selects these memories above others for entry into permanent storage. This may be the way in which our life stories come to contain emotionally meaningful themes and corresponding supportive details.[188]

Could it be that in avoidantly attached children, the lack of emotional involvement keeps the amygdala, orbitofrontal cortex, and other appraisal centers from labeling relationship-related experiences as worthy of recall? In one study, ten-year-olds who had been found to be avoidantly attached to their primary caregivers at one year of age were also found to have a unique and marked paucity of autobiographical narrative detail.[189] They would say things like "I don't know what to say about my life," or "I live at home with my brother; that's about it." Their dismissing parents had this same quality of minimal elaboration of their life stories, especially as these pertained to relationships with other people.

If parents are uninterested in reflecting or unable to reflect upon their children's minds, then we can hypothesize that they may also provide less elaboration via memory talk and co-construction of narrative, both of which appear to be important in making memories accessible. With these diminished mentalizing or reflective functions (thinking about the subjective experience of one's own or another's mind, narrativization, autobiographical memory, and emotional connections with others), it may well be that these individuals' subjective experience of life lacks a certain vitality shared by those in the other attachment groups. Overall, self-awareness and autonoetic consciousness itself may differ as a reflection of these differences in developmental experience.

Avoidant or dismissing attachment can be conceptualized as involving restrictions by the mind on the flow of energy and information. Acquired from emotionally distant communication patterns, this pattern of attachment organizes the mind to reduce access to emotional experience and information in memory. These restrictions impair the mind's ability to develop an integrated sense of the self across time in relationship to others. The view of the self is limited to nonemotional domains, which are seen as quite independent of the influence of interpersonal relationships. Although one can certainly argue that this is just an "adaptation" to prior experience and not an impairment in mental functioning, an organization of the mind that excludes emotion and interpersonal relationships is quite inflexible. If one believes that emotion and relationships play an important role in determining meaning and mental health throughout the lifespan, then such a restrictive approach to living in the world can be seen as an impairment to the healthy functioning of the mind.

## AMBIVALENT ATTACHMENTS

The second form of insecure attachment is called "resistant" or "ambivalent" ("C"). I prefer to use the term "ambivalent," because it denotes the mixed and anxious feelings often associated with this form of relationship. During the Strange Situation, ambivalently attached infants return to their parents upon reunion, but are not easily soothed and do not quickly return to play. They cry, show relief, then cry again; they appear difficult to console.

In their home observations during the first year of life, Ainsworth and colleagues found that the parents in these dyads were inconsistently available, sensitive, perceptive, and effective.[190] Such a parent would have moments of intrusiveness that appeared to be emotional invasions into an infant's state of mind. These were generally not hostile in nature; a parent might suddenly grab a happily playing child and shower him with excited hugs and kisses without warning, disrupting the child's focus of attention and state of mind. That is, the parent would try to be connected, but in a way that was not contingent to the child's communication. In ambivalently attached dyads, the parents' emotions and mental states appear to interfere repeatedly with the ability to consistently and accurately perceive those of their infants. As a result, the infants remain uncertain whether their own emotional states and hence needs will be attuned to and satisfied. Sometimes they will, sometimes they won't. As Mary Main has suggested, this leads to an attentional/representational state that "maximizes" a focus on the attachment system.[191] Mental state resonance or alignment does occur in these dyads, but it is unpredictably available and is at times dominated by the parents' intrusion of their own states into those of the children.

Each of us goes through cycles of needing connection with others and needing to be left alone. These natural oscillations between an external focus with communication to others and an internal focus with periods of solitude are part of what sensitive caregivers perceive in the changing states of their children. Knowing when to go toward a child (or adult) in an effort to communicate, versus knowing when to "back off" and give emotional space to another person, is a fundamental part of attunement. In ambivalent attachments, there appears to be a significant inconsistency in the parents' ability to perceive and respect these natural cycles.

How do interactions with parents create an ambivalent attachment strategy in their children? Examination of AAI findings (see below) reveals that elements of the past significantly intrude into the narratives of "preoccupied" parents, shaping their experience in the present. Is there anyone for whom the past *doesn't* shape the present? Of course not; our brains are always automatically comparing past experiences with present perceptions as we anticipate the next moment in time. This comparing process is a natural outcome of the interplay among memory, perception, and consciousness, and defines the brain as an "anticipation machine." However, the states that children evoke in us as parents create challenges beyond merely cognitively comparing forms of representations and matching our expectations. These parental states of mind are in fact responses to a child's behavior, some might argue. But are they contingent? The issue with "preoccupied " parents is that their responses to the AAI and to their children's behavior are dominated by their entanglements with their own past. Their responses to the external world are shaped intermittently by their internal mental processes, which are independent of the signals sent by their children at the moment.

In this way, an ambivalently attached child experiences inconsistent parental sensitivity and has a degree of distress that is not reliably soothed by the parent. Unlike the avoidantly attached child, who learns to dismiss the mental state of the parent and develops a deactivating strategy, an ambivalent attachment forces the child to be more preoccupied with her own distress[192] and to maximize her attention to the (unpredictable) attachment relationship.

> An ambivalently attached child experiences inconsistent parental sensitivity.

One way of conceptualizing this finding is seen in Aitken and Trevarthen's discussion of "intersubjectivity."[193] In this view, attuned communication has an initial phase during the first few months in which there is a direct form of contingent communication between infant and caregiver. This is called "primary" intersubjectivity. By about nine months, the infant's increasingly complex representational capacities allow for the development of an internal image of the parent, which Aitken and Trevarthen call a "virtual other." This is "secondary" intersubjectivity, in that now the infant (like the parent since the beginning of their relationship) filters perceptions of the other person through the secondary process of a "virtual other" representation. This intermediate step is the typical way in which the mind connects the memory of past experiences with ongoing perceptions. Beyond the first half year of life, we each have a set of "virtual others," which are continually evoked during interactions with other people. If past attachments have been filled with uncertainty and intrusion, then the virtual other—the internal representation of the attachment figure—may interfere with our ability to clearly perceive others' bids for connection. We may (mis)perceive others' behaviors in light of a virtual other that creates caution and uncertainty.

Daniel Stern has described in detail the ways in which such interactions become represented and generalized in the infant's experience.[194] These generalizations form the building blocks of the internal working models. Main has clarified Bowlby's original meaning: Parenting that generates multiple, contradictory models of attachment creates a sense of insecurity,[195] and insecure attachment is generated by multiple "incoherent" models of attachment.[196] In the Strange Situation, the child is not easily soothed by the return of a parent who, in this particular setting, may be acting in a perfectly attuned and comforting manner. The past, encoded within the child's memory, directly shapes both the implicit mental models and the "evocative memory" that creates the image of the virtual other in the child's mind during interactions. We can propose that these processes are state-dependent and can be activated in certain mood states (such as feeling threatened) or within interactions with specific people. The virtual other can be so dominant in an individual's mind that an actual other has little chance of being directly and accurately perceived during a current experience. Informal observations suggest that for the child of such a person, the sense of being "unseen" or "absent" may fill many interactions and create a sense of a "false self." The result is that this attachment history shapes the child's perceptions and expectations of the world, others, and the self in the direction of ambivalence. The result is a confused sense of self.

The ambivalently attached child has learned that his own mental state may be intruded upon by the parent in unpredictable ways. The flow of energy and information within the child will be unpredictably disrupted rather than predictably enhanced by communication with the parent. Nevertheless, the developing child needs to have the attachment figure psychologically accessible in order to feel secure. Ironically, the ambivalently attached child is left with an internal sense of uncertainty, which gives him an even more urgent and continuing need for comfort from external interactions. In this way, the unpredictable and intrusive patterns of communication have established ambivalence in the child's self-regulatory capacities. Combined with the parent's own continuing preoccupations and inconsistent sensitivity to the child's signals, the dance of (mis)attuned communication in such a dyad continues to reinforce the intense, inconsistent, and intrusive nature of the alignment of states of mind.

## ADULT PREOCCUPIED STATE OF MIND
## WITH RESPECT TO ATTACHMENT:
## INTRUSION OF THE PAST UPON THE PRESENT

"We were a close-knit family. We used to play all the time, have fun, walk around. There were never any times when things became too loud, or sometimes they would. But it was OK. One time we went to Disneyland with my uncle. It was a lot of fun. But last week my parents took my brother's kids there and they didn't even call us. Why they do this, I don't know. It doesn't bother me now, but it does. I mean it did. I think. I wish they would stop favoring him over me; but I'm through caring about it, I'm through with the whole thing. When will it stop?"

The person just quoted was responding to the direct request "Tell me about your family from your earliest memories." Her account reveals an adult with an AAI classification of "preoccupied" (coded as "E") state of mind with respect to attachment.[197] The narrative indicates that the past is emerging into this adult's present. The response to the question about early memories begins to include issues about current relationships that contain overt hostility, fear, and passivity. According to Main and Goldwyn, the linguistic analysis reveals the violation of the discourse maxims of quantity, manner, and relevance:[198] The narrative is not succinct and does not directly address the interviewer's queries. Individuals like this woman have easy access to a flood of childhood memories that still actively and profoundly influence their lives in the present. Present reality begins to blend with the past (whether this is directly stated or not).

Preoccupied adults' contradictory models of attachment include concerns that their attachment figures may or may not be able to meet their needs. There is simultaneously a powerful wish for closeness and at times a disabling fear of losing it. This preoccupied state is filled with emotional turmoil centering around attachment-related issues. Mental models of relationships will bias present perceptions and expectations, as we have seen, in such a way that these persons may create their own worst nightmare of uncertainty in their relationships with others, including their own children. The inconsistent emotional availability and intrusiveness of these adults can be seen as resulting from their preoccupation with previous attachments. Using Aitken and Trevarthen's model of the "virtual other," I would propose that one way of conceptualizing this preoccupation is that the virtual other of an adult's attachment figure is so dominant that it distorts the parent's ability to perceive the child directly. In this way, the child may be repeatedly seen through the filter of the parent's preoccupations with the dominant virtual other, and thus may be at risk of developing a sense of inauthenticity within the parent–child relationship. As noted above, such a process may encourage the development of a sense of a "false self" in the child. In this manner, both parent and child become filled with representations of the self and of the other that interfere with contingent, collaborative communication. Their inner worlds may each be dominated by intrusive emotional concerns ("Am I loved enough? Will I be abandoned?"), which will be activated within a variety of relationships.

A parent's emotional turmoil, preoccupations with the past, and preoccupations with his own mental state can create repeated patterns of inconsistent attunements with his child. This may also repeatedly lead to an adult's relating to a child as if the child were a mirror of himself at an earlier age. In this way, entanglements with his own childhood intrude on the way he relates to his child. This may be especially true in one particular subcategory of this adult classification, "preoccupied/overwhelmed by trauma," in which the AAI reveals frequent references to past traumatic experiences.[199] Though these repeated references are not disoriented, they do reveal that the adult continues to have the trauma intrude upon his narrative discourse.

In ambivalently attached children and their preoccupied parents, mental models of the self with others are full of leaky boundaries between past and present. The adults' experience becomes influenced by activations of models of insecure attachment from their own childhoods. As perception and emotional meaning are established through the filter of this uncertainty, a self-fulfilling prophecy is created: New relationships are again experienced as inconsistent and unreliable. Emotional joining or connecting is a longed-for but inconsistently achieved goal in the minds of ambivalently attached individuals.

A parent's preoccupation with her own past—for example, how she felt abandoned by her mother or how her father was disappointed in her—can continually intrude itself into her present perceptions. Being with a child can produce the most intense entanglements with these images and ideas from the past within the parent's mind. The parent enters an old state of mind and can become filled with sensations of fear, rejection, disappointment, or anger, which color her experiences with her own child. The parent often remains unaware of how disabling this preoccupation with the past is to her functioning as an effective parent in the present.

> A parent's preoccupation with her own past . . . can continually intrude itself into her present perceptions.

In memory terms, such parents are being "primed" to recall their childhood experiences. Priming is a normal part of memory, in which elements become more likely to be retrieved following certain contextual cues.[200] For preoccupied parents, the context of being with children who may share some of the features of their own childhoods (e.g., shyness or parental rejection) creates a context in which the parents begin to relive their own childhood struggles. Marital difficulties can also evoke emotional states that tend to reinstate old memories. For example, a father may feel a sense of rejection because of his wife's possibly distant, emotionless pattern of relating, which then creates a mental state within him that resembles the rejected, frustrated state of mind of his youth. His wife's interest in a child may also evoke a sense of rejection resembling the feeling of the birth of a sibling in the father's own childhood history.

"State-dependent" memory is a second fundamental way in which parents' childhood memories are primed. This refers to the way in which events encoded in particular mental states will be more likely to be recalled if a person is in a similar state in the future.[201] This typical feature of memory is prominent throughout life and is particularly relevant to how being a parent can induce states resembling those of one's youth. This happens in everyone, regardless of attachment history. But how these memories are experienced may vary considerably with attachment history. For example, preoccupied parents may be flooded with emotional and behavioral responses within implicit memory. They may begin to remember, both explicitly and implicitly, particular aspects of memories from their own childhoods as they raise their children through the various stages of development. Explicit recollections may return in the form of facts about child rearing or other autobiographical events, or general knowledge from the past. Implicit recall may take the form of many components of "personality," including learned behavioral responses, emotional reactions, mental models, attitudes and beliefs, perceptual images, and possibly internal bodily sensations. The activation of implicit memory by itself does not involve a sense of recollection. When situations activate implicit memories without their explicit counterparts, parents merely act, feel, perceive, or sense in the here-and-now. These implicit recollections are not usually subject to a process of self-reflection, as in "Why am I doing this or feeling this way?" Individuals may sense these experiences as just defining who they are.

There is a direct connection between how past experiences have shaped implicit memory and how they are reactivated in the setting of being with a child. If parents do not recognize this link, then they are at risk of enacting, without conscious awareness, learned behaviors and emotional responses that will dominate their actions and create their children's attachment experiences.

If these implicit memories are of healthy forms of relating, then the outcome will be a secure attachment. If instead the parents had less than optimal experiences, without self-reflective work they may be at risk of passing on either imitated patterns or adaptations to these relationships; these will keep their children from experiencing a dependable emotional closeness (which secure attachments require).

Preoccupied attachment can be described as reflecting an impairment in the flow of information and energy in attachment-related contexts. The intrusion of information (memory) from the past into present situations impairs an adult's ability to have contingent, collaborative communication with a child. We can propose here that one mechanism by which this intrusion of memory influences social communication is within the integrating circuits of the middle prefrontal region, described earlier. As autonoetic consciousness mediates the mind's ability to travel through time—to experience the self in the past, present, and future—then the settings of the AAI, emotional relationships, or ongoing parenting experiences may evoke attachment-related contexts that activate the prefrontal cortex's retrieval of autonoetic representations. For the preoccupied state of mind, autonoetic awareness then evokes a range of intense mental representations that slip easily into this state of roving among past, present, and future preoccupations. This may be how the characteristic AAI pattern is created.

The middle prefrontal region also specifically mediates the perception of emotional signals and social cognition. The dual tasks of the AAI as described by Hesse[202]—to carry out collaborative and coherent discourse while searching for memory—may be particularly challenging to the prefrontal region in insecure states of mind with respect to attachment. For the preoccupied state, such a challenge may lead to a flood of episodic representations, which can be postulated to impair the emotional perception and social cognition functions of this same region. Furthermore, within the context of parenting, such flooding may also impair the capacity of the prefrontal region to mediate sensitivity to the child's signals, to achieve attuned communication, and to regulate emotional states within the parent—the processes that ordinarily allow a child to achieve consistent and predictable social referencing. In an ambivalently attached dyad, these processes, in which the child looks to the parent's often nonverbal responses to "know how to feel,"[203] are inconsistently useful in helping the child learn to regulate her own internal states. Mirror-neuron-related processes may also be at play leading to the child's simulation of her parent's noncontingent emotional response. These transactions may be at the core of the inconsistency and intrusiveness of the ambivalently attached child's experience with the preoccupied parent. Such a distorted "mirror" may add to the child's sense of a confused self.

## DISORGANIZED/DISORIENTED ATTACHMENTS

After reunion following separations, a one-and-a-half-year-old girl sought her father's attention and got on his lap, but continued to cry and did not return readily to play. This behavior was quite distinct from her secure attachment to her mother, in which she sought proximity and then was easily soothed and returned to exploration in the room. Unfortunately, the Strange Situation for this young girl and her father revealed more than these elements of an ambivalent attachment. When he returned to the room, she first got up from playing and moved toward the wall, away from him; then she seemed to walk toward him, but with her gaze focused in the opposite direction from where she was walking. Main and colleagues have classified this type of approach–avoidance during the Strange Situation with a parent as "disorganized/disoriented" ("D"), with a primary or best-fitting alternative classification of ambivalently attached.[204]

During the reunion in the Strange Situation, an infant with a disorganized/disoriented attachment frequently exhibits chaotic and/or disoriented behavior.[205] Examples of this may include first going toward the mother or father and then backing away. In more severe cases, children may go in circles, fall down, enter trance-like states of "freezing," or avert their gaze and rock back and forth. In the first year of life, these dyads are characterized by unusual forms of communication from the caregiver. These have the quality of a "paradoxical injunction."[206] "Come here and go away" is a mild version; they may also involve the parent's frightened, disoriented, or frightening behaviors toward the infant. These communications present a child with an unsolvable and problematic situation. Main and Hesse have proposed that these dyadic interactions are inherently disorganizing.[207] The infant cannot make sense of the parental responses. Furthermore, the child cannot use the parent to become soothed or oriented, because the parent is in fact the source of the fear or disorientation. There is no organized adaptation available for the child. The infant's internal state of mind is thought to lack internal coherence because the attachment system is such that the caregiver is intended to confer safety to the child. Hesse has pointed out that disorganized attachment is seen in many situations that do not involve abuse in which parents exhibit frightened, dissociated, or disoriented behavior.[208]

At another extreme are children who experience physical, sexual, or emotional abuse and develop disorganized/disoriented attachments. In studies of these high-risk, parentally maltreated infants, disorganized attachment was found in about seventy percent of samples; in one such study, in the context of home intervention, the rate was fifty-five percent.[209] In this setting, a child experiences fear or terror of the attachment figure, not just loss of the ability in the moment to use the attachment figure as an orienting, soothing haven of safety. The infant experiences a bind in which the feeling of fear cannot be modulated by the very source of that fear. Without the option to fight or flee, stuck between approach and avoidance,[210] the infant can only "freeze" into a trance-like stillness, which may be the beginnings of a tendency toward clinical dissociation—the phenomenon in which consciousness, states of mind, and information processing become fragmented.[211] The parental behavior of either abuse (frightening) or sudden shifts into mental states independent of the child's signals (frightened or disoriented) are thought to be the mediators of disorganized/disoriented attachment.[212] The child's sense of self can be described as fragmented.

Children with disorganized/disoriented attachment have been found to have the most difficulty later in life with emotional, social, and cognitive impairments.[213] These children also have the highest likelihood of having clinical difficulties in the future,[214] including affect regulation problems, social difficulties, reasoning problems under stress, and (as suggested just above) dissociative symptomatology. Unlike the other forms of insecure attachment, which are "organized" approaches to the pattern of parental communication, this form of insecure attachment appears to involve significant problems

> Children with disorganized/disoriented attachment have been found to have the most difficulty later in life.

in the development of a coherent mind. The sudden shifts in these children's states of mind yield incoherence in their cognitive, emotional, and behavioral functioning. Their social interactions become impaired. Studies have found that these children may become hostile and aggressive with their peers. They tend to develop a controlling style of interaction that makes social relationships difficult. These peer interactions in a school-age child often occur when the child is having continuing difficulties in the home environment that engender unsolvable paradoxes or overwhelming feelings without solution. Disorganized attachment has been associated with serious family dysfunction, such as impaired ability to negotiate conflicts; chronic and severe maternal depression; child maltreatment; and parental controlling, helpless, and coercive behaviors.[215] As the children develop and continue to have such experiences, the recursive aspect of mental development suggests that the very incoherence that is creating their difficulties will be reinforced. Disorienting relationships create internal disorganization that in turn impairs future interactions with others, which disorganize the development of the mind still further.

In these dyadic situations, the child has the double trauma of experiencing terrifying events and the loss of a trusted attachment figure. Terrifying experiences that have occurred early in life, during the typical period of infantile amnesia (before explicit episodic memory is available), will be processed in only an implicit manner. If such experiences occur later in life, then family denial and lack of memory talk can impair explicit recall, which in turn may impair the consolidation process and prevent experiences from becoming a part of permanent explicit autobiographical memory.[216] Instead, these events may remain in an unresolved, unconsolidated form. In this state, they may be more likely to influence implicit recollections automatically, creating elements of emotional, behavioral, perceptual, and perhaps somatic reactions without conscious awareness of their origins.[217] The mind's ability to integrate these aspects of memory is severely impaired in unresolved trauma and in disorganized/disoriented attachments, leading to dissociative tendencies and incoherence of mind.

## ADULT UNRESOLVED/DISORGANIZED STATE OF MIND WITH RESPECT TO ATTACHMENT: INCOHERENT LIFE STORIES AND ABRUPT SHIFTS IN STATES OF MIND

In Main and colleagues' adult attachment studies, episodes of marked disorganization and disorientation in reasoning or discourse during attempted discussions of loss or abuse in the AAI lead to assignment of "unresolved/disorganized" status. As Main and Hesse first discovered, unresolved parents tend to have infants whose Strange Situation behavior is disorganized.[218] A meta-analysis conducted by van IJzendoorn and colleagues has shown that across a full set of existing studies, a child with a disorganized attachment ("D" in Table 3.1, right side) indeed often has a parent with an AAI classification of unresolved (trauma or grief)/disorganized (coded as "U/d").[219] As with the child classification, the adult is also given a primary, best-fitting alternative adult classification (F, Ds, or E; see Table 3.1, left side).

Disorientation or disorganization during an interview may include an individual's referring to a deceased person as if she were still alive (loss) or becoming confused and disoriented when discussing fearful experiences with a parent (trauma).[220] Examples *not* classified as unresolved would be a person's crying during the interview or stating that the subject matter is too painful and wishing not to discuss the topic. These latter two examples reveal that the emotional pain of the loss or trauma can still be active and available to the person's conscious mind, but the person is not showing signs of discourse disorientation or disorganization. In this view, unresolved trauma or loss is reflected in a disruption in the representational processes necessary for coherent discourse.[221] We can propose that the mind's ability to integrate various aspects of representations within memory into a coherent whole is impaired in unresolved states. The middle prefrontal cortex can be hypothesized to be playing a central role in such impairments in integration.[222]

Abrupt shifts in state of mind, intrusive "dissociated" elements of implicit and explicit memory, transient blockages in the capacity to carry out collaborative social communication, and difficulty maintaining a fluid flow in consciousness across these processes may be at the root of unresolved states of mind as assessed in the AAI.[223]

The conditions that elicit abrupt shifts may include questions about the topic (as in the AAI), or relationship contexts that resemble those of the parent's childhood. The latter may include many crucial moments in parenting, such as setting limits, tuning in to a child's distress, responding to a child's testing of limits, and negotiating bedtime and other separations. Hesse and van IJzendoorn have found that in a nonclinical sample of young adults, individuals whose parents had experienced the loss of a child or another loved one within two years of their own birth tended to have higher rates of "absorption," one element of dissociative reactions.[224] Loss in a caregiver around the time of raising an infant may be less likely to have been resolved at that time, and these findings support the view that such lack of resolution may contribute to the development of disorganized attachment and the tendency to dissociate.

If one examines the prevalence of loss or of trauma *alone* (and not the indicators of its lack of resolution), there is little statistical correlation with the disorganized attachment status of offspring or with any other developmental feature.[225] It appears that the AAI is uniquely eliciting this usually unstudied feature of *unresolved* loss, and that unresolved loss, not loss itself, is what leads to disorganized infant response patterns. Lack of resolution of past trauma or loss directly affects emotional regulation.[226] Hesse and Main have emphasized the role of unintegrated fear in the lapses in reasoning or discourse observed in the speaker.[227] Unresolved trauma or grief creates pain and suffering in both these individuals and their children; for this reason, helping people resolve trauma and grief is of vital importance for present and future genera-tions. Failure to identify lack of resolu-

> Lack of resolution of past trauma or loss directly affects emotional regulation.

tion can permit dysfunction to continue across the generations within the devastating effects of disorganized attachment. Again, these children have a marked inability to regulate emotional responses and the flow of states of mind; this establishes a tendency toward dissociation, disruptive behaviors, and impairments in cognition and coping capacities, as well as a vulnerability toward PTSD.[228]

It is clear that there may in fact be many individuals who do have unre-solved grief or trauma, but whose AAI narratives may not reveal disorgani-zation in discourse. It is assumed that the percentages of subjects placed in the unresolved category may actually represent underestimates of the prevalence of lack of resolution. In spite of this unavoidable procedural limitation, the unresolved category has a robust correlation with the group of infants who have disorganized/disoriented attachments.[229]

One father revealed a marked disorientation during discussions about his own father's alcoholism. This incoherence in his narrative suggests unresolved trauma. When asked about times when he may have felt threatened by his parents, he stated:

> "I know I didn't like my mother's depression, but I don't think I felt threatened by it. She would be OK sometimes, other times not. I think I was mostly disappointed and sad. About my father, well, that is a different sort of thing. I try not to think about it much. He is always unpredictable, though I think he can control himself, though sometimes he can't, and I couldn't figure out when he would, so I don't, I mean I couldn't, know how to deal with him . . . [twenty-second pause]. There were things that would happen . . . [seventeen-second pause]. And they weren't very fun, I mean they were scary. Yes, I feel frightened. He is very big, and very threatening. Yes."

Note the use of the present tense to describe the past—a sign of disorientation. The incomplete sentences and prolonged pauses in speech are other signals of cognitive disorganization. During this part of the interview, something was happening in this father's mind that was incompletely processed and was impairing his usual ability to tell a coherent story while searching for memories.[230]

Disorganizedly attached children and their parents with unresolved trauma or grief each have the potential to activate incoherent, conflictual, or unstable mental models. Abrupt shifts in states of mind can occur within these individuals, leading to a disorganized form of behavior externally and to the experience of a dissociation in consciousness internally. AAI narratives such as the one above reveal breaks in the typical flow of communication— both in the extended pauses without explanation and in the incoherent content of discourse. Unresolved traumatic experiences or unresolved grief over loss of a loved one can be revealed through this disorganization in narrative flow.

A young infant, attempting to make sense of the world, is particularly vulnerable to a parent who has abrupt shifts in his own state of mind. These state shifts are primarily functions of the internal processes of unresolved trauma or grief, rather than directly contingent and hence predictable responses to the child's own behavior. The child's capacity to anticipate the parent's behavior is severely impaired, and expectations, mediated via mental models, cannot be created in an organized manner. As the two individuals interact, the child's state attempts to align with the shifting sands of the parent's rapid changes. With these noncontingent shifts, the child's mind may be unable to develop smooth transitions and will continue to have abrupt and at times chaotic shifts in state, which are ordinarily seen primarily during the first year of life. States of mind begin to have significantly smoother transitions by the second year unless mitigating factors, such as frightening or conflictual parental responses, prevent this developmental milestone.[231] Furthermore, the child may begin to take on a disorganized state as a learned, engrained, repeated pattern of neuronal activations. The child learns to re-create the parent's incoherent behavior by attuning to the chaotic shifts in parental state.

Parental lack of resolution may explain the findings that, as Hesse and Main have hypothesized[232] and as several researchers have demonstrated,[233] these parents may behave with fear or fear–inducing actions that are conflictual and confusing.[234] For example, with the father whose AAI was described above, abrupt shifts into dramatically different states of mind would often occur when he initially felt rejected, either by his wife or by his daughter. He described the experience as if something would then happen that would activate a "crazy feeling"—as if "something was about to pop." He would sense a pressure in his head and a trembling in his arms. He would feel that he was going out of his mind, ready to explode, "receding from the world," and drawing away from people as if in a tunnel. At this moment he could no longer stop the process. He knew that his face looked enraged and tightly drawn, and that the muscles in his body were stiff. Sometimes he would hit his daughter. Sometimes he would squeeze her arm. Other times he would just yell at her, at the top of his lungs, filled with a rage he could not control.

The father tried to deny his repeated and sudden shifts into a frightening rageful state. He felt so ashamed of these outbursts that he did not engage in any repair process with his daughter during or after such terrifying interactions. These repeated discontinuities without repair in their communication produced a mental model in her of a confusing and unreliable relationship with her father. Her implicit memories of these frightening experiences might emerge as she grew older and be revealed as sudden shifts in her own state of mind, behavioral responses toward others, bursts of rage, or images of her enraged father. She might have the general sense that whenever she needed something, others might become irritated and betray her.

Such parental behaviors as these reflect parents' unresolved traumatic experiences from their own childhoods. How does this occur?

Traumatic experiences often involve a threat to the physical or psychological integrity of the victim.[235] If the traumatizing individual is someone in a position of trust, such as a parent, relative, friend, or teacher, then the sense of betrayal can play an important role in the meaning of the experience(s). As a child, the father described above was repeatedly subjected to the alcoholic outbursts of a drunk and angry father. His withdrawn mother was unavailable to protect him, and he was vulnerable to his father's unpredictable whims. The son learned that these sudden shifts in his father could be anticipated from the amount of alcohol the father had consumed. He would keep a vigilant eye on how much his father drank each night. If it was too much, his father would pass out. If it were just a little, he would get berated. If it were "just the right amount," he would be at risk of being chased and beaten.

When this man grew up and had a daughter, and the daughter would insist on things being done her way (as children often do), he found it difficult to be flexible. Her irritation with him (also a typical childhood response) was felt by him as a rejection, and set off the patterns of abrupt shifts in his state of mind and the enraged reactions that established the disorganized pattern of attachment. In memory terms, his present perception of her irritation was represented in his mind as a perceptual representation, or engram. This engram became linked with other representations connected with the perception of an irritated face. We can conceptualize these as part of the virtual other from his own childhood. For the father, these linkages included the emotional representation of feeling rejected and the associated implicit memories from past experiences: behavioral impulses to flee, perceptual images of his enraged father or depressed mother, and bodily sensations of tension and perhaps pain. These linkages were made quickly and out of his awareness. He did not feel that he was recalling anything. As implicit memories, they were experienced in the here-and-now, as part of his present reality. These implicit processes created his subjective world and organized his internal experiences.

In those crucial moments in which his perception of his daughter's response initiated a cascade of implicit memory activations, he would become flooded with an emotional response that rapidly shifted his state of mind.[236] This sudden shift could be a sign of a discontinuous experience of the flow of consciousness—in other words, dissociation. At times, such a shift might appear as the entrance into a frozen, trance-like state of mind. At other times, this shift might reveal the sudden onset of explosive rage. The father described the sensation of feeling that he was going out of his mind, that he was about to explode. In this situation, he was overwhelmed with implicit memories and suddenly shifted into a childhood mental state filled with that old and all too familiar sense of rejection, fear, anger, and despair. His sense of impotence and disconnection was experienced as shame. His subsequent perception of his daughter's irritation as anger at him induced a feeling of humiliation within himself. Before he could pull himself out of this avalanche, he would become enraged. In this altered, dissociated state, he would behave in a way terrifying to his daughter, which he would never ordinarily choose to do. He was literally out of control.

Repeated entry into these states of mind as a child had allowed these states to become engrained in this father's neural networks. These were dreaded states, filled with shame and humiliation—painful, despairing, imprisoning, and terrifying. States of mind that are repeatedly activated can become traits of an individual.[237] The unresolved nature of this man's traumatic experiences placed him at risk of uncontrolled entry into these dreaded states. This disorganization in his internal experience was now directly shaping his interactions with his daughter, who in turn was beginning to experience the disorganization of her own internal world. Therapeutic work with this family would require an understanding of these rapid shifts in states and their connection to patterns of relationships from the past. If we can help those with unresolved trauma heal, then we can alter the cycle of intergenerational transmission of relationship disturbances—a cycle that produces and perpetuates devastating emotional suffering.

## RUPTURE AND REPAIR

Repeated and expectable patterns of interpersonal connection between a child and an attachment figure are necessary for proper development. There are always times of disconnection, which can be followed by repair and reconnection. In each of the forms of insecure attachment, there is a problem with connection and repair. In the avoidantly attached dyad, connections are consistently infrequent and unsoothing; there is no repair. In the ambivalently attached dyad, connections are unpredictable and at times overwhelming and emotionally intrusive. There is inconsistent respect for the cycling of needs for interaction versus solitude. Repair in these situations may be overstimulating, such as an intrusive parent's wanting to reestablish a connection and not letting the infant avert his gaze as a means of regulating his level of arousal/ distress. Parents who persist at trying to

> In each of the forms of insecure attachment, there is a problem with connection and repair.

make direct contact or alignment when attunement actually calls for them to back away from such efforts will overwhelm their children and teach them that there is no reliable comfort in connection with the parents.

In a dyad with disorganized/disoriented attachment, interactions can be a source of overwhelming terror and despair, going well beyond misattunement or missed opportunity for connection or repair. In this case, the child is left in an overaroused state of distress without any comfort from the caregiver, who is in fact the source of distress. Disorganized attachment develops from repeated experiences in which the caregiver appears frightened or frightening to the child. As Lyons-Ruth and Jacobvitz have observed,[238] repair in the communication rupture of such a dyad after these interactions does not occur. Often after such frightening encounters, the parent may be so disoriented or in denial that the child is not given the opportunity to experience repair. The child remains frozen, in a state of disconnection, and with the overwhelming feelings of terror that have created such a large and frightening distance between child and parent.

## REFLECTIONS: ATTACHMENT AND MENTAL HEALTH

It is amazing that such a complex process as interpersonal communication and parent–child relationships can actually be understood in a fairly simple manner: Attachment at its core is based on parental sensitivity and responsivity to the child's signals, which allow for collaborative parent–child communication. Contingent communication gives rise to secure attachment and is characterized by a collaborative give-and-take of signals between the members of the pair. Contingent communication relies on the alignment of internal experiences, or states of mind, between child and caregiver. This mutually sharing, mutually influencing set of interactions—this emotional attunement or mental state resonance—is the essence of healthy, secure attachment.

Suboptimal attachments arise with repeated patterns of noncontingent communication. A parent's communication and own internal states may be oblivious to the child's, as in avoidant attachment. In contrast, an ambivalently attached child experiences the parent's communication as inconsistently contingent; at times it is intrusive, and yet at other times there is an alignment of their internal states. If the parent is a source of disorientation or terror, the child will develop a disorganized/disoriented attachment. In such a dyad, not only is communication noncontingent, but the messages sent by the parent create an internal state of chaos and overwhelming fear of the parent within the child.

These characteristics of the relationship with a child are features that emerge in specific relation to each parent. Furthermore, a parent's "state of mind with respect to attachment" is the most powerful predictor of how the parent–child relationship will evolve. The narrative process of the AAI reveals characteristic ways in which parents' coherent or incoherent states of mind are associated with the secure or insecure attachment of their children, respectively. The AAI finding of an "earned" secure/autonomous status—either prospective or retrospective—is an important point for our understanding of coherent functioning. In some cases, therapeutic and personal relationships appear to be able to move individuals from an incoherent to a more integrated functioning of the mind. The fact that these adults are capable of sensitive, attuned caregiving of their children, even under stress, suggests that this "earned" status is more than just being able to "talk the talk"; they can also "walk the walk" of being emotionally connected with their own children, despite not having such experiences in their own childhoods. We may serve a vital role for this and future generations in enabling each other to achieve the more reflective, integrated functioning that facilitates secure attachments.

We can also propose that a transforming attuned relationship would involve the following fundamental elements: contingent, collaborative communication; psychobiological state attunement; mutually shared interactions that involve the amplification of positive affective states and the reduction of negative ones; reflection on mental states; and the ensuing development of mental models of security that enable emotional modulation and positive expectancies for future interactions.

In those adults whose early life probably included a predominance of emotional neglect and rejection, a dismissing stance toward attachment may be found. These adults often have relationships with their children marked by avoidant attachments. Communication appears to have little sensitivity to signals or emotional attunement. The inner world of such adults seems to function with independence as its banner—living free from the entanglements of interpersonal intimacy, and perhaps from the emotional signals from their own bodies. Their narratives reflect this isolation, characterized by the insistence that they do not recall their childhood experiences. Life is lived without a sense that the past or others contribute to the evolving nature of the self.

In those adults who probably experienced inconsistently available caregiving and intrusive emotional communication, there is a preoccupied stance toward attachment filled with anxiety, uncertainty, and ambivalence. The children of these adults experience these preoccupied states as often impairing their parents' ability to perceive their needs consistently. Mental models of others may create a sense of caution about impending loss or intrusion from others. The result for the inner experience of these adults is to be perpetually overwhelmed by doubts and fears about relying upon others. Their AAI narratives are marked by intrusions of these past states upon their ability to focus clearly on the present. These narrative intrusions are reflections of the shifting emotional states that impair their ability to have consistent contingent communication with their own children. In this way, what they may have learned from inconsistent and intrusive experiences is laid down directly within their pattern of relating to others and within their own narrative process.

Finally, we have discussed how parental lack of resolution of trauma or loss has been demonstrated by attachment research to be a major factor associated with the most disturbed child form of attachment, disorganized/disoriented. Examining the nature of memory processes makes it possible to begin to address this basic question: What does lack of resolution truly mean for the functioning of the human mind? Answering this question is of pressing concern, given the impairment that these adults and their offspring may come to experience. These parents appear to enter rapid shifts into states of mind that are terrifying to their children. In studies of PTSD, those individuals who utilize dissociative mechanisms (entering into altered states of mind) during and after a trauma appear to be those most likely to suffer later disability.[239] Understanding how unresolved trauma or loss relates to the disassociation of various processes from one another, including explicit from implicit memory, is essential to gain insight into what later may become terrifying parental behaviors.

The individuals at greatest risk of developing significant psychiatric disturbances are those with disorganized/disoriented attachments and unresolved trauma or grief. From our conceptualization of the developing mind and mental health, these attachments involve the most profound disturbances in how the self is able to organize the information and modulate the energy of emotional states. At a most basic level, these individuals appear to have the most seriously impaired capacity to integrate coherence within the mind. They are not able to create a sense of continuity of the self across the past, present, and future, or in the relationship of the self with others. This impairment reveals itself in the emotional instability, social dysfunction, poor response to stress, and cognitive disorganization and disorientation that characterize both children and adults in this attachment grouping. As we've discussed, children with disorganized attachment tend to become controlling in their behaviors with others and may be hostile and aggressive with their peers. Disorganized attachment in children and unresolved/disorganized attachment in adults has been proposed by a number of authors to predispose these individuals to violent behavior.[240] Finding ways as a society to identify these high-risk individuals and help them to heal their unresolved trauma and repair the devastating effects of such chaotic attachment histories may enable us to help them develop more coherent internal function and more socially adaptive and rewarding interpersonal relationships.

> The individuals at greatest risk of developing significant psychiatric disturbances are those with disorganized/disoriented attachments and unresolved trauma or grief.

It is clear that certain early experiences create a fundamental impairment in self-organization. At one extreme are dismissing or avoidant attachments, which reveal excessively restrictive and rigid processes. At the other are preoccupied or ambivalent attachments, which have chaotic intrusions of past elements onto the present. In unresolved or disorganized attachments, there is a primary difficulty in organizing the self, which leads both to inflexible rigidity and to chaotic internal flooding and disruptions in interpersonal relationships. The inability to integrate a sense of self and of the self with others across time may be due to disorganization in a more fundamental self-organizational process. Studies of early trauma and neglect reveal that neural structure and function within the brain can be severely affected and lead to long-lasting and extensive effects on the brain's capacity to adapt to stress.[241] As we explore the nature of relationships, emotion, and representational processes in the next chapters, we will lay the groundwork for a more in-depth discussion of how the mind regulates its own functioning and how making sense of one's history can cultivate a coherent mind and healthy relationships.

# CHAPTER 4

# Emotion

## DEFINING EMOTION

The study of emotion suggests that nonverbal behavior is a primary mode in which emotion is communicated.[1] Facial expression, eye gaze, tone of voice, bodily motion, and the timing and intensity of response are all fundamental to emotional messages. For example, in the process of "social referencing," a child looks to the facial expressions and other nonverbal aspects of a parent's signals to determine how to feel and to respond in an ambiguous situation.[2] Children also focus on facial expressions and other nonverbal cues from peers and strangers in order to shape their behavior.[3] Social referencing reveals the fundamental way in which nonverbal communication of emotion is the medium in which states of mind are aligned. But what exactly is "emotion"? We can know when others are upset and "emotional," but what does this really mean? This chapter attempts to define emotion and to explore its central role in human relationships and the developing mind.

A much-emphasized universal finding has been that certain types of affective expression seem to be both expressed and recognized in all cultures throughout the world; however, professionals often have quite different notions about what these affective expressions actually represent. There is a wide range of ideas about how to define emotional processes.[4] The definitions that follow incorporate both research and clinical concepts in an effort to outline some fundamental aspects of emotion. The specific purposes of providing these definitions are (1) to attempt to clarify the basic functions of emotions, and (2) to characterize which features of emotions are shared among different individuals and which may be quite distinct.

There is quite a bit of controversy among scientists from various disciplines about what emotions actually are.[5] For example, some physiological and cognitive psychologists view emotions as existing within an individual, whereas more interpersonally oriented social psychologists and cultural anthropologists view emotions as being created between people.[6] Even within the fields of affective and social neuroscience, there is a heated debate about the nature of emotion in the brain.[7] For example, it was generally accepted for many decades that emotions emanate from the part of the brain called the "limbic system." Various authors defined this system as the "primitive" or "old mammalian" brain, and described it as including such structures as the amygdala, orbitofrontal cortex, and anterior cingulate. Research paradigms attempted to delineate the boundaries and specific functions of this frequently cited system, but often failed to identify its functional limits.[8] The essential point here is that emotion is *not* limited to some specific circuit or region of the brain that was once thought to be the center of emotion. Instead, this same "limbic" region appears to have wide-ranging effects on most aspects of brain functioning and mental processes.[9] The "limbic" region is specialized to carry out the appraisal of meaning or value of stimuli. It is also a center for the mental module or information-processing system that carries out social cognition, including face recognition, affiliation, and "theory of mind" (the view that another person has a subjective experience of mind). Some authors use these findings to argue for the socially constructed nature of emotion.[10] These findings also support the idea that emotion is found throughout the entire brain.[11]

Within cognitive psychology, debate exists over the importance of the "discrete" or "basic" emotions: what they are and how important they are in helping us understand emotional experience. Some authors argue that there is little "basic" about these discrete emotions,[12] while others suggest that studying the manifestations of these universally expressed states is crucial to understanding the role of emotions in both cognitive processing and interpersonal relationships.[13] Within the fields of developmental psychology and psychopathology, emotion and emotion regulation are seen as woven from the same cloth.[14] In this manner, emotions both are regulated and perform regulatory functions. Jaak Panksepp views emotion as intricately woven with our basic motivational drives that have evolved over millions of years.[15] Stephen Porges has developed a "polyvagal theory" of emotion, which identifies a reactive state of fight–flight–freeze and a more receptive state that activates the "social engagement system" and makes the individual open to interacting with others.[16] We continually have "neuroception" for assessing the presence of danger, which engages the polyvagal system. One might surmise from these viewpoints that emotions are everywhere in the processes of the mind. For instance, Kenneth Dodge states that "all information processing is emotional, in that emotion is the energy that drives, organizes, amplifies, and attenuates cognitive activity and in turn is the experience and expression of this activity."[17] This view describes the ubiquitous nature of emotion and the way in which the common distinction between cognition and emotion is artificial and potentially harmful to our understanding of mental processes.

Despite these controversial points, most theories of emotion share some common themes. One is that emotion involves complex layers of processes that are in constant interaction with the environment. At a minimum, these interactions involve cognitive processes (such as appraisal or evaluation of meaning) and physical changes (such as endocrine, autonomic, and cardiovascular changes), which may reveal some repeated patterns over time. As Alan Sroufe has described, emotions involve "a subjective reaction to a salient event, characterized by physiological, experiential and overt behavioral change."[18] A similar view suggests that emotion can be seen as involving neurobiological, experiential, and expressive components.[19]

For our purposes, it will be helpful to approach a unifying definition of emotions with an open mind. Let us assume that the familiar end products of emotion—what we usually consider in everyday thinking as the common feelings of anger, fear, sadness, or joy—are actually *not* central to the initial experience of emotion. Let us also assume that emotions do not necessarily exist as we may usually think of them: as packets of sensation that can be experienced, identified, and expressed, as implied in the statement "Just get your feelings out." Instead, let's consider that *emotions represent dynamic processes created within the socially influenced, value-appraising processes of the brain.* Emotion reflects the essential way in which the mind emerges from the interface between neurophysiological processes and interpersonal relationships: It serves as a set of integrating processes linking various systems in a dynamic flow across domains and through time. Emotion readies us for action, for evoking motion of the internal or external sort. Within the brain itself, emotion links various systems together to form a state of mind. Emotion serves as a set of processes connecting one mind to another within interpersonal relationships. In earlier chapters, "integration" has been defined as the linkage of differentiated parts of a system; therefore, *"emotions" are proposed to be "changes in the state of integration."*

> "Emotions" are proposed to be "changes in the state of integration."

When integration is enhanced, our state of well-being is improved, and we move toward a more harmonious way of living. We say that we have "emotional health." When two people feel "emotionally close," both often feel honored for their differences at the same time that compassionate communication cultivates their connection. In contrast, if we've had an emotionally disturbing experience, the degree of integration has shifted downward, and instead of harmony we have moved toward either chaos or rigidity. This is an example of emotional distress or impaired emotional well-being.

"Emotion" and its derivative forms, then, refer to ways in which states of integration are shifted.

Emotion is a process that weaves together the classic notions of thinking and feeling. As Pessoa puts it:

> Complex cognitive–emotional behaviours have their basis in dynamic coalitions of networks of brain areas, none of which should be conceptualized as specifically affective or cognitive. Central to cognitive–emotional interactions are brain areas with a high degree of connectivity, called hubs, which are critical for regulating the flow and integration of information between regions.[20]

Emotion, we are proposing, involves shifts in integration within and between individuals.

As we examine what emotion might be in the individual, let us keep in mind what we have learned about attachment relationships and the alignment of states of mind. This requires that we continue the challenging task of thinking about the individual mind within the context of human relationships, rather than in isolation from social meaning. Emotion in all its myriad manifestations reveals the interplay of the internal and the interpersonal.

## Initial Orientation, Appraisal, and Arousal

In the brain, a signal of heightened activity can be called an "initial orienting response." This expression refers to how the brain and other systems of the body enter a state of increased alertness, with an internal message of "Something important is happening here and now." This initial orienting response activates a cognitive alerting mechanism of "Pay attention now!" that does not require conscious awareness and does not initially have a positive or negative tone.[21] Very rapidly (within microseconds), the brain processes the representations of the body and the external world generated with this initial orienting process. As this occurs, processes that can be called "elaborative appraisal" and "arousal" begin and direct the flow of energy through the system.

Elaborative appraisals assess whether a stimulus is "good" or "bad," and determine whether the organism should move toward or away from the stimulus. There is an evolutionary benefit to having core processes that rapidly assess the value of events in the world; this helps us understand why the appraisal and arousal processes are so central to the functioning of the brain.[22] As the circuits are activated in response to this "good–bad" evaluation, the mind has a further elaboration of the flow of energy through its various mental processes involved in approach or withdrawal.[23] *Emotional processing prepares the brain and the rest of the body for action.* Elaborative appraisal and arousal extend the initial orienting process of "Pay attention!" to "Act!" within a short period of time. The appraisal process evaluates the informational meaning of stimuli; the arousal process directs the flow of energy through the system. Together, they serve to modulate the state of mind by directing the flow of activation of certain circuits and the deactivation of others.

In the field of affective neuroscience, discussions actively focus on whether these appraisal processes are purely serial or whether they in fact occur somewhat simultaneously.[24] Whether they are serial or simultaneous,

> the foundations of orientating and attention are hypothesized to stem from activation of defensive and appetitive motivational systems that evolved to protect and sustain the life of the individual. Motivational activation initiates a cascade of perceptual and motor processes that facilitate the selection of appropriate behavior.[25]

This cascade of responses can be seen as further serial or simultaneous appraisals that illuminate how emotion is a pervasive process within the functioning of the human brain. In this way, initial orientation sets off a cascade of subsequent elaborative appraisal–arousal circuits, which serve to differentiate the unfolding states of mind within the individual.[26]

Appraisal involves a complex web of evaluative mechanisms, in which both external and internal factors play active roles. The specific nature of appraisal incorporates past experience of the stimulus, including emotional and representational elements of memory; present context of the internal emotional state and external social environment; elements of the stimulus, such as intensity and familiarity; and expectations for the future.

Alan Sroufe has described the central role of "discrepancy" in the generation of emotional engagement with the environmental surround.[27] Discrepancy occurs when the external features of a stimulus do not match internal expectations. In Sroufe's terms, the emotional arousal generated in response to such a discordance is called "tension." Emotion and its regulation are examined within a "tension modulation hypothesis": Such tension is not in need of reduction, but is managed within an individual's interaction with the environment, especially with significant others in the social world. Emotional forms of arousal are distinguished from other forms of arousal— such as those arising from exercise or drinking caffeinated beverages—in that they reflect a subjective sense of meaning, which is evaluated in response to engaging with experience (internal or external). The framework offered here is consonant with this view of emotional tension, and I use the general term "arousal" with this emotional engagement frame in mind.

## Primary Emotions

I use the term "primary" emotions to describe the shifts in brain state that result from the initial orientation and elaborative appraisal–arousal processes described above. This concept is distinct from that of "basic" or "discrete" emotions, sometimes also called "categorical," which refer to differentiated emotional states such as anger, fear, or sadness. The term "primary" emphasizes the initial, core, and ubiquitous quality of these essential emotional features. As in "primary" colors, the term also implies that various combinations of primary emotional elements may constitute a wide range of textures within the spectrum of emotional experience.

These primary emotional sensations are without words and can exist without consciousness. They reflect the nonverbal sensation of shifts in the flow of activation and deactivation—the flow of energy and evaluations of information—through the system's changing states. Primary emotions directly reflect the *changes* in states of mind—that is, changes in how a range of differentiated processes become linked. This reveals further how emotions are shifts in integration. These changes may be subtle or intense; they may be fleeting or persistent; they may continue as gentle sensations, like waves lapping on a shore, or they may evolve into larger, global changes, like a storm pounding on the beach. Primary emotions are dynamic processes of change. Again, they are not discrete packets of sensation, but rather are fluctuations in the integration of the energy and informational flow of the mind.

> Primary emotions directly reflect the changes in states of mind—that is, changes in how a range of differentiated processes become linked.

When an event has meaning for an individual, because it is discrepant from prior experiences or because other evaluative processes label it with significance, the brain is alerted: "This is important! Pay attention!" At this initial point, the orientation serves as a kind of jolt to the system. The primary emotional experience is one of increased energy and alertness. Second, the brain must further appraise the meaning of the stimulus and of the aroused state itself. At this moment, primary emotions are being experienced as developing "hedonic tone" or "valence," meaning their internal quality of being positive or negative. For example, the elaborative appraisal and arousal processes may create a sensation such as "This important thing is bad. Watch out! There is danger here." The flow of energy through the system then becomes channeled toward a cautious, hypervigilant stance. In contrast, elaborative appraisal and arousal may assess the initial orientation as good, and thus the stimulus as something to seek more of; this creates a primary emotional state of eager anticipation. In this way, appraisal and arousal create a state of mind that is predisposing the individual to act in a certain fashion. At the most basic level, valence can be labeled as good and involve approach, or can be labeled as bad and involve withdrawal.[28]

In addition to the stimulus, primary emotions themselves can be appraised by the value systems of the brain. In this manner, the mind begins to assess the value of its own evaluative and activation processes. The recursive nature of such a continuing "appraisal of appraisals" is actually quite common in the complex system of the mind (we shall return to this characteristic in Chapter 5). It plays a central role in creating the reinforcing loops that engrain repetitive thoughts and destructive emotional states, such as depression and anxiety. Reframing such states within the setting of a supportive interpersonal therapeutic relationship can alter these reentrant loops and liberate a person from their imprisoning nature and self-defeating narratives.[29] This also raises the issue of how both temperament and learning directly affect core emotional responsiveness.[30] Some individuals may react to their own intense arousal with a negative appraisal and a tendency to withdraw both behaviorally and cognitively from the further elaboration of their own emotional states, as in the case of shy individuals.[31] Others may have learned that certain intense emotional states are not tolerated by others.[32] Such lack of attunement to intense states may lead to the sense that they are "out-of-control" states, and thus "bad" and to be avoided. Such individuals learn to avoid emotional intensity. In contrast, Jerome Kagan has demonstrated that parents who support and encourage shy children to explore novel situations actually enhance the children's capacity to tolerate new experiences.[33] In either of these examples, the appraisal of states of arousal is influenced by interpersonal experience and leads to further elaboration of appraisal–arousal circuits, which directly influence the unfolding primary emotional states.

## Differentiation and Categorical Emotions

Following the first two steps of initial orientation and elaborative appraisal–arousal, a third phase can occur in the experiencing of emotions. This is the "differentiation" or channeling of activation pathways. The more highly specialized and elaborated activations represent the differentiation of primary emotional states. Sometimes we may feel "neutral," unable to identify any particular verbalizable feelings. At other times, our primary emotional states—the flow and change of energy through our emerging states of mind—become further differentiated into more well-defined states as specific circuits become recruited.

The differentiation of primary emotional states into specific classifications of emotions, such as fear, brings us to the more familiar yet debated theory of "categorical emotions."[34] "Categorical," "basic," and "discrete" are terms commonly used for those classifications of sensations that have been found universally throughout human cultures, such as sadness, anger, fear, surprise, or joy.[35] Yet the existence of such clear emotions is still a point of controversy. As Barrett notes:

> People believe that they know an emotion when they see it, and as a consequence assume that emotions are discrete events that can be recognized with some degree of accuracy, but scientists have yet to produce a set of clear and consistent criteria for indicating when an emotion is present and when it is not.[36]

These internal emotional states are often communicated through facial expressions, and each culture seems to have words to describe their unique manifestations.[37] They also appear to have unique physiological profiles in which they manifest themselves. *Categorical emotions can be thought of as differentiated states of mind that have evolved into specific, engrained patterns of activation.* The cross-cultural similarities in the manifestation of categorical emotion suggests that the human brain and body have characteristic, inborn, physiologically mediated pathways for the elaboration of these states of mind.

The brain has a physical reality to its construction through which internal states are expressed via our genetically and experientially created bodies. Throughout the world, human beings share common pathways to the expression of categorical emotions. In every culture, we can identify these characteristic expressions of "basic" emotions[38]—for example, as sadness, anger, or fear. In sadness, the face will show turned-down lips and squinted eyes, together with slower bodily motions. Anger will involve dilated pupils, widened orbital area, raised eyebrows, furrowed brow, and pursed lips. Fear combines raised eyebrows, flattened brow, and open mouth. Though we can categorize emotions within an individual and across cultures,[39] this does not mean that one person's categorical emotion, such as sadness or fear, is identical to that of another individual.

## Affect and Mood

The way an internal emotional state is externally revealed is called "affective expression" or simply "affect." Affect appears within nonverbal signals, including tone of voice, facial expression, and bodily motion. These external expressions can be defined as "vitality affects" or as "categorical affects,"[40] revealing the primary or the differentiated nature of the emotional states, respectively. For many researchers, affect is essentially a social signal.[41] The

purpose of the expression of emotion is considered to be social communication, as supported by the general finding that individuals reveal more affective displays in social settings than they do when alone.

It is interesting how often people consider the categorical emotions the
only emotional processes they can try to know, or attempt to communicate to others. Examining the three phases of emotional response—states
of initial orientation, elaborative appraisal and arousal, and then categorical
emotions—yields a new way of thinking about how to respond to the question "How are you feeling?" The term "feeling" can be used to describe the
conscious awareness of either an emotion or an affect.

We can feel (categorically) "sad" or "mad" or "happy." We may come
to be aware of this by how we sense our minds or our bodies, or by what
we detect on our faces. We may, as children so often do, be aware of just
feeling "bad" or "good," or just "normal" (neutral), reflecting our initial
appraisals without further differentiation into categorical emotions. Often
we may also be aware of only feeling less differentiated primary emotional
states, such as surges of energy, a sense of deflation, images of one sort or
another, diffuse fogginess, or nervous agitation. These flows in our states of
mind—the changes in activations and integration within our brains—are
defined here as our primary emotions, and can be seen externally as what
have been termed vitality affects. Primary emotions are a frequent part of
our basic "feelings."

Parents attune to the subtle changes in a baby's state of arousal, revealed
as the vitality affect, not merely the categorical affect that the infant may be
expressing.[42] In fact, this expression of internal state through vitality affects
is the primary mode of communication between an infant and a caregiver
during the early years of life. These affective expressions reveal the profile or
energy level of the state of mind at a particular moment. The profile contains
within it a picture of how the individual's internal state is being expressed in
a changing state of activation of the face, motion in the body, and tone and
intensity of the voice.

Individuals may attune to vitality affects across sensory modalities. For
example, a facial expression of joy can be mirrored in the response of another
person's tone of voice, with the rising and falling of intensity of the sounds
reflecting those of the muscles of the face. It may be that primary emotional
experience reveals both how we know ourselves and how we connect to one
another. In parent–child relationships in which the parent is depressed, vitality affects may reveal a "depressed" state, with low energy and a global negative hedonic tone. Research also suggests that depression is associated with
abnormalities in the ability to perceive the emotional expressions of others.[43]
The impaired ability to perceive facial expressions has been correlated with

alterations in brain activity in those parts responsible for such perceptual capacities.[44] Studies of dyads with a depressed parent reveal significant effects on the emotional development of the child.[45] *The experience of expressing one's emotional state and having others perceive and respond to those signals appears to be of vital importance in the development of the brain.* This may be why contingent communication in which the internal state of the child is perceived, made sense of, and responded to by the caregiver is found universally across cultures.[46] Such sharing of primary emotions does not merely allow the child to feel "good"; it allows the child to "feel felt" and to develop typically. Some studies suggest that parents' attunement to the internal world of the infant facilitates the child in accomplishing a task and regulates his emotional state in response to stress.[47]

Primary emotions are expressed in a unique manner in the moment, just as an individual's state of mind at a particular time is a one-of-a-kind state. The flow of states moves forward in time and never repeats itself. This flow of states is unique. In contrast, the external expressions of categorical emotions may reflect the very specific routes through which the physical body is able to reveal them. Different categorical emotions, such as sadness, anger, or fear, recruit different characteristic circuits.[48] The view proposed here is that the process from primary to categorical emotion is influenced directly by the unique components of neural processes that form a state of mind. In other words, the mental state active at a given time may shape the elaboration of arousal and meaning from primary to categorical emotions. More often, however, our primary emotions may ebb and flow without necessarily becoming intense, entering consciousness, or becoming further differentiated into categorical emotional states.

The term "mood" refers to the general tone of emotions across time. Mood can be thought of as a bias of the system toward certain categorical emotions. Mood shapes the interpretation of perceptual processing and gives a "slant" to thinking, self-reflection, and recollections. For example, a person who is in a "down" mood may find himself interpreting things as evidence of his failures, think of the future in dismal terms, reflect upon himself as a "loser," and have increased recollections of the numerous times he has made mistakes in his life. The influence of mood upon all of these cognitive functions reveals how general emotional tone reinforces itself in a feedback loop. This may explain the tenacious nature of emotional disturbances such as depression or chronic anxiety, in which a given mood becomes a relatively fixed and disabling state. In certain individuals, the ability to maintain a flexible flow of primary emotional states may be quite impaired and reflect difficulty in their ability to modulate their emotional states.

## THE CONVERGENCE OF SOCIAL PROCESSING AND EMOTION

By clarifying the distinction between primary emotions and the more familiar idea of categorical emotions, we can become more sensitive to the early stages of meaning-making interactions with others. As we'll see in the pages to follow, emotion in general is a complex series of processes and is of central importance in the mind. It involves the essential dual nature of mind: the flow of energy and the processing of information. A brief review of the anatomy involved will help us to visualize how social processing of information and emotion processes converge.[49]

The appraisal centers of the brain are located within the distributed limbic areas, as shown in Figure 4.1. These centers involve such areas as the amygdala, anterior cingulate, and orbitofrontal cortex. External stimuli enter the brain via the sensory systems, such as vision, hearing, and touch. The representations generated from these perceptual processes are then filtered through the thalamus and passed on to the amygdala, where they are appraised and given initial value: "Pay attention: Is this good or bad?" The amygdala can directly affect these basic evaluative and perceptual processes. It also sends these representations on for further evaluation by the anterior cingulate and orbitofrontal cortex.[50] Like the amygdala, these centers are processing information about the social environment: the facial expression, direction of eye gaze, and other aspects of others' nonverbal behavior that reveal their state of mind.[51] *Information about the social context directly affects the appraisal process.*[52]

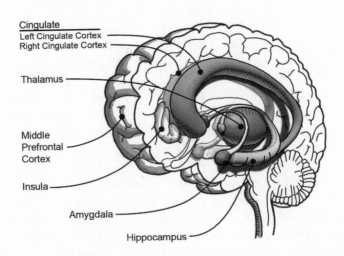

**FIGURE 4.1.** Appraisal centers of the brain in the distributed limbic areas. Copyright 2012 by Mind Your Brain, Inc.

A set of interconnected neural regions I have called the "resonance circuits" enables us to tune in to others and align our internal states with others. This circuit involves the orbitofrontal cortex

> Information about the social context directly affects the appraisal process.

and anterior cingulate, as well as other midline structures that interact with one another, such as the ventrolateral (midline horizontally) and medial prefrontal (midline vertically) cortical areas.[53] Other portions of this resonance circuit involve "mirror neurons," which enable us to perceive the intentional state of another person, and then imitate the other's behavior and simulate the other's internal state. Mirror neuron properties are found in the anterior cingulate, as well as a portion of the ventrolateral region called the anterior insula. The insula has also been shown to be involved in the appraisal of internal visceral states, and plays an important role in our awareness of our own bodily selves via a process called "interoception."[54] The resonance circuits enable us to tune in to others, and even to our own internal states for self-awareness. These areas also register the state of the body and directly affect its states of activation.[55] Information from these areas is passed on to the hippocampus for "cognitive mapping" and, in some cases, transfer into explicit memory. The orbitofrontal cortex and other middle prefrontal regions also play a major role in coordinating these appraisal and arousal processes with the more complex representations of "higher thinking" and social cognition.[56]

This brief review of the neurophysiological coordination of input and brain–body response highlights the general statements made throughout this book about the mind: Neural processes and social relationships both contribute to the creation of mental life. The mind is both embodied and relational. The middle prefrontal circuits function to integrate the processing of social information, autobiographical consciousness, the evaluation of meaning, the activation of arousal, and the coordination of bodily response and higher cognitive processing. These processes emerge as a convergence of information processing and energy flow that directly influences a wide array of both basic and more complex processes of the brain.

## NONCONSCIOUS AND CONSCIOUS EMOTION

Emotions are primarily nonconscious processes. In their essence, they create a state of readiness for action, for "motion," disposing us to behave in particular ways within the environment. Emotional reactions create this disposition by determining the brain's activation of a wide array of circuits, leading to changes in the state of arousal within the brain and other areas of the body. The amygdala is a cluster of neurons that serves as a receiving and sending station between input from the outer world and emotional response. As a coordinating center within the brain, the amygdala, along with related areas such as the orbitofrontal cortex and anterior cingulate, plays a crucial role in coordinating perceptions with memory and behavior. These regions are especially sensitive to social interactions. They nonconsciously assign significance to stimuli; their actions influence a wide array of mental processes without the involvement of conscious awareness. These circuits are extensively connected to other regions that directly influence the functioning of the entire brain as a whole system.

In fact, the middle prefrontal region also registers the state of the bodyand directly influences the body's state of activation via regulation of the autonomic nervous system.[57] In this manner, the middle prefrontal cortex serves as a source of social processing, stimulus appraisal, and body/brainstem/limbic ("emotional") arousal; these may originate within particular limbic and brainstem regions, but there are no clear boundaries to their effects that move throughout the cortex and body as a whole.[58] Once again, emotion is not merely a function restricted to the areas defined as central to the limbic region. Rather, emotion directly influences the functions of the entire brain and body, from physiological regulation to abstract reasoning.[59]

The amygdala has been studied more than any other appraisal center and has been found to play a crucial part in the fight-or-flight response. A range of studies have examined its role especially with regard to fear states.[60] Let's look at the amygdala as an example of the elaborative feedback mechanism of the appraisal process that occurs without the requirement of consciousness. Studies of the amygdala have examined how the initiation of an appraisal leads to subsequent perceptual biases that reinforce the nature of the initial appraisal. The flow of activation of the brain's circuits begins a process of further assembly of various activations, which then ready the individual organism for a particular response. The amygdala receives and sends signals directly from and to the visual system, reacting to visual stimuli without the involvement of consciousness. The amygdala responds to the initial visual representation—say, of a dog—by sending signals back to the same and even earlier layers of the visual processing system, and then by producing initial orientation of the attentional and perceptual apparatus of the brain: "Watch carefully; this is important!" If the amygdala also registers the visual input as dangerous, it can establish elaborative appraisal–arousal processes that create a state of fear in the brain, which then feeds back to the visual system. The amygdala can rapidly bias the perceptual apparatus toward interpreting the stimuli as dangerous. All of this occurs within seconds and does not depend on conscious awareness.

At least with regard to the fear response, the brain is wired to non-consciously create a "self-fulfilling prophecy." If the amygdala is excessively sensitive and fires off a "Danger!" signal, it will automatically alter ongoing perceptions so that they appear threatening. This may be a basis for phobias and other anxiety disorders.[61] For example, if a child encounters a dog that growls and lunges at her, she is likely to have a response of fear. The amygdala directly activates arousal centers (located in the brainstem and forebrain) that create a general state of increased excitability through the release of substances such as noradrenaline in the brain and adrenaline in the body. The whole child becomes hyperalert and ready to deal with the "danger." This process is likely to be mediated by what Stephen Porges has termed "neuroception," which then activates the polyvagal system to engage the fight–flight–freeze set of reactions.[62] If particular mental representations are active at the time of this arousal, then they will become associated in memory with a feeling of danger. This association occurs via Hebb's axiom and Freud's Law of Association: Neurons that fire together wire together (see Chapter 2). Now a learned feedback loop has been established in which a dog can be a source of amygdala activation and brainstem response. The brain learns to anticipate a bodily response of hypervigilance to the animal, and a constellation of fear and avoidance behaviors to dogs can then unfold. Such early experiences of fear may become indelible subcortical emotional memories as well as altering the epigenetic control of gene expression, which may predispose the individual to future difficulties.[63]

How does this rapid, automatic process become conscious? Consciousness is a controversial subject that has long intrigued philosophers and more recently neuroscientists.[64] Though there is no universally accepted explanation for the experience of consciousness, either in the sense of awareness or in the qualities of subjective experiencing, there are some substantiated views that are quite helpful. One such view sees conscious awareness as involving a system in the brain responsible for working memory, the "chalkboard of the mind." In this perspective, perceptual representations from external and internal stimuli are functionally connected within an area of the brain called the dorsolateral prefrontal cortex. It is in this region that attention is modulated, so that an "attentional spotlight" can be focused on particular representational profiles in the brain.[65] Working memory is able to handle only a limited amount of information units, usually in a serial fashion. Neural activation profiles can be linked to the activity of the dorsolateral prefrontal cortex and give the internal sensation of being within an attentional focus of consciousness. The dorsolateral prefrontal cortex is located on the outer side of the front part of the brain, just to the side of the middle prefrontal cortex; it is thought to act by linking items together within conscious awareness, where they can be focally attended to and manipulated.[66]

What exactly it means for neural activation profiles to become "linked" is a central concern for scientists of the brain and mind. How do simultaneously activated processes bind together to form a continuity of experience? One approach to this question comes from studies of the waves of electrical activity sweeping across the brain on a regular basis. A forty-cycle-per-second ("forty-hertz" or "40-Hz") pattern has been noted,[67] in which the brain becomes active from back to front.[68] This activity occurs in both halves of the brain and has been identified as a "thalamocortical" sweep, going from the deeper areas such as the thalamus up toward the higher cortical regions. One view is that representational processes (the neural net profiles activated at a particular moment in time) that are "on" at the time of the sweep are bound together as one seemingly continuous flow of conscious experience. This view allows us to see how the phenomenon of consciousness, as discussed in Chapter 1, creates a sense of continuity out of what is really a set of quite discontinuous representational processes, such as sights, sounds, thoughts, bodily states, and self-reflections.[69] This "40-Hz" view also gives us insight into how the lateral prefrontal cortex may become "linked" to a particular set of representations—those that are active during the sweep. The attentional focus of working memory can select from those representations the limited number it may be able to handle at any one time. Because of the nature of the sweeping, each hemisphere can function to influence conscious awareness quite independently of the other. There are probably left-hemisphere and right-hemisphere forms of consciousness that are quite distinct from each other, based on the unique nature of the representational processes of each hemisphere. This probability is explored briefly below and in depth in the next chapter.

A related view from Edelman and Tononi is that when distributed neural assemblies become active in a rapid and strong manner, so that they can achieve a certain degree of functional clustering, a temporarily stable state of complexity is achieved.[70] Consciousness is then an emergent property of functional clustering of a "dynamic core" that has distributions throughout the brain. When these assemblies achieve a certain level of integration, they can become "linked" to the thalamocortical system and their mental processes become a part of consciousness. As we'll also see, shared awareness between two (or more) people may further stabilize elements in consciousness with increased complexity. This view is compatible with the notion of some core thalamocortical 40-Hz sweeping process and the linkage with the activity of the dorsolateral prefrontal regions. As we shall discuss in more detail in later chapters, these models of consciousness will be useful in helping to understand several aspects of mental life.

One view of how emotions become conscious is when their effects are connected to the activity of the attentional mechanisms of the dorsolateral prefrontal cortex.[71] For example, when we say that we have a "gut feeling" about something, we may be referring, literally, to a somatic representation in our brains of our "gut response"—the body's response—to a stimulus correlated with neural firing in the middle prefrontal cortex.[72] When we have interoception, or awareness of our internal bodily states, the insula and anterior cingulate portions of this middle prefrontal area become active. Interestingly, von Economo neurons (or neural "spindle cells") are uniquely present in this area and connect the anterior cingulate and insula to each other. This integration within the middle prefrontal areas seems to be related to self-awareness in humans and nonhuman primates, as well as in dolphins and elephants.[73] Though the test used to assess such self-awareness is the noting of a mark on the animal's or person's body in a mirror, the larger notion of awareness of a bodily self may depend on the input of bodily states into this middle prefrontal region of the brain. The take-home lesson here is that in humans, awareness of bodily states may be the gateway to becoming conscious of our emotions.[74]

The feedback loop of bodily response leading to emotional reaction has been a perspective long held by researchers with much scientific validation.[75] What is crucial to note, however, is that our brains frequently receive this bodily information without the involvement of conscious awareness. The binding of consciousness may be an "epiphenomenon" in many situations— something that is not essential for other neural reactions subsequently to occur. We may frequently have nonconscious "gut reactions" that profoundly influence our decision-making processes without our awareness of their impact.

We can become aware of a sense that something feels "meaningful." In this case, we have caught a conscious glimpse of emotion as a value system appraising the significance of stimuli. Some aspect of the emotional processing has become bound in consciousness. Another example

> We may frequently have nonconscious "gut reactions" that profoundly influence our decision-making processes without our awareness of their impact.

of emotion's becoming a part of our conscious experience is when we feel ourselves becoming lost in a "sea of emotion." Our minds are capable of being bombarded by a flood of stimuli from emotional processes, which fill us with an overwhelming feeling. These sensations may reflect primary emotions (such as internal shifts in states of arousal) or categorical emotions (such as anger, fear, sadness, excitement, or joy). Emotions are what create meaning in our lives, whether we are aware of them or not.

Some people have very little awareness of their emotional reactions to things. One man was easily conscious of his thoughts about interacting with others, but he had a difficult time letting his wife know verbally "how he felt" beyond simple statements of "good," or "bad," or "I don't know." We could say that for some reason, the representations of his emotional state—things like his bodily response or shifts in his mental state—did not get linked to his dorsolateral prefrontal attentional processes. We cannot say whether they in fact were present or not in his mind. In a sense, this person was emotionally blind. Unfortunately, he was blind to his wife's emotional states as well as his own.

It's important to recognize that emotional processes are primarily non-conscious. Some people, and certainly this man's wife, might say that he "has no feelings." As we've seen in Chapter 3, avoidant attachment fosters an emotional disconnection of the child from the parent. There is some suggestion that this disconnection may also be prominent in this man's lack of conscious access to his own nonverbal experience of primary emotions. The lack of connection between consciousness and the arousal–appraisal system does not mean that there is a lack of emotion, however. Instead, we can state that there is a lack of binding of emotion to consciousness. Consciousness is necessary for an intentional alteration in behavior patterns beyond "reflexive" responses. This may be why every form of psychotherapy that I have reviewed involves conscious awareness as a central aspect of its approach to helping people. Without the involvement of consciousness and the capacity to perceive others' and one's own emotions, there may be an inability to plan actively for the future, to alter engrained patterns of behavior, or to engage in emotionally meaningful connections with others.

## EMOTION AS A VALUE SYSTEM
## FOR THE APPRAISAL OF MEANING

The brain as a complex system of neuronal circuits requires some way of determining which firings are useful, neutral, or harmful. Without such an appraisal mechanism, all stimuli would be evaluated as equally important. The organism would not be able to organize its behavior, to accomplish tasks that allowed it to survive, or to pass on its traits.[76] The brain must have a way of establishing value in order to organize its functions. Value disposes us to behave in particular ways. At the first phase of emotional response, initial orientation lets the organism "know" that it should pay attention to something important. The second phase, elaborative appraisal and arousal, gives the stimulus the value of good or bad. Good things should be sought; bad things should be avoided. *Value systems in the brain function by shaping states of arousal.* Evaluative circuits serve as a neuromodulatory system with extensive innervation throughout the brain and body proper that can lead to hyperexcitability and increased neuronal plasticity. Chemically, this makes the neurons hypersensitive and more readily activated. By initiating attentional mechanisms, arousal enhances the focus of attention on a particular stimulus. In this way, attention is often considered the process that directs the flow of information processing. For perceptual processing, this means, for example, that a person will pay more attention to an object. For memory, arousal leads to enhanced encoding via increased neuronal plasticity and the creation of new synaptic connections and therefore increased likelihood of future retrieval.[77]

As the activations within the brain change, energy flows through the system. Changes in the state of the system are changes in this flow of energy. Many factors in addition to appraisal determine how the system's state changes over time. These determining factors include present input from the external world or from other components of the body, as well as constraints established from prior experience (such as Hebbian connections) and present appraisals. Moreover, there are many forms of arousal, which involve different circuitry. Some of the appraisals that create approach–avoidance distinctions may in fact be hard-wired into the brain. The limbic regions use the input of others' emotions to directly regulate a person's internal state and external responses. Mirror neurons may play an important role in such processes, as we shall discuss shortly.

Some aspects of a value system are inborn, and some are acquired through experience. Some constitutional aspects of a value system include the motivational systems of attachment and novelty seeking. Within the brain are clusters of cells that are designed to fire in response to eye contact and facial expressions.[78] These clusters of socially responsive neurons are located within the resonance circuits of the brain and other areas, such as the amygdala and the perceptual cortex. For example, *the motivational drive to seek proximity to a caregiver and attain face-to-face communication with eye gaze contact is hard-wired into the typical brain from birth.* It is not learned. Similarly, infants are "natural explorers," seeking out new stimuli within their increasingly sophisticated ability to search the environment. Discussions of the genetic determinants of emotional behavior offer helpful insights into the way in which our value systems organize our behavior to increase the chance of survival. Evolutionary theory suggests that those organisms with genetically encoded specificity to their appraisal, such as fearing a snake or becoming aroused by a suitable mate, will have a significantly increased likelihood of passing on their genetic information to future generations.[79] Genes clearly play a large role in the value system of the brain.

The inborn aspects of the value system are in place from the beginning of life, but the system is also shaped by learning from experience. Action, learning, and development can be viewed as interrelated sets of phenomena throughout life.[80] For example, a typically developing child will naturally make eye contact with a parent and appraise this as a "good" interaction. However, if such eye contact results in the child's being overwhelmed and feeling intruded upon by the parent, then such interactions may become associated with a negative value. The child learns that eye contact should be avoided. The brain can learn to modify its response to the evaluative system's initial criteria of what is good or bad, based on past interactions with others. If past eye contact led to a flood of disorganizing activations, the avoidance of such experiences in the future will help keep the self organized. It is possible that the innate neural response of children with autism to eye contact may be so intense that they adapt by avoiding such contact in the future.

*The appraisal of stimuli and the creation of meaning are central functions that occur with the arousal process of emotion.* Incoming stimuli are appraised for their value, and the representations of these stimuli are then linked with a sense of "goodness" or "badness." As the child develops, the increasingly complex representational system becomes capable of more subtle evaluative sensations. These variations on the "good or bad" theme are what lead to the wide variety of emotions we are capable of feeling and the patterns of behavior we enact. We are unique individuals precisely because our value systems and our interactional histories are one-of-a-kind combinations. As the intertwined nature of value system responses and environmental encounters unfolds, each of us continually emerges and defines ourselves.

## HOW "ME" BECOMES "WE": MIRROR NEURONS AND THE SHARING OF INTERNAL STATES

In the mid-1990s, a group of Italian neuroscientists studying the motor cortex in nonhuman primates discovered a property of neuronal firing that revealed a linkage between motor and perceptual processes.[81] A serendipitous finding occurred when a monkey watched a researcher eat a peanut. The neuron that had been activated when the monkey ate a peanut became active when the monkey watched someone else eating a peanut. There was a "mirroring" or "reflection" between the monkey's motor region and perceptual area for the same action. The scientists called these "mirror neurons." This exciting finding revealed the integration of perception and action in a new way. Since that original discovery, numerous research groups have pursued the nature of this neural property and have found its function important for understanding the development of the human mind and the social nature of the human brain.[82] Here I briefly highlight some of these discoveries and show how they relate to our central theme: the interconnectedness of mind, brain, and relationships.

First of all, to be a mirror neuron, a cell must have both motor and perceptual activation. Many neurons may respond to linkages between motor and perceptual processes, but are themselves not considered to have mirror properties. Second, the actions that a mirror neuron responds to are very specific. These are acts with *intention* or purpose behind them—actions with predictable sequences. If I randomly move my hands in front of you, your mirror neurons will not respond. If I have a cup in my hand and begin to drink, your mirror neurons will respond, because you "know" what a cup means: You have seen people drink or have had a drink with a cup yourself in the past. The mirror neuron system learns from experience.

Marco Iacoboni and colleagues have pursued studies of mirror properties in human brain functioning, and have proposed that the mirror neurons in the frontal and parietal regions of the cortex work closely with the superior temporal neurons to create a neural representation of the intentional state of the person being perceived.[83] In this way, firing among mirror neurons and related areas creates a neural image of the *mental state* of another person. Here we see an important third principle: The perception of another's predictable motions is used to create an image of that person's mind. This is a possible way in which mind is imaged by brain at a very basic level. Recently these mirror properties were found in direct studies of single-neuron activity in the living human brain.[84]

> The mirror neuron system learns from experience.

A fourth fundamental concept is that this image of the other's intentional state is then used to initiate behavioral imitation and internal simulation. Imitation enables you to take a drink of water after watching my motion of drinking from a cup. This is the basis of learning behavioral sequences and acquiring language. It is why this learning is so dependent on human interactions, not merely stimulation from the environment.[85]

Mirror properties also enable internal simulation. Though the details of this process are still being formulated, one proposal is that the cortical mirror neurons and related areas influence the state of activation of the lower, subcortical regions (limbic, brainstem, body proper) by way of the insula. With the change in internal subcortical state, these shifts are then sent back upward, also through the insula, and registered in the middle prefrontal regions—especially the anterior insula and cingulate. This is how we come to know what we are feeling, to have interoception. When you see me drink from a cup, you may feel both thirsty and even have a sensation of liquid flowing in your throat.

Finally, a fifth notion is that the mirror properties in our brains enable us to imagine empathically what is going on inside another person. Internal simulation—the process of absorbing and resonating with others' internal states—is thought to be the first stage of compassion, or "feeling with" other persons. This gateway of empathy is clearly dependent on both prior learning and present input. If you are from New York City and I raise my hand in front of you, you may imagine that I am hailing a cab. If you are currently a student, you may imagine that I am intending to ask a question. If you have been abused, you may feel that I am going to hit you. Prior learning shapes the empathic interpretation and the internal simulation.

Overall, the discovery of mirror properties in the brain gives us a window into the profoundly social nature of our nervous systems. Mirror neurons, like any new findings, have generated heated debate, controversy, overenthusiasm, and misunderstanding. Studies of the human brain during surgery have revealed that "multiple systems in humans may be endowed with neural mechanisms of mirroring for both the integration and differentiation of both the perceptual and motor aspects of actions performed by self and others."[86] The initial findings reveal that a human's brain is able to detect the internal states of others by way of their actions, and then to alter both behavior and the human's own internal state in response. Though the details will naturally be revealed with future careful research, these findings help illuminate some of the basic processes that connect mind, brain, and relationships. How we come to understand others is directly related to our awareness of our own internal states. How we come to know "who" we are is shaped by the communication we've had with others. If that communication has been filled with confusion and unpredictable actions—or filled with hostile intention—then our internal sense of a coherent self will be compromised. In contrast, being around caregivers early in life who are attuned to our own internal worlds in a reliable way will provide us with the "mirror experiences" that enable us to have a coherent and flexible sense of our selves in the world.

## RESPONSE FLEXIBILITY, RELATIONSHIPS, AND EMOTION

Central to the process of creating meaning and emotion is the prefrontal cortex.[87] As noted in Chapter 1, this prefrontal area of the brain can be said to include ventral areas, such as the insula, and medial structures, such as the orbitofrontal cortex, the ventromedial prefrontal cortex, and also the anterior cingulate cortex.[88] Overall, the prefrontal areas sit at the interface between the "lower" regions involved in taking input from the body and the senses, and the "higher" parts involved in integrating information and creating complex thoughts and plans. This integrating prefrontal region is involved in stimulus appraisal (the meaning, value, or emotional valence given to a stimulus),[89] affect regulation (the capacity of the brain to modulate its psychophysiological state),[90] social cognition (the complex process by which an individual develops "mindsight" or the ability to perceive the mental state of another),[91] and autonoetic consciousness (the ability to perform mental time travel).[92] Other processes involving the appraisal–arousal structures, such as the orbitofrontal cortex, the anterior cingulate, and the amygdala, include emotional memory (especially fear),[93] empathy (feeling what another feels and understanding the point of view of another),[94] and categorical emotions.[95] The middle of this region—especially the right orbitofrontal area—is postulated to have atypical structure in autism, the major disorder of social cognition.[96] Generally, the more ventral a region is (orbitofrontal, ventrolateral, ventromedial, and the ventral aspect of the anterior cingulate), the more closely interactive it is with lower limbic and bodily processes.[97] More dorsal regions (dorsolateral and dorsomedial prefrontal areas, and the dorsal aspect of the anterior cingulate) play a role in more analytic/cognitive processes related to thought.

The middle prefrontal cortex has also been demonstrated as central in mediating a process we can call "response flexibility." As Nobre and colleagues have demonstrated in visual stimulus experiments, parts of this region appear to mediate the "switching or reversing of stimulus–response associations" and are at the "interface between automatic default-mode operations of the CNS [central nervous system] and neural processes that allow for flexible adaptations to shifting contexts and perspectives."[98] In other words, when there are changing or unexpected conditions, the middle prefrontal region is active in creating new, flexible behavioral and cognitive responses instead of automatic reflexive ones.[99]

In this manner, the capacity for response flexibility may become functionally linked with other prefrontally mediated domains that we have discussed, such as autonoetic consciousness, social cognition, emotionally attuned communication, and working memory. As Mesulam has stated, "The prefrontal cortex plays a critical role in these attentional and emotional modulations and allows neural responses to reflect the significance rather than the surface properties of sensory events."[100] The prefrontal mediation of response flexibility may thus entail a coordinated process incorporating sensory, perceptual, and appraisal mechanisms and enabling new and personally meaningful responses to be enacted. We can propose that such an integrating function may allow an individual, for example, to approach life decisions, relationships, and perhaps narrative responses with self-reflection and with a sense of perspective on past, present, and future considerations. The outcome of such well-developed and integrated functioning can be proposed to play a central role in the individual's ongoing development, subjective experiences, and interpersonal relationships.

Response flexibility enables the mind to assess incoming stimuli or emotional states, and then to modify external behaviors as well as internal reactions. Such an ability can be proposed as an important component of collaborative, contingent communication. The capacity for response flexibility may also be revealed in the coherence of the discourse process of the AAI. As suggested by Main,[101] coherent narratives require the flexible focusing of attention on attachment-related issues. Conversely, the inability to exhibit response flexibility can be proposed to contribute to the incoherent narratives found in insecurely attached adults. Such an impairment may also be revealed in the collapse of a narrative strategy seen in the "cannot classify" adult category described by Hesse.[102] Thus response flexibility may be a contributing link between parent–child attachment and adult narratives. In situations where this function fails to develop, or where its integration with other processes (especially with those mediated by the prefrontal regions) is impaired, we can predict tenacious, global effects on the individual's internal and interpersonal experiences across time. As other mental processes are, response flexibility

> Response flexibility may be a contributing link between parent–child attachment and adult narratives.

is likely to be state-dependent: Internal and interpersonal contexts can promote or inhibit the integrative mechanisms on which they are created. In this manner, response flexibility can be seen as an integrative capacity that is achieved under certain conditions, rather than as a fixed developmental accomplishment. For these reasons, an individual may exhibit this adaptive flexibility in certain situations and not in others. As we'll discuss in the final three chapters, the ways in which emotional states flexibly integrate and organize widely distributed internal and interpersonal processes—the manner in which the flow of energy and information is adaptively modulated—can be seen as having a direct effect on self-regulation, relationships, and development across the lifespan. Future studies will be helpful in clarifying the nature of response flexibility, its mediation by the prefrontal region, its potentially experience-dependent development, and its possible relationship to incoherent narratives and patterns of parent–child communication.

How are response flexibility and other integrative processes influenced by the emotional communication inherent in many interpersonal relationships? Looking toward neurobiological structure and function may shed some light on this question. The middle aspects of the prefrontal cortex sit at a crucial neuroanatomic position at the uppermost part of the limbic region—the center of our basic appraisals, thought to be the origin of our widely distributed emotional experiences. As we can see, the social/emotional/meaning-making processes of the limbic region and related middle prefrontal areas help coordinate a wide range of mental functions. The result of the adaptive integration of these functions may be the proposed process of response flexibility.

The middle prefrontal cortex receives direct input from the sensory cortex, which is responsible for perception; the somatosensory cortex and brainstem, which register somatic sensation; the autonomic nervous system, which controls bodily functions; the dorsolateral prefrontal cortex, involved in attentional processes; the medial temporal lobe, involved in explicit memory; and the associational cortex, involved in abstract forms of thought. Allan Schore has described how the development of one part of the middle prefrontal region, the orbitofrontal cortex, depends on stimulation from the emotional connections of the attachment figure in the form of eye contact, face-to-face communication, and affective attunement.[103] These fundamental aspects of social signals specifically activate these regions of the brain. The orbitofrontal cortex is also crucial in coordinating bodily states and the widely distributed and linked representations that are fundamental to reasoning processes, motivation, and the creation of emotional meaning.[104]

Emotion is a fundamental part of attachment relationships in the early years and throughout the lifespan. The earliest forms of communication are about primary emotional states. This sharing of basic appraisal and arousal processes establishes the fundamental way in which one person becomes connected to another within emotional relationships. We can also propose that the reciprocal collaboration within such contingent communication facilitates the development of a parallel, prefrontally mediated process: response flexibility. This enables the individual to respond to changing contexts in an adaptive, "internally collaborative" manner. Such internal collaboration may be seen as a way in which widely distributed neural processes are recruited into a flexible state of mind—one that is adaptive to a range of internal as well as external factors. In this way, intimate, reciprocal human communication may directly activate the neural circuitry responsible for giving meaning, responding flexibly, and shaping the subjective experience of an emotionally vibrant life. The basic idea is this: Integrative communication leads to the growth of integrative fibers in the brain.

## EMOTION AND SOMATIC RESPONSE

The signals from the body also directly shape our emotions. Our awareness of bodily state changes—such as tension in our muscles, shifts in our facial expressions, or signals from our hearts or intestines—lets us know how we feel. This bodily feedback occurs even without awareness. Perceptions of the environment certainly occur in the brain, but the subsequent reactions of the body may follow very soon after and become the "data" informing us what those perceptions mean to us. In this way, our appraisal mechanisms depend upon bodily reactions to determine the direction of subsequent elaboration. States of mind are created within the psychobiological states of the brain and other parts of the body.[105]

For example, characteristically negative (frowns) or positive (smiles) facial expressions produce corresponding biases in interpreting data.[106] An experiment that illuminated this involved participants' being told to contort their facial muscles in specific patterns. Unbeknownst to them, these config-urations represented the various categories of emotions, such as anger, fear, or sadness. When they were presented with a standardized story, their appraisal of meaning was directly influenced by which facial musculature patterns they had activated. If their muscles were held in a sad way, they interpreted the story presented as sad. If their faces were held in a way to show joy, they had a happy reaction to the same story. Somatosensory data from the face are registered in the brain and directly influence its state of activation, so that information processing is shaped by the effects of these data.

Muscle changes in our limbs and faces are highly sensitive components of emotional reactions, and these send input directly to the brain and are represented in an area called the somatosensory cortex. Of note is that the portion of the somatosensory cortex in the *right* hemisphere has more inte-grated representations of the body, including the face, than that in the *left* hemisphere, suggesting a more direct role of the right brain in the process-ing bodily states. As we'll see in Chapter 6, the brain's asymmetry plays an important role in understanding emotion and the mind. The other form of bodily response takes place in the viscera, such as the stomach, intestines, heart, and lungs. Visceral changes are registered in the middle prefrontal cor-tex, especially in the right hemisphere within the anterior insula and anterior cingulate regions. These are the areas that play a central role in interocep-tion, enabling us to make topical maps of our visceral states as they take in signals from the hollow organs of the body. Interestingly, these regions of the brain monitor as well as regulate these visceral reactions.[107]

Our brains create a representation of bodily changes. These somatic maps are shaped by prior experience and can be independent of the present response. In this view, our knowledge of how we feel is based in large part upon the nature of these somatic maps.[108] This is how implicit somatosensory memory can intrude on awareness of present experience. A thought can be associated with an emotional response containing an implicit somatic reac-tion generated internally. This is a shift in bodily state created by our brains from imagination and past experiences. Memories of emotional experiences evoke automatic, implicit activations, which can feel as real as direct bodily responses and can deeply enliven the associated imagery of the recollection. In some cases (such as when we recall a past frightening event), we will also have the actual bodily changes (such as increased heart rate, sweating, and dilated pupils).

If an adult was scratched by a cat as a child, the state of fear and arousal at the time will be registered in the brain as an implicit somatic memory of fear. It will be associated with the image and idea of a cat. In the future, seeing a cat may activate a similar bodily state of fear, instantiating a somatic recollection similar to that of the initial cat scratch and activating a set of associational memory processes also linked to the original scratch. An implicit bodily memory is how a thought, image, or other memory can elicit a sensory response, which then initiates a cascade of fear-related associations that may be quite debilitating. This may be one way in which unresolved posttraumatic conditions continue to perpetuate frightening reactions from long ago; such individuals feel as if they are being traumatized over and over again.

## INDIVIDUAL DIFFERENCES IN EMOTIONAL EXPERIENCE

Some couples experience a kind of "compatibility" that both members of a pair may have felt when they first met: They resembled each other in certain favored ways of being, in certain needs for play and relaxation, or in preferred times for work. In some of these pairs, there is a discordant match in the partners' attachment histories; the disparity between their individual appraisal systems may lead to difficulty in communicating. For example, a husband with a dismissing state of mind with respect to attachment probably had experiences with his mother that did not reinforce the positive effects of emotional intimacy. As an infant, his encounters with eye gaze and face-to-face contact were probably not associated with a sense of soothing. Recall that studies of avoidantly attached pairs reveal that the body continues to register distress during separation (for children) and in discussion of attachment issues (in adults). This finding suggests that the original value system, which assigned a "good" meaning to affective connections between people, has probably remained intact even after repeatedly disappointing and rejecting experiences. What has been learned is an adaptation. The brain has learned to adapt itself to the experience by minimizing the manifestations of such distress in other aspects of mental functions. The person's development of behavioral and complex cognitive responses, such as memory and narrative, will now serve to minimize conscious access to this persistent distress.

In this couple, the wife's experience of her husband was that in a quiet way he seemed to enjoy her presence. His lack of focus on her emotional states provided her with a sense of first safety and then frustration. She seemed to have had an ambivalent attachment with her own mother and a disorganized one with her father; she now had an unresolved adult attachment status, with a best-fitting alternative classification of preoccupied. On some nonverbal level, she felt that her husband liked being "close" to her, though he would never state this directly. She was probably sensing something real—an intact but frightened social and emotional system in her husband, which did indeed continue to value attachment. Both on the surface of his behavior and in his conscious experience, however, he denied the importance of such connections. In fact, the husband seemed to pride himself on his autonomy, often stating that the sign of healthy development is to "not need anyone, just want them." His wife did not feel needed. She often didn't even feel wanted.

With many couples, the very characteristics that each partner initially found attractive in the other become the qualities that create intolerable frustration and drive them to a therapist for help. In this couple, the wife was attracted at first to the husband's "autonomy and independence." She felt safe and unthreatened by his emotional distance. The husband liked his wife's "sensitivity and ability to express her emotions." She offered him something he had never had. As time went on, however, she began to feel so isolated that his autonomy made her infuriated. He began to sense her emotional response as attacks on his personality. This couple became stuck in an emotional rut.

In this example, the wife's capacity to consciously experience emotion was quite different from that of her husband. She was able to notice changes in her body's sensations, such as a tightening in her muscles, a queasy feeling in her stomach, and a trembling in her hands. She might feel her face beginning to smile, or notice tears on her cheeks. Each of these bodily messages let her know some aspect of her emotional state: anger, fear, sadness, joy. The ability to sense this somatic feedback is the kind of self-awareness that has led numerous researchers to postulate that *the body's response lets us know how we feel.* This can be called "interoception" and seems to involve action of the right anterior insula.[109] As mentioned earlier, the insula is linked directly with another middle prefrontal area, the anterior cingulate, through the neural spindle cells for rapid communication between

> The body's response lets us know how we feel.

these structures, which enables a form of self-awareness. The insula also works closely with the orbitofrontal region, and together they may relay neural processing to the medial prefrontal cortex, wherein a sense of self is further elaborated and the process of self-reflection is created. The ability to be aware of our own internal bodily states and affective arousal—our emotions—directly influences the ability to be in relationship to another.

In this couple, the wife often could sense when she was having an intense "emotional experience" by the way her body felt. For her husband, life was not so full of these sensations. He would make decisions, perceive the world, and recall things (or not) without a sense that any kind of biasing was occurring. But we cannot say that he was any less influenced by his hidden value system than his wife, whose emotions were more readily accessible to her conscious experience.

Working memory is able to contain a number of processes and manipulate them within conscious awareness. These processes include present perceptual representations, items from long-term memory, and states of the body. However, implicit representations can influence perceptual bias, memory processes, and rational decision making without our awareness. To minimize distress and maximize function, the brain of this dismissingly attached husband might have had the challenge of focusing his conscious attention away from attachment-related and bodily generated sensations. This diverting of attention might have concerned external events, such as behaving when he was a child as if his mother didn't return (as seen in the infant separation studies), as well as internal events, such as minimizing the importance of parental relationships (as revealed in the AAI; see Chapter 3). A distressed response is most readily seen in the body's state of increased sweating, heart rate, respiration, and muscle tension. Each of these may become activated in attachment situations with avoidantly attached children and dismissing adults. To avoid impairment of functioning, the representation of these responses must be kept away from working memory. To accomplish such a task means creating a pattern of neural interactions in which somatic representations are not linked to the working memory processes of the lateral prefrontal cortex. Interoception is blocked.

Given the location of these processes, we can hypothesize how this husband might have been affected by such an adaptation. The cortical representations of somatic muscle responses are most highly integrated in the right hemisphere of the brain. Visceral responses are monitored by the anterior insula and the closely associated anterior cingulate, also primarily on the right side. The lateral prefrontal cortex is centered just to the side of the middle prefrontal cortex, with which it receives and sends direct connections. Reduction in input to the right lateral prefrontal cortex would be quite helpful to avoid receiving the representations of the right-sided somatosensory and orbitofrontal cortices.

What would this mean for this man and others with a similar attachment history of distant emotional communication from a primary caregiver? Impaired input of the right-sided sources of somatic representations would functionally lead such individuals to be consciously unaware of their bodies' responses. They would therefore not be able to know easily how they feel. Furthermore, if the right lateral prefrontal cortex had more general blockages, we would predict that the other functions of the right hemisphere might also be less accessible to conscious awareness. In this case, the husband had a difficult time seeing the gist or context of things. He also seemed unable to read his wife's state of mind as expressed through her nonverbal signals. Such difficulties are all problems in functions of the right hemisphere. We shall return to the issue of hemispheric specialization in the mind both below and in Chapter 6.

A common belief is that there is a pattern of gender differences in emotion, especially in the empathic sharing of emotional states between males and females. Developmental studies have focused on the gender differences in relationships among friends during the school years. In general, these studies find "masculine" and "feminine" styles that most boys and girls, respectively, seem to exhibit.[110] The masculine style has been defined as a form of mutual assertion of individuals' talents and skills. Boys' interest in athletic prowess is one example of shared assertion. This strategy leads to a "fight-or-flight" response pattern. The feminine style has been described as one of mutual empathy; girls' interactions with each other tend to focus on shared expression and resonance with each other's emotional experiences.[111] Shelley Taylor has proposed an additional reaction of "tend and befriend" in girls under stress.[112] Clearly, however, many girls have elements of the masculine style, and many boys have elements of the feminine style. Although generalizations of any sort must be carefully examined, it is important to try to understand the genetic, hormonal, developmental, and/or social factors within families and cultures that contribute to such observable gender differences.

Recent discussions of the differences between the male and female brains, exaggerated in the popular media, may mislead us into misunderstanding the fundamental commonalities between the genders. The exposure to male androgens *in utero* will produce a "masculinized" brain, and recent studies suggest that levels of testosterone in both males and females influence the development of the adolescent brain's maturation as well.[113] Genetic and hormonal influences are important. Reinforcement in families and through cultural practices may further elaborate such differences and contribute to the narrowing of how self becomes defined. In other words, social expectations can amplify initial differences between the sexes and limit the freedom that members of each gender can experience during development. Recall that attachment is gender-neutral; this means that both girls and boys are fully capable of making intimate connections with caregivers and of becoming sensitive caregivers themselves. Simply observing girls in active competitive sporting events or boys engaging in artistic pursuits reminds us to avoid overgeneralizations that restrict how we understand the basic needs of all children to develop freely and fully.

# EMOTIONAL COMMUNICATION: EMPATHY AND AFFECTIVE EXPRESSION

An important aspect of emotions is their social function. Emotions, both primary and categorical, serve as the vehicles that allow one person to have a sense of the mental state of another. The capacity to feel another person's experience has many labels, such as "empathy," "compassion," "sympathy," "mirroring," "attunement," and "mindsight." In its essence, the ability of one mind to perceive and then experience elements of another person's mind is a profoundly important dimension of human experience.

Why is this so important? There are several reasons. The ability to perceive another's intentions, attentional focus, and evaluation of events allows us to understand social interactions and anticipate the behavior of other people. Young infants begin to differentiate between animate and inanimate objects in the world, attributing intention and emotional responses to the former and not the latter. With the assignment of intention, our minds are able to compare external behaviors with implied internal motivational states.[114] This ability allows us to detect "cheaters" and note when we are being misled. A further evolutionary benefit is that our ancestors could rapidly sense when a group member was detecting danger by the look on her face, her gestures, or her tone of voice. Those social beings capable of such mindsight escaped danger more often, were less often tricked by the destructive motivations of others, and thus were more likely to survive and pass on the capacity for such state-to-state communication.[115]

From a developmental perspective, the most utilitarian of these benefits is that parents can sense the inner needs of their children and therefore maximize the potential of their offspring's survival. Another benefit of empathic attunement is that it creates an attachment bond between parent and child. This provides increasingly complex layers of external and then internal security for the growing child as he encounters an increasingly challenging world. The experience of being understood develops a mental model or inner expectation that needs are important and goals are achievable. The child's system requires the parent's attunement to help organize the child's own mind. Positive emotional states are amplified and negative ones modulated within these attuned communications. As the child grows, these repeated alignments of mental states allow him to develop a self-organizational capacity for autonomous regulation. Human infants have profoundly underdeveloped brains. Maintaining proximity to their caregivers is essential, both for survival and for allowing their brains to use the mature states of their attachment figures to help them organize their own mental functioning.

The subjective side of these emotional connections is that a sense of belonging grows within the individual. "Feeling felt" is the subjective experience of mental state attunement. The pleasurable response to such a resonance of minds may be built into our brains as a genetic inheritance of evolutionary history. Having such a sense encourages group behavior, which has been of great survival value to our species as we evolved. It may also be the reason why large groups are experienced so differently from smaller ones, in which face-to-face eye contact and other aspects of shared nonverbal communication are readily available. Committees of over a dozen people become unwieldy and inefficient (not that some smaller ones do much better!). Feeling felt for some requires even smaller group settings, with one-to-one situations being the ideal for many people.

As social creatures, we have the capacity for a huge assortment of facial expressions, which are directly controlled by our nervous systems.[116] Our tremendously rich innervation allows for exquisitely subtle and rapid alterations in facial expression. To match this expressive ability, primates have neuronal groups in the brain that are specialized to respond to faces, and also to particular facial expressions. As we've discussed, these neuronal groups often rest in the value system circuits of our brains, such as in the amygdala and orbitofrontal cortex. We are hard-wired to have meaning and emotion shaped by the perception of eye contact and facial expression.[117] We are also hard-wired to express emotional states through the face.

Complex bodily aspects of emotional processes are not easily translated into words. Nonverbal expressions, including those of the face, tone of voice, and gestures, can transfer information about internal states more fully and quickly to the outside world than words can do. Words go only so far. When anyone asks, "How are you feeling?", it is a huge translational challenge to turn such subtle and dynamic neural processes into a verbal statement. Emotion can be seen as an energizing drive toward motion. Seeing what a person does, rather than asking her how she feels, can often be a more direct road into the person's emotional state. Nevertheless, we often feel compelled to ask others how they feel. The social process of "talking about feelings" with each other is much more an interactive event than the mere telling of a linguistic message. Words such as "sad" or "angry" are quite limited and distant symbols we send to each other in response to the query "How are you feeling?" The message is in the medium of how we respond, not in the words alone.[118]

> We are hard-wired to have meaning and emotion shaped by the perception of eye contact and facial expression.

The link between emotion and action is in the appraisal–arousal foundation of these processes. At their core, appraisals define what is good or bad, what should be approached or avoided. Children are often more at ease with the hedonic tone of primary emotional states than with trying to define the categorical emotions they may be experiencing. When children say, "I feel bad," or "I feel good," this may be a very direct statement of their appraisal system and primary emotional experience.

## EMOTION AND THE HEMISPHERES

Affect can be expressed through facial expressions and through modulations in the tone and prosody of the voice. These nonverbal aspects of language communication, in both their expression and perception, appear to be mediated predominantly by the right hemisphere.[119] The body's posture and movement can also blend with the voice and facial expression in sending affective signals that are readily perceived by other people. What is striking is the finding that the input from the body—including signals from the muscles, bones, and viscera (such as the heart and the intestines)—is more highly integrated in the right hemisphere than in the left. In other words, the whole body is represented in an integrated way in the right hemisphere. As we've discussed briefly, even the regulation of the body's autonomic nervous system is primarily mediated by right-brain mechanisms.[120] The right hemisphere therefore appears to play a major role in mediating regulatory emotional processes, as well as in permitting the expression of emotional states and the conscious awareness of emotional experience.

For this discussion of emotion, it is important to provide some background information. Appraisal and arousal occur on both sides of the brain, as do other emotional processes. However, the subjective experience and the nature of emotion on either side of the brain may be quite different. Various theories propose disparate views of emotions and brain asymmetry.[121] One perspective is the valence hypothesis, which suggests that unpleasant emotions are processed on the right side and pleasant ones on the left.[122] Consistent with this suggestion is the view that withdrawal states and processes are mediated on the right side, whereas approach states and processes are modulated on the left.[123] Another view is that socially mediated emotions, such as guilt or the enactment of social display rules, are processed in the left hemisphere, whereas more basic, spontaneous emotions are processed in the right hemisphere.[124]

Furthermore, in studies of patients with blocked communication between the two hemispheres, the left brain appears unable to register the facial expression of others. The right brain both perceives and sends messages through facial expressions and tone of voice.[125] Therefore, it may be fair to propose that the nonverbal right hemisphere may be the primary location for the subjective awareness and expression of primary emotions as we have defined them. The processing of such emotions, however, is likely to be mediated by both hemispheres.

Developmental studies suggest that in fact each hemisphere may mediate quite different processes of engagement with the environment. As noted above, this may mean that approach is mediated by the left hemisphere and withdrawal by the right. For example, behaviorally inhibited (shy) children reveal a dominance in right frontal electrical activity at baseline; more adventurous children demonstrate left frontal activation. Nathan Fox and Richard Davidson have each suggested that such findings support the notion that characteristic emotional styles may reflect profiles of frontal activation.[126] Left frontal activation is associated with active approach, positive affect, exploration, and sociability. The absence of left frontal activation leads to an absence of positive affect and the experience of depression. In contrast, right frontal activation leads to active withdrawal, negative affect, and fear/anxiety. Hypoactivation of the right frontal region leads to disinhibition of approach, with impulsivity and hyperactivity. Such a view can explain some features of shy and of aggressive children and the changes in their states as the context may alter their frontal activation profiles.

Further developmental studies suggest that both constitutional/temperamental and experience/attachment features may directly shape these patterns of frontal activation.[127] In the case of depressed mothers, for example, there is a marked decrease in shared positive affect states, and the infants (and their mothers) are seen as withdrawn. In both parents and children, there is a marked relative decrease in left frontal activation and increase in right frontal activation. If such depression lasts beyond the first year of life, the infants may continue to express this pattern of frontal activity for years in the future.[128]

## SUBJECTIVE EXPERIENCE

Emotion is inherently a subjective and an interpersonal experience, involving interaction with the environment and the evaluation of meaning. Experiences evoke within us textured subjective states that create the fabric of our lives. Music has been described as one of the purest expressions of emotions that exists. It is filled with contours and spacing, varied intensities, and modulations in sound. Studies by Daniel Levitin suggest that music is highly integrative: Melody links the representations in the cortex, and rhythm links the torso with the processes of the cortex.[129] Recall that we have defined emotion as "shifts in integration"; thus this view of music illuminates the fundamental integrative function of emotion. Although the activations elicited by music could be considered categorical emotion, such as joy or sadness, perhaps they more appropriately reflect profiles of arousal parallel to vitality affects. We could call primary emotions the "music of the mind." The process of creating and listening to music is a form of emotional experience and affective communication that is profoundly integrative.

Several studies, and my own informal survey of dozens of children, reveal a common preference among unprofessionally trained individuals for the left ear when listening to music.[130] Sound heard with the left ear may induce a more holistic sensation, a floating with the flow of the music, quite distinct from the sensation produced by music heard with the right ear. How can this be? The left auditory nerve goes primarily to the right hemisphere! Though there is some crossover, the auditory stimulation in the right brain appears to evoke a different sensation from that which goes to the left brain from the right ear. Try it for yourself.

Emotions recruit distributed neuronal clusters that organize the systems of the brain into the emerging states of mind.[131] "Recruitment" can be generally defined here as a process that temporarily links distinct, differentiated elements into a functional whole. In the brain, recruitment involves the binding of the activity of spatially distributed neural circuits at a given moment and across time. Emotion can be proposed to serve this integrative role by way of its involvement of neuromodulatory systems that are themselves widely distributed. These systems have direct effects on neural excitability and activation, on neural plasticity and the growth of synaptic connections, and on the coordination of a range of processes in the brain.

We can suggest that perhaps the most active representations may be the ones that are recruited and then have the potential to enter the spotlight of conscious awareness. Consciousness may in fact be quite distinct on each side of the brain. Some authors have suggested that the right hemisphere is a master at representing social context, whereas the left remains focused on details devoid of contextual meaning.[132] The social context of a situation determines the action of the appraisal systems. Internal context,

> Consciousness may in fact be quite distinct on each side of the brain.

the history of present and recent representational activity, also directly affects the way the appraisal systems work. The impact of representational processes on each side of the brain may create quite distinct contextual influences on the appraisal process and lead to distinct senses of conscious awareness.

We are filled with representations of all sorts: sensations and images in a context-rich form mediated by the right hemisphere, and linguistic symbols in a linear, logical, detail-oriented mode mediated by the left hemisphere.[133] If this view is true, then our daily conversations are filled with a blending of right-sided and left-sided communication. Some authors argue that emotional attunement is fundamentally right-brain-to-right-brain communication.[134]

This view may sound too reductionistic and simple to be either true or useful. But let's take a look at a fundamental notion of attunement: the feeling of another person's experience. Merely to understand another person requires an intellectual grasp of the other's experience. The ability to conceptualize the mind of another, as well as to perceive what the other's subjective world might be like, requires special tools that enable the kind of reflective functioning discussed in Chapter 3. The neurological bases of these tools have evolved over thousands of years and are a fundamental part of the social circuitry of the brain. They are intimately related to emotional experience. These circuits are located primarily in the right hemisphere. To feel another person's experience requires the ability to take in how the other person in fact is feeling by way of specific signals this person is generating. These data then directly affect the receiver's state of mind. Would it be such a big surprise to find that the neural processes of one hemisphere are best expressed externally by that hemisphere, and then perceived best by the same hemisphere, but in another person? After all, words generated by the left hemisphere of one person are best perceived and understood by the left hemisphere of the listener. What we are really talking about are the forms of information that the mind is processing. Information, let us recall, can be considered the swirls of energy flow that have symbolic meaning; they signify something beyond that energy pattern. As we'll discuss more fully in Chapter 6, the types of mental representations—these symbolic swirls of patterns in energy flow—are quite distinct in each hemisphere. Learning about the nature of these differences can give us a better understanding of emotional experience and communication between minds.

By our second year of life, we have learned the trick of showing facial expressions that differ from those that would reveal our true internal emotional states.[135] This form of social deception allows us to act in socially appropriate and sanctioned ways. In a fundamental manner, this behavior creates a division between the private, internally experienced self and the public, externally expressed self. Most of us carry out this dual role every day in our private and public lives. If we spend too much of our time attempting to be "socially appropriate" with a public self, and do not express authentic feelings or thoughts, then we may be vulnerable to developing a "false self" quite distant from our actual primary emotional experience. Of note are findings suggesting that the left hemisphere plays a more significant role in the external communication of emotions that conform to social rules.[136]

As noted earlier, words are often quite limited in their ability to convey our internal states. Attunement to one another's nonverbal means of communicating emotion is a much more direct and satisfying way to join with others. However, we must use words to attempt to understand the nature of emotion and the human mind. Some might argue that without words, we cannot reflect on the conceptual nature of our own minds. As we've seen in Chapter 3, those parents who have the capacity to reflect on mental states are more likely to have secure attachments with their children. This reflective function consists of affective attunement and verbal statements about the importance of mental states in human experience.[137] In fact, the ability to use words reflecting mentalizing concepts, such as beliefs, feelings, attitudes, intentions, and thoughts—"mental state language"—is associated with parents of children who have secure attachments.[138] There is a suggestion from a basic research study that mindfulness traits—the tendency to be aware of present-moment experience, to have an open stance toward oneself and others, to have emotional equanimity, and to be able to describe the inner world of the mind[139]—and secure attachment may go hand in hand.[140] Studies have also shown that in individuals with mindfulness traits, naming an emotion can decrease limbic activations.[141] In other words, they can "name it to tame it." These ideas can inspire an approach to creating "reflective dialogues" with children in order to help them develop emotionally. Using both our nonverbal right and verbal left hemispheres, we can find ways to communicate the important subjective emotional experiences of ourselves and others. One central theme to keep in your own mind is this: Emotion involves shifts in how we link differentiated elements to one another—that is, shifts in states of integration. As we'll see, emotion is regulatory by way of its integrative functions.

## EMOTION REGULATION

Emotion is indeed a complex set of processes. As we've seen in this chapter, emotion is at the core of internal and interpersonal processes that create our subjective experience of the self. The organization of the self is dependent upon the manner in which emotion is regulated. Research reveals that emotion as a set of processes is both regulated and regulatory. That is, emotional processes cannot exist without influencing other such processes and without being influenced themselves by other such processes. Thus the study of emotion and of emotion regulation go hand in hand.[142]

Self-regulation—the manner in which the process called the "self" comes to regulate its own processes—consists in part of the regulation of emotion. Sroufe describes the "twin tasks" of emotion in development as the expression of affect and its management. He states, "The ability to maintain flexibly organized behavior in the face of high levels of arousal or tension is a central aspect of stable individual differences in personality organization."[143]

Susan Calkins has described pathways to emotion regulation as involving both internal and external sources.[144] Internal features include constitutional aspects of neuroregulatory structures (such as neuroendocrine, autonomic, and frontal lobe systems), behavioral traits (such as attentiveness, adaptability, reactivity, soothability, and sociability), and cognitive components (including social referencing, beliefs and expectations, awareness of need for regulation, and ability to apply strategies). External features include interactive caregiving patterns (responsiveness, cooperation, reciprocity, accessibility, support, and acceptance) and explicit training (including modeling, reinforcement, and discipline).

In general, our skills at regulating emotion allow us to achieve a wide range and high intensity of emotional experience while maintaining flexible, adaptive, and organized behavior. The processes of emotion regulation—and dysregulation—can involve any of the basic levels of emotion: physiology, subjective experience, and behavioral change. As we'll discuss in detail in Chapter 7, the regulation of emotion involves the modulation of states of mind. Regulation of the flow of states can involve internal (physiological and cognitive) and interactive (engaging with the social environment) elements.

> The processes of emotion regulation—and dysregulation—can involve any of the basic levels of emotion: physiology, subjective experience, and behavioral change.

For example, alterations in attentional focus, perceptual bias, or the evaluation of meaning can directly change the course of elaboration of primary emotional states into more differentiated categorical emotions. We can utilize the very processes of emotion to regulate their flow.

We've defined emotion as shifts in states of integration. When integration is present, harmony exists. When integration is impaired, chaos and/or rigidity arise. As we will discover, integration within the nervous system is the essential process of internal regulation. Integration between people leads to a social form of regulation. A core aspect of the mind is an embodied and relational, emergent self-organizing process that regulates the flow of energy and information. The mind achieves its regulatory function by way of these integrative, emotional processes throughout life. Healthy emotional development does not move us from dependence to independence; instead, we move from dependence and care receiving to interdependence and the capacity to be both a care receiver and a caregiver. Here is our core proposal: Emotion is central to our well-being, internally and interpersonally, because integration is the essence of health.

Before we can appreciate the details of these complex regulatory processes more fully, we will need to review what is known about how states of mind are created within the complex system of the brain (Chapter 5) and how we construct reality with representational processes (Chapter 6). Then we will be ready to wrestle with the question of how the brain organizes its own functioning, including how it regulates emotional states within itself and in connection with others.

## REFLECTIONS: EMOTION AND THE MIND

An amusing cycle of responses sometimes enters the classroom when a psychotherapy student or teacher asks the question "What is a feeling?" "A feeling," the response sometimes goes, "is an emotion. It is what you feel when you are emotional. Emotions generate feelings." An initial way out of this endless loop comes from the knowledge of how central emotional processes are for human relationships. Emotions are the contents and processes of interpersonal communication early in life, and they create the tone and texture of such communications throughout the lifespan. This view at least brings emotions out of the individual and into the interaction between people. Still, this leaves us with only a bit more clarity about the challenging task of how to define emotions.

Everyday descriptions of emotions may seem more appealing than trying to create seemingly restrictive, scientifically derived concepts and definitions. Emotions are what allow us to fall in love. They are the stuff of poetry, art, and music. Emotions fill us with a sense of connection to others. They link families together; they remind us of who is important in our lives. Emotions make life worth living. For some, becoming scientific about emotions risks reducing the essential and passionate stuff of subjectivity into some neural-circuitry-based explanation that appears cold and useless. However, the application of neural science principles to understanding our feelings can actually expand and enrich the subjective experience of our own emotional minds. Understanding the neuroanatomic convergence of social interactions, appraisal, and emotional arousal helps us to see how the mind creates and is created by interactions with other minds. We can now move beyond circular definitions and embrace the metaphors of emotion in a deeply impassioned and integrated manner.

This chapter has provided a broad set of specific definitions of emotion that can enable us to understand human experience more fully. This view sees emotions as the flow of energy, or states of arousal and activation, through the brain and other parts of the body. This process emerges from and directly affects the further processing of information within the mind by way of the appraisal of meaning. Three phases can be identified. First, a stimulus (internal or external) evokes a state of initial orientation, creating a sensation of "Something important is happening; pay attention now!" This focus of attention is automatic and does not need to involve conscious awareness.

Next, the value systems of the brain continue to appraise the meaning of that stimulus and of that initial orientation itself by means of elaborated appraisal and arousal processes and the activation of certain circuits. At this point, the sensation may become "This is good" or "This is bad." These first two steps of an emotional response contain activation profiles, such as surges of energy, that can be defined as "primary" emotions. In their essence, primary emotions are the beginning of how the mind creates meaning.

Externally, primary emotions can be seen as vitality affects, expressed by the contours of activation of the body, facial expressions, nonverbal gestures, and tone of voice. These vitality affects constitute the primary connection between infant and parent. This finding reveals the exquisite sensitivity of the appraisal centers to social interaction and shows how emotions are initially created within our relationships with others.

A third phase in emotional response is what is more generically thought of as "emotion": the differentiation of initial orientation and elaborated states of arousal and appraisal into categorical emotions. Examples of such emotions found throughout the world in characteristic expressions are sadness, anger, disgust, surprise, joy, fear, and shame. The brain and other body systems appear to have common pathways by which these distinct categorical emotional states are physiologically manifested and expressed as categorical affects.

Generated by the value systems of the brain, these emotional activations pervade all mental functions and literally create meaning in life. *In this way, we can say that emotion and meaning are created by the same processes.*

Information processing involves the creation and manipulation of cognitive representations. Attentional mechanisms direct the flow of information processing. Within perception and memory, the appraisal systems of the brain must label representations as significant or value-laden. In this way, the appraisal and arousal processes—the central features of

> We can say that emotion and meaning are created by the same processes.

emotion—are interwoven with the representational processes of "thinking." *Creating artificial or didactic boundaries between thought and emotion obscures the experiential and neurobiological reality of their inseparable nature.*

Energy flow is a basic aspect of primary emotions. As states of mind emerge within the individual, the changing activations that create them are often experienced as primary emotions. The regulation of emotion, or the regulation of information and energy flow within the brain, creates the experience of the self. The capacity to assess the personal significance of events and to alter automatic, reflexive responses may be carried out by the prefrontal regions in a process we have called "response flexibility." When such an ability becomes integrated with other aspects of emotional and memory processing, the individual may be able to generate a set of internal and interpersonal experiences that enables the self to have a flexible form of regulation. We'll soon dive more deeply into the proposal that regulation itself emerges from the core process of integration. In the next two chapters, we will examine how the mind organizes itself by how it regulates the flow of information and mental states both within itself and with other minds. Emotion and its modulation are in this way a fundamental part of information processing and energy flow.

# CHAPTER 5

# States of Mind

## *Cohesion, Subjective Experience, and Complex Systems*

## DEFINING STATES OF MIND

How does the mind coordinate information processing in order to construct reality in the moment? How do billions of neurons with trillions of interconnections within the brain become activated in organized patterns that influence our mental lives? How is the flow of energy within widely distributed neurons actually regulated? An answer to each of these questions can be found in the idea of a "state of mind." *States of mind allow the brain to achieve cohesion in functioning.*

*A "state of mind" can be defined as the total pattern of activations in the brain at a particular moment in time.* Patterns of activation within distributed regions, called "neural net profiles," reveal the various circuits that mediate information processing. These activated circuits are distributed in a widely interconnected web, with profoundly complex inputs and outputs linking various clusters of cells that carry out particular functions.[1] At a very basic level, for example, we can suggest that a fearful state of mind is the clustering of related processes in a cohesive whole. A state of heightened caution, focal attention, behavioral hypervigilance, memories of past experiences of threat, models of the self as a victim in need of protection, and emotional arousal alerting the body and mind to prepare for harm are all processes that become functionally primed or readied for activity. A state of mind therefore involves a clustering of functionally synergistic processes that allow the mind as a whole to form a cohesive state of activity. Cohesion is the quality of elements' sticking

186

to one another. The benefit of cohesion is to maximize the efficiency and efficacy of the processes needed in a given moment in time. Cohesive states of mind are highly functional and adaptive to the environment. However, "cohesion" is not the same as "coherence," in which there is a fluid and adaptive flow across time.[2] Coherence emerges with increasing complexity—an outcome of integration and mental health.

In Chapter 4, we've seen how emotion can be conceptualized as shifts in the brain's state of integration. Therefore, it is natural to view emotion as central to how a state of mind assembles distinct elements of neural processing into a temporally linked set of firing patterns in the moment. This is the essence of a neural net profile, the set of activated neurons linked together in a given moment of time. To better understand these complex processes— states of mind—we must look at some ideas about how systems function.

## Modules, Modes, and Systems

At a fundamental level, the brain's circuitry creates patterns of activation that serve as symbols (i.e., "representations"). These patterns represent information and cause further mental processes to occur.[3] In turn, these processes themselves represent information. That is, they serve as symbols for something other than the patterns of firing that they are. This is the information processing of the mind. A representation is an active, dynamic process that leads to further neural activations.

The differences between distinct forms of representation lie in the patterns of firing and in the location of the neural circuits being activated. For example, within the circuits linked directly to the outside world and to the body, sensory representations are created. Perceptual representations established by these sensory inputs are then processed and transformed into more complex representations. For example, when you visualize a "table," you activate a representation of the table located in the occipital cortex, which receives signals sent from the eyes. This location helps define the representation's visual quality as a pattern of angles and contrasts. The sensory information is then further processed and transformed into conceptual representations. These more complex and abstract symbols are thought to emanate from the activity of the neocortex, especially toward the front of the brain. Circuits for linguistic representations—words and their various elements and combinations—are primarily located in the left hemisphere in the side or temporal lobes. The expression and reception of nonverbal intonations of spoken language are thought to emanate from the activity of the right hemisphere. Overall, *the localization of processing lends a specificity to our experience of mental representations, directly shaping the content of information and the subjective quality of that content.* An image logically assessed by the left hemisphere's more analytic circuitry will have a very different texture from that of the same image processed in the more receptive, holistic right-hemisphere cortical columns.

Cognitive neuroscience uses the terms "modules," "modes," "systems," and "processes" to describe how mental representations emanating from neuroanatomically distinct sites may be organized into a cohesive whole.[4] This framework is derived from the mind's central function as an information processor. Mental activity stems from basic processing modules. A "module" can be defined as a set of neural circuits carrying a certain type of information and utilizing a similar form of neural signal or code. For example, a module for processing visual input involves the signals sent from the eyes to the occipital cortex. This sensory module may include circuits that detect certain shapes, contrasts, or angles. Another type of module, a visual perception module, may consist of circuits that cluster these sensory representations into perceptual patterns (such as "form of furniture" or "face"). Together, these and similar modules process visual data into more complex representations, forming the visual "mode." If this information is then coordinated with other perceptual modalities (modes), we have the perceptual "system." Examples of other systems of the mind include the various forms of implicit and explicit memory.[5] Within explicit memory, there is a system composed of the modes of autobiographical versus semantic memory. Within the autobiographical mode are the modules encoding specific episodes, gists, and generic autobiographical knowledge. For example, when we ask someone to tell us what he remembers about last year, he will activate his explicit memory system's subcomponent mode of autobiographical memory and its basic modules. As we've discussed, these components have specific neural circuitry involved in the encoding and retrieval functions of autonoetic consciousness.

## States, Traits, and Cohesion

We are using a vocabulary of modules, modes, and systems to describe one way in which the system of the mind can be conceptualized. What is the point? The point is that the activities of the brain become organized in a patterned fashion as these layers of increasingly complex information processing. We experience these patterns of activity as states of mind. The patterns themselves are made of neural firings that contain an electrochemical flow of energy and information. In other words, a "state of mind" arises from a neural net profile of brain activity and is ultimately experienced as an aspect of subjective mental life. I suppose we could call these "states of brain firing" and avoid this mind–brain question. But the reality is that we often use the "state of mind" phrase with its subjective feeling of "mood" or "emotional valence," and so it is naturally a part of our subjective mental lives. Beyond shaping how we feel in the present, a state of mind also does two fundamental things: *It coordinates activity in the moment, and it creates a pattern of brain activation that can become more likely in the future.* That is, a state of mind can become a remembered brain activity configuration or neural net profile. Repeated activation of particular states—for example, a shame state or a state of despair—makes them much more likely to be activated in the future. In this manner, states can become traits of the individual that influence both internal and interpersonal processes.[6]

A state of mind clusters the activity of specific systems of processing. The degree to which this clustering is effective and useful determines the state's cohesiveness. What coordinates a state's clustering process? We can propose here that part of the answer is emotion. The regulation of emotion directs the flow of energy through the brain's changing states of activation. Recall from Chapter 4 that there are convergence zones in the brain, such as the prefrontal cortex, thought to be responsible for the coordination of the activity of widely distributed systems: bodily state, arousal–appraisal centers, attention via the lateral prefrontal cortex, perception from the sensory cortices, abstract representations within the associational neocortex, memory processes via the medial temporal lobe, and motor responses via the basal ganglia.[7] The activation (energy) of these circuits determines their contribution to the brain's overall state at a given point in time. When activated, these circuits create and process representations (information) within their specialized computational modes. The regulation of emotion is mediated in part by the limbic and prefrontal regions of the brain, with their structural interconnections and functional capacity to coordinate a wide range of brain activity.[8]

## Organizing Effects of States of Mind

What does "to coordinate a wide range of brain activity" actually mean? Literally, this means that the various systems that make up the brain—from "lower" or "simpler" ones (such as the registration and regulation of the autonomic nervous system's control of bodily states) to the "higher," more complex ones (such as the neocortical conceptual representations of thought)—can be functionally linked and temporally associated with each other in a given state of mind. In this context, "linked" means that the systems are simultaneously activated and have functional influences upon each other as well as on our interactions with others.[9] This is a state of mind.

*A state of mind can be proposed to be a pattern of activation of recruited systems within the brain responsible for (1) perceptual bias, (2) emotional tone and regulation, (3) memory processes, (4) mental models, and (5) behavioral response patterns.*

A state of mind can have enduring clusters of activation of each of these basic elements. One can discover the elements of an individual's state of mind by focusing on the elements of her perceptions, feelings, thoughts, memories, attitudes, beliefs, and desires—and how these may be influencing her behavior and interactions with others. Also, because states of mind are dynamic processes, trying to understand them also requires that we look at the changes in the individual's mental processes over time.

Each moment brings a combination of activations creating a unique state of mind. However, repeated patterns of activation may become "engrained," meaning that they are made more likely to be reactivated in the future as noted above. Particular states of mind may develop cohesion through their repeated activation, as well as through the functional benefits of their internal linkages.

At times, the mind cannot organize itself effectively in response to experiences. Such experiences are traumatizing, in that they overwhelm the mind's ability to adapt.[10] As we've discussed in the case of disorganized attachment, some interpersonal experiences result in the mind's becoming unable to form a cohesive and adaptive state. In this situation, the mind enters a chaotic, disorganizing state of activations lacking in cohesion. The noncohesive characteristic of such a state may itself become a trait of the individual. Disorganization or disorientation becomes a repeated pattern of activation or state of mind. This may explain dissociation as an adaptation to stress seen in those with histories of disorganized attachments.

If an individual has been exposed to repeated neglect as a young child, a state of despair may have been activated and engrained. In this state of excessively low energy, perceptions of the world are marked by a sense of rejection; emotions are filled with shame and hopelessness; memories may evoke previous experiences of being rejected; a model of the self as unlovable and of others as unavailable may be activated; and there may be a behavioral tendency to withdraw. Because this state of despair has been repeatedly activated, it will be more likely to be activated in response to even minor signs of rejection, such as a friend's or therapist's not returning a phone call on time. The response to this environmental context is a function, in part, of this individual's history. The entire cluster, however, can quickly become the dominant information-processing mode at such a moment, giving the individual a sense of massive rejection and despair far exceeding the initial stimulus and not having any clear, consciously accessible connection to experiences from the past.

Our subjective lives emerge from mental states that are exquisitely sensitive to social interaction. Recall that as open, dynamic systems, we are composed of lower levels of subcomponents, as well as being ourselves subcomponents of the larger systems of social connections in which we live. Our brains have circuits specifically designed to receive and send social signals. Our minds are thus able to process and utilize this information, so that we can be active participants in social communication. In the example above of a despair state, the individual's prior history has engrained a tendency to be excessively sensitive and responsive to social signals containing information about another's lack of interest. In simpler terms, the person can easily feel rejected. When not in such a state of mind, the individual may function perfectly well. However, the regulation of her state of mind—her modulation of emotion—is such that she can quickly (and maladaptively) enter a paralyzing state of despair, which influences the rest of her mind's information processing in the direction of reinforcing that state. She perceives, feels, remembers, conceives, thinks, and behaves in ways that even more deeply engrain the state of mind at that time. Such are the organizing and self-reinforcing effects of a state of mind.

> Our subjective lives emerge from mental states that are exquisitely sensitive to social interaction.

Let's look next at an example of how the state of mind can change rapidly in response to environmental cues.

## Context Sensitivity

If a man is walking with his romantic partner on a beach, enjoying the breeze and the sound of the waves, he will be in a certain state of mind that may be characterized by an attentional focus on the water and sky and on his lover's hand in his own; an awareness of a deep sense of calm and connection; easy access to other similar romantic moments; a mental model of life as simple and rewarding; and a behavioral set of gentle, easy responses to others as he strolls down the sand. He may have a model of himself as a lovable person deserving of such a tranquil and connecting experience.

If someone suddenly grabs this man's shoulder and roughly says, "Hey, give me your money!", his state of mind is likely to be suddenly transformed. This encounter creates a new context. The state of his mind is extremely sensitive to external conditions. This change in the environment creates a shift in his brain. He perceives the sound of the intruder's tone of voice, the content of his message, and the bodily contact. All of his sensory processing systems, including auditory, visual, and somatosensory (bodily sensations), take in the data. At an early, "lower" level—before complex processing and long before conscious awareness—his alarm/defense system, including the amygdala, fires an internal signal of "Danger!" This subcortical processing takes rapid effect in shifting his state of mind. This shift in state leads him to have a perceptual bias to interpret environmental stimuli as threatening. A behavioral response pattern of fight or flight will become activated, with his heart beginning to race and muscles tightening. These sensations may feed back to his emotional processing centers, especially the orbitofrontal cortex, and let his mind know that he is feeling scared and/or angry. His attention may be mostly focused on the intruder's actions, but he may also become aware of his bodily response and altered mental state within working memory, which (as we've discussed) has been proposed as a possible mechanism for conscious experience. Memories, explicit and implicit, of other moments of danger and fear may become more readily accessible via the mechanism of state-dependent retrieval. This is useful in accessing knowledge of what he did and skills he exercised in similar past situations. A mental model that the world is a dangerous place may now become active. A model of the self may include anything from "I can protect myself" to "I knew this would happen to me; I am such a vulnerable and helpless person."

Often the shift between states of mind is not so dramatic as in this example. Context changes can be quite subtle; they may be induced, for example, by alterations in a companion's tone of voice or facial expression. Our minds are continually responding to external cues, especially from the social environment.

A more common situation that generates state shifts occurs when an adult travels "back home" to visit parents for the holidays. Returning to the physical and social environment of one's youth can provide context cues that activate old states of mind. A person may find herself, unwillingly and initially unknowingly, suddenly feeling "like a child" again. Sensations of dependence, inadequacy, or anger may dominate her emotional experience. She may begin acting as if she were a teenager again, taking part in minor (or major) battles with parents. As this person watches herself taking part in these old behavioral patterns, she may notice that her parents are also acting as if she is their renegade adolescent again! Which came first, their treatment of her or hers of them? How does this process occur? To understand states of mind and the rapid and intricate ways they are influenced by our present experiences and past encounters, we need to turn now to the study of complex systems.

## COMPLEX SYSTEMS

### Complexity, Natural Selection, and Connectionism

A single brain functions as an elaborate system that can be understood by examining the "theory of nonlinear dynamics of complex systems" or, more briefly, "complexity theory."[11] This perspective has been applied to a range of inanimate and living systems in an attempt to understand the often unpredictable but self-organizing nature of complex entities functioning as a system. The human brain has been examined by a number of theoreticians as one such nonlinear "dynamic system," also called a "dynamical system." Though a detailed review is beyond the scope of this chapter, some of the basic ideas of this approach are described here. The following discussion also draws on a variety of related theories about systems, complexity, and "parallel distributed processing" or "connectionism."[12] Moreover, I propose that these principles can be applied not only to the single brain or mind, but also to the functioning of two or more brains or minds acting as a single system. These applications allow us to deepen our earlier discussion of states of mind and their fundamental importance in creating internal experience and shaping interpersonal relationships.

The brain is a complex system whose processes organize its own functioning. That is, a complex system has an "emergent property" that arises from the interaction of its basic constituents. This property is called "self-organization."[13] I have proposed from the beginning that the mind emanates from social interaction and from the activity of the brain, and thus it is fair to say that the mind itself is complex and has self-organizing properties.[14] Despite the huge number of neurons involved and the nearly infinite variety of states of mind that can be created, this conceptual approach helps us to make sense of the self-regulating processes of the mind.

Complexity theory is a mathematically derived collection of principles governing the behavior of physiochemical systems, such as groups of molecules or patterns of clouds.[15] The application of this theory to biological systems, including the mind, has some fascinating implications. How can we equate clouds with the human psyche? Aren't inanimate objects and life forms fundamentally different? Remember, however, that biological systems are composed of basic atoms that are not alive. Complexity theory has been applied to an understanding of systems from molecules to societies, with extremely useful and unique applications.[16] What makes living systems unique is that they have evolved through natural selection into the adaptively complex forms that make up life on earth. Evolution has yielded complex designs without a formal designer; the function of the complex forms has allowed them to be open to the external environment and to adapt to it over generations.[17] In this way, *living systems are open systems capable of responding and adapting to the environment.*

> Living systems are open systems capable of responding and adapting to the environment.

What have these complex living systems evolved to do? They have evolved in ways that enable them to survive and reproduce. This is the fundamental principle of natural selection. How well a trait works within a particular environment determines whether a species will maintain the trait in subsequent generations. In this way, a living system is organized to attain goals: to maintain itself and to pass on its genes. The human nervous system, particularly the brain, has evolved to be specialized at solving problems. These problems can range from how to avoid drowning to how to find food or a mate. The adaptive design of the brain allows it to process specific forms of information in the service of achieving the fundamental goals of natural selection: survival and reproduction. The mind, as a product of the activity of the brain and relational interactions, in many ways reflects this evolutionary process.[18]

But the brain has a physical structure of its own that is unique to its evolutionary history. Certain regions, such as those for smell and vision, have become relatively smaller than those of our ancestors. Other regions, such as the neocortex, have become larger. It is clear that the brain itself is composed of an intricately interconnected set of neurons distributed in a spider-web-like fashion.[19] This allows for simultaneous—or parallel—processing of different kinds of information. Studies of this "parallel distributed processing" are part of a perspective called "connectionism."[20] The theory of natural selection does not in any way contradict a connectionist view of the brain. Nor do either of these two views preclude our understanding of the brain as an information processor. In early computer design, information was processed serially, one bit after another. The advent of computers with parallel processors (i.e., simultaneous processing) has resulted in learning capacities far more similar to those of human brains. The issue is that the innate structure of a connectionist set of interconnected processors, such as neurons, yields the ability to remember, compare, and generalize. This helps us understand how the brain carries out these fundamental functions that permit the processing of information.

A "localist view" of information processing proposes that representations may also be embedded in more localized neural assemblies—the simplest being a single neuron, amusingly termed a "grandmother cell." Localist and connectionist views may also work in concert, in that some processing may be locally constructed, whereas other processes may be more widely distributed.[21]

One way in which a connectionist model functions is to place "weights" or "degrees of strength" on the connections among basic elements—such as the neurons, in the case of the brain. When the relative strengths of the synaptic connections are altered, the information contained within the patterns of firing can be modified.[22] Subtle and rapid alterations in synaptic strengths are products of learning; the general ability to have connection strengths is innate and may be influenced by genetics, as well as by a wide range of neural processes in the brain itself.[23] Some of these connection strengths may be predetermined by our genetic inheritance: Our brains may be preprogrammed to create systems that tend to process certain forms of input preferentially, such as the faces of attachment figures in the case of our attachment systems. These innate values are of evolutionary benefit and remain encoded in our genetic endowment.[24] Appraisal systems can have inherited values that imbue emotional meaning in everyday life. But synaptic strengths may also be determined by experience by way of the process of neuroplasticity that allows learning to occur. Here we see how emotional experience may reinforce learning. In this manner, as we've seen, *experience affects the brain by altering the strengths of synaptic connections.*[25]

Complex systems are also believed to have an innate property that creates a sense of order, cohesion, and stability across time. As stated earlier, this emergent property is called "self-organization."[26] Natural selection, connectionism, and information-processing views are all compatible with a complex systems or dynamical perspective on self-organization. Evolutionary theory helps us understand how systems evolved into adaptively complex forms designed to carry out specific problem-solving behaviors. Connectionist theory helps us understand how these skills in processing information can be carried out within the three-dimensional substance of interconnected neural tissue. Our unique patterns of information processing reflect the fundamental components of the mind that are shaped by this evolutionary history and the physical reality of brain structure. Now we will add complexity theory to the conceptual mix in order to understand how the mind organizes its own functioning—and its states of mind.

The theory of nonlinear dynamics of complex systems, or complexity theory, provides several principles that will deepen our ability to understand many aspects of the mind, from emotions to human relationships. As Boldrini and colleagues have stated, "the spontaneity, unpredictability, and self-organizing properties of nonlinear dynamic systems are well suited to explain the notoriously spontaneous, unpredictable, and creative nature of human beings."[27] Dynamical systems are defined by being open to forces from outside of themselves and being capable of chaotic behavior. Dynamical systems have three major features: (1) They have self-organizational properties, (2) they are nonlinear, and (3) they have emergent patterns with recursive characteristics.[28] Let's take a closer look at each of these features.

## Self-Organization: The Movement toward Maximizing Complexity

Within an individual living being, *a driving force of development is the movement from simplicity toward complexity.* Esther Thelen has proposed that in child development, abilities such as reaching, crawling, and walking can be viewed as increasingly complex patterns of a child's behavior.[29] The unfolding of human development throughout the lifespan can be seen as governed by this movement toward increasing complexity. Rather than viewing development as stepwise increments in ability, we can view it as the emergence of increasingly complex interactions between children and their environment. A child responds to the environment with a variety of behaviors, such as trying to grasp a toy. Within a certain context, he then learns that a particular movement is coupled with a specific outcome, such as grasping the toy. When the toy is then covered in similar conditions, the child attempts to find it where it was before. If the effort is successful, the behavior is reinforced. From a dynamical viewpoint, the system is maximizing its complexity and therefore its stability by pushing behavior forward, applying old patterns in slightly new situations. Every moment, in fact, is the emergence of a unique pattern of activity in a world that is similar but never identical to a past moment in time.

Patterns of neural activation emerge in interaction with the environment. Certain patterns become fairly stable under specific conditions or contexts. These reinforced patterns or states of activation are called "attractor states." A state consists of the activity of each component of the system at a given point in time. With unfolding experience, and especially with the value systems of the living brain, certain states become more probable as they are engrained within the system. Those "states of mind" can therefore be seen as "attractor states" of the system. *The probability that a state of mind will be activated is determined by both history and present context or environmental conditions.*

The ability to remember an event from a long time ago is an example of an attractor state. If you try to recall your tenth day in junior high school, you may be unable to remember anything. However, if you try to recall the most embarrassing day you experienced during junior high school, you may become flooded with visual images and bodily sensations of that day. This activation of various components of your brain—the heterogeneous elements of your dynamical system—assemble themselves in a pattern representing your recollection of that day long ago. As elements of your brain become active, they may recruit other neuronal groups to join in the pattern of activation. Your value systems, including your appraisal centers, will have reinforced the strength of such an attractor state in the infinite range of possible patterns of neuronal activation. In this way, the self-organizational properties of the system create a sense of ordered complexity out of the trillions of synaptic connections that can be potentially fired.

*In the brain, we can propose that emotional responses constitute a primary value system that engrains patterns of neuronal firing and shapes the emergent states of activation of the system.* As states become engrained through repeated experience and emotional intensity, they become more likely to be activated. The emotional texture of a state of mind reflects the shifting states of integration (increasing or decreasing) that accompany the assembly and reassembly of states of mind across time. These attractor states help the system organize itself and achieve stability in the moment. Attractor states lend a degree of continuity to the infinitely possible options for activation profiles.

Repeated instantiation (activation) of a particular profile of activations, a state of mind, can make such a configuration a deeply engrained attractor state. What does this really mean? Think of this analogy. A hillside is filled with tall, flowing grass in the springtime. The snow has melted, and you seem to be the first person to take the trail to this spot. As you look out from the top of the hill, you notice that there are no paths toward the pond at the bottom. You wend your way down to the pond, spend a few hours there, and then walk back up the trail that you created earlier, so as to avoid stomping down any more grass. The next day, another hiker comes to the top of the hill, sees the pond, and without much thought follows your path down to the pond. He returns back up the hill the same way. Day after day, other travelers take the same path, carving into the vegetation on the hillside a path that did not exist before. The probability is high that other hikers will continue to take this pathway, further distinguishing it from other potential routes. As the feet keep pounding on the soil, any grass attempting to grow there will be flattened. The trail becomes this year's common pathway from the hill to the pond.

Such is the case for states of mind. With repeated activation, the state of mind becomes more deeply engrained, and the state is remembered. As discussed earlier, according to Hebb's approach as articulated by Carla Shatz,[30] "Neurons that fire together wire together." Shatz also emphasizes how such neural assemblies reinforce their associations with the phrase "out of sync, lose your link." With associated and synchronized neural firing, the brain is more likely to activate this clustering of processes in the future as a cohesive state of mind. As we'll see, the mind as an emergent property of both the embodied nervous system and relationships has a self-reinforcing quality to its organization, which serves as the mechanism for such reinforcement. Post and Weiss have provided a developmental perspective on Hebb's axiom: "Neurons which fire together, *survive together*, and wire together."[31] Thus repeated states of activation at critical early periods of development shape the structure of neuronal circuits, which then form the functional basis for enduring patterns of states of mind within the individual.

*Stability of the system is achieved by the movement toward maximizing complexity.* Complexity does not come from random activation, but instead is enhanced by a balance between the continuity and flexibility of the system. "Continuity" refers to the strength of previously achieved states, and therefore the probability of their repetition; it implies sameness, familiarity, and predictability. "Flexibility" indicates the system's degree of sensitivity to environmental conditions; it involves the capacity for variability, novelty,

> Stability of the system is achieved by the movement toward maximizing complexity.

and uncertainty. The ability to produce new variations allows the system to adapt to the environment. However, excessive variation or flexibility leads toward random activation. On the other hand, rigid adherence to previously engrained states produces excessive continuity and minimizes the system's ability to adapt and change.[32]

Mental disorder can be envisioned in part as restricting the overall movement of the system toward complexity by an imbalance in continuity and flexibility. Pathological states may force the system into disarray or rigidity; either one limits the movement of the system as a whole toward complexity and adaptation to the environment. In fact, as we've discussed earlier, the DSM-IV-TR[33] can be viewed as a collection of syndromes in which the various symptoms represent examples of chaos or rigidity. Integration—the linkage of differentiated parts—is the process that moves a system in a flexible and coherent way, like a choir singing in harmony. Naturally, all individuals, even those with psychiatric disorders, become more complicated as they develop; their brains and their relationships acquire more detail and intricacy as they move through life.

*Complicated is not the same as complex.* The scientific use of the term "complexity" refers to something very different from our everyday notions of something's being "complicated." For example, individuals with manic–depressive illness may have very complicated lives, in that they cannot rely on their own moods to be predictable. They may swing from the rigidity of depression to the chaos of mania. A very complicated set of interpersonal interactions and consequences may ensue, but we would not use the term "complex" to refer to this way of being. Complexity emerges from integration and the self-regulation of adaptive function. Integration is the natural outcome of self-organization in a complex system.[34] I am proposing that the dynamical systems view of self-organization (a mathematically derived emergent property of complex systems) is a process parallel to developmental psychopathology's view of "self-regulation." For a developmental psychopathologist, psychiatric disturbance is often an example of impaired self-regulation. From the consilient approach of IPNB, we can hypothesize that the mathematical emergent property of self-organization is related to, if not identical with, the biological and psychological notion of self-regulation.[35] If this is true, then we can take the next step to propose that the self-organizational movement toward complexity is harnessed to create the most flexible and adaptive self-regulation. Mathematically, when a complex system differentiates its elements and then functionally links them to each other, self-organization moves toward maximal complexity. The system also moves toward harmony when integration is achieved. For a biological system surviving with self-regulation at its core,

we can then ascribe these same notions of integration to the ways it functions. For a living entity, such as a person or a family, when integration is
impaired, self-regulation is compromised and the individual system is prone
to chaos and/or rigidity. We explode in rage, or we shut down in paralyzing
fear. These are both examples of diminished complexity, even though life has
become more complicated for such an individual. Integration, in contrast,
enables coordination and balance as elements of a system are both differentiated and linked. Recent studies of the "default mode"—the state of brain
activity when an individual is given no instructions—reveal the importance
of integration in healthy brain function.[36] When the default mode is studied alongside the functional neuroanatomy of bipolar illness,[37] we see clear
support for the view of impaired linkage in this disorder. Studies of PTSD
suggest that excessive coupling (too much linkage without the necessary differentiation) is present in this condition.[38] Integration is more like making
a fruit salad than making a smoothie: It requires that elements retain their
individual uniqueness while simultaneously linking to other components of
a system. The key is balance of differentiation and linkage. Some researchers
have found that child abuse and neglect impair the growth of the integrative
fibers of the brain,[39] supporting the notion that healthy states emerge from
and also promote integration in the brain.

I am proposing here that integration is the foundation of regulation.
That is, we achieve balanced self-regulation by integrating neural systems
and interpersonal relationships. When a system is regulated, it promotes the
creation of further integration. Integration is both a functional process (the
linkage of differentiated elements) and also a structural feature of the nervous system and relationships. Self-regulation is a process that emerges as a
system moves through time, and thus it is a functional process—one whose
existence may be discovered structurally through the presence of integrative
fibers in the brain. The flow of states of
mind across time may serve as an important measure of the whole system's coherent functioning. An individual may experience relatively cohesive states that, in
isolation, function fairly well. However, the individual's ability to integrate
states of mind across time into a coherent whole may be restricted if these
cohesive states are themselves conflictual.

> We achieve balanced self-regulation by integrating neural systems and interpersonal relationships.

## Nonlinearity

In the second basic principle of complexity theory, dynamical systems are
called "nonlinear," because a small change in input can lead to huge and
unpredictable changes in outcome. Part of this unpredictability is due to the

context–dependent nature of the system's response. The unpredictability also stems in part from the fact that the system as a whole is inherently "noisy"; this means that there will be random activations that may or may not be reinforced by encounters with the environment. Systems have both determinate (predictable) and indeterminate features to their behavior.[40] Because of these features, *small changes in the microcomponents of the system can lead to large changes in the macro-level behavior of the organism.*

In viewing the mind as a complex system, we can see that "dysfunction" at one level of organization may produce large changes in the functioning of other levels and of the system as a whole. Within brain activity, one can envision these changes in the functioning of the mind as emanating, for example, from particular regions responsible for an emotion such as fear. In the case of obsessive–compulsive disorder, an excessive signal, coming from a limbic system that "checks" the environment for danger and finds evidence for fear when in fact there is none, can cause a cascade of responses from other systems in the brain: a sense of panic, with heart rate racing; obsessions composed of complex, abstract thoughts about death; and compulsive behaviors irrationally designed to avoid catastrophe.[41] Though the origin of a dysfunction may emanate from the atypical messages sent from one component of the brain, the cascade of subsequent reactions can be unpredictable, can be huge, and can involve a widely distributed response from other components as well as from the brain and the mind as a whole. This is nonlinearity at its most painful, out-of-control worst.

On the more beneficial side of nonlinearity is the finding that small changes in a person's perspective, beliefs, or mental associations can suddenly lead to large changes in state of mind and behavior. For example, the art of psychotherapy can be seen as finding a way to align oneself as a therapist with a patient in such a fashion as to know what sort of change is needed and what alterations in the constraints on the system might permit such changes to occur. Some of the most difficult kinds of ruts can be reinforced by deeply engrained, inflexible attractor states, including bad habits, intrusive memories, or isolation of information processing. For some people, a small change in behavior or memory processing can yield subsequent changes in mental set (or system state) that produce large changes in behavior and internal experience. The often challenging task is to figure out which system changes are needed in order to alter the constraints on rigidly engrained attractor states.

## Emergent and Recursive Patterns

A third property of the nonlinear dynamics of complex systems is the emergent and recursive properties of their patterns of organization. "Emergent" means arising from the interaction of elements of the system,[42] and one emergent property of a complex system is self-organization. In living systems, there is no programmer, no predesigned formula for the unfolding of experience. As elements are differentiated and linked, as they become integrated, the system self-organizes to maximize complexity. "Recursive" means that the effects of a given state of mind return to further influence the emergence of future states. We are always in a perpetual state of being created and creating ourselves. We will never be the same, and we have never been quite the way we are right at this moment. This emergence of being as we flow from state to state is characterized by an underlying sense that there is an incredible amount of both freedom and cohesion within the system in a given moment. As a person's states of mind emerge in ways determined by the system's own internal constraints and by the external constraints of interpersonal connections with others, the self is perpetually being created.

When we focus on perceiving reality as it is in the present, we can each experience this emergence as a sense of vitality and freshness. Recursive or repeating patterns in states of mind can bring a sense of familiarity to new encounters. This recursive quality reinforces patterns of response learned from earlier encounters with the world. In this way, past events can then have an impact on present moment experience. To use an earlier example, if you were scratched and frightened by a cat as a child, seeing a cat approach now may start your heart pounding and your palms sweating. These are implicit memory reactivations in the limbic regions and brainstem; they are recursive, arising from the past and influencing your present. This quality of having a recursive filtering from past influences can be adaptive in certain circumstances. Sometimes things that have frightened us in the past should continue to be avoided at all costs. In those cases, we need to respond rapidly, long before our cortical thought processes can decide to act. When engrained and restrictive patterns are taken to their extremes and become tyrants, however, the mind can become deadened to the vital and emergent uniqueness of lived experience. If your recursive response to the cat is not a tyrant, then it becomes possible for you to modulate the fear and experience the new cat in the new situation where there is likely to be a new, emergent outcome not imprisoned by the past.

The recursive nature of complex systems is revealed in the increasing specialization of a system's trajectory of states. Early in development, for example, a wide array of states may be possible; as the system or organism evolves, it develops a more limited and more specialized set of possible states. This increases the system's differentiation, based on the coordination of basic elements, into a more highly coupled, integrated system. Such differentiation may be a product of genetically encoded information, the unfolding of developmental processes in transaction with experience, and the ongoing emergence of self-organizing brain states across time. Though at first glance such differentiation with limitations in possible states may appear to limit the system's flow, such a differentiated system actually enables states of activation to achieve more complexity. In this manner, the recursive, self-perpetuating nature of development moves the system toward increasingly differentiated and integrated states. As we'll see later in this and subsequent chapters, when differentiated subcomponent elements become functionally coupled into a larger system, such integration allows for continued movement toward maximizing complexity.

## Constraints

The system attains a balance between continuity and flexibility by having the ability to modify what are called the "constraints" on the system. These constraints are both internal (such as synaptic strength) and external (such as interactions with the environment). The modification of constraints is *not* performed by a hidden designer, a "homunculus," or a "ghost in the machine"—that is, by some mind within the mind whose purpose is to help the organism adapt or organize its functioning. Constraints are modified by the mathematically predictable probabilities of the activities of the subcomponents of the system. The emergent mind organizes itself automatically, based on its ability to modify internal or external constraints. *The mind uses the brain and relationships to create itself.*

Adaptation occurs through modification of constraints. Self-organization is dependent upon the modification of constraints in an effort to achieve maximal complexity. Dysfunctions in self-organization can be conceptualized as due to any pattern of constraint that does not permit movement toward such complexity. As we'll see, patterns of modifying constraints can be effective in adapting to environmental conditions at one time, but can produce later limitations on movement toward maximal complexity. This general process may be the source of psychological dysfunction.[43]

> The mind uses the brain and relationships to create itself.

Within given states of mind, dysfunction may be revealed as an incohesive clustering of mental processes. In PTSD, for example, intrusions of memory, hypervigilance, and excessive arousal are experienced as fragmented mental states. In the states of mind characteristic of other disorders, such as personality disorders or chronic anxiety, there may be a semistable cohesiveness in which the isolated elements of the particular states of mind have a cohesive functional quality within themselves.

## Attachment and Self-Organization

Attachment patterns illustrate how adaptation to the structure of parent–child communication can result in children's modification of constraints in characteristic ways to regulate their states of mind. For example, a securely attached infant uses both (external) communication with her mother and her own (internal) regulatory functions to help organize her self-system. During the first few years of life, this process involves a direct response of each partner to the signals of the other. As we've discussed in Chapter 3, Aitken and Trevarthen have defined this as "primary intersubjectivity."[44] As the child develops into the second half of the first year, her ability to have a representation of the mother, or a "virtual mother," allows for the interaction of the two to have a secondary intersubjective quality in which the child's perceptions of the mother are filtered through her expectations of the virtual, mentally constructed representation of the mother.

In the case of a securely attached infant, the perceptive, sensitive, responsive, and predictable communication from the parent allows a close correspondence between the infant's virtual parent and the actual parent. Cooperative communication involving the parent's capacity to perceive and respond to the child's mental state is the hallmark of a securely attached dyad.[45] These mutually attuned experiences allow the infant to develop a reflective capacity that helps to create a sense of cohesion and interpersonal connection. The other's mental state is a positive element in the infant's life. The securely attached infant is able to use these communicative experiences with the parent to help regulate her internal state. Self-organization is thus achieved through a balance in the infant's use of external constraints (the attachment relationship) and internal constraints (the internal representations of the caregiver and of the attachment relationship itself). In our day-to-day lives, the degree of social support we feel helps modulate our stress response.[46] Holding the hand or seeing a photo of someone you love and trust can actually decrease your brain's anticipatory anxiety, as well as its neural response to a painful shock.[47]

An avoidantly attached infant, on the other hand, must rely primarily upon his own (internal) constraints to keep his system functioning. The emotionally barren and noncooperative nature of the patterns of communication lead to a nonresponsive virtual (representational) parent and to excessive reliance on internal constraints to achieve self-regulation. Reflective functioning is not developed well, in that the parent's mental state is not available to the child. The actual mother provides little sense of mutual regulation; the acquired virtual mother offers little internal regulation. The learned autonomy keeps the individual's system isolated from that of others.

Ambivalently attached infants find themselves excessively responsive to their inconsistent attachment figures and unable to soothe themselves. Their virtual parents are unreliable; their internal working models of attachment are filled with uncertainty; and their capacity for self-regulation is compromised. Their distress becomes a dominant feature in their interactions with others. Though reflective functioning may be facilitated by the (inconsistently) available caregiving, mental states are often experienced as intrusive and not helpful in regulating the self. These children come to experience an approach–withdrawal cycle that leaves them in distress and yet clinging to others in attempts to achieve self-organization.

Infants with disorganized attachments are unable to use either internal or external means to regulate their internal states. They live in a chaotic internal world that reflects the external source of terror in the parents' behavior, which is incompatible with attachment and a sense of security. These infants are prone to have fragmented self-organizational patterns; achieving a coherent state of mind is quite difficult under stressful situations, especially those involving separation and threat.[48] As noted in Chapter 3, these children are vulnerable to developing dissociative disorders and are more likely to develop clinical symptoms in response to overwhelming experiences. Reflective functioning may vary from state to state, as the parents may have been available in certain modes of being and quite threatening in other states. These children's fragmented internal worlds come to resemble the fragmenting interpersonal communication that shapes the development of their minds.

Beebe and colleagues' studies of communication patterns within various mother–child dyads have suggested the following findings. In avoidantly attached pairs, vocal rhythm matching (in which the response of one person corresponds to that of the partner) demonstrates a marked independence of communication signals. Each member communicates almost as if the other hasn't been heard. With ambivalently attached pairs, at the other extreme, there is an excessively matched pattern of response. Each individual acts as a tightly bound mirror of the other. Securely attached dyads have a midrange balance in which there is clearly a correspondence between signals, but each member has the freedom to vary responses, which in turn will be registered and contingently responded to by the partner.[49]

Applying complexity theory, we can propose that the midrange response in communicative contingency is the pattern allowing the maximal complexity to be achieved. In this situation, we can suggest that two systems have become functionally linked or integrated in a manner that allows them to function as a single, complex system. *Maximal complexity* is achieved by the combination of individual differentiation and interpersonal linkage. In contrast, being independent from one's partner (as avoidantly attached children are) is a situation in which the system of one individual acts as if alone, decreasing complexity by way of excessive internal continuity devoid of linkage. Being tightly coupled with another also decreases complexity. Intrusive matching, or paralyzed mirroring of the other, reduces variability between the interacting systems; they are excessively linked, lacking in differentiation.

People may experience a range of rhythm matching with other individuals, often in nonverbal ways. Some people are exquisitely responsive to the most subtle nuances of others' signals—a yawn, a glance out the window, a concerned look. Others seem, at least to an observer, to be oblivious to other persons' signals. This range of matching can be used to gain insight into people's present experience with others and past communication patterns. As an emergent property of a dynamical system, the mind may be restricted in its balanced movement toward complexity either by excessive responsiveness to others or by an intense autonomy and resistance to joining with others' states. Still other people may tend toward dissociative states, in which the overall state of mind can only be assembled by dis-associations of the component parts of mental functioning.

## STATES OF MIND ACROSS TIME

The activity of the brain and the sharing of energy and information within relationships create the mind. We have reviewed how neural activity is composed of the flow of energy through a complex neural network that serves the purpose of carrying and transforming mental representations, or information. The processing of this information allows the mind to solve problems. The specific pattern of energy flow of through the brain activates a particular neural net profile or state of mind. Emotion and its regulation play a central role in determining degrees and localization of neural activation. As we've proposed in this text, emotion reflects shifts in the state of integration. A state of mind is assembled by alteration in how differentiated areas become linked to one another, In other words, a state of mind is created by shifts in integration, and so emotion is at the core of the emergence and maintenance of a state of mind. Emotion in the brain is fundamentally linked to the same circuitry that is responsible for creating meaning and value for mental representations. It is no surprise that particular emotions become associated with particular states of mind: Emotions are a fundamental part of the process that creates a state of mind at a particular moment in time.

> Emotions are a fundamental part of the process that creates a state of mind at a particular moment in time.

Marc Lewis and colleagues have noted that the energy flow within states of mind can be seen as a flow of information through a self-organizing system.[50] Emotions reveal the way in which a system regulates its states of activation in processing information. Woltering and Lewis state that "specific neural 'hubs,' such as the anterior cingulate cortex and the orbitofrontal cortex, which serve as epicenters for the coupling of cortical and subcortical processes," play an important role as the "increasing coordination between brain regions during emotional situations subserves more effective and efficient regulation with development."[51] This self-organization is also dyadic—a part of the interaction between two people—and not only a part of the neural integration within the body. Self-organization reflects the fundamental way in which the mind is created within interpersonal interactions and neurophysiological processes.[52] As Schore has commented, "These transactions represent a flow of interpersonal information accompanying emotion, and critical fluctuations, amplified by positive feedback, lead to disequilibrium and self-organization."[53] The state of the system is dependent upon the induction of alterations, or disequilibrium, in the movement toward self-organization.[54] These alterations are created by emotional transactions with others.

Marc Lewis has suggested:

> Because each episode of real-time cognitive–emotional activity leaves some degree of synaptic change in its wake, we can say that brains develop by elaborating and extending the outcomes of their own activities. And synaptic alterations are recursive, which means that these activities tend to repeat themselves, forming lineages of individual patterning that progressively elaborate their own emergent themes. These features of neural development epitomize self-organization in natural systems. Moreover, because brain activities also change the interpersonal environment (e.g., aggression promotes isolation, independence promotes mastery and admiration), this sequence of self-elaboration occurs in the context of a social world that becomes progressively more shaped to the features of the individual brain. If our minds were not inscribed in flesh, we would not have to worry about the properties of complex dynamic systems. But our minds are greatly dependent on our brains, and brains are designed by evolution to self-organize rapidly under the sway of experiences and the emotions that color them. Therefore, to understand developing minds, we need to understand developing brains, and the principles of self-organization provide a foundation for doing so.[55]

In clinical practice, therapists see a continuity of behavioral and emotional responses that can make people inflexible, nonproductive, dysfunctional, and unhappy. Their minds have lost the capacity for adaptive self-organization and have become stuck in inflexible patterns of activation. These are among the many reasons individuals may come to a psychotherapist for help. Certainly people show unpredictable, spontaneous behaviors that seem to "come out of nowhere." These are "expected" from the nonlinearity of complex systems. As Boldrini and colleagues have stated,

> In chaotic systems, several different patterns of movements are simultaneously present and very small changes in initial conditions can alter the system's trajectory. The system can itself give rise to turbulence and, under some circumstances, this leads to an evolutionary advantage, while, in other cases, it does not yield stability, but leads to intermittent chaos.[56]

Often people who seek psychotherapeutic help feel stuck in patterns of response; they are desperate to change their internal experience but have been unable to do so. To help patients alter such engrained and unhelpful patterns in the flow of states of mind, therapists need to consider how the brain establishes such a continuity across time and what interventions can be designed to change such a process.

Emotion is central to helpful change, but is also central to the process of how we get stuck in certain recursive patterns. Lewis illuminates the dual nature of emotion in dysfunction and transformation in this way:

> The role of emotion in neural self-organization thus functions as a double-edged sword. On one hand, self-*augmenting* feedback, orchestrated by limbic and paralimbic structures with the help of ascending neuromodulators, promotes synaptic activity *and hence initiates synaptic change*. In this respect, emotional processes yield novel synaptic configurations. On the other hand, self-*stabilizing* feedback, orchestrated by the same structures and neuromodulators, but lasting longer and recruiting additional subsystems, consolidates patterns of synaptic activity *and hence minimizes synaptic change*. In this respect, emotional processes are central to the maintenance of synaptic patterning. Thus, emotional processes cut both ways: they generate synaptic change and they maintain synaptic sameness.[57]

Continuity in the flow of states across time is established in part by internal constraints—the neuronal connections that have been established by constitution and experience. In such a model of probabilities, the system moves toward increasing levels of complexity while maintaining elements of continuity, sameness, and familiarity in the face of new and unfamiliar activation patterns. The system by its very structure has a property that maintains some aspect of continuity. As the system produces outputs (behaviors in response to the environment), these too can produce a somewhat consistent pattern of reactions from the outside world, and thus can shape external constraints. For example, shy children may alter their responses to novelty slightly, but their hesitation may continue to irritate their parents, whose frustration continues to reinforce the children's anxiety. The result is that the seemingly "independent" variable of the external (parental) constraints is actually directly influenced by the children themselves. As we will discuss in Chapter 6, some studies suggest that behaviorally inhibited or shy children have a constitutionally active right hemisphere, which produces excessive withdrawal states. Negative responses from parents may reinforce such withdrawal reactions within their children. The system that began with a certain characteristic predisposition establishes continuity through both the internal and external constraints on its flow of states across time.

## Information Processing

One way of viewing a state of mind is that the profile of activation includes *which* modules of information processing are active, as well as *what* they are processing. Of note is that certain circuits that function well in some states appear to be markedly impaired in depressed states—as evidenced, for example, by decreased ability to detect facial emotion and the corresponding brain imaging findings of decreased right-hemisphere blood flow during these tasks. In depression, the circuits for processing facial affect are not functioning normally.[58] The recursive (feedback-loop) nature of states of mind is such that the blockage of this module may reinforce the intensity of the very state of mind that produced the blockage. In other words, the depressed person loses the ability to utilize the facial expressions of others to help modulate his own emotional state. External constraints become unavailable, and the person must rely on the isolated and depressed functioning of the internal constraints alone. Such a person feels and is truly disconnected from others. Here, again, we see an illumination of the embodied and relational nature of the mind.

The selective activation or deactivation of information-processing modules of the mind creates its own continuity in the creation of a given state of mind. As Hofer has stated, "To accomplish various age-specific tasks, the brain must be able to shift from one state of functional organization to another and thus from one mode of information processing to others within an essential modular structure."[59] As clusters of neurons can become rapidly activated or deactivated in the creation of a state of mind, the pattern of neural firing can reflect abrupt shifts in self-organization. The complex system of the brain is inherently capable of abrupt transitions in states. One way of characterizing the nature of the brain's self-organizing properties is through its coordination of such transitions: When a brain remains stuck in a given state, such as depression, or exhibits dysregulated and abrupt shifts in state, such as in dissociation, this may be due to dysfunctional self-organization.

How does the encapsulated episode of experience, the state of mind, become reinforced by the process of self-organization? The characteristic flow of information within a given state helps to define its own boundaries. Being furious can lead to certain thoughts, images, and sensations that reinforce themselves in a rageful state. As this processing begins to become more flexible, the intensity of the state begins to subside, and the state dissolves into a more neutral flow of activations. In this manner, certain states have fairly definable boundaries and characteristics. Others are more adaptive and flexible in the patterns of activation that become clustered as a functional unit. In these more "fluid" and "neutral" states, there may be less easily defined beginnings and endings. Thus the *flexibility* in information-processing modules may help define the flow of states across time, rather than merely the processing by itself.

## Continuity and Self-States

As we've seen in the case of disorganized attachment, unresolved trauma, and dissociation, the mind is capable of clustering its modules and the content of their information within fairly distinct states of mind. But is this the case only in those who have experienced disorganized attachments or childhood trauma? The answer appears to be no. Studies in child development suggest, in fact, that the idea of a unitary, continuous "self" is actually an illusion our minds attempt to create.[60] Childhood is filled with typical examples of the many ways in which a child must "be"—different roles to take, in order to adapt to different social contexts (with parents, siblings, peers, teachers). Adolescence is filled with new challenges to deal with the emergence of new "selves" with seemingly separate identities: a sexual self, a student self, a self independent of parents.[61] Recent brain studies suggest that adolescents utilize more social circuitry in self-evaluations than adults.[62]

> The idea of a unitary, continuous "self" is actually an illusion our minds attempt to create.

Even in cognitive science, the mind is considered as having many distinct "parts" responsible for a wide array of activities, from feeding and reproduction to affiliation and reading other people's minds. As intelligent beings with desires and beliefs, we attempt to achieve our goals by assessing our situations and applying our internal rules to interactions with the environment. Our many layers of information processing have unique sets of rules, as well as specialized problems they are attempting to solve. Dividing these information-processing modules is necessary to carry out efficient interactions with others in the world. We have multiple and varied "selves," which are needed to carry out the many and diverse activities of our lives.

As we are also profoundly connected to others in an ever-changing and interdependent web of social relationships, we can also say that the "self" is not a singular noun, but rather is a plural verb. We are not just an isolated, separate self, but an ever-emerging process of "selfing" linked with other evolving selves over time.

Alan Sroufe has defined the "self" as an internally organized cluster of attitudes, expectations, meanings, and feelings.[63] In his view, the self emerges from an "organized caregiving matrix" that in part determines how the individual responds to and engages with or avoids the environment. Relationships also determine how children interpret experience.[64] An extension of this view, in combination with Susan Harter's research on the many "selves" of typical development, suggests that the "selves" in which we live are dependent upon relationship context.[65] Furthermore, our relationship histories may have shaped particular patterns of feelings, attitudes, and meanings that are more likely to become activated in the future. In these ways, history and present context shape whichever "self" is organized in the moment. As relationship experiences are repeated, these "self-states" become repeatedly engrained and develop their own histories and patterns of activity across time.

As we can see, both developmental studies and cognitive science appear to suggest that we have many selves. Within a specialized "self" or "self-state," as we are now defining it, there is cohesion in the moment and continuity across time. For example, a person's sexual self is made up of all the states of mind that have been clustered over time to deal with sexual information: sexual arousal from within, sexual interaction with others. This sexual self then has a continuity by virtue of its connection strengths or internal system constraints, as discussed earlier. Within this continuity is a sense of cohesion. That is, the various modules of the mind cluster together in the service of specialized activity—processing information in order to achieve a particular goal. Within this cohesion of the specialized self emerges a continuity across time (in that self-state) of feelings, beliefs, intentions, memories, and so forth, which creates a qualitative sense of unity.

A person's mental life as a whole functions as a system that exists across time and is composed of many relatively distinct but interdependent states. As a complex system, it is made up of subcomponent specialized self-states, as well as itself being a subcomponent of a larger interpersonal system. Let's continue to examine this issue of the continuity across states by looking at the selves of the mind.

Here's a bit of vocabulary clarification. We can use the term "state of mind" to refer to the cluster of brain activity (and mental modules) at a given moment in time. This "moment" can be brief or extended, and states of mind can have various degrees of sharpness or blurriness to their boundaries across time. The repeated activation of states of mind as time goes by—over weeks, months, and years—can become a specialized, goal-directed set of cohesive functional units. We can call this a "specialized self" or "self-state."

The most basic division of self-states is into a private, inner self and a public, outer self, which has been described in Chapter 4. Developmental studies have examined how individuals struggle with their various roles in life and how these may be composed of various degrees of "true" or "false" selfhood.[66] Other examples of specialized selves include sexual, affiliative, status-seeking, survival-oriented, and intellectual selves. Clearly the divisions could go on and on, until we get back to our basic unit of the state of mind in a given moment in time. And this is just the point: How does the mind create a sense of continuity across states of mind, if it does at all?

The proposal here is that *basic states of mind are clustered into specialized selves, which are enduring states of mind that have a repeating pattern of activity across time.* These specialized selves or self-states each have relatively specialized and somewhat independent modes of processing information and achieving goals. Each person has many such interdependent and yet distinct processes, which exist over time with a sense of continuity that creates the experience of mental life.

Susan Harter and colleagues' developmental studies suggest that certain self-states may conflict with each other.[67] Such conflicts may be a central source of dysfunction, especially during adolescence. Also, the more extreme the degree of "false selfhood" within specialized selves, the more individuals may experience a sense of disconnection from others and from themselves. How a person resolves such conflicts may be an important determinant of future emotional resilience.[68] The phenomenon of resilience itself may be multifaceted.

For example, children exposed to disorganizing forms of attachment may vary in their response to such developmental forms of interpersonal trauma, according to the genetic variants and changes in epigenetic regulation they have that shape neurotransmitter function.[69] Synaptic shadows created by past experience and innate genetic features can create enduring patterns across the lifespan. The question about well-being and resilience may not be whether there is a sense of unifying *continuity*, but how the mind integrates a sense of *coherence*—of effective functioning—across self-states through time.

*If people become stuck and disabled, if they are filled with adaptive specialized selves without a sense of authenticity, or if they are filled with intense and unresolved conflicts across self-states, then the development of a specific process that integrates the selves across time may become important.* Clinicians often encounter patients who face these dilemmas. Catalyzing the development of such an integrating process may be the central feature of psychotherapy for these individuals. The next chapters will examine how the mind achieves integration and self-regulation, and how interpersonal relationships can assist people in developing the vital capacity to transform their self-organization.

## INTERPERSONAL SYSTEMS AND DYADIC STATES OF MIND

Our review of complex systems and the example of how attachment experiences shape patterns of self-regulation raises the issue of how two individuals come to function as a dyadic system.[70] Various theories of social psychology and psychodynamics suggest that learning, communication, role modeling, internalization, idealization, and identification may each play a role in how children develop.[71] We can also look at the question from the point of view of the mind as emanating in part from the complex system of the brain.

Consider the following. The mind of one person, $A$, organizes itself on the basis of both internal and external constraints. Internal constraints are determined by constitutional features and experience. External constraints include the signals sent from others in the environment. Person $B$ is in a relationship with $A$. $A$ perceives the signals sent from $B$, and $A$'s system responds by altering its state. Two immediate effects are (1) that $A$'s state shifts as a function of $B$'s state (or at least $B$'s signals), and (2) that $A$ sends signals back to $B$. $B$ in turn responds to $A$'s signals with at least these two alterations, and contingent communication is established. If $A$ is an adult and $B$ is a baby, then the pattern of responses will shape the function and the developing structure of $B$'s immature brain, not merely $B$'s present state of mind. So what's new about this view?

What's new is that the *patterns* of $A$'s response to $B$ and $B$'s response to $A$ can begin to shape the states that are created in both $A$ and $B$. $A$ and $B$ come to function as a supersystem, $AB$. One can no longer reduce the interactions of $A$ and $B$ to the subcomponents $A$ and $B$; $AB$ is an irreducible system. Systems theory provides a hierarchical understanding of interpersonal relationships. For some people, sharing an "interpersonal state" is one of the most rewarding experiences in human life. For others, such dyadic states are occasionally welcome, but a hefty dose of isolation is preferred to the feeling of "disappearance" that such an $AB$ state may create. Still others long for such a union, but feel they can never truly achieve it. Even when they are "almost in it," they fear it will disappear; that very fear can itself destroy the dyadic experience. Is this just another way of talking about the different attachment patterns? Certainly the attachment approaches may represent variations on the fundamental "I–thou" theme. There are selves, others, and their relationships together. But systems theory offers us a perspective and vocabulary on the constraints that help the system organize itself. These internal and external factors provide a new framework for understanding how one mind joins with others to form a larger functional system.

The imprint of a parent's patterns of self-organization is manifested within a child's own patterns of self-regulation. In this way, the joining of two systems into a single supersystem may continue to show its effects even when the child is away from the adult, or when the child has grown up. For example, in children with disorganized attachments and in dissociative adults, their chaotic and terrifying experiences with caregivers may have become not only a part of

> The imprint of a parent's patterns of self-organization is manifested within a child's own patterns of self-regulation.

their memories, but a part of the very structure of their self-(dys)regulation. Even the epigenetic regulation of gene expression in neural regions involved in the stress response may be negatively altered.[72] Neural structure, abnormal stress response, and epigenetic changes interact to maintain impediments to the healthy regulation of states of mind. Such is the effect of early trauma on the developing mind.

Understanding the behavior of complex systems can provide insights into the sometimes automatic ways in which relationships with others seem to evolve. Looking toward the interpersonal state as the fundamental unit of "self-organization" for a relationship can be very helpful. For example, relationships that become stuck can be envisioned as unable to move in a balanced way toward increasing complexity in their interpersonal states. Rigid styles of communicating and unwillingness to enter into intense sharing of primary emotional states may lead to a sense of "deadness" in a relationship. The states of an emotional relationship may reflect elements of here-and-now communication and remnants of past patterns of relating. Individuals join with each other in creating a system larger than the individual self.

Often the shift between states of mind within a dyadic relationship may be quite subtle. Context changes can be hidden—induced, for example, by alterations in a companion's tone of voice or facial expression. The ways we join with another person in forming an interpersonal system with its own emerging dyadic states can often be quite rapid and nonverbal.

Let's look at the example from earlier in this chapter of how an adult can experience a shift in her state of mind when she returns home for the holidays. If a family is viewed as a supersystem, a cluster of the smaller systems of its individual members, then we can begin to make sense of this common phenomenon. As we've seen, a state of mind includes the assembly of various processes via reentry loops, each of which may emanate from the activity of relatively distinct circuits in the brain. A state of mind involves the recruitment of these various subsystems into activity together—in other words, the coupling of disparate processes into a simultaneous set of reentrant, coassembled activating components. The adult child has her own developmental history in which her genetics and repeated encounters with the environment have reinforced her states of mind—specific patterns of clustered neuronal activations that are sensitive to initial, specific environmental conditions. Her parents also have their own developmental histories, part of which includes having her as their child. Their histories have created specific states and patterns of response. They may have been quite happy during the years since their daughter has moved away, but somehow on these holiday visits things for them, and for her, fall back into old patterns.

The context shift of the grown child's returning home—possibly sleeping in the same room, eating meals with her parents, having siblings present, and experiencing other old and familiar conditions—reestablishes a fertile setting in which each family member's mind can respond. The new contextual frame evokes old attractor states. Literally, what this means is that each of their brains is responding to this new setting with an alteration in its individual constraints to make old patterns of states of mind more likely to occur. The recruitment or coassembly of components of the individuals within the family allows us to see how the larger framework of a supersystem contains its own developmental history, with attractor states and coupling processes of its own. Recruitment is often automatic, without conscious awareness or intention. The family now functions as a whole system, reinstating its old attractor states. For the adult child, the experience may be one of being drawn back into old sensations and patterns of behavior without her initial awareness or sense of control.

Recall that states of mind contain the clustering of perceptual biasing, behavioral response patterns, emotional tone and regulation, memory processing, and mental models. For the adult child's parents, all of this may involve interpreting her behavior as oppositional, being harsh and critical in their own behavior, feeling scared and distrustful of her, recalling various conflicts she's had with them, and having a mental model of her as an impulsive, uncooperative teenager. Their shift in state probably occurs simultaneously with their daughter's. She may view their behavior as controlling and insensitive to her needs; she may find herself responding to them with impatience and disrespect; she may feel angry and disappointed, and challenged to keep these feelings from overwhelming her; she may have easier access to the memories of the painful years of her adolescence; and she may have a mental model of her parents as being unsupportive and of herself as a victim of their shortcomings.

The rapidity with which these virtually simultaneous and instantaneous shifts in state can occur once the daughter arrives back at her parents' home is astonishing. Neither part of this supersystem is to "blame" for such changes. Each subset of the larger system is taking part in a shift in state based on present context. Subsequent, often subtle, responses of one component to another reinforce the "appropriateness" of such shifts for adaptation. The daughter may find herself saying, "I knew I shouldn't have come home. They never change. This is hopeless." She may be right. Or she may be experiencing the tenacity of old attractor states, both within herself and within her parents, and especially within the relationship system. As her sense of helplessness continues, and the rapid interactions return to their old patterns, the old and painful mental state configurations are reinforced yet again. At this moment, she is in desperate need of a "change"—a way of healing old wounds and lifting herself out of engrained and dysfunctional patterns of dyadic self-organization.

Each of us needs periods in which our minds can focus inwardly. This process can be called "time-in" and constitutes a part of what might be considered a daily mental nutrient to promote well-being. Solitude is an essential experience for the mind to organize its own processes and create an internal state of resonance. In such a state, the self is able to alter its constraints by directly reducing the input from interactions with others. As the mind goes through alternating phases of needing connection and needing solitude, the states of mind are cyclically influenced by combinations of external and internal processes. We can propose that such a shifting of focus allows the

> Each of us needs periods in which our minds can focus inwardly.

mind to achieve a balanced self-organizational flow in the states of mind across time. Some forms of mindfulness practice may be examples of time-in training of such internally attuned attention.[73] The inspiring poet and philosopher John O'Donohue has written: "When you acknowledge the integrity of your solitude and settle into its mystery, your relationships with others take on a new warmth, adventure, and wonder. . . . If you bring courage to your solitude, you learn you need not be afraid. . . . Human solitude is rich and endlessly creative."[74] Respecting the need for solitude allows the mind to "heal" itself—which in essence can be seen as releasing the natural self-organizational tendencies of the mind to create a balanced flow of states. Solitude permits the self to reflect on engrained patterns and intentionally alter reflexive responses to external events that have been maintaining dyadic dysfunction.

We are all nonlinear dynamical systems. This means that small changes in input can lead to large, often unpredictable changes in response. It also means that good portions of human behavior and the human mind are unpredictable in the long run. If the adult daughter in our example becomes aware of these old patterns and decides, consciously, not to take part in them, she may find that they begin to change a bit. Solitude may permit the reflection necessary to enable her to initiate such changes. If she then makes a deliberate effort to alter her state—and especially her behavioral responses and patterns of communication—major changes in interpersonal interactions may occur. It takes diligence, but for many people, pulling out of the automatic reflexes of old family patterns is worth the effort. The daughter's changes in response, her internal awareness of her own and the family's processes, and her willingness to give up old beliefs that "I am right and they are wrong" can each bring about an alteration in system constraints, which can shift the patterns of the family system's trajectory, its pattern of state shifts, and subsequent behavioral patterns.

We have noted throughout this chapter that repeated activation of states, especially those involving significant emotional intensity during the early years of development, makes them more likely to be repeated in the future. In this manner, historical patterns of states of mind, both within an individual and within a family system, may become characteristic traits. It is in this way that attractor states become engrained within us and allow old interpersonal states to continue to influence our individual patterns of self-organization.

Rigidly engrained states reduce variability in the system, which diminishes its adaptability to the environment and its capacity to maximize the system's complexity. Self-organization is always attempting to move us toward increasing levels of complexity, and it is inhibited if flexibility is reduced. When states have become so engrained as to inhibit exploration of new possibilities, the people affected can no longer grow and develop.[75] The subjective experience of such a condition is one of stagnation and malaise. Bringing new life to stuck patterns means infusing energy into a system, destabilizing old states, and establishing a new balance between continuity and flexibility—one that will allow for emergent states of increasing complexity. Such emergent states of mind within responsive interpersonal relationships can create an electrifying sense of vitality.

## REFLECTIONS: THE FLOW OF STATES

Emotional growth is based on the movement of dynamical systems toward a balance between continuity and flexibility in the flow of states across time. A balanced flow of energy within the system is a goal of emotional development. This balance is without rigid constraints on which neuronal groups will be recruited and without chaotic activations. Either excessively rigid or excessively disorganized self-regulation limits the stabilizing movement toward increasing levels of complexity of the system. These conditions reflect emotional dysregulation.

The attainment of maximum complexity is a function of the system's balance between flexibility and continuity. Flexibility is based on the generation of a diversity of responses and variation in the flow of states; it allows for a degree of uncertainty that leaves room for novel adaptations to changing environmental conditions. In contrast, continuity emerges from the system's learning processes, which establish a degree of certainty in response patterns as determined by an engrained set of constraints. This balance between flexibility and continuity, novelty and familiarity, uncertainty and certainty, allows a dynamical system to recruit increasingly complex layers of neuronal groups in maximizing its trajectory toward complexity. As the mind is both embodied and relational, this recruitment process also involves our interactions with others in the world around us as we evolve and grow.

Over time, cohesive states achieve enduring continuity as self-states. Each self-state is created and maintained in order to carry out specific information-processing tasks. As environmental conditions change, the context-dependent nature of states leads to the instantiation of a particular self-state required at the time. The healthy, adaptive mind is capable of entering a range of discontinuous (but minimally conflictual) self-states, each with its own coherence and sense of continuity.

There are various ways in which cohesion and continuity may be impaired. Excessive rigidity in a state of mind leads to an inability to try new configurations and to adapt flexibly to changes in the environment. Such rigidity may be seen in those with avoidant attachment histories, in which input from other people is adaptively blocked in order to maintain self-organization. Homeostasis is achieved at the expense of connections with others and with primary emotional states of the self. In this manner, right-hemisphere information processing may be dis-associated from that of the left hemisphere in order to maintain functioning. Such a person faces the challenge of learning to create some tolerable level of disequilibrium, in order to allow the system to try new pathways toward balanced self-regulation. In such a case, we can envision strategies of moving toward growth and development as initially involving right-hemisphere-to-right-hemisphere communication between two people. Eventually, further internal change may be brought about by a process facilitating integration of the right and left hemispheres within the individual. Within a psychotherapy setting, such techniques as journal writing, guided imagery, and exercises for "drawing on the right side of the brain" have proven helpful to catalyze a new form of bilateral resonance.

In ambivalently attached individuals, states may be somewhat fragile and easily disrupted. Cohesion may have a semistable quality that is particularly vulnerable to perturbation from social nuances. Some such individuals may be quite sensitive to subtle nonverbal cues and inadvertent misattunements; these disconnections may lead rapidly to states of shame from which it may be difficult to recover. For other people, past histories of parental intrusion make their semistable cohesion hypervigilant to the intrusion of others' internal experiences into their own. In this manner, they may defensively guard against the perception of others' minds, creating interpersonal disconnection.

In individuals with disorganized attachments, two major forms of dis-association can occur. One is within a state of mind at a given time, in which there is a "strange attractor" state of widely distributed activations. In the second form, cohesive states are dis-associated from one another across time; that is, there is a functional isolation of information transfer across states. Cohesion is achieved only through the restriction in complexity achievable by this particular configuration of self-states.

Complexity theory suggests that self-organization allows a system to adapt to environmental changes through the movement of its states toward increasingly complex configurations. We've explored the proposal that the linkage of differentiated elements (i.e., integration) enables the system to achieve the most flexible, adaptive, and energized patterns. Moving with a balance of flexibility and continuity, the system's flow across time is shaped by the internal and external constraints that define the trajectory of state changes. Internal constraints include the strength and distribution of synaptic connections within neural pathways; external constraints include social experiences and attuned emotional communication between people. By regulating these internal and external constraints, the self-system evolves through an emerging set of self-states that have coherence and continuity within themselves. Our subjective mental lives are also quite capable of abrupt shifts in constraints, which lead to the instantiation of distinct, discontinuous self-states. The mind's creation of stable systemic coherence across these self-states is one of the central goals of emotional development and self-regulation. Within the swirls of energy and information flow regulated by the mind are representational processes shaped by the neural circuitry of the brain. These circuits have genetic and experiential influences that continually mold the way we come to know our moment-to-moment experience. In the next chapter, we turn to these fundamental ways in which we filter reality and perceive our inner and interpersonal worlds.

# CHAPTER 6

# Representations

## Modes of Processing
## and the Construction of Reality

Our perception of reality is shaped by the activity patterns of neuronal groups within the brain that, as we've seen in Chapter 5, help form a "state of mind." These groups are clustered into functional units capable of representing experiences in different modalities, such as sight or taste, words or sensations, abstract ideas or perceptual images. The ways individuals assemble particular neuronal activations within themselves or in interaction with other people determine the nature of their subjective experiences of reality. We can view communication within human relationships in part as the ways in which these mental representations are shared. The patterns of this communication within early relationships directly shape the development of the mind.

A frustrated wife looked at her confused husband and said, "You never understand what I am talking about. All you know is what you have learned in books. You couldn't read my face if your life depended on it!" To this challenge, the man responded, "I can tell from what you say that you're probably not happy with me. But, you know, there are two kinds of people in this world: those who are too needy, and those who aren't." The wife got up and left the room.

How do people ever communicate with each other? How does one mind "read" the signals sent by another? How are words and nonverbal modes of communication, such as tone of voice and facial expressions, processed differently by the brain? Why couldn't this husband respond to the emotional content of his wife's message? Answers to these questions come from insights into the ways in which people's minds construct reality. In this chapter, we explore these ways by examining how the mind creates representations and processes information. The couple described above clearly had a major problem in how each partner constructed and therefore experienced reality. By examining the different mental modules responsible for representing the world and other people, we can begin to understand the foundations of this couple's profound difficulties.

As discussed briefly in Chapter 4, the individual brain is divided into two halves that have distinctly different mental representations and modes of processing. Asymmetry of the brain exists in almost all mammalian species, as well as in reptiles and birds. Asymmetry is present in the human fetus, and is functionally evident in the behavior of the human infant long before complex cognition is available.[1] The developmental origins of bilateral differences in the brain are deeply rooted in our evolutionary and genetic history. The ways in which such asymmetries influence our experiences—both internal and interpersonal—are explored throughout this chapter. The anatomic and functional separation between the two hemispheres permits their processes to be quite independent at times, and it directly shapes the construction of subjective experience. Repeated patterns of neuronal activations help to establish a continuity in the individual's representations of reality across time. How two individuals come to share their individual representational worlds is a fundamental part of "feeling felt" and establishing a sense of interpersonal connection.

This chapter proposes that the *different attachment patterns involve the recruitment of unique patterns of neuronal group activations*. For example, the emotionally distant connection of avoidantly attached children with their dismissing parents can be understood as involving primarily the linear, logical, linguistically based mode of communication of the left hemisphere. Persons in whom the left-brain mode of processing predominates have been shown to be markedly deficient in the ability to read others' nonverbal communications and to sense the emotional expressions of others or of the self. Imagine what being in an interpersonal, emotional relationship with such a person might be like. This may in part have been what the wife in the example above was encountering in her marriage. The experiential reinforcement of particular representational processes can become an engrained pattern in the way an individual comes to experience the world. As we shall see, new forms of experiences within interpersonal relationships may evoke new representational processes. This would be one of the aims of therapy for this couple's mismatch in representational processes.

## INFORMATION PROCESSING
## AND MENTAL REPRESENTATIONS

Though there is much debate about what the mind is, there is little controversy about the mind's innate ability to process information. The elaborate circuitry of the brain is reflected in the many elegant ways in which it can process information: We can learn, note similarities and differences, make generalizations, categorize, associate, analyze, and create new combinations of information within the intricate firing patterns of our brains. These patterns are not random, but emerge from the arrangements of neural connections that are able to carry out specific kinds of processing. For instance, we have circuits responsible for visual processing and others for processing the more abstract representations of ideas.

Cognitive science has provided a conceptualization of how particular information processing systems within the mind give rise to some fundamental building blocks of internal experience. Within a simple but powerful computational model, the nature of the brain's processing of information is captured by two fundamental ideas: *A mental symbol (and its neural correlate, a pattern of neuronal group activation) contains information, and it creates an effect.*[2] Recall that information is a pattern of energy flow that stands for something other than itself. We experience desires and beliefs that emanate from the meaning of mental representations. What is the nature of this representational language of the mind? At a very basic level, one perspective on cognition suggests that the patterns of firing serve as codes or symbols that carry information and cause events to happen in the brain. These events themselves are patterns of neuronal group activation, which in turn carry further information.[3] The processing of the codes or symbols—the essence of information processing—is based on both the representational and causal properties of the symbols themselves. This chain reaction of symbols and events cascades into "cognitive processes" such as memory and abstract thought. In other words, the brain creates symbols whose actions are themselves symbolic— they carry information.

> The brain creates symbols whose actions are themselves symbolic— they carry information.

How does the brain do this? By altering the firing rates of neurons, the brain is able to establish a set of signals or codes that serve as symbols as defined above. The term "mental representation" has been used to designate a mental symbol as created by neuronal firing patterns.[4] Changes in the rate of firing (increases or decreases in the baseline firing rate of a given neuron or clusters of neurons) create a pattern of activation at a given moment. A representation is itself a dynamic process in the brain. Firing patterns initiated by these representations further alter their form and shape subsequent neural activity within the brain. Such complex transformational patterns are called "cognitive processes." These processes can make new associations among representations, identify similarities and differences, or extract global themes and principles from patterns of representations over time. In this way, the brain generates new combinations and features of representations, which are further acted upon by specific processes. This is the fundamental framework for the computational mind; it takes place within specific neural pathways in the brain.

Recall that no one "knows" how the physical property of neurons firing and the subjective mental experience, say, of a thought, mutually co-create each other. Correlation is not causation: We actually do not know yet—and perhaps we will never know—how these correlated "subjective" mental experiences and "objective" firings of neurons arise from one another. Why shouldn't we say that mental experience is "simply" the activity of the brain? One reason is that we do know that the mental process of intentionally focusing attention—with imagery, for example—can get the brain to fire in specific ways, even changing the structure of the connections among neurons. Another reason is that the subjective quality of what we are aware (e.g., the image of a sunset) and the physical property of activated neurons are not the same phenomenon. Furthermore, awareness itself has the subjective experience of a sense of knowing. In other words, there are two dimensions to subjective mental life: our experience of knowing, and our experience of that which is known. These aspects of subjectivity are not the same as neuronal firing. Even the brain's regulatory self-organizing properties and processes are not the same as the related but different objective findings of neural structure and function. We now know that mind can change brain as much as brain can change mind.[5]

It bears repeating here that we are not making these two dimensions of energy and information flow into separate "domains of reality." We are not saying that the brain and mind are independent of one another. We are instead noting that they are two facets of one reality. Brain is the embodied mechanism through which energy and information flow; mind is the embodied and relational process that regulates that flow; relationships are the sharing of the flow. Our main focus, then, is on the nature of energy and information flow in human development—and so we focus deeply on all three facets of this one reality by examining the triangle of mind, brain, and relationships.

One perspective on information processing comes from evolutionary psychology.[6] Evolutionary pressures have required the brain to become specialized in its problem-solving skills. We inherit the genetically preprogrammed capacity for information processing of a particular sort. This means that the brain cannot process all types of information; a given module of the mind is only able to handle certain kinds of information in specific kinds of ways. For example, one requirement of living in the physical world is to be able to navigate the three-dimensional space in which we live. One evolutionary purpose of explicit memory has been to represent objects in space and time—a capacity that allowed our ancestors to find hidden food or recall where an enemy might be lurking. Autobiographical memory may reflect this temporal and spatial representational ability of the self in the physical world. At the other extreme, the mind must be able to transform these particular events and facts into more generalized representations, in order to allow learning and adaptation to repeated experiences with the world. This is seen in memory systems as implicit mental models, general autobiographical knowledge (e.g., "When I was seventeen I was unhappy"), and semantic concepts or categories of objects. These properties of the specific versus the general can be seen in various aspects of the mind's specialized problem-solving skills. As we come to generalize and abstract features from the original perceptually based, input–driven representational process, our representational processes become more complex. For example, we can have ideas of "freedom" and "justice," which have their origins in physical reality but contain far more complex and abstract features than spatial and temporal representations permit.

We have distinct modules of the mind, from sensory and perceptual processing to abstract reasoning and the conceptualization of other minds. This view of cognition suggests that these processing strategies are each designed to solve specific kinds of problems. They do this by creating and handling specific kinds of representations. Interaction among specific modules and among modes allows for the transfer of information, as in the coordination of sight and hearing or the influence of implicit on explicit memory processing. Artists and poets can extract meaning from sensory experiences, which they then translate back into powerful symbols through visual or literary media. In this way, various layers of representational processes, from perceptual images to abstract concepts, can become linked within a single experience. The mind is governed by the ways in which these information-processing modules function and interact with one another. We need to consider these differing forms and layers of information as we experience our sense of knowing in the world. The brain's structure in the present moment directly shapes our subjective experiences in life.

## FORMS OF REPRESENTATIONS AND SUBJECTIVE EXPERIENCE

The subjective experience of information processing can help to illustrate its relevance for understanding the mind. The information contained within representations can be about many things. For example, Steven Pinker and colleagues describe a four-part division of representations as follows: visual images containing a two-dimensional pattern or mosaic; phonological representations as a stretch of syllables in a string-like display; grammatical representations carrying the information of nouns and verbs, phrases and clusters, stems, roots, phonemes, and syllables; and "mentalese," the language of conceptual knowledge and the medium in which the gist of an idea is contained.[7] Within this framework, one can see that the mind may include codes for objects, words, and other complex entities. Other researchers have proposed a three-part division of representations into sensory–perceptual, conceptual (or categorical), and linguistic forms.[8]

Whatever perspective one takes, it is clear that the mind has distinct information that it symbolizes, as well as different modes of processing these specific forms of representations. The activation of each of these types, their interaction with each other, and their accessibility to various states can help illuminate some basic aspects of subjective experience. With a wide array of mental processes, individual differences in experience, and a fundamental limitation in how one person can know the subjective experience of another, it may seem an impossible task to define how the mind represents information and therefore constructs reality. We need to be able to have a common language for communicating some of what is known about the basic aspects of the mind's processing of information. For the purposes of this book, then, let us use a basic vocabulary of representational processes as described below.

> The mind has distinct information that it symbolizes, as well as different modes of processing these specific forms of representations.

## Sensation and Perception

A "sensory representation" contains information representing sensations, including input from the outside world, from the body, and from the brain itself. External sensory data include sight, hearing, olfaction, taste, and touch. These enter the body through sensory receptors in their respective areas. The signals then travel to the brain, where they are usually processed first in the thalamus at the top of the brainstem and then in their particular sensory areas in the cerebral cortex. At the level of the sensory cortices, the brain analyzes and compares incoming information with memories from prior experience in order to categorize the sensations into a perception. Internal sensations include bodily motion and physiological status of the body (such as states of arousal, temperature, and muscle tension). These are passed upward in the spinal cord in a layer called Lamina I and by way of the vagal nerve. This energy flow is distributed to the brainstem, the hypothalamus, and then on to the anterior cingulate and insula, especially on the right side. In general, a sensory representation is thought to have a minimal amount of categorization; that is, input is registered in the brain with relatively little "top-down" processing. A blast of sound, a bright light, and a pressure on the skin of the arm are all examples of stimuli that we may sense but may be unable to classify into a previously experienced representation, which we can then compare and contrast to prior experiences (top-down). We "sense" such stimuli, but we do not (yet) have a category or name for what they are.

In the strictest sense, even a sensory representation meets the literal definition of a "symbol"—something that carries information about something other than itself. The sensory neural input we have from putting our hands in cold water are signals generated from the firing of our neurons connected to our temperature receptors in the skin of the hand. This firing pattern is not the "cold" itself; it *stands* for "cold," because it comes from receptors that detect temperature in our skin. This pattern is a basic code directly related to the sensory medium. In an extended definition, however, some scientists refer to a more direct code as a "presymbolic" representation: It is as close to the thing itself as we can get before the mind does a lot of top-down categorizing and manipulating of incoming data based on preconceived ideas and past experiences. The term "presymbolic" is useful because it will help remind us of the nature of information processing within the mind, and also because it is often useful to distinguish these forms from those representations that are more easily translated into words.

Some might argue that this brain activity is not part of the "mind," since it is often at a nonconscious level and is thought by some to be merely an "automatic" function of the brain. However, these presymbolic representations, these less complex codes, serve a vital function in influencing all other information-processing aspects of the mind. From a regulation perspective, these sensory representations can be seen to influence self-organization, subjective experience, and, at times, awareness, and so, from an IPNB perspective, we would consider these to be building blocks of mental functions.

A "perceptual" representation is a more complexly processed unit of information than a sensory one. In contrast to a "basic" sensation, a percept is "symbolized"; it represents a constructed bit of information created from the synthesis of present sensory experience with past memory and generalizations contained within experientially derived mental models. This is the essence of top-down processing.

The flow of processing from sensation to perception is influenced by the state of mind at the time of sensing something. This is sometimes described as how bottom-up input is filtered by the top-down processes of memory, expectation, emotion, and mood. Mindful awareness—the effort to be "in the present moment" with an open stance toward oneself—may involve training the mind to distinguish between sensory and perceptual streams, and learning not to get swept up in the ubiquitous top-down filtering of daily life.[9] Mental states profoundly influence our construction of reality at this emerging symbolic representational level. The mind constructs perceptual reality from bits of selected information it receives through the senses, in combination with extremely subjective and context-sensitive mental processes, such as mental models and the influence of emotion.[10] Some may ask, "Does the outer world exist in any accurate and direct way in the mind?" A good question! Internal mental experience is not the product of a photographic process. Internal reality is in fact constructed by the brain as it interacts with the environment in the present, in the context of its past experiences and expectancies of the future. At the level of perceptual categorizations, we have reached a land of mental representations quite distant from the layers of the world just inches away from their place inside the skull. This is the reason why each of us experiences a unique way of "minding" the world.

## Conceptual (or Categorical) Representations

We may be aware of sensing or perceiving various things without the ability to describe them in words. These elements of awareness are sensory and perceptual symbols, which are considered "prelinguistic" representations. Another type of prelinguistic symbol is a "conceptual" representation. It is this form of encoding that carries information about more highly processed entities, such as the gist of an idea, "reading between the lines" of a story, or notions of freedom and justice. These complex conceptual representations are an important part of the mind's information processing. They are not directly related to the external world and the derived sensory and perceptual representations, but are created by the computations of the mind in its interactions with the world and other people within it. In this sense, sensory–perceptual representations attempt to symbolize the physical world (external or internal); conceptual representations symbolize the mind's creation of ideas and notions of the mind itself. We can create complex representations of the self, others, and the relationships we have. These conceptual representations are nonverbal. They form the fundamental building blocks of our thoughts, beliefs, and intentions, and aspects of our explicit memories. We will see later in this chapter how this ability to form complex representations allows the mind to create the concept of the minds of other people.

Although the word "concept" does not fully capture the range of representations falling under this divisional framework, it is a useful term in contrast to "percept." These conceptual representations appear to have no direct three-dimensional correlates in the external world. How, for example, would the concept of "freedom" or "justice" be simply represented in the world? An artist may be able to portray these concepts in a visual form, but their status in the mind may not be so easily linked to perceptual representations.

Another way of thinking of this is that the mind utilizes a categorical structure in which to classify and organize perceptual representations. (In fact, as described below, some authors use the term "categorical" representations rather than "conceptual.") For example, we can generate a list of mammals that live in the ocean, or fish, or living creatures that swim, or plants that live in water. In each of these categories, there is no single entity in the world that constitutes the category. For instance, there is no such animal as a "mammal"; there are many individual species that fit into the overall classification. These groupings certainly come from patterns observed by the human mind. But in this way, they are abstract top-down creations of the mind, not direct perceptions of actual things in the world.

## Linguistic Representations

"Linguistic" representations contain information about sensations, perceptions, concepts, and categories within the socially shared packets called "words." Words themselves have physical properties; they can be seen, heard, felt, spoken, and written. But words move beyond the physical world and link the mental representational worlds of separate people. We can throw mental representations out of our minds and into the air or onto a printed or electronic page, where they can be detected by a receiver whose mind in turn activates "similar" packets of verbal representations. Human language permits information processing to be shared across individuals. The evolutionary benefit of such an innate ability has been that it has allowed us as social beings to create complex cultural history and pass on knowledge across generations, across time, and across the huge space that exists between the minds of two people.

Information processing is often automatic. Most of it occurs without the participation of conscious awareness and often is not translatable into linguistic representations. However, some people are more aware of certain layers of information than other people are. For example, the capacity to conceptualize the "nature of a relationship" will vary quite a bit. Some individuals may take the phrase and expound for hours on the patterns of their relating with others. Others will hear the phrase and may only be able to respond with "It is good" or "It is bad." These individuals may have the ability to form complex representations of relationships, but these representations may not be accessible for translation into words. That is, such persons may be able to form very sophisticated reactions to intricate social interactions, but may be unable to describe the internal processes which have led to them. Still others may be quite "concrete" and be unable to make such abstract representations.

Awareness of the body is another example of how people may differ in their awareness of internal information processing. The importance of bodily responses in determining emotion and meaning makes awareness of this form of information vital to grasp. Awareness of the body—interoception—is correlated not only with enhanced self-understanding, but also with empathy and compassion.[11] The ways our functionally distinct modes of representational processing interact with one another may be keys to understanding the blockages in information processing that are a part of mental dysfunction. Such impairments in the flow of information can be seen, for example, in the memory disturbances of individuals with PTSD. Altering the flow of information processing may be a fundamental part of psychotherapy for these individuals. Also, being able to put some of these representations into words may enable such an individual to reflect on personal history and alter the future outcome of the representations' effects on the self.

> Awareness of the body—interoception—is correlated not only with enhanced self-understanding, but also with empathy and compassion.

## CONSCIOUSNESS AND REPRESENTATIONAL PROCESSES

Gerald Edelman has described a process by which the mind functions through positive feedback loops that reinforce their own patterns of firing.[12] This is called "reentry" and is based on the principle that loops of reciprocal firing—in which one group of neurons activates another, which then in turn activates the original group—constitute a major organizing process of the brain. We can visualize this as a form of interneuronal group "resonance." Reentry stabilizes a neuronal firing pattern that allows for the subjective experience of the processing in that moment At certain times, this stabilizing process permits the activation of consciousness.[13] As Edelman and Giulio Tononi put it, "Reentry leads to integration . . . integration is achieved not in any place but by a coherent *process*."[14] By linking functionally and anatomically segregated areas of the brain to one another, integration enables them to operate coherently as a unit. Edelman has described a form of "primary consciousness" as occurring when our basic sensory–perceptual processes resonate with our conceptual ones (which he terms "categorical" processes). This is the "remembered present," giving us a sense of awareness and familiarity with something without our being able to name it or to see it from a distanced temporal perspective involving past and future.

In Edelman's model, there are three major forms of neuronal groups that function as representational processes; he describes these as "perceptual," "categorical," and "linguistic." Perceptual groups are activated in response to sensations from the environment or the body. If the mind has experienced these sensations before and has categorized them with larger informational meaning, then the neuronal groups for that category will also be activated.

For example, if a child has never seen a dog before, the child's visual sensation of the canine will be experienced without a connected sense of "what it is." If the child has seen pictures of dogs or actual dogs before, the child will have remembered these and created a general category, or "schema," for such a sight. In this case, she will also have neuronal groups activated representing the category or concept of "dog." The *simultaneous* activation of perceptual (seeing the dog) and categorical (having a category for "dog") neuronal groups is thought to produce the internal sensation called "primary consciousness." There is an awareness of the sight as a familiar animal, a "being in the moment" with such a sight, which heightens an internal conscious sensation. This is the remembered present.

With the development of language, Edelman argues, the neuronal groups responsible for linguistic processing allow a different form of consciousness to emerge. When a more experienced older child with language sees the dog, the perceptual groups are activated along with the simultaneous activation of the categorical and linguistic neuronal groups. This yields a "higher-order consciousness" in which the child is freed from the prison of the remembered present and is able to reflect both backward and forward in time. In this view, it is our unique language capacity as humans that allows us to be both historians and actuaries, reflecting on the past and consciously planning for the future.

Edelman and Tononi have elaborated this view by further suggesting that elements in awareness achieve a certain degree of complexity in their assembly that temporarily stabilizes their presence in consciousness.[15] Others, such as Wheeler, Stuss, and Tulving, might argue that such a form of cross-time representation is a fundamental part of autonoetic consciousness, or self-knowing awareness.[16] We might go on to suggest that such a form of mental time travel is not dependent upon linguistic representation, but rather on the mind's capacity to represent the self as experienced. For example, the developmental acquisition of autonoetic consciousness may be more a function of the child's developing self-awareness and understanding of perceptual processes that permit experiential awareness than of linguistic abilities alone.[17] In this way, autonoetic consciousness is a function of an individual's understanding of minds—linking it, as we've discussed in earlier chapters, to the integrating processes of the prefrontal regions, including social cognition, response flexibility, and working memory. As Buckner suggests, however, the specific circuits of the prefrontal area of the brain may carry out quite distinct processes mediating aspects of autonoetic consciousness.[18] In general, the capacity to reflect on the self across time—with or without linguistic representations—may be considered as an extremely evolved, "higher-order" form of consciousness. As we'll see, the development of such a capacity may be intimately influenced by early interpersonal relationships.

Consciousness, as we've discussed in Chapters 1 and 4, is a subject of great interest and impassioned debate among academicians ranging from philosophers to neuroscientists. Recall from Chapter 1 that consciousness has two dimensions: *access* to information, and the *phenomenal* or subjective quality of an experience. In both of these realms, information processing and mental representations play a central role in determining the nature of our conscious experience. For example, consciousness can access within it the awareness of sensation or perceptions, as well as focal attention to aspects of the internal world, including the experience of emotional processing and our beliefs, wishes, and intentions. The sentience or phenomena of these representations will depend upon the nature of their integration and the information they encode, whether we associate from memory and with conscious awareness tones of music, the rough surface of a sheet of sandpaper, or memories we have of learning to swim.

We can gain a deep appreciation of the differences between people in the qualitative ways in which life is experienced within awareness. For example, those with a history of avoidant attachment seem to have minimal access to the nonverbal signals that reflect primary emotional states. Such an absence is seen in their frequent lack of awareness of others' emotions, and of their own emotions as well. By examining which representational processes are utilized to perceive such states in others and in the self, we can begin to understand what may be missing or impaired in these individuals. Internal subjective experience may vary, depending upon which systems of representation are activated at a particular time. By definition, subjective experience implies the unique, internal quality of an experience. To understand more deeply how individuals may differ in this fundamental way, it will help to understand how these representational processes are integrated to achieve higher complexity and then bound to the 40-Hz sweeping process and the activity of the lateral prefrontal cortex, discussed in Chapters 1 and 4. Our very sense of self—our autonoetic consciousness, which creates our awareness of the self across time and space—is shaped by our experiences within our families and our culture. During college, for example, a close friend from Vietnam said that he saw himself as a tree that was a part of a large forest. I, American-born, first saw myself as an individual tree, noting my roots, trunk, and branches before identifying with the forest in which I grew. Culture shapes the very perceptions we have of our selves in the world.[19]

## DEVELOPMENTAL PROCESSES AND BRAIN ASYMMETRY

We have seen how mental experience correlates in time with the activation of different circuits within the brain. "Emotion" has been defined as a set of processes involving, most importantly, the appraisal of information and the arousal of energizing activations, as well as being a fundamental element of how we communicate with one another. How the mind creates representations and places value on them is inextricably linked with emotional processes within us and among us. The flow of information and energy moves fluidly within individuals, between two or more people, and within entire cultures. We are synaptically, semantically, and societally interconnected. Though I use these terms for didactic purposes, there is no true dichotomy between "cognition" and "emotion." Brain structure and function and our interwoven social relationships give rise to the integrated complexity of mental life. In fact, infant studies suggest that we can examine how the intrinsic features of the developing brain may create specific forms of representations via neural specialization present at birth, such as brain asymmetry.

Colwyn Trevarthen, who has studied infants and brain asymmetry for decades, suggests:

> Psychology and brain science come together in the scientific analysis of cerebral localization of function. Asymmetries of function, correlated with the deeply separated left and right cerebral hemispheres, have particular value in the opening up of an approach to mental activities at the highest level. Cognitive and voluntary processes that attain maturity only after many years and that have special importance in cultural life tend to be asymmetric in the brain. The basis for this asymmetry seems to be set down very early, probably in fetal stages. It becomes elaborated in the subsequent development of the brain. Throughout childhood, as the brain takes up the lessons of experiences, and even in the moment-to-moment adjustments of adult consciousness, structures beneath the cortex continue to exercise their regulations. They assist in the development of a bihemispheric system in which the two sides have complementary roles.
>
> Finally, completing the picture, we find evidence that the intrinsic regulators of human brain growth in a child are specially adapted to be coupled, by emotional communication, to the regulators of adult brains of people who know more. This seems to be the key generic brain strategy for cultural learning that takes place not in single brains, but in communities of them. Developmental brain science will have great importance in future efforts to understand the growing human mind, and the life of ideas and beliefs in human communities.[20]

Trevarthen proposes an "intrinsic motive formation," which emerges in the embryo brainstem and regulates asymmetries in the development and functioning of the cerebral cortex.[21] Within the brainstem are interneuronal systems that carry out aspects of sensory integration; that coordinate motivational states and motoric action patterns; and that develop linkages to the important regulatory structures of the hypothalamus, basal ganglia, and amygdala. These are the brain circuits that constitute the intrinsic motive formation, which is proposed to exist even before cortical neurons develop. These essential and asymmetric elements of the emotional, motor, and motivational systems are in place long before the "higher" representational neocortex is formed.

Indeed, the cognitive systems exhibiting the most distinct asymmetry are thought to exist between intake and output circuits and the emotional processing limbic region of the brain; again, this view emphasizes the interweaving of emotion and cognitive processing. Trevarthen goes on to state:

> Human cerebral asymmetry at the level of neocortical cognitive processes that take up and store experience develops from a deeper and more ancient asymmetry in regulatory motive structures that both control morphogenesis of the brain in the embryo and guide the infant into skilled action and an understanding of the motives and ideas of other members of the cooperative community. Expression of motives and emotions between young children and their caregivers and companions regulates the acquisition of sense in the human world.[22]

Numerous lines of research suggest that the hemispheres differ in the predominance of those neurotransmitters that regulate attention, motor behavior, approach–withdrawal, and self-regulation.[23] From the embryonic stage onward, there appear to be remarkable differences in "intrinsic motives," the driving forces behind both in-the-moment processing and developmental trajectories. Trevarthen proposes that *the left hemisphere tends to have an "assertive" motivational state* governing active engagement with the world of others, as seen in the finding of the infant's right-hand gestures and cooing vocalizations in response to the mother's speech (each of which is left-hemisphere-mediated). *In contrast, the right hemisphere is proposed to be more "acceptive"*—that is, receptive and self-regulatory—as evidenced by the infant's left-handed self-touching and the right hemisphere's being better developed than the left and more responsive to the prosody of "motherese" (nonverbal, sing-song quality of tone of voice). These findings are supported by the notion that the left hemisphere is more active in motor expression and "approach," mediated by activity of the neurotransmitter dopamine. The right hemisphere, in contrast, focuses on and responds to novelty and can be seen as mediating a "withdrawal" response in certain new situations; it is also more involved in attentive and reflective states, mediated by activity of the neurotransmitter noradrenaline.[24]

> The left hemisphere tends to have an "assertive" motivational state . . . In contrast, the right hemisphere is proposed to be more "acceptive."

Moreover, the hemispheres appear to play distinct roles in the process of attention itself. The right hemisphere appears to be dominant in various aspects of attention, including vigilance, sustained attention, and alertness. In contrast, the left is dominant for focused attention—the ways that we select what we will pay attention to, our discriminatory attention.[25]

Tucker, Luu, and Pribram offer a complementary view of the relation between circuitry and representational asymmetries. These authors review the development of two "streams" of information that have evolved between the cortex and deeper structures via the frontal lobes. In an "archicortical trend" or "dorsal pathway," there is an emphasis on certain types of cells and on noradrenergic activity. In a "paleocortical trend" or "ventral pathway," there is the involvement of different regions and a predominance of dopaminergic activity. Though each of these trends is present on both sides of the brain, *the dorsal pathway appears to be predominant on the right side of the brain, and the ventral pathway on the left side.* Tucker and colleagues suggest that

> these two limbic–cortical pathways apply different motivational biases to direct the frontal lobe representation of working memory. The dorsal limbic mechanisms projecting through the cingulate gyrus may be influenced by hedonic evaluations, social attachments, and they may initiate a mode of motor control that is holistic and impulsive. In contrast, the ventral limbic pathway from the amygdala to orbital frontal cortex may implement a tight, restricted mode of motor control that reflects adaptive constraints of self-preservation. In the human brain, hemispheric specialization appears to have led to asymmetric elaborations of dorsal and ventral pathways. Understanding the inherent asymmetries of corticolimbic architecture may be important in interpreting the increasing evidence that the left and right frontal lobes contribute differently to normal and pathological forms of self-regulation.[26]

Tucker and colleagues review the findings that the ventral pathway (dominant on the left side) has a motivational bias toward specific details of objects and involves a feedback system whereby representations of present perceptions have a high degree of tight monitoring of the generation of behavioral output. Such a feedback process lends itself to object perception and competence in analytic processing, which may "be especially involved in object memory and the fine-tuning of the neocortical representation of objects whether the objects are conceptual or perceptual."[27] In contrast, the dorsal stream of information (dominant on the right side) involves spatial and context representations that rely on a "feedforward" or projectional mode of motor control, which activates arousal of attention and memory processes in response to novel situations and favors "impulsive" or spontaneous behavioral output. Such a projectional mode is also thought to involve representations of the future. This dorsal stream incorporates information from the body itself (autonomic activity and the state of viscera and smooth muscles), which makes it "well suited to evaluate stimuli for their motivational significance in relation to internal states."[28]

We can therefore see a parallel in viewpoints that the right hemisphere plays a dominant role in autonoetic consciousness, which involves a sense of self (internal states, state of the body), context, and time as these can be represented in the past and projected into the future. The predominance of the dorsal stream in the right hemisphere in this way establishes the motivational formation that drives the creation of autonoetic representations of the self through time. These views allow us to understand the notion of "cognitive representations" in a developmental light: Neocortical capacities to represent reality between perception and action emerge in the setting of powerful and asymmetric intrinsic motivational factors built into the structure and function of the brain. These motivational systems influence embryonic growth and postnatally depend on interpersonal experiences for their continued differentiation. We shall see that these genetically driven asymmetries create their own subjective and interpersonal effects on human experience.

## MODES OF PROCESSING:
## CEREBRAL ASYMMETRY AND "DICHOTOMANIA"

Literature on the two hemispheres of the brain reveals the fascinating origins of the awareness of our distinct ways of knowing about the world.[29] An early form of research into these modes focused on the experiences of some patients with epilepsy, who had to undergo a procedure that cut the connections between the two hemispheres in order to control their seizures. In these people, called "split-brain patients," the corpus callosum was severed, resulting in the functional isolation of the left and right halves of the brain. Researchers were then able to present either half of such a patient's brain with stimuli and study the patient's responses. A second prevalent source of information has been research on patients with anatomic lesions (tumors, strokes) in one hemisphere or the other. Their deficits demonstrate patterns of disrupted functioning implicating the central importance of processes specific to a particular side of the brain. A third source of insights has been ingenious experimental designs devised to expose only one hemisphere of the brains of nondisabled subjects to stimuli. The "unilateral" response in these situations has provided more data supporting the notion of hemispheric specialization.

A fourth type of research utilizing brain imaging studies has contributed to the examination of hemispheric laterality by following the activity of nondisabled subjects' brains during various procedures. Some of these studies have revealed patterns of activation that tend to confirm the original findings; others have revealed a lack of differences between the two sides. We need to interpret these findings carefully, as these more recent discoveries are quite complex: Increased blood flow as measured in a functional magnetic resonance imaging scanner may actually reveal the inhibitory efforts of one hemisphere as the other is becoming more active, with its own enhanced blood flow in response to a specific task. The overall result of such inhibitory firing may make it appear as if both hemispheres are "contributing" to a cognitive task when in fact they are not participating equally. Equivalent blood flow changes do not mean that the two sides are performing similar information processing. This challenging situation may explain the fascinating finding that in the new millennium, a number of neuroscientists shy away from stating that the left and the right sides are distinct in their functions. The biological reality, however, is that we have had asymmetries in our nervous systems as vertebrates for over 300 million years. These findings are supported by the other sources of data—from clinical studies of individuals with lesions on one side, for example, that for over one hundred years have revealed distinct processes on each side. We will need to rely on a broad range of scientific and clinical findings beyond the understandably limited technologies in order to formulate a deep understanding about the truth of asymmetry and its importance in illuminating the developing mind.

Iain McGilchrist has reviewed the scientific studies of bilaterality, examining the methods and results from an array of approaches in order to offer the data prior to any unwarranted generalizations. He, like Springer and Deutsch in earlier years,[30] cautions against the trend some call "dichotomania," in which popular writers have extended the scientific findings far beyond even the implications of the data. For example, whole cultures have been accused of being only "left-brained" or "right-brained," without an acknowledgment of the usual bilateral participation of the hemispheres in the vast array of mental processes. The temptation to focus on two distinct modes of processing has its historical roots. Philosophers have long noted the differing styles of knowing and being in the world; they have contrasted creative, synthetic, emotional, intuitive, and nonconscious patterns with those of critical, analytic, intellectual, rational, and conscious modes of thought.[31] There may be a very basic reason for this long history of seeing dichotomies in human experience. As we've discussed, the anatomic structure and neurochemistry of the two halves of the brain are somewhat distinct.[32] But even more than mere anatomy and physiology, the processes that have now been identified to be dominant in the functioning of each hemisphere generally support the philosophers' observations.

The brain—including the amygdala and orbitofrontal cortex (responsible for the assignment of meaning to stimuli), the hippocampus (the major center for integrating declarative, explicit memory processing), and the lateral prefrontal cortex (thought to be a primary center for focal, conscious attention)—is divided into two halves. At various points, bands of tissue, including the corpus callosum and the anterior commissures (and, indirectly, the cerebellum), connect the left and right halves of the brain. The uppermost part of the brain is called the cerebrum and includes the area called the neocortex, where complex thinking is believed to be correlated with neural firing. Each half of the upper brain can be referred to as a "cerebral hemisphere." In this book, the terms "right" or "left" as applied to brain, cortex, hemisphere, side, or mode refer in general to the specialized anatomy or functions of that side of the entire brain: from the abstract processes at the top of the brain, to the more basic physiological and sensory ones lower down, emanating from the brainstem. These intrinsic differences may have direct effects on the unfolding of asymmetric representational capacities, including the more abstract processes of the neocortex. The predominance of the ventral or dorsal pathways within each hemisphere may shape the motivational bias of attention and memory within that stream of information flow. Although certain functions appear to be specialized in each half, the typical functioning of the mind involves "cross-talk" between the two sides of the brain. The connecting tissue between the hemispheres appears to be important for both mutual activation and inhibition of corresponding

> The typical functioning of the mind involves "cross-talk" between the two sides of the brain.

("homologous") cerebral centers on either side of the brain. Mental life can "flow" along with activation in these differentiated and at times linked neural circuits on each side of the brain.

Our ways of being in the world, as well as our subjective perceptions, are shaped by the emergent processes in these differentiated regions of the brain—the right and the left sides. Rather than simply stating that this or that side "does" something, it is perhaps better to view laterality as an overall way of being. For example, both the left and the right side of the brain "handle" language, not just the linguistically "dominant" left. Likewise, the left hemisphere can process some forms of nonverbal pantomime—an analogic form of information processing that may previously have been assigned solely to a right-hemisphere role.[33] Interestingly, these researchers also found that spontaneous (vs. intentional) nonverbal communication was processed predominantly by the right hemisphere. Nevertheless, ongoing findings suggest that it is true that certain overall processes are dominant on one side or the other—and so we can use the notion of a right or a left "mode" of information processing. The way in which modes of processing interact with each other cooperatively, interact conflictually, or remain rigidly dis-associated may play a large role in the qualitative experience of mental functioning and well-being. These are the lenses through which we perceive the world; they shape our inner sense of being and of being aware.

The following is a generally accepted description of the processes in which each cerebral hemisphere specializes. In the *right* hemisphere are fast-acting, parallel (simultaneously active), holistic processes. The right side specializes in representations such as sensations, images, and the nonverbal polysemantic (multiple) meanings of words. These nonverbal and often spontaneous representations are often called "analogic." Visuospatial perception is an example of such an analogic function specialized on the right side. As mentioned above, the strict, traditional verbal–nonverbal distinction between the left and right hemispheres is not completely accurate. Examples of this include the contribution of the right hemisphere to understanding metaphor, paradox, and humor embedded in language. Also, the reading of stories activates both left- and right-hemisphere processes more readily than the reading of scientific texts, which primarily activates the left hemisphere.[34]

On the *left* side of the brain are slower-acting, linear, sequential, temporal (time-dependent) processes. Verbal meanings of words, often called "digital" representations, are a primary mode of processing for the left side. The left hemisphere is thought to utilize monosemantic "packets" of information as basic representations, which are then processed in a slower, linear mode. Examples of linear processing are reading the words in this sentence, aspects of conscious attention, and determining the sequence of events in a story. Our linguistic communication is dominated by this linear mode of expression and reception of "bundled" bits of symbols, which carry restrictive definitions and are relatively clearly demarcated. This is quite distinct from the analogic representations seen, for example, in an artist's painting or in a photograph. We can translate these analogic components of the world into digitalized forms within words, but the translation is never complete. In this way, some authors argue that the right hemisphere more fully "sees the world for what it is," whereas the left hemisphere must reduce the world much more into mentally defined, often socially constructed chunks of information.

These distinctions have their developmental origins in infancy, as we've discussed above. The right hemisphere is dominant for the prosodic aspect of "motherese" and appears to be more involved in acceptive, receptive, and self-regulatory activity. In contrast, the left hemisphere is involved in actively asserting communications via the right hand; these are more outwardly oriented, approach/assertive motor activities.[35] One can propose a perhaps simplistic but useful generalization here that the left hemisphere is motivated for externally focused attention and action, whereas the right is motivated for internally focused attention and action. As neocortical representations emerge between perception (input) and action (output) in the form of thought and memory processes, we can see that *such core asymmetries in motivational factors will bias each hemisphere to develop distinct capacities for complex representations.* On the left are the semantic memory representations of objects in the world, which can be manipulated and communicated to others as distinct packets of information. On the right is the internal world of the mind—both of the self and of the other—as the primary subject of memory representations within episodic memory and social cognition. The "theory of mind," or capacity for "mindsight," is likely to depend upon right-hemisphere representations. Intentions, beliefs, attitudes, perceptions, memories, and feelings are represented in analogic forms that are not easily reduced to digital packets of information.

Studies of laterality, which have involved somewhat fewer participants and therefore have fewer available data supporting their results, have suggested the following findings. The right hemisphere is considered to work as a pattern recognition center, assessing the gestalt and context of input from a synthetic mode of processing. The left, in contrast, uses logical and analytical processing to construct its detail-based representation of reality. Because of these differences in processing, writers have often summarized the contrast between right and left as that between the intuitive and the rational, between context and text, and between the polysemantic and the monosemantic meanings of words.[36]

Michael Gazzaniga and colleagues suggest that the left hemisphere is primarily responsible for "syllogistic" reasoning, in which the mind searches for causal explanations about events and reaches conclusions based on limited information.[37] The right hemisphere lacks such a drive to explain; rather, it "sees things as they are with little alteration."[38] Gazzaniga has used the term "the interpreter" to describe the process of the left hemisphere's attempts to use reason to explain cause–effect relationships in the limited pieces of information with which it is provided. In split-brain patients, the left hemisphere has been shown to weave fanciful tales to explain its perceptions. Such narratives, Gazzaniga and colleagues argue, are driven by the interpreter's need to create an explanation even in the face of quite limited data. Under typical conditions, such sustained syllogistic reasoning allows us to try to explain how things function and why the world is the way it is. In this manner, the left hemisphere is the center of the cognitive machinery that attempts to explain events and therefore, in Gazzaniga's view, is the primary motive for narrative thinking. In later chapters, we will return to this notion of an "interpreter" and its contribution, together with that of right-hemispheric processes, to the production of autobiographical narratives and attachment patterns.

More fanciful authors have extended these general dichotomies to less well-accepted philosophical notions, such as that of the right hemisphere as the origin of Eastern thought and the left hemisphere as the source of Western philosophical views. Psychological works have suggested that the right hemisphere is the center of the "unconscious" and that the left hemisphere is the origin of "consciousness."[39] Although these views indeed may be useful and perhaps have an essence of truth, their uncritical acceptance can limit a more careful application of the scientific findings to understanding subjective experience. An important example is in the generalizations of laterality and emotion.

## ASYMMETRY AND EMOTION

The most common (and oversimplified) notion in the popular literature on psychology is that the intuitive, nonverbal right hemisphere is the source of all emotion. If this idea is taken literally, it does not leave much room to explore the various shades of emotional response woven throughout all internal processes on each side of the brain. Emotion exists on both sides of the brain. Research on emotion, for example, demonstrates the intimate influence of emotion on all cognitive processes, from attention and perception to memory and moral reasoning.[40] Examination of the actual scientific data available on the nature of emotion and laterality can shed some fascinating and useful light on the topic, and can help us move further in understanding the development of the mind.

> Emotion exists on both sides of the brain.

In the various studies of emotion and hemispheric specialization, the right hemisphere appears to be primarily responsible for the reading of social and emotional cues from other people, and for the external expression of affect by an individual. For example, the left side of the face, controlled preferentially by the right side of the brain, has been shown to express more emotion than the other side.[41] Studies of patients with right-hemisphere deficits also suggest that many attentional mechanisms may be dependent on the right prefrontal cortex.[42] Recall that appraisal and arousal, which constitute the second and central phase of emotional response, alert the brain to focus attention on stimuli labeled as "important." Anatomically, the right side has a slightly higher density of neuronal interconnections than the left. As discussed earlier, what is particularly fascinating is that the right cortex also contains a more integrated somatosensory representation of the whole body, including the state of tension in the body's voluntary muscles and positions of the arms and legs. In addition, somatic "maps"—representational input from the body's viscera (heart, lungs, intestines)—are present in the right middle prefrontal cortex. These two findings suggest that the right hemisphere is more capable of having a sense of the body's state. These somatic inputs can influence limbic appraisal and shape how the cortex regulates attentional focus. It may indeed be the right hemisphere that is capable of sensing a "gut reaction" or "heartfelt sense" that something is important.[43] Emotions are directly influenced by the right brain's representations of the body's changing states. The interoceptive sensations experienced as visceral representations in the right hemisphere may be quite difficult to translate into the words of the left hemisphere. The "language of the right hemisphere," the nonverbal representations, may be a more direct means of both being aware of and expressing primary emotional reactions.

The right hemisphere, via the middle prefrontal cortex, also appears to be more capable than the left hemisphere of regulating states of bodily arousal.[44] This suggests that factors directly impinging on right-hemisphere processing, such as bodily input or others' nonverbal emotional expressions (especially when negative), may have a direct impact on the person's emotional state before the involvement of a linguistically based consciousness.[45]

The right brain will thus be more readily involved in the registration of the somatic input that makes up part of an emotional experience and the regulation of attention. Control of the body's response will also be located primarily on the right side. For these reasons, primary emotions—the textured emotional states resulting from initial orientation, appraisal, and arousal— are likely to be experienced more immediately on the right than on the left. However, appraisal and arousal circuits, the value centers of the brain, are located on both sides. For these reasons, it is fair to say that both sides of the brain are filled with meaning and emotional processes. *The qualitative ways in which each hemisphere is influenced by these neuronal activations—the essence of primary emotions—may be quite distinct because of the representational processes that are unique to each side.*

Studies of emotion and bilaterality have led to several different theoretical models. At this point, there is no clear view of some simple way in which emotion is asymmetrically processed. One view is based on emotional *intensity*: It holds that the right hemisphere is able to generate and experience more intense emotion than the left. States of high arousal, ranging from intense joy to rage, are sometimes thought to be products of the right hemisphere. Clear research data supporting this proposal are not presently available—perhaps because the notion of "intensity" is not well defined, nor are arousal or activation levels limited to one side of the brain or the other.

Instead, we can propose as one possibility that the waves of "emotional experience" may be more varied on the right side of the brain, giving the internal subjective feeling of a wider, more spontaneous sense of inner textures than those on the left. Positively valenced emotional states and more regulated, even states of mild interest and calm, are thought to be the left hemisphere's range of affective experience.[46]

The model of emotion and asymmetry based on *hedonic tone* or *valence* has had mixed support from emerging brain imaging research. This view, debated in the literature, suggests that negative, uncomfortable emotions are the products of the right hemisphere and are more readily perceived by this side of the brain.[47] For example, patients with overactive right-sided functioning may experience intense sadness, anger, or anxiety and may become more aware of negative expressions in others. Left-sided overactivation, in contrast, yields states of happiness and contentment. Popular extensions of these studies might call the right hemisphere pessimistic and the left optimistic. There is much controversy over this distinction, in that studies suggest a role of inhibition of the asymmetric corticolimbic dorsal and ventral pathways, rather than merely an activation of one side or the other.[48] For example, Alfano and Cimino state:

> There appears to be accumulating evidence for asymmetries in perception/identification of emotion that are not consistent with existing valence models and which need to somehow be reconciled. . . . The mechanisms underlying these asymmetric valence effects in perception of emotional stimuli are, as yet, unexplored. It may be that each hemisphere exerts an enduring affective bias that subsequently influences individuals' appraisal of stimuli in their environment. That is, like affective *experience* and *expression*, the *perception* and even *recall* of emotional stimuli may also be differentially mediated by anterior (or other) regions of the cerebral hemispheres.[49]

Future research will be needed to illuminate how the many layers of arousal, valence, perception, expression, and memory each contribute to the asymmetric ways in which emotion is processed in the brain.

Furthermore, each hemisphere may be involved in contralateral inhibition—and thus lesion studies that have been interpreted to reveal, for example, negative affect on the right side may actually be demonstrating release of the inherent emotion of the opposite side of the lesion. It is indeed quite complicated.

Nevertheless, there is some agreement that emotions eliciting *approach* behaviors are experienced on the left side, and that emotions producing *avoidance* or *withdrawal* are processed on the right.[50] This dimension of asymmetry may be most evident in frontal regions. The distinction helps illuminate the nature of seemingly contradictory findings. For example, the emotional state

> There is some agreement that emotions eliciting approach behaviors are experienced on the left side, and that emotions producing avoidance or withdrawal are processed on the right.

of anger for many people is considered "negative," and one might predict that an angry state of mind would be associated with right-hemisphere activation, according to the valence hypothesis described above. However, as Harmon-Jones and colleagues note,

> Results of several studies revealed that anger is associated with greater relative left frontal activation. Moreover, manipulated increases in the approach motivation of anger cause even greater relative left frontal activation. These results support the idea that greater relative left frontal activity is associated with approach motivation and not positive affective valence.[51]

When we move toward rather than withdraw from something or someone, we may be harnessing the approach state of the left frontal regions.

Another often initially counterintuitive finding is the important "left shift" revealed in individuals participating in research on mindfulness meditation. Mindful awareness is often filled with sensory and nonverbal immersion in here-and-now experience, and therefore it could be considered a "right-hemisphere activity." However, it is actually thought to involve a mental training that enables individuals to approach, rather than withdraw from, challenging stimuli.[52] This increased left frontal activation (also associated with enhanced immune function) does not mean that other left-dominant components of information processing are increased with mindful awareness. Rather, mindfulness is thought to be associated with an increased ability to stay present with moment-to-moment experience—to approach life fully, rather than withdrawing or avoiding life's challenges. These studies remind us that both the left and right sides of the brain have a wide array of processes specific to certain regions. It is not only possible, but probably very common, that we utilize different regions on the two sides of the brain simultaneously in a variety of life's tasks. This view is supported by the notion that motivational factors are asymmetric from prenatal development onward, and that the value systems on each side of the brain push experience and development in specific directions.

Another view is based on a distinction between "social" and "basic" emotions."[53] Social emotions—adaptations of emotional states to meet the needs of social situations—are thought to be functions of the left hemisphere. In this model, basic emotions include both primary and categorical emotions as these have been defined in Chapter 4; they are the value-based responses to internal or external events and are thought to be products of the right hemisphere. In this view, sadness, anger, fear, disgust, surprise, interest/

excitement, enjoyment/joy, and shame are all part of the right hemisphere's processing. Display rules—the culturally transmitted lessons about which, and how, emotions can be expressed in social settings[54]—determine the social appropriateness of affective expression and are presumably mediated by the left hemisphere. This view is consistent with the notion proposed earlier that the left hemisphere has an inherent external bias toward our focus of attention, whereas the right is biased toward reflecting on internal subjective experience.[55] Spontaneous motor output, the direct expression of internal states via affective signals, is a product of the right hemisphere. In this model, the tightly controlled, routinized output of social display rules is a product of the left hemisphere, which some studies suggest more readily controls the lower face with intentionally mediated, socially engaged emotional expressions. In contrast, the right hemisphere regulates upper facial expressions that are more spontaneous and reflective of "authentic" internal states.[56]

## CONSCIOUSNESS AND LATERALITY

Though the popular literature and other publications sometimes call the right hemisphere the "seat of the unconscious," *each hemisphere may have its own conscious and nonconscious processes.* Both hemispheres may sometimes function in a quite distinct and isolated fashion; at other times there may be an integration within bihemispheric functioning. Consciousness in general may be qualitatively different on the left and on the right, because the connection of working memory within the lateral prefrontal cortex and the 40-Hz thalamocortical sweeping process will recruit and have available to it representations that are distinct in character within each hemisphere. The associational processes thought to underlie conscious experience may also be quite different on each side of the brain. It is therefore reasonable to suggest that there may be a right-brain and a left-brain form of consciousness. Both hemispheres can become involved as a "supersystem," in which consciousness recruits various neuronal groups across the hemispheric connections, leading to a bihemispheric form of consciousness. We can call this a form of "interhemispheric resonance."

The left hemisphere is the center of logical, linguistic, linear processing. (It may help your explicit memory to notice all the L's in this left-sided list. Some say that the left is also quite literal.) It is sequential, with one representation leading to another and then another. This is inherently slower than the rapid, parallel processing of the right side. The basic form of conscious representation in the left hemisphere is the word: Thoughts filled with linguistic representations fill our consciousness from left-hemisphere activity. What we call "thinking" often refers to the conscious verbal processing of the left hemisphere. When we are conscious of sensations and images, these are likely to emanate from the right hemisphere.

Of note is that *the left hemisphere appears not to be highly skilled at reading nonverbal social or emotional cues from others.* Facial recognition centers are primarily in the right hemisphere. What this suggests is that *right-hemisphere "reality," its constructed representational world, will contain the information derived from the internal states of others.*[57] The right hemisphere's language is one of nonverbal sensations and images. In sum, the general impression of the right hemisphere as being "more emotional" is somewhat oversimplified; it is more accurate to state that the emotional experience in the right hemisphere may be more attuned to the emotional states both of others and of the self. The right hemisphere's nonverbal representations involve the essence of affect, whereas the left hemisphere may have little innate ability to construct or be conscious of such a nonverbal, nonlogical view of the world. However, the left hemisphere is able to mediate social display rules and can assess complex social situations to some degree.[58] Emotional processes are a fundamental part of both hemispheres and are not restricted to only one side or one area of the brain. Our abilities to perceive primary emotional states, to become conscious of them, and to express them directly to others may be at the heart of the qualitative difference in the experience of emotion between the hemispheres.

## ATTACHMENT, LATERALITY, AND REPRESENTATIONAL PROCESSES

Because emotions are fundamentally linked to appraisal–arousal mechanisms in both the right and left hemispheres, they influence all aspects of cognition, from perception to rational decision making. As we've seen, attachment experiences early in life appear to have direct influences on various basic processes, including forms of memory, narrative, emotional regulation, and interpersonal behavior. Studies suggest that the left and right hemispheres may experience different aspects of emotional response. We can then ask how intimate affect attunement—the resonance of states of mind between child and caregiver—might influence the two hemispheres in unique ways. The proposal being made here is that the different patterns of attachment relationships can be understood in part as differentially involving communication between one hemisphere of the parent and the similar hemisphere of the child. The conceptual basis for this proposal is that the more mature adult state of mind will tend to recruit similar brain processes in the child. If this occurs repeatedly during the crucial early years of development, it is plausible that these shared states may become engrained as traits within the child.

What is the evidence that parent–child relationships may involve asymmetric effects on the developing child's brain? Studies by Geraldine Dawson and colleagues, Tiffany Field and colleagues, and others suggest that the left hemisphere's involvement in positive emotions such as joy and excitement make it particularly vulnerable to dysfunction in cases of maternal depression.[59] In studies of mother–child dyads with prolonged maternal depression, EEG findings were suggestive of dampened left-hemisphere functioning, with relative increases in right-hemisphere activation in both mothers and children. If a mother's depression lasted beyond one year, then the child was more likely to have prolonged impairment in left-hemisphere activation in the future. Maternal depression involves decreased affective attunement and diminished sharing of heightened moments of state-to-state resonance around positive feelings, such as excitement, interest, and joy.[60] The right hemisphere, in this view, is involved in negative emotions, such as fear, sadness, and anger. Overall, these findings are consistent with the valence-based view of emotional laterality, in which asymmetry generally determines the hedonic tone of emotional experience. Interestingly, one study revealed that with a continuity of breast feeding with depressed mothers and their infants, these effects on the brain were not seen. The authors suggest that these enhanced positive dyadic interactions may have partly ameliorated the potential negative effects of the mothers' depression.[61]

Other types of studies suggest that the form of parent–child communication during the early years of life may directly shape the lateralization of brain function. Newman, Bavelier, and their colleagues have revealed that the mediation of American Sign Language (ASL)—a visual display of signals used for communication with and by many hearing-impaired individuals—is carried out in different areas of the brain, depending on when it was learned.[62] For example, congenitally deaf individuals who have learned ASL utilize the left-hemispheric regions usually involved in spoken language, in addition to harnessing aspects of the right hemisphere. Newman and colleagues also elected to study hearing children raised by deaf parents who learned sign language as their first "language" and to compare them to individuals who learned ASL later in life. In individuals who learned to communicate with ASL early, the left-hemisphere centers that usually mediate "spoken" language subsumed this role. However, in hearing adults who learned ASL after adolescence and not early in life, the left hemisphere did not subsume this role. Early ASL users harness both sides of the brain.[63]

A study comparing deaf children raised by experienced users of sign language with deaf children of parents new to its use also revealed important developmental findings. The ability to think in mental terms—to perceive the mind or have "theory of mind"—was found to be well developed only in those children of parents who could sign in a sophisticated manner. The conclusions of that study are that children need to experience communication about internal mental life using mental-state language, such as feelings, thoughts, and memories, in order to develop this important mindsight capacity.[64]

These studies suggest that the brain responds to experience by altering its neural circuitry; that it is capable of devoting its circuitry to alternative sensory modes depending on stimulus input; and that the timing of exposure to stimuli has a direct influence on how "plastic" the brain is in adapting its circuitry. We can further propose that the social nature of information processing—the form in which interpersonal communication takes place—may be an important determinant in brain differentiation. This latter possibility highlights the notion that whether language is mediated by visual or by auditory means early in life, similar brain regions will take on the task of language processing. Could it be that forms of emotional communication (or the lack of them) that involve nonverbal aspects of communication can also directly shape brain development in these lateralized ways by experience-dependent developmental processes as well? Future studies will need to explore this possibility.

> The brain responds to experience by altering its neural circuitry.

The right hemisphere is dominant in its activity and development during the first three years of life.[65] Children who experience severe emotional deprivation during this period may be at most risk of losses in the structural components that link the right and left hemispheres, with reduced volume of the connecting fibers of the corpus callosum.[66] The vulnerability from such impaired neural integration may be understood as a function of the primary role of integration in mediating the affect attunement that serves as a major form of connection and communication between the child and caregiver. This view also supports the notion that primary emotions, which give rise to vitality affects, may be closely linked to integrative neural function. When we examine the functional properties of each hemisphere, especially the right hemisphere and its connection to both affect regulation and social communication, we gain insights into the differences between individuals with different attachment experiences.

These issues also raise the point that the timing of experience, be it optimal or traumatic, may have the largest impact on those parts of the brain that are in the most active phase of development.[67] These are times of maximal opportunity as well as vulnerability. As Robert Thatcher and colleagues have demonstrated, the brain may undergo a cycling of phases throughout childhood, in which one and then the other hemisphere is in an active phase of growth and development.[68] Clinicians and researchers may benefit from awareness of the possibility that the correlation of overwhelming experiences with the natural oscillations in hemisphere maturation may lead to differing outcomes for development.

If a child has had little interpersonal right-hemisphere resonance with his caregivers during the first three years of life, underdevelopment of that hemisphere and of its linkage to the left hemisphere may result. Nonverbal communication, facial expressions, subtleties in tone of voice, and emotional attunements will all be minimal in the "experience-dependent maturation" of this child's right hemisphere. These are the experiential food for the right hemisphere during early development, as well as in adult life. A parent's attachment model may directly influence the nature of her emotional attunement, selectively reinforcing the activity of certain emotions and disavowing (by nonattunement) other ones.[69] These studies support the view that integrative communication links the differentiated selves of infant and caregiver and promotes the growth of the integrative fibers of the brain. These circuits link differentiated neural regions in the body and link different people to one another. They are regulatory: They help coordinate and balance the functioning of the child in an embodied and relational world. The right hemisphere (especially the middle prefrontal region), plays a dominant role in integration and regulation throughout our lives, as it links social, somatic, brainstem, limbic, and cortical into one functional whole.

Fonagy and colleagues found that certain attachment dyads do not foster the development of elements of the "theory-of-mind" module of processing information.[70] These findings can be extended here to support the idea that attachment has lateralized effects. We can propose that "reflective function," in which the mind of one person is able to "mentalize" or create representations of the mind of another, is probably dependent upon processes mediated primarily via the right hemisphere. Carrington and Bailey's metaanalysis of forty theory-of-mind studies suggests an active role for a core network of neural regions with a general dominance in the right hemisphere.[71] The reflective function also serves as the substrate for self-awareness and for the ability to process information about the self and the self with others—processes mediated in adjacent regions of the prefrontal areas. Recognizing facial emotional expression, having cognitive representations of others' minds, having self–other relationship representations, and having the capacity to respond to the mental state of others can all be proposed to be mediated by the social-emotional processing of the right hemisphere.[72] However, the integration of these modules of processing into a coherently functioning reflective mode may require a well-developed coordination of right-hemisphere and left-hemisphere processing, as discussed below. Attachment studies by Fonagy and his coworkers support the notion that interpersonal experiences within early caregiver–child relationships can facilitate, or impair, the development of such reflective capacity.[73]

Adults who have insecure states of mind with respect to attachment can be proposed to reveal, within their AAI narratives, frames of mind in which such integration of the hemispheres has not been achieved. Such a restricted state of mind may impair a parent's ability to achieve resonance of states with a child. Specifically, the parent will be unable to foster the activity of each hemisphere and will have difficulty enabling the child to achieve some form of interhemisphere integration. We can further suggest here that the coherent AAI narratives of securely attached adults reveal a coordinated functioning of the "mentalizing" right hemisphere and the "interpreting" left. We shall see how the integration of right- and left-hemisphere representational processes and motivational states leads to a "bilateral form of coherence" and can be revealed within coherent life narratives. The ways in which the mind may come to integrate these processes and achieve such coherence are explored in greater detail in Chapter 9.

The right hemisphere has a nonverbal "language" of its own, focusing on the gist, context, or social meaning of experiences. Just as the left hemisphere requires exposure to linguistically based language in order to grow properly, one can propose that the right hemisphere may require emotional stimulation from the environment in order to develop properly. Attachment research clearly demonstrates that communication between caregiver and infant shapes the ways in which the child's developing mind learns to process information. As Aitken and Trevarthen have stated,

> Human cognition developments, and their pathologies, are regulated, from birth, by highly specific motives in the child's brain for engaging with motives in other brains. Emotions constitute an innate system by which functions of attending, purpose, and learning may be coordinated between subjects.[74]

In this manner, emotional communication and affective attunement become the medium in which the child's cognitive capacities develop.

The organization Zero to Three's logo reads, "To grow a child's mind, nurture a baby's heart." This view is supported by the writings of Stanley Greenspan and Berry Brazelton, who suggest that early emotional relationships form the building blocks for the development of all other representational processes.[75] Aitken and Trevarthen also suggest this view:

> Subjective and intersubjective processes are mutually regulating, and, in early infancy, before manipulative investigation of objects is under efficient volitional control, the regulations of communication with a caregiver who offers affectionate, emotionally available company appear to dominate in the

discovery and learning of reality. . . . There is abundant evidence now that neonatal brains are embarking on changes in organization that are highly responsive to stimulation from caregivers. The effects of this experience, while demonstrating the adaptive plasticity of the newborn brain, also give proof of highly elaborate and highly selective systems in the infant for engaging with the processes that motivate expressive behaviors in caretaking individuals.[76]

In other words, the infant both responds to the world of others and plays an active role in influencing how others respond. This process can be seen as a form of "recruitment," in which neuronal processes selectively activate patterns of firing of other neural pathways—in this case, within other brains.

Recall that when neuronal circuits become activated, they create and reinforce their connections with each other. With this in mind, we can see why an avoidantly attached child's conscious experience of life, his subjective sense of

> Emotional communication and affective attunement become the medium in which the child's cognitive capacities develop.

daily living, may be quite different from that of a securely attached child whose right hemisphere has been encouraged to develop. Once established, such a pattern in neuronal activations will tend to recruit similar patterns in the future. Within the avoidantly attached individual, there may be a disconnection in the integrative functioning of the two hemispheres that parallels the emotional disconnection within the attachment relationship. Studies of avoidant mother–child pairs have shown that words are used without correlation with nonverbal components of communication.[77] Such an interactive disconnection becomes repeated within a child's own mind. In this way, one hemisphere may begin to act as an autonomous subsystem of the brain. At the extreme, one might predict that such a person may feel more comfortable with abstract ideas and the sharing of intellectual views about the world than with intense emotional exchanges involving the sensation of "feeling felt" or the content of others' minds. Over time, the relative dominance of one hemisphere over the other and the functional isolation of the lateralized modes of processing may begin to dominate the subjective experience of life for that individual.

## GENETICS, GENDER, AND EXPERIENCE

The proposal being made here is that certain attachment experiences preferentially reinforce the development of one hemisphere over another and therefore lead to impaired bilateral functioning. Before we can accept this idea, we need to take a more global perspective on what is known about the effects of innate, nonexperiential factors on the developing individual. Studies have found, for example, that gender plays a large role in determining hemispheric strengths.[78] Some findings contradict common assumptions, however; for example, one study showed that men may actually use right-hemisphere middle prefrontal areas more preferentially in mediating social cognition than women do.[79] Oversimplification of gender findings should be carefully avoided. Nevertheless, a range of studies suggest that, on the average, females are better than males in a broad range of skills involving the use of language, such as verbal fluency, articulation speed, and grammar. They are also superior to men at tasks involving perceptual speed, manual precision, and arithmetic calculations. Males, in contrast, are generally better at tasks that are spatial in nature, including picture assembly, block design, mental rotation, maze performance, and mechanical skills. Men are also superior to women in mathematical reasoning, in intercepting a moving object, and (believe it or not) in finding their way along a route. As you can see, these differences demonstrate a trend that may be surprising: Women have more facility in classically left-hemisphere processes, and men in right-hemisphere ones. In fact, it is important to note that attachment categories are distributed equally across the genders. Both males and females need and can give empathic, sensitive, and nurturing care to their offspring and their romantic partners.

Exposure to hormones such as testosterone during fetal growth is felt to be one factor that directly influences the specialization of hemispheric function and may explain some of the initial differences across the hemispheres as children grow. As mentioned in Chapter 4, testosterone levels also influence the modeling of the adolescent brain.[80] Studies have found that lateralization probably occurs before birth, reinforcing the notion that innate genetic and other constitutional factors (produced by conditions *in utero*) may play a large role in the initial differentiation of the two hemispheres.[81] As the newborn grows, specialization appears to continue and now experience may directly play a role in how each hemisphere grows and learns to integrate with the other. The role of socialization in hemispheric specialization has not been clarified as yet, but it is clear that experiences within families and in the larger culture are important in how children's brains develop.[82] In general, these social experiences may be formative in shaping not only neural connections, but also the epigenetic regulation of gene expression.[83] The known distinctions in various cultures in the rearing of boys versus girls may serve to elaborate and reinforce these initial inborn gender-based differences, and to shape the epigenetic factors and synaptic connections of the developing brain. These are important issues to be illuminated in future research.

One general view is that females tend to have more processes that are *bilaterally* distributed. For example, women often have words represented in the (usual) left hemisphere and also in the right hemisphere. This finding of more integrated functions across the two sides is supported by anatomic studies demonstrating a number of differences between women and men that support, but do not prove, the notion of increased similarity and accessibility of the left and right hemispheres to each other in women.[84] Not all studies support this view, and caution is advised. Men and women may be quite similar as individuals, even in the face of differences in general group trends.[85] Cerebral blood flow findings often support the view that men have greater asymmetry in function than women do. One way of summarizing these suggestions is that women are "less lateralized" than men. For both men and women, however, the left and right hemispheres are anatomically quite distinct.[86]

Why do women and men differ in their laterality? One view is that proposed by Jerre Levy, who suggests that the greater lateralization in men would have been necessary to preserve the high level of visuospatial skills necessary for hunting. In women, the role of child rearing would have necessitated more bilateralization of such functions as the use of language for communication of internal states, as well as social sensitivity and facility with nonverbal modes of communication.[87] This hypothesis combines an anthropological view of gender roles with cognitive findings on the relationship between sex and asymmetry. It speaks directly to the idea of how generations of humans exposed to evolutionary pressures may have been selected for particular patterns of hemispheric specialization. It does not focus on how an individual's experience will "pull" for particular functions. Gender differences in cognition may change as cultural roles in future generations continue to evolve.

Other studies, however, suggest that there are no consistent population differences in laterality across the genders.[88] Testosterone in males, and alterations in estrogen and progesterone in females, may play a role in how mental processes and behavioral interactions unfold across the lifespan. Stress levels with increased cortisol secretion may also influence cognition by inhibiting the functioning of the hippocampus in integrating explicit memory and altering the capacity for learning. Perhaps the most parsimonious view is that whatever the genetically and hormonally induced differences across the genders may be, they reveal a wide range of possible outcomes in development for any individual. Given the high degree of plasticity of the human brain, as well as the wide array of experiences and expectations that children encounter as they grow, a great deal of freedom and flexibility is possible. This enables us to view a child, whether male or female, as having a wide range of potentials that are limited more by our expectations than by our XX or XY chromosomes.

Why would the brain be genetically programmed in either males or females to differentiate left from right in the first place? Why do we have two hemispheres with differential functions anyway? There are many speculative answers to these questions. One view holds that the functions of one hemisphere can conflict with those of the other. This is called the "cognitive crowding hypothesis" and specifically highlights the idea that if each hemisphere performed the same function, then the ensuing competition would lead to cognitive dysfunction.[89] Having two separate hemispheres with distinct forms of processes allows for the preservation of the functions of each side. Those organisms that developed bilateral specialization had increased survival ability and were able to pass on the trait to later generations. Asymmetry actually appears to have a long history in many species of animals.[90]

## HOW DOES EXPERIENCE INFLUENCE HEMISPHERIC SPECIALIZATION?

There are developmental phases in which primarily one, then the other, hemisphere grows and expands.[91] In the first few years of life, as described earlier, the right hemisphere is both more active and growing more rapidly. After these first years, the left hemisphere becomes more dominant in activity and development. By the end of the third year of life, the corpus callosum allows for the transfer of information between the two hemispheres. The mind is created, in part, from the whole brain within the activity of its disparate circuits, their interactions with each other, and their interactions with the body as a whole. As we've seen, the intrinsic motive formation system may exist before the neocortical capacity to construct representations even begins. The developing mind of the child reflects the manner in which it is anatomically predisposed to processing information. After four years of age, children usually become much more facile at using words to describe their inner states and impulses. Preschools take advantage of this developmental capacity in helping children learn to socialize with their peers by utilizing language to express what they feel and want. Such accomplishments require the joint cooperation of both hemispheres and may not be possible at an earlier age in most children.

We know from studies of children and adults with neurological lesions that the brain can adapt to experiential pressures.[92] For example, in young children with severe forms of epilepsy who have had to undergo treatment involving removal of an entire hemisphere, the remaining half of the brain appears to be able to take on the functions (such as language) of the now missing hemisphere. In adults suffering from strokes, however, the brain may not be so "plastic" or able to adapt to loss of specialized functions.[93] Through lengthy rehabilitation efforts, however, experience can result in the emergence of needed old functions within new circuits. The same appears to be true in cases of congenital impairment of certain sensory modalities, such as sight, in which other modalities (such as touch) utilize the anatomic zones usually specializing in the impaired mode.[94]

In professional musicians, the study of music appears to involve the growth and development of parts of the brain in a different manner from their development in the casual music listener. Specifically, some studies suggest that the left brain's language-based, analytic mode becomes a more dominant part of the music experience with education and formal training. This appears to involve judgments about duration, sequence, and rhythm. In contrast, the right side's ability appears to be stronger in the areas of tonal memory, melody recognition, and intensity. The complexity of how various forms of musical training affect brain organization, however, makes it difficult to make global lateralized conclusions, especially when developmental age is taken into account.[95] One view of music and the brain suggests that rhythm links the body proper with the functioning of the higher neural regions of the cortex; melody builds on the anticipatory functions of the neocortex in integrating the familiar with the novel in the capturing of the musical imagination.[96]

The repeated activation of specific neuronal pathways reinforces the strength of connections between groups of neurons. Those neuronal circuits that are not activated do not get reinforced and can die away. Some researchers suggest that there are "windows of opportunity," during which the activation of specific functions is essential for continued development in that area. If kittens are not exposed to horizontal lines during a certain critical period, for example, the visual cortex may lose the ability to process such input later in life.[97] Infants who are not exposed to any spoken language may lose the ability to acquire typical linguistic functions after the first few years.[98] Similarly, infants who have no attachment relationships (e.g., ones who are in orphanages with so few staff members that attachments do not develop) before the end of the third year of life, at the latest, may have extreme difficulty forming attachments later in life.[99] The motivational system of attachment—its circuits and potential for development—may have became not readily available for maturation in the future.

How "plastic" is the brain after the early years of childhood? Recent findings in the field of neuroplasticity reveal that the human brain remains open to changing in response to experience throughout the lifespan. It can grow new synaptic connections, make new myelin, and even grow new neurons from neural stem cells that develop into fully mature integrative neurons within several weeks.[100] This issue has important implications for our understanding of the developing mind across the lifespan. For example, if it is true that certain attachment experiences lead to the underdevelopment of the right-hemisphere processing of nonverbal aspects of emotional signals, and of the two hemispheres' ability to coordinate and balance their asymmetric processing, how much can new experiences alter such a condition in an adult? We could use future studies, say, of the brain's default mode of activity—its resting state of functioning when not given specific tasks to accomplish—to examine whether there is impaired integration following suboptimal attachment experiences. Impaired integration has been found in some preliminary studies of disorders that are not experientially induced, such as bipolar disorder, schizophrenia, and autism.[101] Outcome studies might then look for improvements in the integrative intrinsic functioning of the brain following appropriate therapeutic intervention, no matter what the etiology of the condition being treated might be. Research suggests that there is far more plasticity in the adult brain than was previously believed possible, even in the face of neurological impairments.[102] These studies suggest that alterations in input from the environment, such as those resulting from inability to move a limb, lead to restructuring

> The human brain remains open to changing in response to experience throughout the lifespan.

of the representational processes in certain regions of the brain. Even in an adult, therefore, the brain appears to be capable to some degree of responding to changes in experience with further development of brain structure and function.

Another reason for optimism about further brain development in adults is that some psychiatric disturbances may be due to impairments in integrative functioning among widely distributed, sometimes bilateral processes.[103] These impairments may be due to the failure to develop associative neural pathways linking relatively autonomous modules of processing. This is consistent with our proposal over the last two decades that mental health emerges from integration and that psychiatric disturbances are due to impediments to integration. There is preliminary support for clinical assessment aimed at identifying such integrative impairments (as revealed in the states of chaos or rigidity), and then focusing interventions on promoting integration.[104] The creation of new neural integrative links is part of a learning process that remains possible throughout adulthood. Addressing the issue of the emergent properties of neural systems in development, Post and Weiss suggest:

> The synaptic networks are in a state of continual rearrangement on both a micromolecular basis at the level of neurotransmitter and receptor subtype, as well as on a larger integrative basis for the synthesis of objects in the environment, including food and individuals such as self and others.[105]

Our brains may retain the ability to continually reshape, in some fashion, emergent properties that allow us to learn and grow with new experiences.

For example, informal clinical observations suggest that some individuals do remain capable of activating the inherent capabilities of the right hemisphere well into adulthood.[106] Learning to integrate these nonverbal functions into an active contribution to both internal and interpersonal experience can be a major challenge, however, especially for those with avoidant attachment histories. Other individuals seem much less able, or at least less willing, to experience such transformations. One question is how impairments in integrative functioning may be a result of underdevelopment or an adaptive underutilization. For example, allowing the mind to begin to process the less definable, predictable, and controllable information inherent in nonverbal representations can be frightening for some people. At times, having unilateral dominance may be a defensively adaptive function. In this situation, attempts to improve bilateral functioning may involve efforts both to catalyze new development and to support the lowering of defensive avoidance tactics.

The blockage of right-hemisphere processes from consciousness and from engaging with others may be an adaptive "defense" against feeling anxious and out of control. Moving toward the left hemisphere's more detail-oriented, routinized, top-down processing and its "even-keel" emotional style may be a mental system that is eagerly welcomed if the world is otherwise filled with uncertainty and excessive overstimulation. Such may be the case for individuals with certain highly reactive temperamental styles or for those raised in chaotic homes.

In fact, bilateral asymmetries have been associated with certain temperamental, affective, and cognitive styles.[107] For example, as discussed in Chapter 4, right-hemisphere dominance has been found in young infants who later are found to have shy temperaments.[108] The behavioral inhibition that accompanies such a constitution can be thought of as due to an excessive reactivity of the right hemisphere, which has been proposed to mediate withdrawal behavior. In the face of novelty, such activation may lead to a turning inward and avoidance of engaging in the world. Recall that the dorsal corticolimbic pathway is dominant in the right hemisphere, and that this pathway is involved in orienting to novel stimuli, the activation of internal self-regulatory mechanisms, the representation of the self and the body, and the "feedforward" representation of the future.[109] As we put these elements together here, we can propose that an individual with an overly active dorsal pathway/right hemisphere early in life may experience not only increased attention and reactivity to novel situations, but also engrained representations of the self in distress, which may create further caution and withdrawal. As such a child matures, the active representation of the future within the dorsal stream may extend such a cautious stance as the mind attempts to anticipate the world of uncertainty by matching actual experiences with well-elaborated fearful expectations. Such an attempt to anticipate the world can be seen in the behavior of the slow-to-warm up, shy child clinging to a parent's side at a friend's birthday party. What has begun as an initial overdominance of right-hemisphere functioning may now have blossomed into a significantly impairing behavioral inhibition. Interactions with parents and other caregivers during the early years of such a constitutionally shy child's development can help ameliorate such a trajectory. As discussed earlier, research has demonstrated that interactions with others supporting a shy child's emotional experience, but nurturing attempts to "push the envelope" into tolerable levels of uncertainty and exploration, may be the most helpful in enabling the child to grow and develop.[110]

## WAYS OF KNOWING

What are the implications of asymmetry for our experiential ways of knowing about reality? One view is that with the advent of language, the brain has to preserve a way to continue to process things quickly and more directly in relation to the body and the external world. This becomes the continued work of the right hemisphere. The left, in contrast, has fewer inputs from the body and is able to use the abstract manipulations of linguistic representations to allow us to experience a "higher-order consciousness": Linguistically, we are able to reflect on the past and the present, and to plan for the future. Such abilities also allow us to create new combinations of things, both in our minds and in the world. We can build buildings, fly airplanes, and write books of poetry (or books about the brain). The logical, linear, detail-focused, linguistic left brain is crucial for human creativity as well as technology. It is essential for getting the message into shareable packets of socially transmissible information. What is the right brain for?

The right brain appears to be able to perceive patterns within a holistic framework, noting spatial arrangements that the left is unable to sense. The right brain is able to create the gist or context of experiences and the overall meaning of events. The nonverbal codes of the right hemisphere are predominantly based on sensations and images. These rapidly associated images give us a more direct and immediate representation of the world and of ourselves. This gives us a perceptual advantage: We can perceive the world for "how it is" from a bottom-up perspective. The left hemisphere, in contrast, is able to categorize perceptions based on prior experience from a top-down view. In their essential features, Levy argues, the spatial abilities of the right hemisphere are directly conflictual with the linguistic representations of the left.[111] According to this "cognitive crowding hypothesis," *keeping the right mode separate from the left allows for the existence of two extremely different but vital and important ways of knowing.* In this manner, the isolation of the two hemispheres is required in order to achieve the unique information-processing modes of each side of the brain.[112]

Memory processes are also specialized in each hemisphere.[113] The memory researcher Daniel Schacter notes:

> Neurologists and neuropsychologists have known for over a century that language and verbal abilities are heavily dependent on the left hemisphere, whereas nonverbal and spatial functions are more dependent on the right hemisphere. Memory is similarly lateralized. Patients with damage to the left hippocampus and medial temporal lobe tend to have difficulties explicitly remembering verbal information but have no problems remembering visual designs and spatial locations. Patients with damage to the right hippocampus and medial temporal lobe tend to show the opposite pattern.[114]

Goldberg and Costa extend this argument by suggesting that the functional and anatomic studies of specialization support the view that the right hemisphere is better equipped to deal with *interregional integration.*[115] That is, the right hemisphere has more associational links, integrating information within the right brain in a "horizontal fashion" across modalities and attaining a contextual pattern of the world. The right hemisphere has a greater capacity for dealing with context and informational complexity and for integrating data across various modes of representations (such as sight, sound, and touch) within a single effort or task. Some consider that the right hemisphere is in this way better equipped to perform parallel processing.

> Keeping the right mode separate from the left allows for the existence of two extremely different but vital and important ways of knowing.

The left hemisphere, in contrast, is built for "vertical integration" within the cortical columns of this side, with *intraregional* linkages allowing for detailed assessment of a single mode of representation. For example, when a perceptual representation matches a linguistic category, it allows the left hemisphere to move deeply into routinized responses in its top-down processing. These linear relationships are well established and link specific inputs with particular outputs. The left hemisphere is therefore said to be built for a categorical response to routine stimuli. In other words, the left hemisphere's experience of reality is literally created by the more rigidly established definitions of its linguistic packets of representations: words. The right hemisphere, in contrast, is designed for newly assembled responses to novel stimuli. This asymmetry of the brain creates a functional contrast between familiarity on the left and novelty on the right.

A practical and intriguing example of experiencing the difference in these two modes of seeing reality is provided by Betty Edwards's book *The*

*New Drawing on the Right Side of the Brain.*[116] In this practical workbook, the educator/author introduces the reader to the notion of cerebral lateralization and provides exercises in which the differences between the two ways of knowing can be personally experienced. Essentially, when the left brain is told to "be quiet" and is not allowed to categorize what it sees, the right brain is able to assert its bottom-up mode of constructing visual reality. The results can be staggering; for instance, those who have forgotten since childhood how to draw may be happily shocked at how active their right hemispheres can still be. As Edwards's book demonstrates, many individuals have found a way to live primarily in a left-hemisphere mode of top-down categorizations with routinized perceptions and behaviors. The timeless and direct quality of experience that the book facilitates—the right hemisphere's mode of knowing the world—can make the reader feel quite alive.

Such an experience often leaves the individual with a clear view of how distinct these two ways of knowing are. Though supported by a wealth of research data on laterality, the issue of "left brain or right brain" is not even really important in the final analysis. What we are concerned with is the subjective experience of minds—different ways of being and perceiving, not merely the functional anatomy of the brain. It is indisputable that there are two profoundly different general modes in which the mind processes information. One or the other mode can dominate our conscious experience at various times. The finding that these modes of the mind do indeed have robust correlations with the sides of the brain just helps us to understand the probable neurophysiological mechanisms underlying what has been known for hundreds of years.[117]

Neuroscience can also help us avoid excessive generalizations about bilaterality. Our different ways of knowing intermingle in our daily lives. Creativity does not come from only one mode or the other. Happiness or other emotions do not emerge from living only in the timeless, nonverbal mode of constructing reality. Success does not emerge solely from the linguistic, controlled, and well-defined rules of the other mode. What research findings can be synthesized to suggest and what we can propose, in fact, is that an emergent quality of living a vital and flexible life may come from an openness to bilateral functioning involving many ways of knowing. The brain is designed to integrate its functioning.[118]

## THE DEVELOPMENT OF MINDSIGHT:
## MINDS CREATING MINDS

One of the basic forms of information that the mind constructs and processes is that of the sense of mind itself. The "mind-creating" capacity of the mind develops early in life. Many studies point to a special role of the middle (ven-tromedial) prefrontal cortex on the right side of the brain in creating maps of self and other.[119] Recall that the right hemisphere is dominant in both its activity and its growth for the first years of a child's life.[120] Children dur-ing the first years of life are able to detect the difference between animate and inanimate objects and to attribute qualities of mind, such as intentions, attentions, and feelings, to the former ones. By their third year, they are able to engage in symbolic play, in which they can invest inanimate objects with animate qualities of intentionality and emotional response.[121] This immer-sion in pretend play involves the creation of social interactions and stories that involve the subjective, mental lives of the interacting characters. As Fon-agy and Target have noted,

> The child's development and perception of mental states in himself and oth-ers thus depends on his observation of the mental world of his caregiver. He is able to perceive mental states, to the extent that his caregiver's behavior implied such states. This he does when the caregiver is in a shared pretend mode of playing with the child (hence the association between pretend and early mentalization), and many ordinary interactions (such as physical care and comforting, conversation with peers) will also involve such shared men-tation. This is what makes mental state concepts such as thinking inherently intersubjective; shared experience is part of the very logic of mental state con-cepts. . . . We believe that most important for the development of mentalizing self-organization is that exploration of the mental state of the sensitive care-giver enables the child to find in his mind an image of himself as motivated by beliefs, feelings, and intentions, in other words, as mentalizing.[122]

The initial sharing of mental experiences therefore lays the groundwork for the rest of mental development, including the acquisition of complex cognitive abilities. How does this occur? As with other aspects of mental functioning, looking toward information processing helps us to understand the "mentalizing" ability of the mind.

A typical child's brain is able to take in information about the subjective men-tal state of another person. These sig-nals are those of the nonverbal realm, which we've discussed: eye contact, facial

> The initial sharing of mental experiences therefore lays the groundwork for the rest of mental development.

expression, tone of voice. An important aspect of communication involves "joint referencing" signals (such as looking at a third object or pointing), which contain the information that the sender is focusing her attention in a certain direction or on a particular object. During the first year of life, joint referencing becomes a shared form of communication. It is during this phase that the child begins to sense the intention of another person; this permits jokes, such as pretending to jump in a sink or to eat a book, to be understood and enjoyed. During this phase of life and onward, *the mind has the ability to detect that another person has a mind with a focus of attention, an intention, and an emotional state*. To put it simply, the child has a concept of others' minds. This is also referred to as the child's "theory of mind." As we've discussed earlier, the theory-of-mind module is a component of the larger capacity of "reflective" functioning hypothesized to be an essential parental feature of secure attachments.

In the pervasive developmental disorder of autism, one sees the dysfunction in this mind-creating ability of the mind.[123] Simon Baron-Cohen has used the term "mindblindness" to refer to this inability to see others' minds, a view that has raised many questions and important debates.[124] We have used the opposite term, "mindsight," to refer to this innate capacity for perceiving the minds of others and of the self. Baron-Cohen discusses the central role of the right orbitofrontal cortex in mediating this fundamental process, which is constitutionally atypical in children with autism. Some researchers have found that the mirror neuron system does not seem to work well in individuals with autism and related disorders.[125] But the finding that these building blocks of social cognition are not functioning well does not necessarily imply their dysfunction; there may be alterations in the motivations to utilize the neural machinery that initiates the mapping of others' minds, or even of one's own mind.[126] When a neural process is not engaged, it does not necessarily mean that this circuit is innately compromised in its structure or function. We can say that, whatever the mechanism, not processing the mental side of human interactions is accompanied by social impairment and difficulties for all concerned.

In a mind that does not have the capacity to process the signals from another person, or to create the mental representations of another's mind, there is literally an absence of such a reality. In this case, the mind of the other does not exist. Within the perceiver's mind, the other's mind has not been created by the necessary representational machinery of the mind itself. It may also be that the perceiver lacks the ability to reflect upon her own mind because of this impairment in the ability to form representations of minds.

But how can a mind not be able to conceptualize a mind? If we view the mind as a processor of information, the answer is straightforward. Without the representations of mind within the neural symbols of the mind, there exists no information about the mind within the mind. Others' subjective experiences, their minds, do not exist. However, we can use the information-processing framework to suggest more universally what mindsight means for the mind and mental health. Within individuals, developing mindsight enables them to identify domains of their lives that are filled with chaos and rigidity, and then to promote the growth of integration in those areas. This process is elaborated in a series of texts that go into greater depth in the science and application of this concept.[127]

In most individuals without autism, the mind-creating or mindsight mapping process is presumably neurologically intact. We would be advised to remember that mindblindness, though, is not like being pregnant: There appear to be mild degrees of impairment in mindsight that may have neurologically constitutional underpinnings.

Can impairments to the mentalizing aspects of mindsight be created by experience? Fonagy and Target suggest that the answer is yes: Specific forms of insecure attachment, in which the parent does not focus on the mental states of the child and in which parental states are intrusive or disorganizing, can lead to an impairment in the acquisition of theory of mind.[128] How is such impairment to mindsight mediated? Are the dulled mindsight abilities of a dismissing adult a form of such impairment? Is it established by their lack of activation during childhood? Does such a developmental impediment respond to future interventions? These are questions that researchers of the future may attempt to answer.

## ADAPTIVE IMPAIRMENT OF MINDSIGHT

Psychosocial context can permit the activation or deactivation of reflective function.[129] To mediate this context-specific use of the reflective, mentalizing function, we can propose here that the mind may be capable of dis-associating component modules by impairing the integrative function of essential associative neural pathways. Relationship histories can impair the development of the integrative reflective function. This impairment can be pervasive and can lead to a child's generalized inability to mentalize, as revealed in impaired symbolic play and joint referencing.

We can also suggest that an impairment to mindsight may be state-dependent. That is, under specific conditions, a child (or adult) may be able to disengage the components essential for reflective function, shutting down this important capacity. How does the mind achieve this? In this instance, we can propose that blockage of the corpus callosal fibers interconnecting the two hemispheres, and of interconnections within the right hemisphere itself, may be a mechanism that allows mindsight to be impaired as an adaptation to certain overwhelming situations. Developmentally, this may be the situation in avoidant or disorganized attachment, in which communications are emotionally empty or terrorizing, respectively.

> Relationship histories can impair the development of the integrative reflective function.

In either of these situations, a child adapts to a particular relationship context with the inhibition of reflective function.

This finding may help explain why some individuals, such as those who commit war crimes or genocide, are capable of empathic relationships with their families and friends but can enter cold, disconnected states when involved in crimes against individuals or humanity. This ability to dis-associate thinking and behavior from the creation of the subjective mental experiences of others within our own minds may help us to understand various aspects of antisocial behavior. The fact that such state-dependent impairment or more pervasive lack of development of mindsight exists is too often revealed by the violence in our society.

The impairment in reflective function, in the setting of limited but functioning logical, language-based thinking, reveals how the separation of the hemispheres can allow for the dis-association of normally associated modes of processing information. Under certain conditions it may be prudent to develop at least partial impairment of one's mindsight abilities. An example is the phenomenon of intellectualization seen within some members of the medical profession, especially during training. A medical student working for the first time with acutely ill patients may use a nonmentalizing mode of processing—an adaptive inhibition of empathic, interpersonally connecting processing. This allows the student access to the linear, logical sequences of factual knowledge and the ability to focus on the details of patient care, while avoiding the mulitlayered emotional meaning of a patient's illness. At the oversimplified level, this could be explained by a shutting down of the right hemisphere's capacity to reflect on mental experience, while at the same time maintaining the syllogistic reasoning of the left hemisphere's mode of cognition.

If the medical student can't reintegrate the information-processing modules of her right hemisphere after a work day, or after a week, month, or year, then we can predict that certain features may become missing from her life. These adaptations can be seen as a function of the student's present hemispheric adaptations, but they may be shaped in part by the patterns from an earlier attachment history. That is, these learned adaptations may result in part from patterns of disconnection that may have been established and made readily accessible by prior experience. For the student, the present disconnection may lead to a loss of readily accessible autobiographical memory and of spontaneous primary emotional states whose appraisals create a sense of meaning in life. Personal relationships may become strained as communication becomes dominated by context-independent details and logical, linguistically based talk, rather than also including emotional messages between two relatives or friends. For this medical student, or for others engaged in emotionally challenging work, shutting down the right hemisphere temporarily may be a needed adaptation in order to perform a job efficiently. Living in an isolated, left-hemisphere-dominated internal world, however, can be experienced as filled with highly categorized routines or top-down processes that lack a feeling of spontaneity and vitality. If the right hemisphere does not become integrated with the left later, then such adaptations may prove to be dysfunctional and lead to serious problems outside, or even inside, the workplace. The medical student, and others learning to cope with overwhelming experiences, may be aided by understanding this adaptive dis-association of integrative processes.

In this example, the adaptive need under stress to diminish (at least conscious) access to the representations of others' minds may lead to the isolated restriction of the mindsight module of the right hemisphere. As with any form of dis-association, anatomically dispersed processes can become functionally isolated if the integrating neural pathways making associations become blocked. Such a process may occur either at the level of the inter-hemispheric transfer of information or in the form of dis-associations within the information processing of one hemisphere—in this case, that of the right. As with other forms of dis-association, blockage of certain modes may also involve the impairment of related functions. In this example, the middle pre-frontal cortex is the primary site for integrating a wide range of fundamental processes, including mindsight, stimulus appraisal, somatic representation, autonomic activity, affect regulation, and autonoetic consciousness. The adaptive blockage of mindsight representations may tend to be associated with the unintentional impairment of a number of these anatomically and functionally related prefrontally mediated processes.

Just as the mind can isolate implicit recollections from explicit ones, so too can it isolate right- from left-hemisphere functions. Hemispheric dis-association can be understood as a domination of one mode over the other. The monosemantic, linguistic left hemisphere—filled with modes of information processing that rely upon the rules of logic and reason, and able to negotiate in an external world of symbols and language—can often find its place in interacting with the outside world. The left hemisphere's experience of consciousness may be better equipped to deal with the world in abstract concepts independent of emotional context. The right hemisphere, in contrast, is filled with polysemantic images of the world, perceptions of others' emotions, sensations of the body, and holistic patterns of intuitive insights that often defy words. These mental representations are context-dependent, filled with horizontal, multilayered associations to a wide array of bodily sensations, sense of self and other, autobiographical memories, and emotional meaning. There is often no easy way for the right hemisphere to "speak," especially if only the left hemisphere (of oneself or another) is listening.

## REFLECTIONS: REPRESENTING REALITY
## AND PSYCHOLOGICAL WELL-BEING

The mind constructs its own experience of reality. Emanating from the interface of the brain and human relationships, the mind creates connections among the various elements of representations, ranging from sensations and images to concepts and words. The connections we have within our relationships and among the layers of neural activity within our bodies weave a fabric of subjective life: They enable us to feel, behave, think, plan, and communicate.

> The mind constructs its own experience of reality.

Living in a world constructed by our own minds makes knowing about these representational processes essential in deepening our understanding of human experience. Patterns of representations differ markedly between the left and right halves of the brain. Often underrecognized within the fields of clinical psychiatry and psychology is the important distinction between the modes of representation within the two hemispheres of the brain. The left hemisphere has been described as having a logical "interpreter" function that uses syllogistic reasoning to deduce cause–effect relationships from the representational data it has available to it. The right hemisphere specializes in the representation of context and of mentalizing capacities. It is therefore uniquely capable of registering and expressing affective facial expressions, developing a "theory of mind," registering and regulating the state of the body, and having autobiographical representations.

How are these bilateral processes relevant to relationships? Communication is crucial in establishing neural connections early in life and involves the sharing of energy and information. Levels of arousal (energy) and mental representations (information) are very different on each side of the brain. The sharing of arousal and representations from one brain to another—the essence of connecting minds—will thus differ between the hemispheres. We can propose, in fact, that the right brain perceives the output of the right brain of another person, whereas the left brain perceives the left brain's output. In intimate, emotional relationships, such as friendship, romance, parent–child pairs, psychotherapy, and teacher–student dyads, what does this look like? The left brain sends out language-based, logical, sequential interpreting statements that attempt to make sense of things. The left brain receives these messages, decodes the linguistic representations, and tries to make sense out of these newly arrived symbols. At the same time, the right brain is sending nonverbal messages via facial expressions, gestures, prosody, and tone of voice, which are perceived by the other's right brain. OK. So what?

The "what" is that the right brain takes this information and uses its social perceptions of nonverbal communication to engage directly in a few very important processes. It creates an image of the other's mind ("mind-sight"). It regulates bodily response while at the same time registering the somatic representations of shifts in bodily state. It creates autobiographical representations within memory. It appraises the meaning of these events and directly affects the degree of arousal, thus creating primary emotional responses. Spontaneous and primary emotional states are therefore likely to be mediated via the right hemisphere.

When we examine these findings alongside the independent set of data from attachment research, certain patterns are suggested. The early affect attunement and alignment of mental states can be seen as a mutually regulated hemisphere-to-hemisphere coordination between child and parent. In this view, we can propose that avoidant attachment involves a serious lack of this form of communication between the right hemispheres of child and parent. The extension of this finding to laterality research raises the possibility that the left hemisphere serves as the dominant mediator of communication between an avoidant child and a dismissing parent. As noted in Chapter 3, a preliminary study by Behrens and colleagues is consistent with this view of left-hemisphere dominance in avoidant/dismissing attachment.[130] In further support of this perspective, it turns out that in 1989, Main and Hesse examined exactly this hypothesis in two large-scale samples of Berkeley undergraduates, each of whom were asked about their degree of right-handedness (or left-handedness), as a rough approximation of brain dominance.[131] At the same time, Main and Hesse had devised a set of self-report items that they considered indicative of a "dismissing" state of mind. This type of scale was not ultimately able to predict AAI classifications statistically,[132] and therefore these findings were never published; in keeping with the hypothesis, however, both studies found that the degree of right-handedness was significantly correlated with elevated scores of the scale for "dismissing" state of mind.

Further extensions of these ideas to relationships allow us to look more deeply into why certain couples may be "unable to communicate" with any emotional satisfaction. When we know about the different languages of the right and left hemispheres, it is possible to make hypotheses about why interactions may be frustrating: Individuals may not know how to understand the particular language being expressed by their significant others. If we then integrate past attachment history in understanding the pattern of these difficulties, it is possible to create a framework of understanding that can help the partners in such relationships escape their well-worn ruts.

If this laterality–attachment hypothesis is correct, then a logical implication would be that any experiences that help to develop the processing abilities of each hemisphere and/or the integrated activities of the two hemispheres may improve certain individuals' internal and interpersonal lives. Such movement toward more coordinated interhemispheric functioning would be quite welcomed by many people (especially by the lonely and frustrated spouses of dismissing individuals).[133] The developmental and experiential histories that have led to a lack of integration of the functioning of the two hemispheres may leave individuals vulnerable to emotional and social problems. Unresolved trauma and grief, histories of emotional neglect, and restrictive adaptations may each represent some form of constriction in the flow of information processing between the hemispheres. This proposal of the central role of dis-associated hemispheric processing in emotional disturbances is supported by the finding that insecure attachments in childhood may establish a vulnerability to psychological dysfunction.

Emotional relationships that enhance the development of each hemisphere and its unrestricted linkage with the activity of the other are thus likely to foster the development of psychological well-being. In this way, a secure attachment can be seen as a developmental relationship that provides for an integration of functioning of the two hemispheres, both between child and caregiver and within the child's own brain. At the most basic level, right-hemisphere-to-right-hemisphere communication can be seen within the affectively attuned communications that allow for primary emotional states to be shared via nonverbal signals. Left-hemisphere-to-left-hemisphere alignment can be seen in shared attention to objects in the world. Reflective dialogues, in which language is used to focus attention on the mental states of others (including the two members of the dyad), may foster bilateral integration between the two hemispheres of both child and parent. The resilience of secure attachments can thus be proposed as founded in part in the integration that these relationships foster. Ultimately, integration creates self-regulation and the movement of our lives toward flexible, adaptive, and coherent ways of being. In the next chapter, we'll turn to the process of the mind's self-organizing movement toward regulation; we will further examine the role of the brain and relationships in creating this important aspect of human life.

# CHAPTER 7

# Self-Regulation

## THE CENTRAL ROLE OF EMOTION IN SELF-REGULATION

The self is created within the processes that organize the activity of the mind in its interactions with the world. As we've seen in Chapter 5, such self-organization is a fundamental way in which complex systems function. At a given moment in time, the array of mental activity becomes organized within a mental state that functions to create a coherent set of goal-directed processes. Across time, we can understand how continuity is created within a given self-state through the various principles of complexity, connectionism, and information processing. Integrating these processes is emotion.

As Luc Ciompi has described, emotions function as "central organizers and integrators" in linking several domains: providing all incoming stimuli with a specific meaning and motivational direction; participating in state-dependent memory processes; connecting mental processes "synchronically" and "diachronically" (within one time and across time); creating more complex interconnections among abstract representational processes that share emotional meaning; and simultaneously attuning the whole organism to current situational demands on the basis of past experience through neurophysiologically mediated peripheral effects.[1] Such organizing features intimately link what are traditionally considered the mental, social, and biological domains. As Alan Sroufe has pointed out, then, emotions are inherently integrative in their function.[2]

As we further explore the nature of the mind, we will find that understanding the creation of the self at the interface of brain and human relationships focuses our attention on the fundamental ways in which emotion is experienced and regulated. As many researchers have suggested, emotion is both regulated and regulatory. In its manifestations as neurophysiological events, subjective experiences, and interpersonal expressions, emotion interconnects various systems within the mind and between minds. Focusing on emotion regulation allows us to explore how the mind becomes organized and integrated.

In this chapter, we'll explore some ways of viewing the regulatory processes that organize the mind. From a developmental perspective, an infant's first challenge is to achieve internal homeostasis via the activity of deep structures of the brainstem, which mediate sleep–wake cycles and other basic bodily functions (such as heart rate, respiration, and digestion). Myron Hofer has described how even at this early stage, the parent provides "hidden regulators" that directly facilitate these basic functions in the infant.[3] As maturation unfolds, "dyadic regulation" becomes important in enabling the child to monitor and modify more complex states of mind.[4] Attachment serves as a crucial way in which the self becomes regulated. As the child's evaluative mechanisms become more active, and memory processes enable the child to respond to discrepancies, subjective meaning is created in engaging with the social surround. Intimate attunements permit a resonance of states of mind that are mutually regulating. Misattunements lead to dysregulation, which requires "interactive repair" if the child is to regain equilibrium.[5] Achieving emotion regulation is dependent upon social interactions. At this early point, according to Sroufe, the child has become an emotional being—not merely a reactive one—in that arousal or tension is created via evaluative appraisals that create subjective meaning in engagements with the environment.[6] As infancy gives way to the toddler period, dyadic regulation is supplanted by "caregiver-guided self-regulation," in which the adult helps the child begin to regulate states of mind autonomously.[7] As the child's brain matures into the preschool years, the emergence of increasingly intricate layers of self-regulation becomes possible.

> Attachment serves as a crucial way in which the self becomes regulated.

As emotion continues to function in integrative ways throughout life, it reveals the continuing process by which our minds carry out intersystem integration: within our own modes of processing, across various modalities, and between our own minds and those of others. As Antonio Damasio has noted,

> Emotion, and the experience of emotion, are the highest-order direct expressions of bioregulation in complex organisms. Leave out emotion and you leave out the prospect of understanding bioregulation comprehensively, especially as it regards the relation between an organism and the most complex aspects of an environment: society and culture.[8]

From our discussion of complexity, we can see that emotion and the development of emotion regulation move the self into more complex states of intra- and intersystem functioning.

*Integration leads to optimal regulation.* As we've discussed in Chapter 4, emotion can be seen as "shifts in integration." In essence, "emotion regulation" is how we use our minds, bodies, and relational processes to enhance integration. To achieve regulation, the mind both monitors and modifies the flow of energy and information internally and interpersonally. What this means is that processes linking differentiated elements of a system—within or between individuals—can produce the integration at the heart of regulation. In this manner, we utilize both the nervous system and relationships to regulate the "self." Emotion regulation that allows the mind to emerge in a flexible manner in interaction with the environment reflects optimal state regulation. As we've also discussed in earlier chapters, the prefrontally mediated capacity for response flexibility may be a central component to such a balancing skill. These regulatory prefrontal regions link widely separated areas to one another. That is, these are regions that create neural integration linking the differentiated input from cortex, limbic areas, brainstem, the body proper, and even the social signals from other nervous systems. Emotion "dysregulation" can be seen as impairments in this capacity to allow flexible and organized responses that are adaptive to the internal and external environment. When integration is impaired, coordination and balance cannot be achieved, and the system moves toward chaos, rigidity, or both. As we'll discuss, repeated patterns of such dysregulation can have their origins in constitutional elements, interactional experience, and the transaction between these two fundamental components of the mind.[9] The mind is the process that regulates the flow of energy and information, and it is both embodied and relational. Self-regulation entails this continual emergence of regulation at the interface of the neural and the interpersonal.

## DYSFUNCTIONAL PATTERNS OF SELF-REGULATION

The structure of the brain gives it an innate capacity to regulate emotion and to organize its states of activation. Sometimes referred to as "affect regulation" or "emotion regulation," this capacity is crucial for the internal and interpersonal functioning of the individual.[10] A number of psychiatric disturbances can be viewed as disorders of self-regulation.[11] As mentioned earlier, varied symptoms and syndromes described in the DSM-IV-TR[12] can also be seen as examples of impaired integration, revealed as chaos, rigidity, or both. Recent work by Marcus Raichle and colleagues on the default mode of brain activity supports this proposal by noting that integrative brain functioning is impaired in a range of psychiatric disturbances.[13] Among these are the mood disorders, in which emotional state is massively dysregulated, producing states of depression or mania. Within these states of mind are characteristic dysfunctions in perception, memory, beliefs, and behaviors. These are disorders where the unique feature is a profound instability in mood. Anxiety disorders also reveal the flood of arousal that evokes a dysfunctional state of mind. Individuals with these difficulties may be excessively sensitive to the environment and may also have autonomous signals of impending disaster, as in panic disorder and obsessive–compulsive disorder. Here, too, there is a marked incapacity to regulate one's state of mind. As individuals with these and other disorders (see below) develop, the instability of their states may become a characteristic feature, or trait, of their self-regulation. Indeed, in studies of patients with bipolar disorder, the untreated swings between mania and depression can begin to create a "kindling effect" that makes their onset more frequent and intense, with rapid cycling. In this way, the instability can become a repeated, "stable" feature of the individual's self-organizational dysfunction.[14]

In many of these disorders, a combination of pharmacological and psychotherapeutic interventions may be indicated. Even if the origin of the dysfunction is seen as the neural instability of some neuronal circuit in the deep or limbic regions of the brain, the mind of the individual is inextricably created in part by the brain's activity. As we've seen in Chapter 5, dysfunction of a subcomponent in a system can have profound and unpredictable effects on other subcomponents, as well as on the system as a whole. To help the individual achieve a more balanced and functional form of self-organization, it may be essential to aim interventions at many layers of the individual's functioning, including the brain, the body as a whole, and relationships. For this reason, even approaches that harness mental training, such as mindful awareness practices, are now being explored in the treatment of individuals with bipolar disorder.[15] Focused attention can mobilize neural circuits of self-regulation as the individual uses awareness to modulate the "internal constraints" of the brain.[16] Within the clinical setting, the relationship of therapist and patient can become the "external constraint" that can help produce changes in the individual's capacity for self-organization.

The developmental origins of impaired self-organization can be seen in those with insecure attachments. With the experience of avoidant attachment, the mind learns to adapt to the barren psychological world by decreasing awareness of socially generated emotional states. The rigidity of such a constrained pattern is revealed in the ways that the significance of social interactions is cognitively blocked, despite continued physiological responses. In disorganized attachment experiences, the child acquires the ability to respond to stress with a dis-association of processes, leading to dissociative states. Some of these states are quite disorganized and incohesive, whereas others have the appearance of functional cohesion. Closer examination of even these latter dissociated states reveals a marked cognitive blockage restricting the over-

> The developmental origins of impaired self-organization can be seen in those with insecure attachments.

all processing of information and flow of energy through the mind as a whole. The apparently divergent avoidant and disorganized attachment patterns actually share the characteristic of restriction in the flow of states of mind. This convergence is supported by the finding in the Minnesota Longitudinal Study of Parents and Children that during the early years of life, before adolescence, children with disorganized and avoidant attachments have the greatest degree of dissociative symptoms.[17] This finding supports the proposal that impairments to mental well-being may be understood as adaptations that impair the balanced flow of energy and information in the formation of emerging states of mind.

As noted above, many psychiatric disturbances involve affect dysregulation. In addition to mood disorders (such as depression and bipolar illness) and the anxiety disorders (including panic disorder, phobias, obsessive-compulsive disorder, and PTSD), these include dissociative disorders and certain personality disorders, such as borderline and narcissistic character structures.[18] Rather than reviewing all of these disorders in detail, let us look at a single case example to gain additional insight into the nature of emotion dysregulation.

> "I couldn't help myself. He made me so furious with his mistakes that I told him to go jump in a lake. Not in those friendly words, of course. I was so angry. I wasn't going to let him get away with that kind of stuff again. Maybe for others it's OK, but not with me. Why is everyone in this world so stupid?"

This thirty-five-year-old attorney was fired by her client of ten years after screaming and apparently threatening a colleague at a meeting for missing a deadline in mailing a document she had given to him. This was not the first time her emotions had "taken over"; she had lost several boyfriends in the past for her "instability" and was now at risk of being alone again, in addition to having lost her most important client. For this patient, the inability to regulate her emotions was a major problem in both her personal and professional lives.

This woman's interactions with other people had historically evoked "sudden outbursts of intense emotion." Let's examine what this phrase may have meant for her within our framework for understanding emotional processes. "Sudden" refers to the notion that something seems to occur with-out some warning or clue that a process is about to occur or is even occur-ring. At a minimum, we can suggest that she was not consciously aware of the impending external expression of her emotional response. "Intense emo-tion" is a common term that we can now interpret in the language of the mind. "Intense" probably signifies a strong degree of activation or arousal, which became expressed in this woman's case as the categorical emotion of rage. So we have taken this a bit further, but not much. Is this just the use of new words to describe the familiar notion of an emotional "hijacking" or "outburst," in which rational thinking is suspended and anger or other emo-tions cloud perceptions and influence behavior?[19] It is much more than this, as we'll see later in the chapter.

But, you may say, perhaps it was just this woman's "genetic legacy" to have uncontrolled outbursts of anger. Perhaps so. But in any psychiatric con-ditions that may have a large genetic component, understanding the mecha-nisms of the mind and the contributions of interactive experiences can help provide interventions that can alter the way the brain functions.[20] Recall that the reduction of human behavior into an "either–or" condition of "genet-ics versus learning" or "nature versus nurture" is unhelpful and clouds our thinking about the issues, especially when it comes to designing interven-tions. We will return to this example of the attorney toward the middle of this chapter, to examine ways of understanding how constitutional and experiential factors can lead to certain kinds of emotion dysregulation.

## A CONCEPTUAL FRAMEWORK OF EMOTION REGULATION

The remainder of this chapter provides a conceptual framework for under-standing some basic components of emotion regulation. These include regu-lation of intensity, sensitivity, specificity, windows of tolerance, recovery processes, access to consciousness, and external expression. This is not an exhaustive review of emotion regulation in its myriad manifestations; such reviews can be found elsewhere in a number of useful texts.[21] Rather, this is a practical framework that draws on our study of the mind in order to illus-trate how individuals achieve a flexible and adaptive capacity for the regula-tion of emotional processes.

The brain has developed a rich circuitry that helps regulate its states of arousal. The nature of this process of emotion regulation may vary quite a lot from individual to individual and may be influenced both by constitu-tional features and by adaptations to experience. "Temperament" describes some of the aspects of inborn characteristics, including sensitivity to the environment, intensity of emotional response, baseline global mood, regularity of biological cycles, and attraction to or withdrawal from novel situations. These inborn features of the nervous system, which are the results of both genetic and intrauterine factors, probably have powerful shaping effects throughout the lifespan. Temperament can evoke particular parenting responses and create its own self-fulfilling reinforcements, which further amplify the inborn neural proclivity. The example of a slow-to-warm-up or shy child whose mother has little patience for his hesitancy illustrates how the response of others can engrain temperamental features.[22]

Attachment studies support the view that the pattern of communication with parents creates a cascade of adaptations that directly shape the development of the child's nervous system. Both longitudinal attachment studies and early intervention research support the idea that what parents do with their children makes a difference in the outcome of the children's development.[23] It is important to realize that temperament, attachment history, and other experiential factors each contribute to the marked differences we see between individuals in their ability to regulate their emotions.

If emotions influence the flow of states of mind that dominate so many of our mental processes, how do we keep them in some form of balance? The mind's ability to regulate emotional processes is dependent in part on the brain's ability to monitor and modify the flow of arousal and activation throughout its circuits. Primary emotional processes, categorical emotions, affective expression, and mood can each be regulated by the brain. "Emotion regulation" refers to the general ability of the mind to alter the various components of emotional processing. The self-organization of the mind in many ways is determined by the self-regulation of emotional states. How we experience the world, relate to others, and find meaning in life are dependent upon how we have come to regulate our emotions.

Why should emotions and their regulation be considered so central to the organization of the self? As we've discussed in Chapter 4, emotion reflects the fundamental way in which the mind assigns value to external and internal events and then directs the allocation of attentional resources to further the processing of these representations. In this way, emotion reflects the way the mind directs the flow of information and of energy. The modulation of emotion is the way the mind regulates energy and information processing. With this perspective, emotional regulation can be seen at the center of the self-organization of the mind.

From the wide range of research on emotions, it is possible to propose here at least seven aspects of emotion regulation that can illustrate these ideas.[24] These are derived from a synthesis of scientific concepts and clinical observations. Other aspects of regulation could also be proposed, but these seven areas provide a practical framework for understanding the various ways in which the mind regulates its own functioning—how it shapes energy and information flow within the brain and within our relationships.

## Intensity

The foundation of emotional processing is the appraisal–arousal system, which can respond with various degrees of intensity. The brain appears to be able to modify the intensity of response by altering the numbers of neurons that fire and the amounts of neurotransmitters released in response to a stimulus. Degrees of arousal have a wide range. If initial appraisal and arousal mechanisms minimally activate the body and brain, then the elaborating appraisal–arousal response will also be minimal. For example, studies have shown that participants who are asked to meditate or who are given pills to reduce bodily responses and physiological arousal will interpret a stimulus as "not so important," and the primary emotion will not be as intense, as in participants without such inhibitors of bodily reaction.[25] The body's state of arousal is mediated by the brain through the autonomic nervous system. As discussed in Chapters 4, 5, and 6, the brain in turn monitors the state of the body and incorporates emotional meaning from the somatic maps of the body's change in physiological state. These maps are represented in the prefrontal regions and experienced as interoceptive awareness.

An individual's characteristic pattern of high- or low-intensity responses may be a product of both constitutional and experiential factors. People with shy temperaments may have an inborn tendency to respond intensely to new situations and to withdraw when confronted with novelty. Geraldine Dawson and colleagues have found that *intensity* of emotional response appears to be related to bilateral frontal activation, in contrast to the quality or *valence* of response, which is asymmetric (involving left activation for approach and right for withdrawal states).[26] Shy people have a more intense right-hemisphere response to novelty. Other individuals may experience milder degrees of intensity of emotion in response to novelty.

As noted in Chapter 6, Dawson's group and other researchers have also found in studies of infants of clinically depressed mothers that the infant's capacity to experience joy and excitement is markedly reduced, especially if the maternal depression lasts beyond the first year.[27] Experience can thus directly shape the general intensity and valence of emotional activation in children. In particular, the sharing of positive emotional states may be missing from the experience of children with depressed parents. The sharing of such states under typical conditions permits an amplification of these pleasurable emotions, which sends both child and parent "into orbit" with waves of intensely engaged positive affect.[28] If such shared amplification of positive

emotional states is missing, as in depressed dyads, then the capacity to tolerate (i.e., to regulate in a balanced manner) and to enjoy these intense states
may be underdeveloped. Interactive experiences enable the child not only
to experience high levels of "tension" or emotionally engaged arousal,[29] but
to entrain the circuits of the brain to be able to manage such states.[30] Feeling comfortable with intense arousal and engagement with others may have
its origins in both constitutional and experiential features of the individual.
Secure relationships can be seen to involve the caregiver's ability to stay with
the infant in times of intense distress to provide a soothing presence, as well
as to amplify states of joy for shared experience of positive joining.

As we'll see, intensity of arousal can be masked. It is often when emotion
becomes most intense that we seem to have the greatest need to be understood and the most intense feelings of vulnerability. This sense of exposure
may make many individuals, especially those who have had unsatisfying past
experiences with communication, reluctant to reveal openly what they are
feeling. At a moment of intensity, a failure to be understood, to be connected
with emotionally, can result in a profound feeling of shame.[31] The shame
generated by missed opportunities for the alignment of states—for the feeling of emotional resonance, of "feeling felt"—can lead to withdrawal. Even
with less intense states, not being understood may lead to a sense of isolation.
Recognizing this vulnerability and the fact that moments of unintended disconnection are inevitable can allow us to repair such ruptures in alignment.
Such interactive repair experiences allow us to learn to tolerate new levels
of emotional intensity and the feeling of vulnerability that may accompany
them.

## Sensitivity

Each of us has a "threshold of response," or the minimum amount of stimulation needed in order to activate our appraisal systems. Those with a hair-
trigger response mechanism will find life filled with challenging situations.
Their brains will frequently fire off messages of "This is important—pay
attention!" Those with "tougher skins" will not readily respond with arousal
and will be less emotionally sensitive to the same stimuli.

Sensitivity, like intensity, may be both constitutional and modified by
experience. Both variables may also be dependent on an individual's state of
mind at a particular moment in time. We can have times in our lives when
our "nerves are raw" and we react quickly to previously innocuous events.
When we are preoccupied by something else or emotionally defending ourselves, we can be less sensitive than we might otherwise be. Alterations in
our threshold of responding may be an important way our brains regulate
emotional responses.

How can a mind alter sensitivity? Turning to the foundation of emotions in appraisal, we can make some educated hypotheses. By increasing the amount of stimulation a value center needs to become activated, the brain can directly decrease its sensitivity to the environment. Modifications in the appraisal system itself can also decrease or increase sensitivity. For example, if you have recently seen a violent movie with gunshots and murders, your mind may be sensitized to loud sounds and dark alleys. If, upon returning to your car in a dark parking lot, you hear a sudden loud sound, you may be more likely to become aroused and to appraise such a situation as dangerous. If you had just been to a party with a lot of noise and fireworks, your mind would be less vigilant for signs of danger and would be less sensitive to those same sounds in the dark parking lot. Recent experience primes the mind for a context-specific change in sensitivity.[32]

Repeated patterns of intense emotional experiences may engrain chronic alterations in the degree of sensitivity. For example, overwhelming terror, especially early in life, may permanently alter an individual's sensitivity to a particular stimulus related to the trauma. If a cat scratches and bites a young child, the sight of even a distant cat may evoke a strong emotional response of fear in this individual for years into the future.

> Recent experience primes the mind for a context-specific change in sensitivity.

Furthermore, early trauma may be associated with abnormalities in cortisol release in response to daily life experiences.[33] Studies have revealed, too, that the regulation of genes responsible for the HPA axis may also be negatively affected by early life stressors.[34] These findings, along with other studies, suggest that early neglect and abuse may lead to damage or impaired growth in the integrative fibers of the brain.[35] Since regulation arises from integration, these studies support the view that regulation can be severely hampered following early trauma and neglect. Early alteration of the circuits and epigenetic regulation of specific regions of the brain involved in the stress response and in evaluative processes can deeply influence the appraisal mechanisms that directly influence emotional experience and its regulation.

Some early experiences that sensitize the arousal system to fire off may never be fully desensitized.[36] Patients may remain in a chronically hypersensitized state. However, specific appraisal of the excessively sensitive general arousal stage can be changed. Let us look at an example of this "cognitive override" mechanism.

As a young child, a forty-year-old man had been mauled by a dog; in the incident, he lost part of his left ear and sustained deep wounds to his arms and chest. Throughout his youth, he naturally avoided dogs. As a young father, he dreaded the day when his own children would ask to have a dog as a pet.

He came to therapy when that day indeed arrived. What could be done? Every time he saw a dog, his heart would pound; he would sweat profusely, clutch his chest, and feel a sense of doom. This panic was once treated with medications, which were effective but excessively sedating for him. The man wanted to get a dog for his children, but he couldn't live with his fear.

Some might appropriately say that parents should let children know about the limits of what can or can't be done. They might feel in this case that the father's need to have a canine-free house should have been communicated and respected. Another possibility—the one that this man preferred—was to try to "deal" with his fears. The original accident had happened when he was two years old. He had little explicit recall of anything from that period. We know, of course, that this was a typical part of his childhood amnesia; that is, explicit autobiographical encoding was not yet available to him, due to the immaturity of his hippocampal and orbitofrontal regions. And so his primary form of memory for this event was implicit: He exhibited emotional (fear and panic) and behavioral (avoidance) memories of the accident. Fortunately, he knew about the experience from the stories he had been told by his parents and from his own semantic memory. This knowledge was in a noetic form: He knew the facts, but he did not have a sense of himself at this point in the past, so it was not autonoetic. Seeing his mauled ear in the mirror also reminded him each day that something terrifying had occurred.

This patient's amygdala was probably exquisitely sensitized to the sight of a dog. As we've discussed in Chapter 4, a preconscious feedback loop involving the perceptual system and the amygdala would have allowed for the fight–flight response to be initiated even before he became aware that he had seen a dog. These functional circuits have been evolutionarily helpful to us as human beings: Once we are hurt, our amygdalas will do everything they can to keep us from allowing it to happen again.

Teaching this man about the nature of the fear response and the neural circuits underlying it was relieving for him. Relaxation techniques and guided imagery with exposure to self-generated images of dogs were provided. Nevertheless, he still had an initial startle response to dogs. A "cognitive override" strategy was then tried. That is, this patient learned to acknowledge the relevance of his amygdala's response to the present dog and the past trauma (the initial arousal mechanism). He then would say to himself, "I know that you are trying to protect me, and that you think this is a dangerous thing" (the specific appraisal stage). What he would say next was what eventually allowed him to buy his children a (small) dog: "I do not need to see this sense of panic as something to fear or get agitated about." He would then imagine his amygdala sighing with relief, having discharged its duties to warn, and the sense of doom would dissipate. After several weeks of performing these internal override discussions, he felt ready to proceed with the purchase of the pet. Six months later, he and his family were doing well with the new addition to their household.

This example illustrates that even if the sensitivity to particular stimuli cannot be changed, a person's response to the initial arousal can be diverted in ways that lead to a more flexible life. In this case, this may have been made possible by the development and involvement of the patient's prefrontally mediated response flexibility process. This individual's past trauma had led to a rigid pattern in the flow of information processing and energy (the sight of a dog led to massive arousal and the sense of fear). By altering the engrained patterns of information and energy flow, the patient became more flexible in his behavior, and he was able to move forward more adaptively in his life. As we shall continue to explore, impediments to mental health may often be seen as blockages in information processing and energy flow. Experiences that allow these fundamental elements to achieve a more flexible and adaptive flow or "circulation" through mental life can contribute greatly to emotional well-being.

## Specificity

Emotion regulation can also determine which parts of the brain are activated by arousal. By determining the value and meaning assigned to a stimulus—specificity of appraisal—the brain is able to regulate the flow of energy through the changing states of the system. For example, being awakened by a sound while taking a nap will probably lead your body to enter an aroused state of initial orientation. As your brain begins to process this stimulated state, it can assign meaning to various aspects of the sound. If you are expecting the arrival of your spouse while you are resting, the context of anticipating your spouse's return will be represented, and you may interpret the sound as a source of excitement. If instead you aren't expecting anyone, the sound may be interpreted as a possible intruder and a signal of danger, and you may feel fear. The representations activated at any particular moment, including the context of the situation, help shape the specific direction of stimulus appraisal elicited. The specificity of elaborated and differentiated appraisal directly shapes arousal and thus determines the specific type of emotional experience that unfolds.

Through its shaping of arousal, the specificity of appraisal directly influences the differentiation of primary emotions into categorical emotions. Characteristic differences among individuals in their appraisal mechanisms can directly determine the kinds of emotions generated and can influence the general "nature" of their moods and personality. This may be one way that some more entrenched aspects of temperament for certain individuals persists into adulthood. Specificity of appraisal creates not only the meaning we attribute to stimulus events, but the meaning of the self–environment context and the form and meaning of the emerging emotional processes themselves. Specificity is thus a complex, recursive process of evaluation that appraises the meaning of events and the ongoing appraisal–arousal processes. The specificity of appraisal may be influenced by several elements of the evaluation of the stimulus, such as the individual's assessment of its relevance to the achievement of current or future goals, its threat to the individual's capacity to cope and to maintain the self as the locus of control, and its meaning to global issues regarding the self and the self in relation to others.

As a child develops, the differentiation of primary emotions into categorical ones becomes more and more sophisticated. In this manner, there is a progression from the earliest states of pleasure or discomfort to the basic or categorical emotions, such as fear, anger, disgust, surprise, interest, shame, and joy. Sroufe has described the "precursor emotions" of pleasure, wariness, and frustration/distress as preceding the development of the more discrete emotional states of joy, fear, and anger, respectively.[37]

As the child continues to develop, more complex and "socially derived" emotions, such as nostalgia, jealousy, and pride, become differentiated. Linda Camras has suggested that dynamical systems theory may be useful in examining the development of emotional expression.[38] From this perspective, the infant's mind functions to integrate internal processes with interactional responses from parents. The emerging differentiation of emotional processes arises within the interacting domains of neurophysiology, subjective experience, interpersonal relationships, and affective expression. The more differentiated, discrete emotions come to function as attractor states that have internally and externally determined constraints. As described by Carol Malatesta-Magai, such a process is a form of "emotion socialization," which reflects the fundamental way in which affect serves as a social signal and develops in part as a reflection of interpersonal history.[39] Such emotion socialization occurs both within the child–caregiver relationship and in peer–peer interactions, and it may have significant variation across cultures.[40]

The experiences children have within their families and within the larger culture directly shape the ways in which rules of social interaction are established. The sharing of internal states, then, is one aspect of communication that can be learned through these moment-to-moment emotional interactions with significant others. For example, one study revealed that children from the Brahman caste in India were less likely to communicate negative emotion than children from the United States were.[41] These interactive social behaviors may also become differences in the internal experience of mental life, as Lev Vygotsky noted; that is, social communications can become the template for internal processes we call "thought."[42] Other studies have suggested that people from individualistic nations other than the United States were also more likely to communicate negative affect and to be more externally focused on solving problems. In contrast, those from collectivist nations were found to have less self-reflective emotions.[43] We are shaped by our culture, and our culture shapes who we are.

The specificity of emotional experience is determined by the specific complex layers of appraisal activated in response to a stimulus. These evaluative processes, mediated by our socially sensitive value circuits in the brain, emerge within our individual constitutions and interactional histories. It is for this reason that two people often have qualitatively different reactions to the same situation. Unique personal meaning is created by the specificity of our emotional responses.

Researchers have named a wide range of emotions in various categories.[44] Some of these include interest/excitement, enjoyment/joy, surprise/astonishment, sadness, anger, disgust, contempt, fear, anxiety, shyness, and love. Other types have also been described, such as the "self-conscious emotions" of embarrassment, pride, shame, and guilt, as well as a sense of exhilaration and humor. Individuals may have experienced many or all of these emotions at some point in their lives. They may also

> Unique personal meaning is created by the specificity of our emotional responses.

have noticed that each time they experienced a given categorical emotion (e.g., sadness), it has both unique and universal aspects. As a state of the system is assembled, it has unique features of both inner processes and external contexts.

The differentiation of primary emotional states into categorical emotions is a rapid process illustrating how various layers of the brain are influenced by the unfolding state of mind. In its essence, emotion is a set of processes involving the recruitment of various circuits under the umbrella of one state of mind. Thus the appraisal and arousal processes create a neural net activation profile—a state of mind—whose characteristics in turn directly shape subsequent appraisal and arousal processes. This intricate feedback mechanism helps us to see why patterns of emotional response can be so tenacious in a given individual. The elements of continuity in specificity are self-reinforcing.

Creating change within rigid patterns of specific appraisals requires a fundamental change in the organization of information and energy flow. As we have seen in the example of the man who eventually bought the dog for his children, the alteration in sensitivity to the image of a dog took place at the level of altered specificity of appraisal. The specific appraisal response to both "dog" and "panic" needed to be revised before a new pattern of emotional reaction could be achieved.

Value circuits determine specific appraisal, creating the basic hedonic tone of "this is good" or "this is bad" and the behavioral set of "approach" or "withdraw." Value circuits also continue to assess the meaning of these initial activations as they are elaborated into more defined emotional states, including the categorical emotions. What determines the nature of the appraisal/value process itself? How does the mind "know" what should be paid attention to, what is good or bad, and how to respond with sadness or anger?

From the perspective of human evolution, the organization of this complex appraisal process is likely to have had survival benefits for our ancestors. According to the principles of evolution, the genes that now shape the appraisal process are likely to have helped early humans survive, and so were passed on to be present today. This is one explanation, for example, of why some people are frightened of snakes even though they may never have seen one before. This may also explain why infants have a "hard-wired" (inborn) system to appraise attachment experiences as important. In other words, there is a hard-wired, genetic aspect to the appraisal process.

A second crucial evolutionary influence on the appraisal mechanism is that it can learn from an individual's experience. For example, individuals who could not learn that touching a flame hurts would have been more likely to be repeatedly injured, and therefore less likely to survive and pass on their genes. Those individuals whose brains could alter their evaluative mechanisms would have been more likely to survive. Hence *the appraisal system has a genetic basis and is also responsive to experience; it learns. Emotional engagement enhances learning.*

## Windows of Tolerance

Each of us has a "window of tolerance" in which various intensities of emotional arousal can be processed without disrupting the functioning of the system. For some people, high degrees of intensity feel comfortable and allow them to think, behave, and feel with balance and effectiveness. For others, certain emotions (such as anger or sadness), or all emotions, may be quite disruptive to functioning if they are active in even mild degrees. The intensity of a specific emotional state may involve arousal and appraisal mechanisms outside awareness. As we've seen, these nonconscious activities of appraisal influence how the brain processes information. *One's thinking or behavior can become disrupted if arousal moves beyond the boundaries of the window of tolerance.* For some persons, this window may be quite narrow. For such individuals, emotional processes may only become conscious when their intensity nears the boundaries of the window and is on the verge of disorganizing the functioning of the system. For others, a wide range of emotion may be both tolerable and available to consciousness—from pleasant emotions including joy, excitement, or love, to unpleasant ones such as anger, sadness, or fear.

Recent research suggests that parts of the middle area of the prefrontal cortex we have been discussing are actively involved in how we appraise the meaning of events and keep our emotional lives in balance.[45] Wager, Oschner, and colleagues have concluded: "In sum, this study shows evidence for a distributed set of lateral frontal, medial frontal, and orbitofrontal regions that together orchestrate reappraisal of the meaning of emotional events."[46] One aspect of this middle prefrontal area, the ventrolateral prefrontal region (especially on the right side of the brain), plays an especially important role in this process as it links cortical activities with the firing of subcortical regions, such as the limbic amygdala and parts of the brainstem. Wager et al. state:

> If our emotions are woven into the fabric of human life, then our ability to regulate them keeps us from coming unraveled. In the best of circumstances, successful regulation leaves us feeling frayed around the edges. In the worst of circumstances, regulatory failures take a severe toll and contribute to the genesis and symptomatology of many psychiatric disorders.[47]

The important integrative functions of the prefrontal cortex can be seen to play a central role in the coordination and balance of emotion-generating subcortical neural activity with the cortical functions of thought and reflection. Both genetic and experiential factors influence the way this integrative prefrontal region develops. Without the coordination and balance of such prefrontal neural integration, the states of activation driven by emotion-generating subcortical firing can lead to dysfunction.

The width of a given individual's window of tolerance may vary, depending upon the state of mind at a given time, the particular emotional valence, and the social context in which the emotion is being generated. For example, many of us may be more able to tolerate stressful situations when surrounded by loved ones with whom we feel secure and understood. Within the boundaries of the window, the mind continues to function well. Outside these boundaries, function becomes impaired as we move toward chaos or rigidity.

At its most basic level this can be understood in terms of the activity of the autonomic nervous system's branches, to be discussed in detail in the next chapter. Outside the window of tolerance, excessive sympathetic branch activity can lead to increased energy-consuming processes, manifested as increases in heart rate and respiration and as a "pounding" sensation in the head. At the other extreme, excessive parasympathetic branch activity leads to increased energy-conserving processes, manifested as decreases in heart rate and respiration and as a sense of "numbness" and "shutting down" within the mind. Other autonomic combinations are possible, with the most common being simultaneous activation of both branches; this creates the internal sensation of an "explosion" in the head and tension in the body, as if one were driving a car with the brakes and the accelerator on at the same time. Some individuals refer to such a state as "explosive rage."

Under these conditions, the "higher" cognitive functions of abstract thinking and self-reflection are shut down. The prefrontal circuits linking these cortical processes with the highly discharging limbic centers are functionally blocked, and rational thought becomes impossible. In states of mind beyond the window of tolerance, the prefrontally mediated capacity for response flexibility is temporarily shut down. The "higher mode" of integrative processing has been replaced by a "lower mode" of reflexive responding. The integrative function of emotion, in which self-regulation permits a flexibly adaptive interaction with the environment, is suspended. We can propose that under such conditions, the dynamical system appears to shift away from movement toward maximizing complexity by entering into states characterized by either excessive rigidity or randomness. These states are inflexible or chaotic, and as such are not adaptive to the internal or external environment. The mind has entered a suboptimal organizational flow that may reinforce its own maladaptive pattern. This is now a state of emotion dysregulation.

A window of tolerance may be determined by constitutional features and by experiential learning. Present physiological conditions, such as hunger and exhaustion, may also markedly restrict individuals' windows of tolerance and make them more vulnerable to irritability and "emotional outbursts." Windows can be shaped by individuals' constitutional qualities. People with shy temperaments may find emotional intensity of many sorts very uncomfortable, and seek environments that are familiar to them and that do not evoke such disturbing and disorganizing inner sensations. Such individuals may feel safe enough to move toward novel situations when they are with attachment figures

> A window of tolerance may be determined by constitutional features and by experiential learning.

with whom they have secure relationships. Without such a context, they may withdraw and become socially isolated. For others with more adaptive sensitivities, novelty may be quite pleasurable, evoking a feeling of excitement that is not disruptive to their sense of balance. In these bolder individuals familiarity may sometimes become quite boring and create an internal sense of restlessness. Children with "easy" temperaments are characterized by such open approaches; on the whole, they make life for their parents less demanding. Those with more irritable, unpredictable, and "difficult" temperaments are "moody" and have frequent reactions outside of their windows of tolerance. The resulting outbursts create challenges for many parents. As such children mature, many of them find more sophisticated ways to regulate their emotions, with a subsequent decline in the frequency and intensity with which they break through their windows of tolerance.

Windows of tolerance may also be directly influenced by experiential history. If children have been frightened repeatedly in their early lives, fear may become associated with a sense of dread or terror that is disorganizing to their systems. Repeatedly experiencing out-of-control emotions, without a sense of others' helping to calm them down, can lead such persons to be unable to soothe themselves as they develop. This lack of self-soothing can lead directly to a narrow window of tolerance. When such a person breaks through that window, the result is a very disorganizing, "out-of-control" sensation, which in itself creates a further state of distress.

A person's present state of mind can also narrow or widen the window of tolerance. Being emotionally worn, physically exhausted, or surprised by an interaction can each narrow the window of tolerance. In such cases, an individual may become emotionally wrought up or visibly upset by an encounter that, under other conditions, would have occasioned only mild arousal.

Let's return to the example of the attorney offered earlier in this chapter. We cannot take the interaction with her colleague out of the temporal and social context in which it occurred. The document the attorney had given her colleague was addressed to one of her most important clients, a woman executive in her late sixties whom the attorney saw as a mother figure. She had always wanted to please this woman, because she felt (as she later revealed in therapy) that her actual mother had never been supportive of her or able to be pleased with her. Despite being reminded before the attorney left for a vacation, the colleague failed to mail the document on time, jeopardizing their legal case. The colleague's mistake created the sense in the attorney that "yet again" she would be unable to please her mother. This activated in the attorney an internal image, a cognitive representation, of herself in relationship to an angry mother. She had experienced as a child, and was now experiencing again as an adult, the state of mind that wanting to please but being unseen creates: shame. What was worse, the mother (and the business client's image, in the attorney's mind) had frequently expressed anger and hostility toward her, creating a sense of both shame and humiliation.

Some might ask how much of this patient's recollection was accurate, and, if it was accurate, how we can distinguish genetic from experiential

effects. This patient's memories of these early events were independently supported after the patient entered therapy by the recollections of a cousin who
had lived across the street and personally witnessed some of these humiliating
interactions. In an even more uncommon type of corroboration, the therapist
was able to interview the mother herself, at the request of the daughter. The
mother reflected on these incidents very much as the patient had reported
them; she also stated that her own mother had "practiced" such a style of parenting, in order to "harden" her for the "real world." Her treatment of her
own daughter, she said, was intentionally a "watered-down version" of the
treatment she herself had received. Such single clinical case examples are not
the same as research data, but they do offer us in-depth examples of how
early experiences of dysregulated dyadic states can be associated with the
development of individual dysfunction later in life. Still, "association" does
not mean "causation." After all, the mother passed on her genes and possibly
even her epigenetic regulatory mechanisms, as well as providing a particular
parental experience for her daughter. Having an explosive temper—a form
of emotion dysregulation—can certainly be an inherited or acquired trait.
The mixture of two individuals, mother and daughter, each with a constitutional tendency to break through their windows of tolerance, might help
explain some of this patient's experience. The transgenerational passing of
patterns of humiliating parenting could also explain such a finding. In any
case, this woman found herself with the reality of dysregulation.

   The repeated activation of these configurations of mental representations
and a state of mind of shame/humiliation can be seen to have engrained this
state as a repeating pattern of neural activation. We could almost say that
the activation of this state had become a personality trait. The attorney was
prone to entering this state of enraged humiliation at "inappropriate" times.
In this manner, she entered an inflexible state that was no longer adaptive
and inhibited new behavioral responses in interaction with the social environment. We can view this state as induced by the massive activation of the
parasympathetic branch (the sense of not being understood or listened to
when the colleague failed to mail the document on time, despite a reminder)
and the sympathetic branch (the internal state that she was being yelled at by
her client and feeling anger toward her colleague) of the attorney's autonomic
nervous system. The brakes and accelerator were being applied simultaneously. The car, her mind, could not be regulated. The cues that set her off
were rationally related to the earlier states, but the logic of these reasons was
of emotional and historical value only. Her colleague and her client couldn't
care less about the "meaning" of her frightening rages. She was removed
from all of the client's cases immediately after this last incident.

   When the intensity of an aroused state moves beyond the window of
tolerance, a flood of energy may bombard the mind and take over a number

of processes, ranging from rational thinking to social behavior. At this point, emotions may flood conscious awareness. Some have called this an emotional "hijacking," "breakdown," or "flooding."[48] In such a situation, one's behavior may no longer feel volitional, and thoughts may feel out of control. Images may fill the mind's eye with visual representations symbolic of the emotional sensation. For example, when angry, some people may "see red" or visualize doing harm to the target of their rage. They may lose control of their behavior, performing destructive acts that would not be part of their behavioral repertoires under "normal" conditions. In this "lower mode" of processing, the state of mind has pushed beyond the window of tolerance. Such a person has "flipped his lid."

As we've seen, emotion, meaning, and social interactions are mediated via the same circuitry in the brain. Information in the brain is not handled independently of the biological reality of how the brain is in fact structured. For example, within the convergence zones of one of the central regions of emotional processing, the prefrontal cortex, we can see the way in which brain structure shapes the mind's functioning. In this neural region, inputs from anatomically distinct areas converge: Neural firing patterns transmitting the "information" from these regions are sent directly to the prefrontal cortex. This information includes social cognition, autonoetic consciousness, sensation, perception, various representations (such as words and ideas), somatic maps representing the physiological state of the body, and the output of the autonomic nervous system (which allows for "affect regulation" via the balancing of sympathetic and parasympathetic branch activity, often shaped by the "polyvagal system").[49] As we've discussed earlier, the capacity to respond adaptively to the personal significance of an event, not merely with an automatic reflexive reaction, may require the capacity for response flexibility as well as its integration with these other prefrontally mediated processes.

It has been suggested that in states of excessive arousal, the "higher" processing of the neocortical circuits is shut down. In addition, the direction of the energy flow within the brain, usually coordinated and balanced by the prefrontal regions, is then determined more by input from the "lower" processing centers of the brainstem, sensory circuits, and limbic structures. In this way, the beyond-tolerance state of hyperarousal leads neurologically to the inhibition of higher perceptions and thoughts; more basic somatic and sensory input is favored. In this situation, people don't think; they feel something intensely and act impulsively. What this means is that an individual who enters a state outside the window of tolerance is potentially in a "lower mode" of processing, in which reflexive responses to bodily states and primitive limbic and brainstem input are more likely to dominate processing.

## Recovery Processes

In the attorney's interaction with her colleague, she went beyond the boundaries of her window. She entered a state in which self-reflection, thinking about her emotions, achieving some distance from her reflexive reactions, and considering other options for behavior beyond her immediate impulses were not possible. All of these cortical processes are thought to be shut down when a person is emotionally flooded in this way. A first step in helping this patient was having her learn the boundaries of her window of tolerance— that is, the points at which interactions with others began to generate intense responses that moved her to the edge of control. Becoming aware of the state of her body (tension in her muscles, tightness in her stomach and throat) and sensing images of anger in her mind were the first stages in learning to monitor her internal state more effectively. This is one aspect of "mindsight skill" training. Its aim was to enable her to modify the flow of energy and information toward integration as she progressed in her treatment. Prevention of ruptures exceeding her tolerance was the most helpful strategy for her. She also needed to learn techniques for increasing the speed at which she could recover, once she was outside her window.

How does the mind ever recover from this state of suspended cortical processing and thinking about thinking (metacognition)? The recovery process may vary from person to person, again depending on present context, constitution, and personal history. Certain states may be easier to recover from than others; specific contexts may activate a particular cluster of neural net profiles from which it is especially difficult to recover, whereas others may be more readily repaired. For example, if a person feels betrayed by a close friend who has never been suspected of being disloyal, then recovering from a flood of anger and sadness may be particularly difficult. On the other hand, being let down by an acquaintance of dubious reliability may create anger that is relatively easy to bring back into the window of tolerance.

*Recovery means decreasing the disorganizing effects of a particular episode of emotional arousal.* Recovery may be a primary physiological process in which appraisal mechanisms bring the degree of activation to tolerable levels. This modulation may involve a dampening in the intensity of arousal, as well as a restriction in the distribution of neuronal groups activated within the state of mind at that time. Recovery may also involve the reactivation of the more complex and abstract reasoning that the cortex mediates. This will then allow for the metacognitive processes of self-reflection and impulse control. The capacity to reflect on mental states of self and others, and to integrate this knowledge, may be important in enabling this

> Recovery means decreasing the disorganizing effects of a particular episode of emotional arousal.

aspect of emotion regulation. Studies of children reveal that those who use private speech or self-talk are better able to soothe themselves.[50] Reinstated cortical processes may help by altering the characteristics of the elaborated emotion and permitting an individual to begin to tolerate arousal levels that previously would have been flooding. For instance, the person engulfed in rage at a close friend may find that activating old memories of the friend and engendering a feeling of loss and sadness may allow the emotional experience to be transformed. With intensive work, the attorney in our case example began to become aware of the sadness and profound disappointment she had experienced as a child within her interactions with her mother. She also began to connect the meaning of her present interactions with what she (her value system) had learned through these repeated experiences of her childhood. This process apparently has allowed her to widen her window of tolerance. For some, sadness is more easily tolerated than rage.

Some individuals have extreme difficulty recovering from emotional flooding of any sort. For these people, life may become a series of efforts to avoid situations that evoke strong emotional reactions. These avoidance maneuvers are defensive, in that they are attempts to keep the individuals' systems in balance. For those whose windows are quite narrow for certain emotions, such avoidance behaviors can shape the structure of their personalities and their ways of dealing with others and the world. If recovery processes are unavailable, then such individuals become prisoners of their own emotional instability.

Emotions are central in the self-regulation of the mind. It is inevitable that at times emotional arousal will be too much for any of us to tolerate. At these moments, the flood of emotions without an effective recovery process will result in prolonged states of disorganization that are ineffective and potentially harmful to ourselves or to others. Recovery allows us to move back within the boundaries of our tolerance and to "push the envelope" but not to break it. In essence, recovery allows the mind's self-organizational processes to return the flow of states toward a balance that maximizes complexity—that is, to move the system between the extremes of complete predictability or rigidity on the one side and excessive randomness or chaos on the other. The system becomes more adaptive by tuning itself to both internal and external variables in a more flexible manner, thus enhancing complexity, which allows the mind to achieve stability.

How can recovery occur? Looking toward the two fundamental elements of the mind—energy and information—can help us to answer this question. Let's return to the example of the attorney. In her interaction with her colleague at the meeting, she remained in a state of hyperarousal, agitation, and rage, in which her cortical processing was surely suspended. The internal representations of the colleague's deadline error were probably linked, as we've discussed earlier, to the attorney's sense of shame and humiliation from interactions with her mother. "Linked" means that the situation created within her a humiliated state of mind, with excessive arousal of both branches of the autonomic nervous system. This familiar state quickly flooded her beyond her window of tolerance. Her higher reflective processes were suspended. She began yelling at the top of her lungs, feeling misunderstood, demeaned, and enraged. She stated in retrospect that the colleague's attempts to calm her down were interpreted as condescending (like her mother) and further irritated her. For hours after she had yelled at him, she remained in a seething, agitated state.

Recovery from that episode was long in coming. As time wore on, she seemed to calm down, but was easily agitated by thoughts of the experience and of the eventual call from her client. As therapy progressed, the therapist and patient began to examine what had occurred in terms of these ideas about windows of tolerance, emotions, memory, and states of mind. She was very motivated at this point to understand how her own mind was "betraying" her. She was eager to change this pattern of emotional outbursts.

Within the sessions, she would again enter these hyperaroused, beyond-her-tolerance states. But now her experience of being "out of control" was joined by the reflective and supportive dialogue with her therapist. She was able to listen in her agitation, but remained hyperaroused. However, she now had two objects for her attention—her internal state and the external dialogue. This "dual focus" of attention may be an important feature of psychotherapy. As time went on, she began to reflect on the nature of her own mental processes. She could picture her circuits with an excessive flooding of activity; she could notice her tense muscles contributing the feedback to her mind that she was furious; and she could begin to see how the deadline error meant something to her and her past, beyond what the colleague and the mistake in reality were about.

This woman learned to enhance her recovery processes by learning to use the energy flow and information processing of her mind in a new way. Therapy allowed her to experience emotionally flooded states, and *within that state of mind*, she was then able to apply her newly acquired abilities. She could use relaxation and imagery to "lower the energy of her circuits" and the tension in her body. Her metacognitive cortical capacities were strengthened and made more accessible *during her rages* in ways that were not possible before. Such capacities allowed her to use previously inhibited pathways during this state of mind to alter the way she processed information. What had been a blockage in information processing and an inhibition in the flow of energy now became more adaptive states of mind. Her capacity for emotion regulation, and thus for self-regulation, became more flexible and more effective. She could say to herself, "This interaction is more about my feelings of shame than about my colleague," and focus her experience in a different way.

## Access to Consciousness

As our appraisal mechanisms operate, and as our primary emotions are further differentiated at times into categorical ones, our minds are influenced by our value systems in every aspect of their functioning. These influences occur without the necessity of conscious awareness. The idea presented in this book is that emotion is a central set of processes directly related to meaning, social communication, attentional focus, and perceptual processing. Emotion is not just some "primitive" remnant of an earlier reptilian evolutionary past. *Emotion directs the flow of activation (energy) and establishes the meaning of representations (information processing) for the individual.* It is not a single, isolated group of processes; it is an integrative process that has a direct impact on the entire mind. By defining emotion in this way, we can begin to make sense of the wide-ranging interpretations of research findings on emotion, thinking, and social processes. Discussing the relationship of emotion to consciousness provides a useful opportunity to delineate our ideas about emotion further.

Huge amounts of evidence support the view that the "conscious self" is in fact a very small portion of the mind's activity.[51] Perception, abstract cognition, emotional processes, memory, and social interaction all appear to proceed to a great extent without the involvement of consciousness. Most of the mind is nonconscious. These "out-of-awareness" processes do not appear to be in opposition to consciousness or to anything else; they create the foundation for the mind in social interactions, internal processing, and even conscious awareness itself. Nonconscious processing influences our behaviors, feelings, and thoughts. Nonconscious processes impinge on our conscious minds: We experience sudden intrusions of elaborated thought processes (as in "Aha!" experiences) or emotional reactions (as in crying before we are aware that we are experiencing a sense of sadness). So we can say that for the most part, the self is not divided by some line between a conscious and a nonconscious self. Rather, the self is created by nonconscious processes, as well as by the selective associations of these processes into something we call "consciousness." To put it another way, we are much, much more than our conscious processes.

But what does it mean to have consciousness? Why do we even have consciousness at all? One answer to these questions, among many possibilities, is that *when processes become linked within consciousness, they can be more strategically and intentionally manipulated, and their outcome can be adaptively altered.* Consciousness may allow us to become free from reflexive processing and introduce some aspect of "choice" into our behavior. In this way, individuals may be able to get themselves off "automatic pilot," stop reacting with top-down constraints, and tap into the spontaneity of bottom-up incoming sensations. The practice of mindful awareness may enhance this capacity to "come to our senses."[52] Having awareness gives us choice to make a change.

For example, a soon-to-be-married man has a nonconscious fret about who will sit where at his wedding. By making

> Having awareness gives us choice to make a change.

this into a conscious concern, he can raise the issue with his fiancée, and they can then examine the options together. They can gather new information and consider alternatives, which can result in a more satisfactory seating arrangement. A process made conscious can be directly shared across individuals, and the outcome can be strategically altered. The strategic manipulation, the introduction of choice, and the sharing of information are made possible by consciousness. If the groom is unable to be conscious of the meaning of his sensations of discomfort or thoughts about the wedding, it is likely that he will not bring up the issue for examination.

What is a neuroscientific explanation for how consciousness occurs? Consciousness is important for focal attention and working memory, which allow information to be processed into long-term, explicit memory storage. As noted throughout this book, working memory is considered the "chalkboard of the mind"; it allows us the ability to reflect on several (seven, plus or minus two) items simultaneously. Such reflection allows us to manipulate these representations, to process them (e.g., to note similarities and differences, create generalizations, and recognize patterns), and to create new associations among them. Working memory allows self-reflection and creates cognitive "choice." In other words, it introduces the possibility of personal intention and strategic, deliberate behaviors that are independent of automatic reflexes.

At the most fundamental level, consciousness involves the selective linkage or binding of representations, which then can be intentionally manipulated within working memory. As discussed earlier, some researchers suggest that neural firing patterns achieve a certain degree of complexity as they become integrated and then become incorporated as aspects of "conscious experience." Once stabilized, they can be "intentionally" manipulated within the space of conscious attention. The idea of intention is itself a philosophical puzzle.[53] What we can say is that with consciousness, new information can be introduced or new manipulations can be attempted for a strategic purpose determined by the individual. Consciousness itself is not necessary for information processing, but it is necessary at times to achieve new outcomes in such processing.

From this vantage point, we can say that emotional processing—the initial orientation, appraisal, arousal, and differentiation mechanisms—usually occurs without consciousness. An individual's consciousness of these processes allows for the qualitative sensation of emotion, experienced as a sense of energy, meaning, and categorical emotion. Any and all of these sensations can be called a "feeling," which explains why people of many different ages respond with a range of reactions to the common query of "How are you feeling?" "I feel . . . up . . . down . . . excited . . . that this means the end of our relationship . . . like I want to run and hide . . . that he didn't understand my intentions . . . that I am bad . . . sad . . . angry . . . happy." "Feelings" can therefore involve energy, meaning, behavioral impulses, or the discrete categories of emotion. Why do emotional processes enter consciousness at all? What information processing does this permit when we become aware of a shift in integration?

The ability to involve conscious processing with something as fundamental as the creation of meaning, social relatedness, and perceptual processing certainly does give us an increase in the flexibility of our responses to the environment. Having a consciousness of emotions is especially important in the social environment. Without it, we are likely not to be aware of our own or others' intentions and motives. Awareness of emotional processes, our shifts in integration, has value for our survival as a social species: We can know our own minds as well as those of others, and can negotiate the complex interpersonal world with increased skill and effectiveness at meeting our needs.

Recall that consciousness may involve an integration of distributed neuronal activities that achieves a certain degree of complexity.[54] Effective processing within consciousness can thus be seen as the furthering of such an integrative process. Consciousness is more than the mere activation of representations in working memory that have become linked via the thalamocortical system and the lateral prefrontal cortex. Active, executive functions that direct the integrated flow of energy and information play an important role in the coordination of mental processes and response. These executive functions are possibly mediated also by nearby middle prefrontal regions (including the orbitofrontal cortex, the medial prefrontal cortex, and anterior cingulate) and other areas (including the parietal and temporal lobes).[55] For example, Nobre and colleagues suggest that findings regarding the orbitofrontal cortex indicate that its activity may be important in

> inhibiting prepared motor programs [and in] the tasks of motor selection and preparation requiring withholding of responses. The orbitofrontal cortex participates both in the redirection of the response based upon a violation in stimulus contingencies and in possible changes of emotional state. . . .

Activity in the orbitofrontal region is recruited as stimulus contingencies change, interacting dynamically with the basic neural–cognitive system that directs attention. The anatomical connections of the lateral orbitofrontal cortex support this ability.[56]

Earlier we have called such a capacity "response flexibility" and have suggested that such a process may be an important element in self-regulation and in the behavioral and attentional flexibility seen in the contingent, collaborative communication and coherent adult narratives revealed in secure attachments.

What role does consciousness itself play in the regulation of emotion? *Consciousness can influence the outcome of emotional processing.* Conscious awareness allows for self-reflection, which can enable the mobilization of strategic thoughts and behaviors and can therefore enhance the flexible achievement of goals. This can be seen as the achievement of new levels of integration. For example, if a person realizes that she is feeling sad about a friend who has left town, she can then write or call that person and reestablish contact. If, instead, her

> Consciousness can influence the outcome of emotional processing.

sadness remains nonconscious, she may never reach out to her friend in this way. Given the fundamental role of the appraisal system in distinguishing what is good and should be approached from what is bad and should be avoided, emotions that are accessible to parts of cognition can consciously mobilize behavior. This can be crucial if emotion is to be effective in certain adaptive ways as a value system. Consciousness allows emotion to play a more adaptive role in an individual's behavior. But how does it help regulate emotion?

Let's return again to the example of the attorney in psychotherapy, to illustrate how consciousness can permit two fundamental elements of emotion regulation: the modulation of energy flow through the brain, and the adaptive modification of information processing. After her "explosion" with her colleague and her dismissal from the case, the attorney's motivation to understand her social difficulties reached a peak. Though she had had a number of brief encounters with therapists in the past, this was the first time she felt driven to examine what role she was playing in these difficulties. Earlier, she had focused on how troubled the world and other people were. For the first time, she now became consciously aware of the possibility that the source of her difficulties was within her own mind.

Such a change in attitude was itself quite an accomplishment; in this woman's case, it was brought about by "hitting bottom" with her job. This new openness was a window of opportunity for therapy to provide her with some new tools. In the therapy sessions, therapist and patient began a dialogue in which they examined the patient's memories of experiences in both the recent and distant past. The patient was also coached to reflect in the present on her own internal processes—in other words, to begin the development of her metacognitive abilities. The therapist strongly encouraged this self-reflection, knowing that it would be an essential tool for the patient to learn in order to regulate her emotions.

Specific skills of reflecting on the internal nature of experience may be acquired within psychotherapy, using mindsight training techniques such as the "Wheel of Awareness" practice.[57] The Wheel of Awareness is a reflective, "time-in" practice that uses the metaphor of a wheel as a visual image for the mind. The hub represents the experience of being aware. Points on the rim signify anything of which we can be aware. The rim itself is divided into four segments. The first includes the five senses that bring in data from the outside world. The second segment represents the input from the body—the "sixth sense." The third segment of the rim represents our mental activities, such as emotions, thoughts, images, and memories. A final segment signifies our sense of connection to other people and to things outside our bodily selves, such as our relationship to our community or our planet. The Wheel of Awareness practice enables an individual to gain the skill of differentiating the elements of the rim from one another, and to distinguish the experience of knowing (the hub) from that which is known (the rim). Through the systematic focus of attention, this practice is designed to integrate consciousness.

Metacognition begins to develop within the second year of life and appears to enable children to link different representations from memory within present-moment experience.[58] This capacity probably changes the subjective nature of consciousness and permits children to begin developing new levels of self-regulation. Metacognition gives the developing minds of children (and adults) the ability to perform a number of unique processes: thinking about thinking itself; forming a representation of one's own mind; becoming aware of sensations, images, and beliefs about the self; and reflecting on the nature of emotion and perception.[59]

In formal terms, the mind develops the metacognitive capacity for the "appearance–reality distinction," which allows an individual to comprehend that what something looks like may be different from what it actually is in the world.[60] The notions that one's perceptions and ideas can change over time, and can be distinct from the equally valid ones of other people, are called "representational change" and "diversity," respectively. Metacognition also includes the awareness that emotion influences thought and perception, and that one may be able to experience two seemingly conflictual emotions about the same person or experience. In the attorney's case, each of these areas became vital for this patient to develop a more adaptive capacity for emotion regulation.

Metacognitive abilities often, but not necessarily, involve consciousness. In this patient's case, her lack of metacognition required that it become a part of the focus of the therapeutic dialogue. Not having metacognitive ability at this point in her development also necessitated that she make it a conscious part of her processing of intense emotions. With time, these new capacities, which had to be initiated intentionally and with mental effort, might become more automatic for her and might not require as much exerted conscious effort.

Before therapy, this patient's orientation, appraisal–arousal, and differentiation processes were often out of her conscious awareness. At some point, her rage became expressed externally as her screaming. Internally, she might first become aware of her emotional state through a burning sensation in her head and an intense focus of her attention on the "evil" of the person with whom she was interacting. Her consciousness was linked to the elements of emotional processing only when they burst through her window of tolerance in the form of uncontrolled fury and perceptual distortions filled with suspicion. In this state, she literally viewed others as "out to get her." Some might say that she was projecting her anger onto others. Another view might be that she was entering a state of shame and humiliation in which she was implicitly recalling an angry and betraying mother. Whatever the explanation, her conscious awareness began in a state of rage when self-reflection was impossible. Recall that in states of excessive arousal, higher cognitive functions, including metacognition, are shut down. The key to this woman's development was to bring such "lower-mode" states into a more balanced modulation. Conscious awareness of emotional processes is always a beginning; in this case, metacognitive reflection on these processes was essential to enhance response flexibility and self-regulation.

Therapy includes various aspects of an attachment relationship, as well as the co-construction of stories, bearing witness, teaching, and role modeling for patients. Each of these was essential in taking the next step with this frightened individual. Giving her a conceptual framework for how her emotions worked and influenced her experience of herself and interactions with others was vital in allowing her not to feel "accused" of being defective. The shame state involves a sense that something is wrong with the individual, and this emotion is often at the root of why patients have not developed the ability to reflect on their own contribution to their troubles. They may have an inner belief that they are defective, and they seek to hide this "truth" from others.

As therapy permitted the patient to tell the story of her life, the therapist could bear witness to the pain and vulnerability of her having been a child in a hostile family world. Linking of these emotional experiences to her present encounters, both with people in her daily life and with the therapist, allowed the patient to experience firsthand these emotional processes at work. She became sensitive to the subtle sensations of primary emotions long before they were elaborated into the categorical states that so often burst through her window of tolerance. These primary sensations allowed her to become aware of what was arousing to her ("This interaction now has some meaning for me—watch out!"). They also permitted her to reflect on how the specific meaning of an interaction had dual layers: her appraisal of its significance in the moment ("What is happening now with this person?") and its parallel historical meanings for her ("How does this relate to my emotional issues from the past?"). The important step for her was to associate primary emotions with consciousness.

At first she continued to have outbursts, but these were less intense and less frequent, and it seemed easier to recover from them. Her feeling of success at actually stopping such an outburst was exhilarating. This allowed her to consciously alter her bodily response by reducing the somatic feedback that was automatically reinforcing the cascading cycle of appraisal and arousal. This clearly empowered her to intentionally alter the flow of activation (energy) through her mind.

Simultaneously, she began a metacognitive analysis of the meaning of these interactions and emotional experiences. She could recognize that something "significant" was occurring, and was then able to connect the recurring themes of being ignored or misunderstood with her prior history of shaming and humiliating interactions with her mother. That is, she became able to note similarities and to work with generalizations within working memory. She was then able to examine the meaning of a representation (e.g., the interaction with her colleague was associated with shame) and compare it to those from the past (e.g., her interactions with her mother had been humiliating and shameful). Such a nonconscious linkage in the past had created an explosion. Now, with conscious reflection, the same comparison permitted the outcome to be quite different: She altered the appraisal process to highlight a different aspect of the meaning of these representations. Previously, her mind would have nonconsciously responded to the similarity in the interaction and created a state of humiliation and outburst. This was an automatic component of the synaptic memory process, in which past states were reactivated by similar retrieval cues without an awareness of their origins from the past.[61] Now, consciously, she was able to add the dimension of metacognition. This allowed her to state to herself, "I am becoming agitated because of the similarity of this interaction to my earlier ones, filled with feelings of shame. I am not a slave to the past, and I do not have to react in a similar way." Instead of the nonconscious, reflexive response, consciousness permitted response flexibility and a more adaptive reaction. By acquiring the ability to reflect on the relationships among past, present, and future, this patient was developing her capacity for autonoetic consciousness. She could choose not to become explosive. She could decide that what was best for her was to alter her initial impulses and try to achieve her professional goals in a more productive manner.

Appraisal processes, operating even without consciousness, recruit new neuronal groups into their active state of mind. The addition of consciousness to such a recruitment effort permits further mobilization of a new set of processes: Consciousness allows for the manipulation of representations in new combinations within working memory, the chalkboard of the mind. Consciousness involving the linguistic system and autonoesis allows for reflections on the past and future, moving us beyond the lived moment.[62] We are also able to be motivated by our awareness of emotions, which then facilitates more strategically focused achievements that are not likely without the involvement of consciousness.

> Consciousness allows for the manipulation of representations in new combinations within working memory, the chalkboard of the mind.

## External Expression

From the beginning of life, emotion constitutes both the process and the content of communication between infant and caregiver. Simply put, a baby's inner state is perceived by parents, who in turn feel in a parallel manner themselves. The baby perceives the parents' contingent response, and the affect is mutually attuned. Later, in addition, parents use words to talk about feelings and direct a shared attention to the infant's state of mind. The parents may state directly that the baby is feeling sad or happy or scared, giving the infant the interactive verbal experience of being able both to identify and to share an emotional experience. This earliest form of communication in a setting of safety and comfort provides the child with a sense that her emotional life can be shared and be a source of soothing from others.

By the second year of life, the infant has learned the adaptive behavior of not showing how she might be feeling. The social context in which an intense emotion is experienced may motivate the child to "hide" her inner experience. For example, if the toddler wants something but has learned that she will be yelled at if she shows an interest in that object, it will be best if she keeps a "poker face" and does not show her true emotion. For us adults, complex social situations repeatedly teach us the essential ability to mask our inner states from the criticism and harsh reactions from others. Culture and family environments play a central role in a child's experiential acquisition of these often unspoken laws of emotional expression, called "display rules."[61] Culture shapes how we come to feel "right" or "comfortable" in how we express our internal states to others—and perhaps even to ourselves. Some researchers use the terms "collectivist" and "individualistic" to contrast the social or private focus of a culture's emphasis. In general, these studies reveal that the display rules of a given society have important impacts on how people communicate with one another and on the role emotional expression plays in their lives.[64]

Studies of children and adults in various cultures demonstrate that people may show emotions quite differently if they are with unfamiliar people or if they are by themselves. For example, one study showed that in the Japanese culture, facial expression showing emotional response to a stimulating film was quite evident if a participant believed that he was alone in the room. With the experimenter present, facial expression was quite flat.[65] If display rules tell people not to show emotion, does this affect how conscious they may become of their own emotional response? This may in fact be the case: We use our own facial responses to become aware of how we are feeling. This fits in with the general view that the brain has a representation of the body's state, including states of arousal, muscle tension, and facial expression, which it uses as interoceptive information to register "how it feels."[66]

In another study, Japanese-born individuals perceived emotional expressions as being aspects of a social world, in contrast to Western-born individuals' seeing emotions as expressions of an individual. Social context—a perceptual ability of the right hemisphere—can then be postulated from these findings to be more engaged in the perception of emotion.[67] In contrast, a noncontextual, nonsocial view of emotional expression may involve a more dominant left-hemisphere response. This finding would be consistent with the finding mentioned in Chapter 2 that Japanese-born individuals perceived the marine environment of an aquarium within its larger (right-hemisphere-perceived) gestalt, whereas American-born Japanese perceived the individual details, a more left-hemisphere form of response.[68]

*The self is capable of at least two contextual states or ways of being: a private, inner, core self and a public, external, adaptive self.*[69] Some authors have used the parallel notions of a "true" and a "false" self. This terminology, however, suggests that it is somehow false to adapt to social requirements; instead, it may be more useful to accept that different contexts evoke different states in each of us. Indeed, we have "relational selves" that emerge naturally as we continually recreate our selves in different settings and with different people.[70] Repeated patterns of social interactions can make a specific state, such as the masking of internal emotions from the outer world, an important and persistent adaptation. There is nothing "false" about a mechanism of survival. However, if the brain often relies on the expression of emotion as a signpost of what the individual truly feels, then this masking process certainly can create a challenge to knowing one's "true" response.

The regulation of expression may assist the mind in modulating its states of arousal by social and intrapsychic mechanisms. Socially, masking internal states can permit the individual to avoid an experience of interpersonal resonance, in which the response of the receiver at times can amplify or distort the initial state of the sender. Masking inner states can also enable an individual to avoid being misunderstood, and so avoid the painful state of shame that would be induced. Within the individual, regulating affect can dampen the positive feedback loop in which an internal state is expressed externally as facial expressions and bodily responses, which then are perceived by the mind and heighten the initial emotional state. In both the individual and social feedback processes, regulating external expression of an internal state can help to keep the state of arousal from breaking through the window of tolerance.

A very difficult situation arises when an aspect of this form of emotional modulation—the inflexible and "nonexpressive" regulation of affect—is so engrained that it becomes a rigidly and repeatedly evoked state, or trait, of the individual. If there are no contexts available in a growing child's life when the inner, private self can be fully engaged in interactions with others, then the adaptive, external, public self may perpetually mask internal states even from the individual. This condition may be experienced by the person as a sense of not knowing who she is. There may be a feeling that life is meaningless. In emotional terms, this person's conscious access to her own emotions has been repeatedly blocked.

The danger of chronically blocking general affective expression is that it may also repeatedly inhibit the access of emotions to an individual's consciousness. The exact mechanism that blocks expression is unknown, but perhaps involves a temporary shutting down of the circuits that control affective expression. As we've seen, these appear to be primarily located in the right hemisphere, especially in the prefrontal cortex and the amygdala. Individuals with right-hemisphere lesions, for example, may have a reduced ability to perceive others' emotions, as well as to express and gain conscious access to their own. Furthermore, imaging studies of depressed individuals (who show reduced facial expression) have revealed a functional abnormality in the activation of right-hemisphere facial perception centers.[71] The implication here is that the expression and perception of facial affect may be neurologically linked processes.

People vary widely in their ability to express affect. One way we can begin to make sense of these variations is to conceptualize nonverbal signals as the external expressions of internal states of mind. Primary emotions are expressed as the vitality affects described as the profiles of activation, including "crescendo" (increasing energy) and "decrescendo" (decreasing energy) states. A person reveals such vitality states in facial expression, tone of voice, activity of the limbs, gestures, and the timing and fluidity of these signals in interactions with another person. These signals may enter the person's own awareness, and may also directly influence the adjustment of his own state to that of the other person. Becoming aware of the external signals from another person and those being given off by the self can be crucial. Reflection on internal sensations may be an essential aid in knowing how another person may be feeling.

"Feeling felt" may be an essential ingredient in attachment relationships. Having the sense that someone else feels one's feelings and is able to respond contingently to one's communication may be vital to close relationships of all sorts throughout the lifespan. Such attachments foster the interactive sharing of states, which facilitates the amplification of positive, enjoyable emotions and the diminution of negative, uncomfortable emotions. The attuned communication within attachment relationships allows such interactive amplification and diminution to occur. The outcome is that each member of the pair may "feel felt" by the other. For the developing child, the secure attachment relationship provides the amplification that heightens pleasurable states and allows the child to engage in the self-regulation needed to diminish unpleasurable ones.

> Such attachments foster the interactive sharing of states, which facilitates the amplification of positive, enjoyable emotions and the diminution of negative, uncomfortable emotions.

The challenge of communicating internal states may be a bit less demanding when it comes to the expression of categorical emotions. These more elaborated states of activation, with their cross-culturally similar patterns of expression that are probably embedded within the brain's physiological response patterns, seem to involve a different form of communication. The studies cited above suggest that some aspects of categorical affect are mediated by social display rules. People sometimes mask certain intense feelings in the presence of strangers; in other situations, people only reveal certain responses (such as smiling or laughing) in the presence of others. These findings, combined with the developmental acquisition of masking categorical affects, support the social communication aspect of this form of categorical emotion. The sharing of these states has a more "distant" quality and can involve more of the classic sense of empathy as a state of understanding another's experience rather than feeling another's feelings. We can feel sad when other persons feel sad, and we can rejoice in their excitement and joy. In this way, categorical affects can certainly be shared as well. But categorical emotions allow us to become more actively verbal within the communication with others. That is, we can use words with roughly shared definitions to encapsulate the shared experience: "It must have been so sad to have that happen," or "It is great to see you feel so excited about that event." In this way, the expression of a categorical emotion permits more linguistic distance from a shared moment in a relationship than the "feeling felt" of a primary emotional state attunement alone.

Of course, categorical expressions are usually accompanied by all the undefinable nonverbal signals of vitality affects that are reflections of the ongoing primary emotional processes. But the point here is that the perception of a classic categorical affect, such as anger, sadness or fear, often overshadows the less classifiable and often more subtle aspects of vitality affects. The "risk" of a predominantly categorical emotional communication is that one may begin to use only one's intellect in linguistically classifying what this particular emotional experience means, rather than attending to the unique meaning of that moment, both for the other person and for the relationship itself.

## PERSONALITY, MENTAL TRAINING, AND THE TRANSFORMATION OF SELF-REGULATION

Patterns of self-regulation can be seen within what we often consider as our "personality." We have seen how the seven components of emotion regulation shape our patterns of thinking, feeling, and interacting, and how they emerge from an amalgam of inborn proclivities (sometimes called "temperament") and our experiences (including our attachment relationships) early in life. Research to date using existing measures suggests that, for the vast majority of individuals, there is no clear and predictable pathway between childhood temperament tendencies and adult personality characteristics. As nonlinear dynamical systems, we humans naturally have a range of outcomes that can emerge with small inputs internally and externally that make us quite unpredictable creatures as we develop in our formative years. Yet as we move through and beyond adolescence, some of our persistent innate tendencies and our learned responses may coalesce within our synaptic sculpting such that we do have a personality pattern, a recurring way that we regulate our emotions and interact with the world. And for some individuals, these adult features may have had their origins in early childhood. There are certain tendencies we may have had from our earliest days—ones that exist especially at the extremes, like the intense behavioral inhibition also known as extreme shyness—that may persist in our neural functioning even if we've learned externally to overcome them.[72] But a pioneer in the field of affective neuroscience, Richard J. Davidson, suggests that even if we are born with some innate tendencies, these generally can and do change over the course of development.[73] During his career carving out a path in the neural study of emotion, Davidson has come to view a range of patterns of self-regulation that have observable neural correlates. This approach offers a different way of envisioning self-regulation and extends and broadens our discussion of the seven components of emotion regulation: intensity, sensitivity, specificity, windows of tolerance, recovery processes, access to consciousness, and external expression. As you'll see, these patterns in many ways reflect the mind as both an embodied and a relational process that regulates the flow of energy and information.

Here is how Davidson describes the six dimensions of what he calls our "Emotional Style," which are each revealed within fundamental aspects of brain function that he and his colleagues have been able to observe using scans of neural activity:

> Resilience: how slowly or quickly you recover from adversity; Outlook: how long you are able to sustain positive emotion; Social Intuition: how adept you are at picking up social signals from the people around you; Self-Awareness: how well you perceive bodily feelings that reflect emotions; Sensitivity to Context: how good you are at regulating your emotional responses to take into account the context you find yourself in; Attention: how sharp and clear your focus is.[74]

In Davidson's view, personality and temperament reflect different combinations of these dimensions. As mentioned above, Davidson emphasizes that what we may think are "fixed traits of temperament" are actually quite changeable in our childhood years. But these patterns of emotional style can become persistent in our adulthood even if they did not come directly from our childhood tendencies. He offers as one example a discussion of the "big five" personality traits[75] from the field of psychology that involve the aspects of openness to new experience, conscientiousness, extroversion, agreeableness, and neuroticism. Here is how Davidson describes how he would assign the emotional style dimensions to these big five personality descriptions:

> Someone high in openness to new experience has strong Social Intuition. She is also very self-aware and tends to be focused in her Attention style. A conscientious person has well-developed Social Intuition, a focused style of Attention, and acute Sensitivity to Context. An extroverted person bounces back rapidly from adversity and thus is at the Fast to Recover end of the Resilience spectrum. She maintains a positive Outlook. An agreeable person has a highly attuned Sensitivity to Context and strong Resilience; he also tends to maintain a positive Outlook. Someone high in neuroticism is slow to recover from adversity. He has a gloomy, negative Outlook, is relatively insensitive to context, and tends to be unfocused in his Attention style.[76]

Emotional style dimensions can be used in everyday descriptors of personality. For example, an optimistic person would be one who is Fast to

Recover on the Resilience scale and has a positive Outlook; a chronically unhappy person would be both Slow to Recover and have a negative Outlook and so could not experience positive emotions for long and would be filled with a negative state in the face of challenges. A shy person would have a combination of low Sensitivity to Context combined with a Resilience dimension of being Slow to Recover from an upset. These repeated internal experiences of distress would then become generalized across experiences because of the low context sensitivity and there would be a broad wariness even in appropriate settings. In contrast, people with a lot of patience would be high on Sensitivity to Context (they'd be very specific in their learning about the importance of setting and response) and also high on the Self-Awareness dimension of emotional style.

Personality in many ways is an amalgam of our experiences and our temperament. Davidson and colleagues' research has shown that in childhood, these various traits are generally quite malleable. At the extremes they may be persistent, as discussed earlier, but for the most part there is a great deal of change during our developmental years. This is why it is so difficult to predict, for the vast majority of children, how they ultimately will "turn out" even in the face of observable patterns of behavior we may call "temperament" that during the adolescent years and into adulthood simply do not continue. Ongoing experiences in life continue to shape our neural circuits as a part of our neuroplasticity.[77] But even in the face of the tenacious habits of mind that we find ourselves trapped in as adults, there is a great deal of hope that, with intentional effort, deep changes can be created. The developing mind does not have to become fixed with one pattern of traits or another. An important lesson that comes from Davidson's pioneering work is that an individual does not have to "settle" for some innate temperament or personality that is unchangeable. In fact, Davidson's work has shown just the opposite: Mental training can alter the dimensions of emotional style. Because his and others' work has revealed how the prefrontal circuits help coordinate and balance the lower subcortical states, it becomes possible to see the mechanisms by which processes like meditation can alter prefrontal fibers and their connections to the lower structures. This change in the linkage of differentiated areas alters how an individual coordinates and balances the information and energy flow in his or her body. In essence, the focus of the mind can change the integrative fibers that regulate emotion and shape what we call "personality."

In Davidson's own words:

> The seat of reason and higher-order cognitive function in the brain plays as important a role in emotion as the limbic system does. My research on meditators has shown that mental training can alter patterns of activity in

the brain to strengthen empathy, compassion, optimism, and a sense of well-being—the culmination of my promise to study meditation as well as positive emotions. And my research in the mainstream of affective neuroscience has shown that it is these sites of higher-order reasoning that hold the key to altering these patterns of brain activity.[78]

The great news of these discoveries is that self-regulation can be enhanced through skills that build the foundation for sensing and shaping the internal flow of energy and information within the brain. Monitoring energy and information flow and modulating that flow toward integration is the outcome of mindsight. These mindsight skills offer hope of cultivating integration in our brains, in our relationships, and in our mental lives. Such mental training includes mindful awareness practices and other forms of meditation that have been shown to transform the functioning of the prefrontal cortex and to actually alter the structural interconnections it has within itself and with other regions.[79] As this important "seat of reason and higher-order cognitive function" links widely distributed and differentiated neural regions—and even the neural functioning of other people, of "other brains"—to one another, the prefrontal cortex is one of our most integrative circuits. Transforming self-regulation is possible because we can develop mindsight skills that enhance the integrative functions and structure of the prefrontal cortex throughout our lives.[80] As Davidson and others have revealed, we can intentionally use the focus of energy and information flow with our minds to change the function and structure of our brains. Personality is not fixed. Temperament is not destiny. When we come to realize that the brain develops across the lifespan, we can see that we can use our relationships to "inspire to rewire" our own and others' brains toward integration to cultivate more well-being and compassion in our lives.

## REFLECTIONS: EMOTION REGULATION AND THE MIND

The capacity to regulate the appraisal and arousal processes of the mind is fundamental to self-organization; therefore, emotion regulation is at the core of the self. The acquisition of self-regulation emerges from dyadic relationships early in life. Attachment studies suggest that the type of interpersonal communication that facilitates autonomous self-regulation begins with healthy dependence. Such relationships involve sensitivity to the child's signals, contingent communication, and reflective dialogue that permits the child to develop coherence and mentalizing capacities. Achieving self-organization occurs within emotionally attuned interpersonal experiences. At the emotional core of attachment relationships are the amplification of shared positive states and the reduction of negative affective states. As these dyadic states are experienced, the child comes to tolerate wider bands of emotional intensity and shared affective communication.

A proposed model of emotion regulation includes seven components: intensity, sensitivity, specificity, windows of tolerance, recovery processes, access to consciousness, and external expression. As we've seen, early attachment experiences and constitutional variables such as temperament help form these emotion regulation processes. "Epigenetic" factors—especially the social experiences that shape genetic expression and the experience-dependent maturation of the brain—directly influence how neuronal connections are established. In early childhood, such epigenetic attachment experiences influence the development of the neuronal pathways responsible for emotional modulation. Continuing emotional development within adult relationships can utilize the same attachment elements in helping to develop new paths to self-organization.

Lack of mental well-being may often be a result of emotion dysregulation. This may be experienced as abrupt ruptures of emotion through the window of tolerance, such as episodes of rage or sadness, from which it is difficult to recover. In these ruptured states, the mind loses its capacity for rational thinking, response flexibility, and self-reflection. Waves of intense arousal and sensations of "out-of-control" emotion, such as anger or terror, may flood the mind. In these states, the individual is both internally and interpersonally unable to function. The integrative role of the prefrontal region can be temporarily disabled in such states. Helping such an individual requires the development of a more effective self-organizational process. Metacognitive processes and mentalizing reflective functions embedded in mindsight skills may be important in the development of an integrative mode of processing, which is essential to achieve a more flexible and coherent experience.

If constitutional features, traumatic experiences, or severely suboptimal attachments have produced maladaptive emotion regulation, then individuals may be restricted in their ability to achieve emotional resilience and behavioral flexibility. In some situations, a form of "cortical override" mechanism may be useful. If there has been excessive parcellation (pruning) of corticolimbic structures, then the brain's ability to monitor and modify states of arousal may be quite compromised. Learning to use neocortical reasoning abilities to observe and then intervene in reflexive initial dysregulatory responses is often a helpful approach. What does this mean? When people move beyond their windows of tolerance, they lose the capacity to think rationally. This initial response may be difficult to alter if it is engrained within deep circuits, such as those encoded early in life in the limbic and brainstem regions. However, the neocortex can override these responses and bring the deeper structures into a more tolerable level of arousal. This can be accomplished by any number of "self-talk" strategies in which imagery, internal dialogue, and evocative memory (e.g., evoking the soothing image of an attachment figure) can be activated. Mental training, including mindful awareness practices, has been demonstrated to enhance the function and structure of these regulatory prefrontal circuits. Over time and with continued practice, the frequency and intensity of breakthroughs into the "lower mode" of reflexive states beyond the window of tolerance can be significantly decreased, and the speed of recovery can be greatly enhanced.

Why is self-regulation seen as fundamentally emotion regulation? Emotion, as a series of integrating processes in the mind, links all layers of functioning. In fact, the study of emotion itself is essentially the study of emotion regulation. Though emotion can be defined as a subjective experience involving neurobiological, experiential, and behavioral components, it is in fact the essence of mind. Early in life, the patterns of interpersonal communication we have with attachment figures directly influence the growth of the brain structures that mediate self-regulation. "Emotional communication" is the fundamental manner in which one mind connects with another. It is to interpersonal connection that we now turn.

# CHAPTER 8

# Interpersonal Connection

This chapter explores more fully what is known about how the relationship between parent and child enables the child's brain to develop the circuits responsible for healthy emotion regulation. The intention here is not to imply that all or even most individuals' troubles with self-regulation stem from attachment difficulties. Instead, the aim is to review what is known about the emotional communication inherent in attachment, in order to guide our understanding of emotion regulation within interpersonal relationships. Such an exploration allows us to look more deeply into the ways in which one mind directly shapes the development and function of another—the essence of interpersonal connection.

How can one mind influence another in this way? By viewing mental life as composed of the flow of information and energy, we can envision the complex neural systems from which it emanates as involving various dimensions: the parts of a single neuron, neurons in synaptic connections, groups of neurons organized within specific circuits, or systems such as the left or right hemisphere of the brain. The patterns of information and energy flow through such systems allows them to form more and more complex layers of systems.[1] But how can the system of one person directly interface with that of another to create a "supersystem"? Just as we can receive information in various forms—from oral to written to digitally transmitted via facsimile or electronic mail—so too can the energy and information of the mind be relayed via means including the electric action potentials of single neuronal axons, the patterned release of neurotransmitters, the physiological neuroendocrine milieu, and the complex neuronal activation of a neural net profile.

The human brain has evolved with one such system that has been shown to be vital in interpersonal connection. As discussed in Chapter 4, certain neurons have "mirror" properties that link the perception of others' activities to one's own behavioral imitation or internal state simulation. These mirror neurons not only allow us to "sponge up" what we see others do and feel; they also shape our own actions and even feelings.[2] These neurons directly influence our motor actions (imitation) or shifts in our subcortical states (internal simulation), so that we feel inside our bodies a state similar to that of another person.[3] These internal shifts are driven upward along the insula to create interoceptive maps that reflect—or mirror—what is going on inside of someone else. In essence, we come to "resonate" with the other person, and two "me's" become a "we." This whole set of connections—from mirror neurons to middle prefrontal maps enabling compassion and empathy—is called the "resonance circuitry."[4]

> We come to "resonate" with the other person, and two "me's" become a "we."

The linking of minds occurs via different modalities of the transfer of energy and information. The physical proximity of one individual to another has direct effects that may serve as "hidden regulators" conveying, for example, warmth and tactile stimulation.[5] Touch is an extremely important part of parent–child relationships.[6] Some studies suggest that close physical proximity also directly shapes the electrical activity of each individual's brain.[7] But even at a physical distance, one mind can directly influence the activity—and development—of another through the transfer of energy and information. This joining process occurs via both verbal and nonverbal behaviors, which function as signals sent from one mind to another. Words and the prosodic, nonverbal components of speech contain information that creates representational processes within the mind of the receiver. Other nonverbal signals, including facial expression, tone of voice, gestures, and timing of response, have a direct impact on the socially sensitive value circuits of the brain. The expression of these emotional elements of social signals serves to activate the very neuronal circuits that mediate the receiver's emotional response: orienting attention, appraising meaning, and creating arousal. This emotional engagement with another person creates a cascade of elaborated and differentiated appraisal–arousal processes, which serve to direct the flow of energy and information processing within one's own brain. It is in this manner that the emotional state of the sender directly shapes that of the receiver. In complexity terms, such "external constraints" as the signals sent from another person have a powerful and immediate effect on the trajectory or flow of one's own states of mind. Two differentiated individuals can become linked as a part of a resonating whole. This is interpersonal integration.

As we'll explore in this chapter, childhood patterns in the transfer of energy and information between minds can create organized strategies in relationships. These are revealed within characteristic behavioral responses in attachment-related situations. The minds of children learn to adapt specifically to the emotional communication they receive from their caregivers. Over time, such relationship-dependent patterns may become engrained as strategies that are employed in more general contexts. Aspects of children's emotion regulation (such as adaptation to stress), cognitive processes (such as memory and attention), and social competence (including peer interactions) have been related to attachment history.[8] In adults, one may see characteristic approaches to interpersonal intimacy and the organization of autobiographical narrative reflected in generalized states of mind with respect to attachment.

Alan Sroufe and colleagues have been conducting an important longitudinal study over the last thirty-five years—the Minnesota Longitudinal Study of Parents and Children, mentioned in earlier chapters. This study's important findings reveal how early interpersonal relationship experiences shape the unfolding of developmental pathways.[9] As Alan and I recently wrote in an article titled "The Verdict Is In":

> Those with secure histories had a greater sense of self-agency, were better emotionally regulated, and had higher self-esteem than those with histories of anxious (insecure) attachment.
>
> In general, attachment predicted engagement in the preschool peer group, the capacity for close friendships in middle childhood, the ability to coordinate friendships and group functioning in adolescence, and the capacity to form trusting, non-hostile romantic relationships in adulthood. Those with secure histories were more socially competent and likelier to be peer leaders. Each finding holds true controlling for temperament and IQ.
>
> As Bowlby's theory indicated, security of a child's attachment predicts the reactions of peers and teachers to that child. Children describe peers with avoidant histories as aggressive or "mean." They frequently victimize those with resistant or ambivalent attachment histories, who tend not to be socially competent, and are the least liked by others. Those with secure histories are liked best. This finding can be best understood by recognizing that early attachments create social expectations in children, and may incline them to see the present in terms of negative past experiences. For such children, their attachment history can become a self-fulfilling prophecy as they behave toward new people in their lives—like peers or teachers—in ways that reproduce old, negative relationships.
>
> Teachers, too, with no knowledge of the child's history, treat children in the different categories of attachment differently. Coders, who were blind to the child's history, but who watched videotapes of interactions between teachers and each child, rated teachers as treating those with secure histories in a warm, respectful manner. They set age-appropriate standards for their behavior and had high expectations for them (indicated by actions such as moving on to take care of other tasks after asking the child to do something). With those having resistant histories, the teachers were also warm, but highly controlling. They didn't expect compliance, set low standards, and were unduly nurturing (taking care of things that 5-year-olds should do for themselves). Teachers were controlling and had low expectations with the avoidant

group, but displayed little nurturing and got angry at them most frequently. Thus, the reactions of teachers tended to support the attachment assessment of the children that had been made through other observations.

Anxious (insecure) attachment doesn't directly cause later disturbance, but it initiates a developmental pathway that, without corrective experiences, increases the probability of psychopathology. In fact, anxious/resistant (ambivalent) attachment increases the probability of anxiety disorders and avoidant attachment increases the likelihood of conduct problems. However, the strongest predictor of pathological outcomes, including dissociation, is "disorganized attachment." This "disorganized" infant attachment pattern predicts later dissociative symptoms up to age 26 (and even borderline personality symptoms at age 28).[10]

We can see, then, that our early imprint of relational experiences probably creates synaptic shadows that reflect ways we have adapted to these important interactions at the very time our regulatory circuits have first been developing. Now, shaped by these early effects, we carry these neural proclivities out into the world, and we interact with others in ways that then induce the others to give behavioral responses that mimic exactly the social world in which we grew. This is the developmental neural mechanism by which we can become "lost in familiar places" and have ongoing life experiences that repeatedly reinforce earlier learned patterns of being in the world with others. Ultimately, these deeply felt experiences evoke in us emotions that are at the heart of our subjective sense of being connected—or disconnected—from others in life.

## ATTACHMENT AND EMOTION REGULATION

The biological system that helps organize the self is crucial in determining our subjective experiences in life. One reason is the important role of emotions in creating meaning. The view proposed earlier, and explored further here, is that human emotions constitute the fundamental value system used by the brain to help organize its functioning. The regulation of emotions is thus the essence of self-organization. Communication with and about emotions between parent and infant directly shapes the child's ability to organize the self.

Allan Schore's work on affect regulation provides an extensive review of the neurobiology of emotional development.[11] This section highlights some of Schore's views and integrates them with the framework for emotion regulation proposed in Chapter 7. Children need to be able to regulate their bodily and mental states. They respond directly to their parents' neural activation patterns through the processes of emotional communication and the alignment of states of mind. A child's response to a parent's patterns can be described as the child's "internalization" of the parent. From a basic biological perspective, the child's neuronal system—the structure and function of the developing brain—is shaped by the parent's more mature brain. This occurs within emotional communication. The attunement of emotional states is essential for the developing brain to acquire the capacity to organize itself more autonomously as the child matures.

Reaching out from the brain to the body proper, the autonomic nervous system helps to control the body's state of arousal. This system can induce excitatory, arousing, energy-consuming bodily states, which are produced by the activation of one of its two branches, called the "sympathetic" branch. Examples of physiological responses to the sympathetic branch are increases in heart rate, respiration, sweating, and states of alertness. The autonomic nervous system also includes an inhibitory, de-arousing, energy-conserving portion called the "parasympathetic" branch. The parasympathetic branch mediates such responses as decreases in heart rate, respiration, and states of alertness to the outside world.[12]

The sympathetic branch's development predominates during the first year of life. The parasympathetic branch comes online during the second year. This timing is helpful because as the infant becomes ambulatory, it is important to have some way in which the primary emotional states mediated by the sympathetic branch—interest/excitement and enjoyment/joy—can be modulated in order to inhibit potentially dangerous behaviors.[13] The sharing and amplification of these positive emotional states, so common during infancy, can be seen as a resonance of the sympathetic branch activity of the two individuals. These upbeat states are a major part of the emotional communication between infant and parent during the first year of life. By the second year, when a child becomes able to walk, prohibitions from the parent must be able to inhibit such activating emotional states in order for the child to remain safe. The baby must learn to stop moving in the face of danger. For example, if a child is climbing up the stairs, it is useful to have him learn what "No!" means: "Do not do that; stop what you are now doing." Before the first birthday, most parental communications are alignments with the aroused, positive or negative emotional states. After that time, inhibitory comments from the parent become more prominent.

How does the need for contingent communication—for the alignment of states of mind between parent and child—influence the nature of parental behavior and prohibitions? How can these alignments occur if the child is learning that the parent may not share his excitement about doing something? Balancing the needs for mental state alignment and for parental prohibition is one aspect of how the child acquires a healthy capacity for self-regulation. Let's look at one view of the biology of this process.

Schore, Colwyn Trevarthen, and others have described shame as the emotion evoked when a child's aroused state is not attuned to by the parent.[14] Shame in certain degrees is actually an essential emotion for children to experience, in order to begin to learn to self-regulate their state of mind and behavioral impulses. However, Sroufe has noted that although this form of shame is inevitable and necessary, parents do not need to use shame intentionally as a strategic form of parenting.[15] Shame is thought to be based on the activation of the parasympathetic system (to an external "No!") in the face of a highly charged sympathetic system (an internal "Let's go!"). It's as if the accelerator pedal (the sympathetic branch) is pressed down and then the brake (the parasympathetic branch) is applied.

Schore has proposed that not connecting with a child's active bid for attunement leads to shame.[16] These types of transactions are necessary for a child to learn self-control and then to modulate both behavior and internal emotional states in prosocial ways. Shame, in this very specific sense, is not damaging. Emotional states emerge from the patterns of changes in states of activation. Parasympathetic states alone do not produce the feeling of shame. *Shame requires the dynamic profile of high sympathetic tone (a "crescendo" state) followed by onset of the parasympathetic system (a "decrescendo" state).* Shame is different from humiliation. Shame-inducing interactions coupled with sustained parental anger and/or lack of repair of the disconnection lead to humiliation, which Schore and others have proposed to be toxic to the developing child's brain.[17] This view has been confirmed by others and offers insights into how misattunements and hostility can be traumatic for a young child's developing sense of self.[18] Shame and potentially related social anxiety may also be experienced differently across cultures.[19] Nevertheless, numerous studies suggest that the findings from attachment research of the importance of the parental state of mind with respect to attachment, as revealed in the AAI, is a powerful predictor across cultures of how the parent will provide sensitive parenting to the child.[20] Making sense of our lives seems to have powerful influences on how we can move beyond implicit echoes of our past experiences. Central to this process of making sense is the mental time travel that enables us to reflect on the past, live fully in the present, and become the active creators of our potential future. The middle prefrontal areas play a major integrative role in how we come to make sense of our lives and become the authors of our own life stories.

The orbitofrontal cortex—the part of the middle prefrontal area of the brain just behind the eyes and located at a strategic spot at the top of the limbic area, next to the "higher" associational cortex responsible for various forms of thought and consciousness—plays an important role in affect regulation.[21] This area of the brain is especially sensitive to face-to-face communication and eye contact. Because it serves as an important center of appraisal, it has a direct influence on the elaboration of states of arousal into various types of emotional experience. Schore's detailed conceptualization of this region's role in attachment relationships helps describe the steps involved between emotional attunement and affect regulation.

A brief word on terms may be useful at this point. Researchers have used the term "affect attunement" to refer to the ways in which internal emotional states are brought into external communication with each other within infant–caregiver interactions.[22] Schore uses the term *"attunement"* in this manner, highlighting the importance of this communication in the interactive experiences upon which the brain's development depends. He, Tiffany Field, and others have suggested that *what are attuned are psychobiological states in both members of the interacting pair.*[23] In this book, I am suggesting three related terms: "tracking," "alignment," and "resonance." When we *track* the signals of another person, we focus our attention on his communication and stay present with his changing states from moment to moment, in an open and receptive way. Tracking permits us to alter our own state of mind—to align with the other person. *Alignment* is one component of affect attunement, in which *the state of one individual is altered to approximate that of the other member of the dyad.* Alignment can be primarily a one-way process, in which one individual's state changes to match and anticipate that of the other; or it can be a bidirectional process, involving movement by each member of the dyad. As an example of the former, imagine that a parent is preparing an excited child to get ready to go to sleep. The parent is likely to be more successful if he gets closer to the child's state and then brings the child down to a calmer state than if he simply expects the child to calm down suddenly on her own. Such tracking of a child's state creates an initial alignment that allows the child to feel that she is being attuned to by the parent. This "feeling felt" and alignment then enables the mutual change into a calmer state to be more readily achieved. Such alignments occur frequently, but of necessity they cannot occur all the time. Attunement requires times when individ-

> Alignment is one component of affect attunement, in which the state of one individual is altered to approximate that of the other.

uals are in nonalignment—when they are not directly attempting to match or anticipate each other's states. In this way, attunement is a broader concept than alignment: It includes sensitivity to times when alignment should not occur.

The overall process of attunement leads to the mutual influence of each member upon the other—a characteristic described earlier in the book as "resonance." Emotional resonance, for example, involves more than the alignment of states; it also includes the ways in which the interaction affects the individuals in other aspects of their minds. Resonance also continues after alignment has stopped. The mutual influence of the alignment of states persists within the mind of each member after direct interaction no longer occurs. Attunement yields moments of both alignment and nonalignment, and it also permits emotional resonance to occur between two people even after they are no longer in direct communication.

Healthy attachment relationships—and indeed all close relationships—involve tracking, alignment, attunement, and resonance between people. In everyday life, ruptures in this interpersonal connection are inevitable. Sometimes we miss the opportunity to track because of our distractions or our misunderstanding of the other person's need for connection. These common forms of disconnections are actually quite frequent, if not the norm in our daily lives.[24] But at other times, our own internal preoccupations or distortions can make us misinterpret the meaning of communication, and we may not respond in as sensitive and connecting a manner as is needed in that moment. Still other forms of painful ruptures involve more toxic outcomes, in which we "flip our lids" or "go down the low road" and lose the integrative functions of our middle prefrontal regions. At those times, any of the middle prefrontal functions may become impaired, from our balanced emotions and bodies to our attuned communication, empathy, self-understanding, and even moral judgment.[25] The key to healthy relationships that involve such ruptures is repair—repair, repair, repair. It is of central importance in healthy, secure attachments. Repair is an interactive process in which the rupture is recognized, reconnection is established, and attunement and resonance are experienced as a soothing process that enables the relationship to continue on a supportive path.[26]

The effects of attachment relationships and the process of attunement on the mind have been postulated by Schore to have direct impacts upon the orbitofrontal cortex.[27] Others have found empirical evidence that supports this region's role in attachment.[28] This region of the brain plays an important role in associating sensory input with reward, cognition with emotion, and the appraisal of interpersonal interactions with internal states.[29] The orbitofrontal cortex works with other areas of the middle prefrontal cortex to facilitate the regulation of bodily arousal by pushing down a kind of emotional "clutch" that disengages the sympathetic "accelerator" and activates the parasympathetic "brakes." The parasympathetic system is later deactivated with realignment, and the proper adjusted or regulated level of arousal is established through reactivation of the sympathetic system. In other words, the brakes are applied with the disconnection; the repair process allows the child's energies to be redirected; and then the accelerator is applied again with resumption of the emotional connection during the repair process. The child essentially learns this: "My parents may not like what I am doing, but if I change my activities, they will then connect with me; things in the end will be OK." There is a balance between the accelerator and the brakes. This is the essence of affect regulation.

The band of tolerable activation levels of the autonomic nervous system—of either the sympathetic or parasympathetic branches—may vary widely among individuals. Levels outside a person's window of tolerance, in either direction, may be accompanied by diminished ability to function in an adaptive and flexible manner. Neither excessive, nonregulated arousal (sympathetic activity) nor excessive inhibition (parasympathetic activation) is healthy for the development or the ongoing functioning of the brain.

## The Circuitry of Connection

This section outlines two views of the social nature of the human brain. Jaak Panksepp has proposed a view of affective neuroscience suggesting that the brainstem and limbic areas serve as the source of emotional life and motivational drive in human beings.[30] These subcortical areas influence cortical function revealing how emotion and cognition are inseparable processes of the nervous system. In particular, specialized circuits are involved in seven basic emotional systems: seeking/desire, fear/anxiety, rage/anger, lust/sex, care/maternal nurturance, panic/separation distress/grief, and playfulness/physical social engagement. These are basic mammalian systems; they can influence our temperaments or constitutional, innate neural proclivities,[31] and they shape our motivational drives for attachment, play behavior, exploration, mastery, resource allocation, and reproduction. Clearly, attachment is a central aspect of our lives as mammals. In fact, the evolution of the mammalian limbic areas is associated with the emergence of attachment behavior in which the infant mammal requires the close care of a parent in order to survive. As we've seen throughout this book, human attachment has elaborated this basic mammalian system in response to more complex cortical development that requires even longer care of the young.

Panksepp has proposed the following in reference to the epigenetic construction of our social brains:

> A focus on the social/cultural environments of developing human beings is more important than past evolutionary dynamics for understanding human cognitive tendencies. The growth and maturation of higher aspects of human social brain functions depend more on developmental/epigenetic progressions than on the gene sequences that are critical in construction in our brains and bodies. Family/social/cultural dynamics are more important than Pleistocene evolutionary dynamics for programming higher brain regions that bring forth our uniquely and fully human social qualities. . . . Most of the

higher social brain [may be] epigenetically constructed through the use of basic social-emotional tools, especially the CARE, PANIC, and PLAY systems, rather than through genetically prescribed "adaptations."[32]

A related finding is that the more intricate our social environments, the more complex our cortical structures.[33] For us as mammals, this means that after birth our social experiences will directly shape the intricate connections established within our growing cortical structures. Because the regulation of the subcortical areas appears to depend upon the coupling of prefrontal areas to them, it is natural, then, to see how interpersonal interactions shape both the growth of connections and the epigenetic regulation of brain regions responsible for control of these emotional systems.

> The more intricate our social environments, the more complex our cortical structures.

Stephen Porges has proposed that one aspect of our social brains is the "social engagement system," which utilizes a recently evolved branch of the polyvagal nerve, the myelinated ventral vagus.[34] When activated following evaluations by the prefrontal areas assessing for conditions of safety, the social engagement system relaxes the facial muscles and muscles controlling the tympanic membrane, so that a person becomes more receptive to engaging with others in the world. When a sense of danger is evaluated, the prefrontal regions, in conjunction with the subcortical limbic and brainstem areas, can shut off the social engagement system and activate the sympathetic branch of the autonomic nervous system. This releases catecholamines (adrenaline and noradrenaline), which "rev up" the body to prepare for fighting, fleeing, or activated freezing. If the individual's prefrontal region assesses a situation in which there is felt to be no strategy of escape from harm, a portion of the parasympathetic branch, the unmyelinated branch of the dorsal vagal nerve, is activated; the individual then experiences a "dorsal dive," in which blood pressure and heart rate are dropped and fainting may result. This is the helpless/hopeless state, or a "flaccid freeze" response, sometimes attributed to a dissociative reaction. This is Porges's "polyvagal theory" and it expands on the simpler notion of the brake–accelerator model of the parasympathetic and sympathetic autonomic branches, presented earlier in this chapter. Our reaction to threat is actually composed of two different elements: the activated sympathetic fight–flight–freeze response and the parasympathetic shutdown state of collapse.

Utilizing this view, Porges identified a subset of children with autistic features who were acoustically sensitive, and offered an intervention: headphones with sound modification that eliminated the low-frequency vibrations associated with a sense of danger, and only permitted midrange frequencies. When they used these headphones, the children had a marked decrease in their avoidance of social interaction.[35] Although many children with social communication difficulties may not have acoustic sensitivity, this finding raises the important conceptual issue that a child who is not participating in expected social engagements may be experiencing a sense of threat that others do not sense in the same environment.

Studies of autism and related disorders of social communication are filled with emerging and controversial findings. Recent studies of individuals with these disorders suggest that their mirror neuron areas do not become active in response to social stimuli—a situation typically associated with high activations.[36] One interpretation of this finding is that these individuals have "dysfunctional" or "nonexistent" mirror neurons. But another point of view is that the motivational circuits do not appraise social engagement as rewarding, and so they do not engage the mirror neuron system—or that these circuits are shut down temporarily in response to being overwhelmed and having a feeling of lack of safety.[37] It is clear from these various studies that in persons with these disorders, social interactions and neural activity are not functioning as they do in other people; future research will need to clarify both the origins and specific mechanisms for these disparities. Clinicians and educators devising interventions to help individuals with social communication challenges may benefit from keeping an open mind about creative strategies for helping introduce and maintain growth-promoting interpersonal connections.[38]

## Parenting Approaches

Children challenge parents continually. How parents respond to these challenges will set the tone of their interactions and will shape their children's capacity to regulate their states of mind and emotions. Research suggests that the ways parents respond to their children reflect the parents' early life experiences, the sense they have made of their past,[39] and their genetic makeup.[40] Children, too, come with their own genetic differences that influence their temperament and how responsive they will be to their environment, including how their parents interact with them.[41]

Take, for example, a fourteen-month-old boy who wants to climb onto a table with a lamp on it. One possible parental response would be to yell "No!" and then take the boy outside, where his drive to climb can be "attuned to." Another response would be not to notice the attempt to climb, to hear the lamp come crashing down, to pick it up, and either to tell the boy quietly not to do it again or just to ignore him the rest of the evening. A third response would be for the parent to yell "No!" and reprimand the boy, hug him out of guilt, then distance herself from him because he has disappointed her. A fourth approach would be to become enraged and throw the lamp to the floor next to the boy, to teach him never to do that again. Which attachment pattern would be associated with each form of prohibition/disconnection and repair? Think of how the child over time would learn to regulate his baseline emotional state as well as his aroused state in each case, if each pattern of interaction were to be repeated many times. Naturally the child's innate sensitivity will shape the exact degree and nature of his response, but parental input will influence the learned regulatory patterns that will develop over time. Recall that temperament does not predict the form of attachment the child develops with a caregiver.[42] These four parental responses would be associated with the attachment patterns of security, avoidance, ambivalence, and disorganization, respectively.

## Security

The first year of life is filled with the attunement of infant and attachment figure, which often centers on the upbeat, high-vitality affects of interest/excitement and enjoyment/joy. The sympathetic system is being activated and developed at a high level during this period. Children who become securely attached to their parents are likely to have a good baseline autonomic tone. They are capable of tolerating high-intensity emotional states. Specifically, if a pattern of attunement like the first one described above is chronically repeated, the securely attached child will experience an aroused state (excited about climbing) that is responded to by the parent with a prohibition (inducing parasympathetic activation and a sense of shame), rapidly followed by a repair (attuning to the gist of the initial aroused state and redirecting it in socially acceptable ways). This child's prefrontal cortex "learns" that even high-arousal states (in need of connection) can be modified, and *then* connection will be reestablished. We can propose that such connection–disconnection–repair transactions are one means by which patterns of parent–child communication promote the prefrontally mediated capacity for response flexibility.

In addition to repairing ruptures, having reflective dialogues is an important part of secure attachment. They focus the child–parent dyad on the internal experience of each member. Joining at the level of the mind and developing communication around mindsight help develop a coherent narrative of the shared experiences in the family. A parent's capacity to be sensitive to a child and provide contingent communication is based on her ability to perceive the child's signals, make sense of them, and respond in a timely and effective manner to them. As mentioned earlier, studies of memory talk and of the parent's capacity for mentalizing experience—for seeing the mind beneath behavior—support these important mindsight skills at the heart of security.[43]

## Avoidance

The avoidantly attached child is not so fortunate and learns little about the emotional state of the parent, with no warning about the parental response, which in fact may be quite uninvolved (neglectful) or severe and misattuned (rejecting). In such a dyad, it is likely that the general level of shared emotion is quite low, possibly resulting in an underdevelopment of the child's capacity for normal levels of interest/excitement and enjoyment/joy. Prohibitions may be behaviorally severe and emotionally disconnected. This, coupled with the generally low levels of attunement and sensitivity to the child's signals, may produce an excess in overall parasympathetic tone. The child's early experience may have a significant impact on the expression of affect and access to conscious awareness of emotion. Overall, the avoidantly attached child may develop an internal and interpersonal sense of disconnection. The child learns to minimize the expression of attachment-related emotion, which may serve to reduce the disabling effects of overwhelming frustration in the face of continuing interactions with the caregiver.[44]

## Ambivalence

In the third approach, parental facial expressions of continued disapproval, eye gaze aversion, and body language of disconnection or anger are all perceived by the child. The child's high-arousal states may be attuned to sometimes, but if they are not, disconnection and shame may be associated with humiliation and may thus become toxic, especially if disconnection is prolonged or associated with parental anger.

At times, parents may be unable to track and align with the child, producing excessive arousal in the disconnection. At other times, the parent may intrude her own state of mind, leading to the introduction of a "not-me" experience in which the child absorbs the internal subjective world of the caregiver, which is not contingent with the child's initial communication. Either of these situations may produce an internal state of confusion. The child's range of tolerable emotional arousal may be broad, but uncontrollable swings beyond the window of tolerance may occur. Inconsistent attunements and repair may lead to excessive arousal, so that the sympathetic system may often be unchecked because of a diminished parasympathetic system response. Alternatively, prolonged despair may result if the parasympathetic system is excessively activated. Anticipatory anxiety and fear of separation may be evident. Separation in the ambivalently attached child means having to rely on the self for ineffective emotion regulation. Repeated experiences of going beyond tolerable levels with excessive arousal or despair teaches such children that they themselves are unreliable affect modulators; this is the reason for their paradoxical excessive reliance on the inconsistent attachment figures. Such experiences may produce an apparent increase in a child's sensitivity, especially in relationship to interactions with others and to situations of loss and separation. Overall, there is a maximizing of the expression of attachment–related emotions, which some authors suggest may serve as an attempt to enhance the chances that the inconsistent parent will pay attention to the child.[45]

### Disorganization

In the fourth pattern, the child's behavior elicits a rageful parental response, producing terror in the child. This is not simply the child's fear of consequences, but a fear for safety induced by the attachment figure. The child's adaptation to this suddenly induced fear state (high levels of both sympathetic and parasympathetic discharge) is a conflictual one: The accelerator and the brakes are being applied simultaneously. This is an example of a disorganized form of attachment.[46] The ensuing dissociation may involve the collapse or "flaccid freeze" response, in which the dorsal branch of the vagal nerve becomes active in a recurring state of helplessness. The parent, who often has unresolved trauma or loss (as described in Chapter 3), may unintentionally and unknowingly be providing the child with a set of responses that are disorienting and disorganizing. As an attachment figure, such a parent has become a source of fear and confusion, not of safety and security. This can be a result of active aggression or of exhibiting a fearful or confused state of mind. The intense and frightening moments of disconnection with the parent remain unrepaired. As the parent disappears into rage or panic himself, the child becomes lost in terror. These disorganizing and disorienting experiences become an essential part of how the child learns to self-regulate behavior and emotional states. The child has the double insult of becoming engulfed in confusion and terror induced by the parent, and of losing the relationship with an attachment figure that might have provided a safe haven and sense of security. Dissociation can be an outcome of these experiences and produce an internal sense of fragmentation of the self.

## RELATIONSHIPS AND SELF-REGULATION

The lessons from attachment research can guide our understanding of the powerful effect interpersonal relationships can have on the development and ongoing functioning of self-regulation. Studies suggest that the regulating prefrontal cortex remains plastic throughout life; that is, it is able to develop beyond childhood.[47] This region mediates neurophysiological mechanisms integrating several domains of human experience: social relationships, the evaluation of meaning, autonoetic consciousness, response flexibility, and emotion regulation.[48] The nonverbal social signals of eye contact, facial expression, tone of voice, and body gestures communicate the state of mind of each member of a dyad. The interactions that occur have direct effects on the emotional experience *in that moment*. Within the context of an attachment relationship, the child's developing mind and the structure of the child's brain will be shaped in such a way that the ability to regulate emotion *in the future* is affected.

The proposal being made here is that interpersonal relationships can provide attachment experiences that allow integrative neurophysiological changes to occur throughout life. Integrative communication honors differences and cultivates compassionate connecting and is likely to induce the growth of integrative fibers in the brain. The hypothesis is that integrative sharing of energy and information flow between people leads to the activation of the integrative embodied mechanisms of energy and information flow in the nervous system. The opposite is also a natural implication—that suboptimal experiences of impaired communication, as in neglect or abuse, will produce impediments in the growth of integrative fibers in the brain. Indeed, recent research supports this proposal: Individuals with extreme cases of trauma, such as neglect or abuse, have been found to have damaged integrative structures in their brains.[49] Such impediments to integration would explain how the coordination and balance of the nervous system would be affected and adaptive functioning would be impaired.[50]

> Interpersonal relationships can provide attachment experiences that allow integrative neurophysiological changes to occur throughout life.

Even in these situations, however, the principles learned from attachment research may perhaps still prove useful in helping people adapt to life's stresses. In many cases of disorganized attachment and clinical dissociation, for example, therapeutic relationships can facilitate effective movement toward well-being and adaptive self-regulation.[51] In less extreme cases, the integrative structures of the brain may have developed well, but maladaptive states of mind may have been engrained. For these people, therapy may help to move their minds toward more adaptive modes of processing information and regulating its flow. The patient–psychotherapist relationship may provide a sense of proximity, a safe haven, and an internal model of security. These elements of an attachment relationship within therapy (or other emotionally engaging relationships, such as romance and friendship) may possibly facilitate new integrative development and enhance the regulation of emotion throughout the lifespan. Specific techniques within a psychotherapy relationship are sometimes needed to alter engrained patterns of emotion dysregulation.[52]

The following example illustrates the use of psychotherapy to enable the mind to develop flexible self-regulation. A five-year-old girl was referred for "impulse control" problems in school. A review of the child's history revealed that she had severe visual problems, which had remained undetected until she was three and a half years of age. Even after she received proper glasses and could see objects in focus, however, she continued to have "outbursts of emotion" and impulsivity at school. In the therapist's office, it was clear that she did not look to other people's faces to "check in" with how they might be responding to her. She seemed to have an impairment in the typical process of social referencing, which is usually evident during the first year of life.[53] At school, she seemed oblivious to the reactions of her teachers and her classmates. This social disconnection gave her the outward appearance of being oppositional and perhaps of having a basic deficit in social cognition—the ability to perceive and process social signals. Face-to-face communication is one route by which attunement and social referencing enable the emotional state of one individual to be perceived by another. Such abilities allow for emotionally contingent communication, which is at the developmental heart of emotion regulation.

In therapy, the child was encouraged to look at the therapist's face. Her parents and teachers were counseled about the nature of attachment, social referencing, and the use of face-to-face communication in the development of emotion regulation. The impairment in her vision, now corrected, was offered as a working hypothesis for why this girl exhibited such social difficulties. Over several months of intervention, she began to look more frequently at others when she spoke. In play, she engaged more in identifying dolls' internal states, and their emotions became a more active part of the stories that unfolded in therapy. With the development of these capacities for facial perception, "theory of mind," and social referencing, she began to engage more appropriately in social interactions. The use of reflective dialogue—talking about feelings, thoughts, memories, beliefs, and perceptions—in conjunction with the nonverbal face-to-face communication enabled her to develop previously unstimulated abilities in her mind. Her ability to regulate her emotions seemed to improve: Her explosions became less frequent and less intense, and her impulsive behavior diminished significantly. One could hypothesize that each of these developmental accomplishments was mediated by the interactive maturation of her prefrontal cortex in response to these integrative communication-based experiences.

In theory, this therapeutic approach enabled this young girl to use the nonverbal signals that she had generally missed because of her visual difficulties. The possible role of her mirror neurons and larger resonance circuitry in such social experiences may help us to understand how communications lead to more adaptive internal regulation. Other modalities that can allow two individuals to communicate their states of mind, such as hearing and touch, are also important in communication during childhood. The use of this approach allowed this child to take in the vital information of other people's minds instead of living in isolation, where her frustration level was high and her behaviors appeared "impulsive" because they were so independent of the signals and needs of others.

## Romantic Attachments and Interlocking States

Knowing the attachment histories of each member of a couple can be essential in clarifying how micromoments of misattunement can blow up into major battles and become interlocking, dysregulated dyadic states of despair and distancing. Small changes in input, such as subtle shifts in the emotional expression of one member of the pair, can produce large and rapid alterations in output in the nonlinear complex systems of each individual and of the dyad. These dysregulated interlocking states often have their origins in the attachment models of each member of the pair.

"Interlocking" in this context means that the separate states of mind activated by these repeated patterns reinforce their respective historical models of relationships. The partners keep continually reexperiencing lack of attunement, misattunements, and repeated verification of the lessons learned from their own individual attachment histories. These repeated ruptures in connection are rarely repaired. Interlocking states strengthen earlier maladaptive self-organizational pathways. They create a rigid or a chaotic pattern of interaction that prevents the partners from joining together into a larger system capable of moving toward dyadic states of increasing complexity. At one extreme, these ruts can be experienced as a sense of malaise or deadness, which each member of the pair may feel but cannot articulate; at the other extreme, these ruts may be filled with anxiety, a sense of intrusiveness, and uncertainty. To remain healthy, a dyadic system, like an individual, must find a balance between flexibility and continuity in its perpetual move toward increasingly complex states of existence. Couple therapy may sometimes be necessary for the partners to recognize and then to alter these profoundly frustrating and deadening interlocking states.

As early models of attachment are activated within a couple's relationship, the opportunity emerges to learn about how early experiences shaped implicit reality. In interlocking states, both partners' private selves may be hungry and in pain, fearing annihilation, abandonment or intrusion (as in ambivalent attachments) or be adapted to emotional distance and rejection (as in avoidant attachments). Nurturing their private selves requires that the members of the couple join together in supportively reflecting on how their public selves have struggled to adapt to these experiences of disconnection without repair. Growth emerges as reflective and resonant dyadic states become achieved within the attuned relationship. Such a process can then allow the couple to achieve more fulfilling and adaptive levels of dyadic self-organization.

## PATHWAYS OF EMOTIONAL GROWTH

This section integrates many ideas about memory, attachment, and emotion in exploring some insights gleaned from therapeutic work with adults and children. These illustrations are offered not as scientific data, but as clinical impressions to further our discussion of how interpersonal experiences may shape the developing mind across the lifespan.[54]

### Avoidance and Dismissing States of Mind

Emotional relationships of all sorts can be healing and promote healthy maturation. At times, however, the unique configuration of psychotherapy is needed to facilitate movement toward an "earned" secure/autonomous adult attachment status.[55] For Main and Goldwyn's dismissing adult,[56] without awareness of "what life could be like," promoting this growth may be quite a challenge for his therapist and his partner alike. On the one hand, the individual has the right to remain as he is; there are no definitions of absolutely "normal" ways of relating that some "objective" therapist can push onto others. However, isolation and emotional distance take their toll—within the person's romantic relationship; within relationships with others, including his children; and within the self. His intense emotions and enjoyment in life may be severely muted. Part of this neutral emotionality may be attributable to the proposed parcellation of the sympathetic (accelerator) branch of the autonomic nervous system, which is responsible for heightened states of arousal. His mindsight—the ability to sense the subjective mental life of others, or of himself—may also be severely restricted. The result is that his basic emotional needs are not met by anyone. However, the avoidantly attached individual does not believe this, because his approach to survival has seemed successful thus far. His private self remains highly underdeveloped and consciously unaware. A therapist working closely with such individuals is especially challenged to remain fully present so that attunement and resonance can ultimately occur.[57]

The avoidantly attached (dismissing) adult often comes to therapy at the insistence of his securely or ambivalently attached romantic partner. The partner feels that the relationship is too distant and emotionally barren to tolerate. Ironically, the partner may have been initially attracted to the patient because of his "independence and autonomy—he didn't have to rely on any-one." This autonomy gives the ambivalently attached mate a feeling at first that intrusion (the dreaded experience of the mate's own childhood) need not be feared. As adult development progresses, however, the ambivalently attached part-ner may change and come to feel the need for more emotional intimacy. The avoidantly attached partner is less likely to develop as quickly toward models of security, because he often lacks aware-ness of internal pain or dissatisfaction with the relationship, which might otherwise serve to motivate change.

> The avoidantly attached (dismissing) adult often comes to therapy at the insistence of his securely or ambivalently attached romantic partner.

Logical discussions, which are so natural for avoidantly attached indi-viduals, only go so far. Gentle and unintrusive attunements to their shifts in states begin to open up new possibilities. These are right-hemisphere-to-right-hemisphere connections between a therapist and a patient. In addition to these affect attunements, activation of right-hemisphere processes can be helpful. For example, by encouraging imagery and other nonverbal processes (such as "drawing on the right side of the brain" art techniques,[58] aware-ness of bodily sensations, dance, and music), psychotherapy can facilitate the emergence of new ways of experiencing the self. Such self-awareness often facilitates the development of new ways of seeing the world, especially the subjective mental lives of others. This process may be helpful for many other individuals besides those who have a history of avoidant attachment.

Guided imagery provides direct access to prelinguistic symbolic imagi-nation and processes driven by implicit memory. The results can be deeply moving, though often initially derided by some avoidant/dismissing patients as "weird" and useless. As time goes on, emotional states become accessible to these patients in the form of images that they can come to respect. These nonverbal, nonrational, right-sided processes begin to influence the patients' behavior and make them more aware of similar states in others around them. In some cases, psychotherapy can catalyze the development of new conscious awareness of the self's and others' emotional processes. As the attuned and resonating emotional communication within psychotherapy continues, new models of the self and of the self with others can gradually begin to develop. These right-hemisphere models facilitate the promotion of emotional con-nections with others. As such resonant experiences unfold, an integrating process emerges and a more coherent narrative evolves, coupled with a more complex and enriching sense of meaning in life. The nature of such an inte-gration is explored in depth in Chapter 9.

In one case, a man who had a dismissing state of mind with respect to attachment was introduced over time to the techniques of guided imagery and asked to do the drawing exercises outlined in Betty Edwards's art book.[59] At first, this man seemed very reluctant to consider these new experiences as important in any way. He had come to therapy at the insistence of his wife, who stated that he was "too cold and intellectual." As the imagery continued over several sessions, however, the emerging stories became more and more complex and compelling to him.

For the therapist, this imagery process revealed a previously quiet, non-conscious, and dormant right hemisphere's construction of reality. It was filled with sensations, intense emotions, visual scenes, thematic struggles, and new perspectives on dilemmas of which this left-side dominant individual was quite unaware. For example, he experienced the notion that he had better let his "wilting" marriage "blossom" by buying his wife roses when she didn't expect them. He had never done such a thing as buying flowers for her without a particular "reason," such as a birthday or anniversary. He got the roses simply because it "felt" right. He couldn't explain it at the time, but he just followed his gut instinct. As we'll see in the next chapter, this is a form of integration involving the linkage of his lower bodily processes with his higher cortical awareness. His right hemisphere took his wife's internal world into account, provided him with a metaphor for her needs, and enabled him to feel her feelings. This revealed how he could now resonate with his wife. Though there was no logic to the act, this man learned—from his own gut (literally: sensations from the intestines are represented in the right middle prefrontal region)—the importance of letting another person fill him.

Over many months of therapy, as this man continued to allow his innate right-hemisphere processes to "blossom," he found himself slowly becoming aware of new types of internal sensations. He would feel his body more in response to interactions with his wife; he also began to become aware of shifts in her facial expressions, and found himself responding more to these internal and external emotional cues. What was particularly striking to him was that his internal experiences seemed to shift. He stopped being so concerned about goals and outcomes, and became more focused on the process of things, both at home and at work. These changes at first were quite subtle. Though this man would not openly admit it, he seemed to feel very vulnerable experiencing and expressing these new sensations. His life seemed to be opening up to a new mode of experiencing both himself and his wife.

## Ambivalence and Preoccupied States of Mind

For an individual with a history of ambivalent attachments, inconsistency and the intrusion of parental emotional states have led to an intense sense of vulnerability and loss of the self. As this individual struggles to connect, she feels perpetually at risk of losing her connections to others, or to herself.

Retreating into chameleon-like imitations of meeting others' expectations is a learned, reflexive public adaptation to these intrusive assaults. In psychotherapy, this may lead to an attempt to be the "perfect patient." As this individual tries to define herself, there may be patterns of withdrawal and approach similar to those in her childhood history of attachment—a form of the psychoanalytic concept of transference—which lead to fluctuations in openness to being understood in psychotherapy.

As this person's inner, private states of mind become slowly accessible, the therapist must be ever vigilant to the critical micromoments of interaction, where attunement is crucial. Responding to the patient's nonverbal signals, including tone of voice, facial expressions, eye gaze, and bodily motion, can reveal the otherwise hidden shifts in states of mind. Resonating with these expressions of primary emotions requires that the therapist feel the feelings, not merely understand them conceptually. Resonance involves the alignment of psychobiological states between patient and therapist.

One aspect of this attunement is the recognition that everyone seems to go through naturally oscillating cycles of internal versus external focus of connection. There are times when an individual needs to have self-focus, perhaps reflecting the internal self-regulation of emotional states. Within moments, however, there may be a noticeable shift to an other-focus, in which external connections are used for dyadic self-regulation. These natural oscillations suggest the use of modifications of the internal versus external constraints of the individual's system, in order to regulate the flow of states and self-organization. These ideas also remind us of the important concept that self-organization is a result of both internal individual processes and dyadic processes. Another implication of such oscillations comes from the findings on hemispheric specialization discussed in earlier chapters, in which the left hemisphere mediates approach states and the right hemisphere facilitates states of withdrawal. This relates to a form of integration that links the differentiated sides of the nervous system, left and right, as we shall see in the next chapter. The changing focus of processing, mediated via a cycling of left- versus right-hemisphere dominance and of external versus internal focus, may be a part of what we sense when others have a cycling need for external versus internal connection.

Misattunements and missed opportunities for attunement are unavoidable, whether these occur in psychotherapy, parenting, or other emotional relationships. Unless repair is undertaken, toxic senses of shame and humiliation can become serious blocks to interpersonal communication. These dreaded states are not merely uncomfortable and disliked; they can feel like a black hole, a bottomless pit of despair, in which the self is lost for what seems to be forever. Repair requires the recognition that a rupture has occurred in the attunement process, and then the realignment of states between the two individuals involved. The repair process is an interactive one, requiring the openness of both people in attempts to reconnect after a rupture.

The public self strives to avoid the dreaded states of shame and humiliation; it scans the social environment for clues of connection, but is often unable to prevent the activation of these states. The anxiety accompanying the emergence of these dreaded states into one's consciousness can induce defensive adaptations. Fears of annihilation and abandonment are the origins of the desperate withdrawal and anxious approach common in ambivalently attached individuals. The excessive parcellation of the parasympathetic "brakes," proposed to be one adaptation to inconsistent and intrusive parenting, may make these states especially vulnerable to dysregulation. An adaptive, public self may emerge at these times to avoid the dreaded state by meeting the needs of others. The adaptive defenses of such a public self vary greatly and can include primitive modes, such as denial and the projection of the sense of disconnection onto other people or life events. In contrast, some individuals may utilize more mature approaches, such as seeking emotional connection with others or sublimating their painful experiences into efforts to help others through professional work (e.g., teaching with an emphasis on supporting others' self-esteem, working in the government to establish laws protecting the rights of children, or becoming a therapist and emphasizing the importance of understanding others and respecting their individuality).

> Fears of annihilation and abandonment are the origins of the desperate withdrawal and anxious approach common in ambivalently attached individuals.

From primitive, "nonproductive" defenses to mature, "socially helpful" ones, an ambivalently attached (preoccupied) individual may experience any of a wide range of adaptive modes within differing emotional and social contexts. The relative distance of a work setting may permit sublimation to flourish; the close quarters of a romantic relationship or a parent–child relationship may periodically activate an intense sense of intrusion or other forms of misattunement, and yield a sudden emergence of the dreaded states of shame and humiliation. To avoid these painful states, activation of more primitive modes of defense may occur, filled with fear, anger, and associated perceptual distortions and misinterpretations of others' behavior. These are moments of intense vulnerability and risk for dyadic dysregulation.

## Disorganization and Unresolved States of Mind

Unresolved parental trauma or loss can lead to disorganized/disoriented attachment, which is a much more chaotic form of dyadic system than either avoidant or ambivalent attachment.[60] For the person who has experienced disorganized attachment, the experience of parental fear or fear-inducing behavior has often been associated with the parent's lack of resolution of trauma or loss. That is, the incoherence of the parent's life narrative has been behaviorally injected into the child's experience by way of the parent's own disturbance in self-organization and the resultant dysregulated states and disorienting actions. Epigenetic research may reveal in the future how the stress of these unresolved states may negatively influence gene expression in both parent and child. Preliminary studies have revealed, for example, that a gene variant (an allele) for a neurotransmitter transport system, when combined with an epigenetic regulatory control change, has a higher degree of association with unresolved trauma and loss.[61] Our experience does not occur in a vacuum: We live in bodies with vulnerabilities both in nucleotide sequencing (genes) and in gene expression control (epigenetics). Given these vulnerabilities, an overwhelming event can make it more difficult for us to overcome adversity in the future. For some individuals, however, adversity in later years may serve as a seed of "posttraumatic growth" rather than vulnerability.[62]

Parents with disorganized or unresolved states of mind with regard to attachment may have a negative effect upon their children without intervention. Unresolved parental behaviors, which are incompatible with providing a sense of safety and cohesion, are "biological paradoxes" that activate approach and avoid circuits of survival in a child's brain.[63] They directly impair the developing child's affect regulation, shifts in states of mind, and integrative and narrative functions. The result is that the child enters repeated chaotic states of mind. From a dynamical point of view, these can be considered "strange attractor states"—neural net configurations that are widely distributed throughout the system. They become engrained states of dissociated and dysfunctional activation. From a polyvagal perspective, they may involve the sympathetically driven fight–flight–freeze activations and the dorsal vagal initiation of the flaccid freeze response of collapse.

When a patient has a history of disorganized attachment, the therapist is faced with the especially crucial challenge of providing the essence of a secure attachment: a predictable emotional environment in which the patient can learn to depend upon the therapist for regulating state shifts. The therapeutic relationship and the dyadic self-regulation subsequently become "internalized" through the development of a mental model of the self with the therapist, and through the acquisition of new capacities for autonomous emotion regulation. As we'll discuss in the next chapter, achieving this new level of self-organization is often facilitated by an integrating narrative process that facilitates a deep sense of internal coherence.[64]

## Unresolved Trauma and Grief

In addition to the influence of repeated patterns of communication within attachment relationships, specific overwhelming events may produce marked effects on the developing mind. Psychological trauma can overwhelm affect regulation mechanisms, and various forms of adaptation may be required to maintain equilibrium. The flood of stress hormones can produce toxic effects on the development of brain systems responsible for self-regulation and epigenetic factors may impede the way gene expression regulates a child's response to stress. Integrative function is compromised. In this way, early, severe, and chronic trauma may create impairments in a child's ability to adapt to future stress.[65] The individual's developmental stage at the time of a trauma—be it loss of a loved one, an abusive experience (especially those involving a sense of betrayal), or the witnessing of a violent event—markedly influences the adaptive responses available. In general, loss or trauma can have a negative impact on a child's expectations for the future, directly shape his anticipational models and prospective memory, and disrupt his narrative process. Trauma may produce a narrowing in the windows of tolerance for certain emotional states (such as anger, fear, or sadness) or particular social interactions (such as sexuality or assertive behavior). An individual may thus have very specific patterns of dysfunction that relate only to a relatively narrow set of internal or external conditions. Avoidance of such states in order to maintain functioning may severely restrict a person's life when trauma remains unresolved. This is an example of how chaos (eruptions of excessive arousal) or rigidity (avoidance of certain experiences) can dominate a person's life. This nonintegrated condition is called "lack of resolution." These synaptic shadows of prior events that remain unresolved produce impairments to achieving self-regulation and integration of self-states, and in these ways damage the individual's deepest sense of the self and the ability to regulate the flow of internal states.

It is important to realize that challenging life events, like trauma, divorce, or loss of a loved one, can overwhelm an individual's ability to cope but also can serve as significant sources of strength when they are integrated into the person's life.[66] Research on the lack of resolution of trauma or loss in adult attachment studies, for example, reveals that having experienced such events does not by itself produce a parent with negative functioning and offspring with insecure attachment. The key issue is whether these events have been incorporated into a coherent narrative of the adult's ongoing life story.[67] Resilience in life may emerge as relationships and self-reflection facilitate the integration of memory, emotion, and a wide array of neural processes.

In some cases of engrained patterns of dysregulation, psychiatric medications may be needed to help the brain achieve the capacity to regulate the flow of states of mind. Direct biochemical effects can alter the synaptic strengths determining the internal constraints of the system. A positive response to medications does not confirm some "genetic disorder." For example, some of the symptoms of PTSD respond well to medications. Furthermore, studies of laboratory animals that have experienced maternal deprivation and reveal subsequent behavioral disturbances find that these animals respond well to selective serotonin reuptake inhibitors, but relapse when these medications are removed.[68] It may be the case that certain individuals—whether because of genetic and epigenetic factors, early traumatic experiences, or some combination of inherited vulnerability and stressful environmental conditions— have developed such maladaptive brain structures and self-organizational capacities that intensive psychotherapy and/or medications are essential. It is important to keep in mind, however, that the regulating regions of the brain (especially the prefrontal cortex) may remain open to further development throughout the lifespan, and thus to experience-dependent maturational processes. Psychotherapy can utilize this potential in helping to facilitate the further development of the mind.

If severe trauma occurs early in life, or if a form of divided attention (such as entering a state of intense imagination or trance) is utilized during an overwhelming experience, explicit memory for the traumatic experience(s) may be impaired. Intense and frightening elements of implicit memory will be encoded and may later be automatically reactivated, intruding on the traumatized individual's internal experience and external behaviors without the person's conscious sense of recollection or knowledge of the source of these intrusions.

In the case of loss of a loved one, especially an attachment figure, the mind is forced to alter the structure of its internal working models to adjust to the painful reality that the self can no longer seek proximity and gain comfort from the caregiver. Loss, especially early in childhood, can have a deep impact on the growing mind. The extent of the impact may be related in part to how well the family can meet the child's ongoing attachment needs. The child's developmental stage at the time of the loss will also influence the nature of the grieving process. As the child continues to develop, grieving may need to be revisited so that the new developmental capacities can process the loss. For both a child and an adult, dealing with loss takes time and a nurturing environment. John Bowlby's view of the grieving process is that the attachment models must be deeply altered to take the loss into account.[69]

> Loss, especially early in childhood, can have a deep impact on the growing mind.

Delayed or pathological grief can be seen as the impairment in the ability to make such alterations within the attachment system. States of mind continue to be activated in which connection to the actual attachment figure is expected. Prohibitions to sharing the grieving process may result in impaired grief, as can be seen in a family whose members are unable to communicate about painful issues or to recognize the different emotional needs of individuals within the family. If conflictual feelings toward a deceased attachment figure were present, then grieving may also be difficult.

The effects of unresolved loss or trauma in relation to specific overwhelming events can be powerfully disorganizing and often hidden from conscious awareness. At the most fundamental level, such a lack of resolution involves disturbances in the flow of energy and information in the mind. As the mind emerges at the interface of neurophysiological processes and interpersonal relationships, such disturbances can be seen within neural pathways and within dyadic communication. Given the devastating effects of unresolved trauma and grief on the individual, and its potential to impair attachment with future offspring, it is vital for help to be offered to those who remain in an unresolved state following overwhelming experiences. Attachment disturbances in the children of parents with lack of resolution result directly from the impairments to contingent, collaborative communication As suggested above, the flow of energy and information between parent and child—the essence of attuned relationships—is disturbed in cases of parental unresolved trauma or loss.

Prospective memory allows us to "remember the future." In memory-related terms, lack of resolution means that the mind has a tendency to create repeated patterns of disorganizing states, often without conscious awareness of their origin. These states may be created by sudden and unwanted activations of implicit elements of memory, such as flashbacks of traumatic events or mental models of a deceased attachment figure as if the figure were still alive. These activations can seriously impair functioning, especially in the realms of response flexibility, emotional modulation, and contingent communication with others. Unresolved trauma or loss leaves the individual with a deep sense of incoherence in autonoetic consciousness, which tries to make sense of the past, organize the present, and chart the future. This lack of resolution can produce lasting effects throughout the lifespan and influence self-organization across the generations.

Making the connection within psychotherapy between these aspects of memory and past experiences allows patients to understand the origins of their disturbances. Such reflections must take place within the therapeutic attachment setting, which allows the mind to experience intensely dysregulated states and learn—dyadically at first—to tolerate them, then to reflect on their nature, and eventually to regulate them in a more adaptive manner. This expands the windows of tolerance and may promote the growth of integrative fibers.[70] Much of this emotional processing is in its essence nonverbal and is probably mediated initially via right-hemisphere processes (both those within the patient and those between patient and therapist).

Bringing conscious reflection to such unresolved reactivations permits the consolidation process of explicit memory and the integration of traumatic experience within autobiographical narrative. As we'll explore in Chapter 9, this process may allow for cooperative processing in both hemispheres of what may have been only unilateral representations. The attuned resonant relationship with the therapist allows patients to make left-hemisphere, verbally mediated, interpreter-driven sense out of their right-hemisphere autobiographical representations. This integrative process probably has direct effects on the right hemisphere's capacity to regulate primary emotional states. This is how we "name it to tame it." The patient's mind is prepared for such a process by the development of a secure attachment with the therapist. Furthermore, the elaboration of autonoetic consciousness permits patients to reflect on the past, understand the present, and help actively shape the future. Such mentalizing reflective dialogue is also a fundamental component of secure attachments. Individuals with histories of disorganized attachments can thus become freed from the "prison of the present," in which they were repeatedly trapped with no words to reflect on their rapidly enveloping and terrifying states of mind.

## REFLECTIONS: EMOTIONAL RELATIONSHIPS AND THE JOINING OF MINDS

We all need contingent communication. Our history of being close with others, having affective attunements and resonating states of mind, allows us to connect with others and to have a sense of coherence within our own internal processes. Adaptations to patterns of misattunements without repair, and to the subsequent states of shame and humiliation, shape our subjective experience of self, others, and the world. These patterns of relationships can lead to a large disparity between our adaptive, public selves and our inner, private selves. The attachment models that reflect these early, pre-explicit-memory experiences influence our emotions and their regulation, response flexibility, consciousness, self-knowledge, narrative, and openness to and drive toward interpersonal intimacy.

At times, engrained dysfunctional patterns of self-organization may require the specialized interpersonal relationship of psychotherapy to alter the emotion dysregulation that has come to be the source of pain in some individuals' lives. Psychotherapy establishes a safe environment in which present and past experiences can be explored. A therapist and a patient enter into a resonance of states of mind, which allows for the creation of a co-regulating dyadic system. This system is able to emerge in increasingly complex dyadic states by means of the attunement between the two individuals. The patient's subtle nonverbal expressions of her state of mind are perceived by the therapist and responded to with a shift in the therapist's own state, not just with words. In this way, there is a direct resonance between the primary emotional, psychobiological state of the patient and that of the therapist. These nonverbal expressions are mediated by the right hemisphere of one person and then perceived by the right hemisphere of the other. In this way, the essential nonverbal aspect of psychotherapy, and perhaps all emotional relationships, can be conceived as beginning with a right-hemisphere-to-right-hemisphere resonance between two individuals.

The left hemispheres of both members of the dyad are also important and active in the verbal exchanges and logical reflections on the patient's present life, past history, and the therapy experience itself. The left hemisphere's interpreter function attempts to "make sense" of experiences and therefore can be seen as a motivational force in the narrative process. As we'll explore more fully in Chapter 9, coherent autobiographical narratives—a primary focus of therapy of all sorts—probably involve a resonance of left- and right-hemisphere processes in both the teller and the listener. In this way, the joint construction of narratives reflects the interhemispheric resonance within both members of the therapeutic relationship.

The flow of states within the dyadic system is allowed to achieve increasing degrees of complexity as the individuals themselves achieve increasingly coherent states of interhemispheric resonance. Such a state is achieved via the right-to-right and left-to-left attunements that emerge from the nonverbal and verbal communication between patient and therapist. The emergent sense of flow, of connection, between two individuals in such a state of resonance is deeply compelling.

As self-states emerge over time, the mind has the challenge of integrating these relatively autonomous processes into a coherent whole. Psychotherapy can catalyze the development of such a core integrative process by facilitating dyadic states of resonance: right hemisphere to right hemisphere, left hemisphere to left hemisphere. In such a process, the mind of the patient (and that of the therapist) can become immersed in primary emotional states while simultaneously focusing on reflective narrative explorations. Such affect attunement and reflective dialogue catalyze an internal, bilateral form of resonance within each member of the dyad. As we'll explore in the next chapter, this form of resonance may be at the core of an integrating process that permits emotion regulation across time and across self-states. It is from this state of cooperative activation that coherent narratives emerge, and through this process that the mind is able to achieve integration and thus stable self-organization.

Psychotherapy is a complex process. The brain can be ravaged by inter-actions between genetically influenced mental storms and experiential his-tories of family strife. Both inherited disturbances and adaptations to trau-matic experiences can have complex effects on the neurophysiologically constructed reality of our subjective lives. Our minds are complex systems constrained in their activity by neuronal connections, which are determined by both constitution and experience. Different therapeutic tools—including medications, mindsight-skill-building practices, and specific psychothera-peutic techniques—may be useful at various times in helping patients achieve self-organization and live balanced and enriching lives. Whatever tools or techniques are used, the relationship between patient and therapist requires a deep commitment on the therapist's part to understanding and resonating with the patient's experience. The thera-pist must always keep in mind that inter-personal experience shapes brain structure and function. It is from this interaction between the interpersonal and the neural that the mind emerges.

> It is from this interaction between the interpersonal and the neural that the mind emerges.

It is a challenge, and a profound privilege, to keep an objective focus on a patient's emotional needs while at the same time allowing oneself as the therapist to join with the patient's evolving states of mind. This resonance of states bonds patient and therapist. By joining, they become part of a larger system that develops its own self-organizational processes and coherent life history. In many ways, therapy reflects the challenge of all human relation-ships: understanding and accepting people as they are, and yet nurturing fur-ther integration and growth. These connections within ourselves and with others are the essence of living vital lives and remaining open to all layers of our own emerging experiences.

# CHAPTER 9

# Integration

One of the mind's most robust features is its capacity to connect a range of processes within its present activity, as well as its functioning across time. Researchers studying diverse aspects of mental life—from social psychology to the neurosciences—have focused on the collaborative, linking functions that coordinate various levels of processes within the mind and between people.[1] This linkage of differentiated elements is called "integration." This chapter explores various ways in which integration can be understood as a fundamental aspect of interpersonal experience, health, and the developing mind.

As mentioned throughout the book, integration is postulated to be the central mechanism by which health is created in mind, brain, body, and relationships. We've seen that from the view of science, the linkage of differentiated elements of a system produces a harmonious flow of that system. The characteristics of this flow are that it's *flexible, adaptive, coherent, energized, and stable* (FACES). When a system is not differentiating its parts, and/or is not linking them, then the system is not integrated and tends to move toward either chaos or rigidity, or some combination of the two. We have also proposed that the field of mental health can reframe its compendium of disorders as revealing the chaos and rigidity of nonintegrated conditions. Assessment of symptoms and their clustering as syndromes can thus be organized through the lens of this integration framework: Problems with differentiation and/or linkage may be at the heart of nonintegrated states across a range of "domains of integration."[2] In this view, therapeutic, preventative, or educational measures would be aimed toward promoting integration—in the body and brain, in relationships, and in the regulatory functions of the embodied and relational mind.[3] This is the fundamental approach of IPNB in a nutshell, and the fine details of this view are explored in this final full chapter of the book. The Epilogue presents a framework for cultivating integration within nine domains.

# INTEGRATION AT THE HEART OF HEALTH AND RESILIENCE

A number of scientific disciplines support the proposal that integration is the core mechanism in well-being and optimal living. In these empirical studies, the examination of brain networks, the subjective experience of emotion, or the ways in which people communicate with one another are the focus of investigation. Olaf Sporns highlights the neural systems approach succinctly:

> Network interactions can be formally described by using concepts from statistical information theory, for example, mutual information, integration, and complexity. Some of these measures allow us to characterize statistical interactions in a network as a whole. When structural connections are arranged in such a way as to maximize some of these informational quantities, it appears that complexity is uniquely associated with structural patterns that resemble those of brain networks. This result is consistent with the theoretical idea that brain networks balance *segregation* and *integration*, which we defined as complexity. High complexity allows networks to integrate efficiently large amounts of information, a capacity that has been linked to consciousness.[4]

The notion underlying this approach is that differentiation comes from segregation and specialization. Linkage is the resultant integration of these segregated, differentiated elements. In these terms, the movement toward complexity is achieved by balancing differentiation and linkage. The most adaptive flow of a system arises when it moves toward maximizing complexity, a state achieved with the integration of the system's elements.

Building on this perspective, we can view Barbara Fredrickson's "broaden-and-build" model of positive emotion as exploring the inner positive states that both arise from and support integration:

> The broaden-and-build theory describes the form and function of a subset of positive emotions, including joy, interest, contentment and love. A key proposition is that these positive emotions broaden an individual's momentary thought–action repertoire: joy sparks the urge to play, interest sparks the urge to explore, contentment sparks the urge to savour and integrate, and love sparks a recurring cycle of each of these urges within safe, close relationships. The broadened mindsets arising from these positive emotions are contrasted to the narrowed mindsets sparked by many negative emotions (i.e., specific action tendencies, such as attack or flee). A second key proposition concerns the consequences of these broadened mindsets: by broadening an individual's momentary thought–action repertoire—whether through play, exploration or similar activities—positive emotions promote discovery of novel and creative actions, ideas and social bonds, which in turn build that individual's personal resources; ranging from physical and intellectual resources, to social and psychological resources. Importantly, these resources function as reserves

that can be drawn on later to improve the odds of successful coping and survival.[5]

Our earlier discussion of emotion as an emergent process reflecting shifts in integration is consistent with this view, in that a positive emotion arises with increases in integration, whereas a negative emotion occurs with decreases in integration. With positive emotional states, the individual is both internally and interpersonally more integrated; the results are a broadening of perspective and a building of increased differentiation and linkage.

> A positive emotion arises with increases in integration, whereas a negative emotion occurs with decreases in integration.

The capacity to solve problems is greatly enhanced when we work collaboratively in groups with an integrated process. Compare this with situations in which one individual asserts his own perspective to the exclusion of other viewpoints. In this nonintegrated, uncollaborative group state, linkage is dampened and differentiation heightened; the group's intelligence reaches only to the level of the assertive individual. In contrast, groups with cooperative members achieve a "group intelligence" that far exceeds the intellectual problem-solving ability of any of the individuals. Here we see the honoring of differences, the drawing upon each individual's unique strengths, and the collaborative use of these for the benefit of the group's task. Such integrative collaboration enables far more to be achieved than any single individual could do, either alone or by dominating the group process.[6] Interpersonal integration increases the IQ of the group!

Integration not only increases our intelligence, but it also makes life feel good. We accomplish more; we connect more; and we are more flexible, creative, and adaptive. With increased meaning and efficacy, our integrative living fills us with positive emotions. The outcome of positive emotional states is enhanced resilience, which is also consistent with Fredrickson's view:

> The association between resilience and positive emotions is supported by the network of correlates of resilience discovered across a range of self-report, observational and longitudinal studies. This converging evidence suggests that resilient people have optimistic, zestful and energetic approaches to life, are curious and open to new experiences, and are characterized by high positive emotionality. . . . Strikingly, resilient people not only cultivate positive emotions in themselves to cope, but they are also skilled at eliciting positive emotions in others (i.e., caregivers early in life and companions later on), which creates a supportive social context that also facilitates coping.[7]

When we link these empirical findings with the discoveries of attachment research and the new findings from studies of the resting state of brain function—its default mode[8]—we come away with a consilient view that integration is at the heart of health. From the IPNB perspective, developmental experiences that enable individuals in a relationship to be differentiated and then to become compassionately connected in caring communication are those relationships that help people thrive. Integration can be seen as the heart of health, even in emerging new studies of the nervous system itself. Well-being seems to be an outcome of integration. If we see these positive states as reflecting shifts in integration, then positive emotion becomes the natural outcome of enhanced integration. Barbara Fredrickson's concluding remarks about this aspect of positive emotion in her broaden-and-build theory reflect this perspective:

> The broaden-and-build theory underscores the ways in which positive emotions are essential elements of optimal functioning, and therefore an essential topic within the science of well-being. The theory . . . suggests that positive emotions: (i) broaden people's attention and thinking; (ii) undo lingering negative emotional arousal; (iii) fuel psychological resilience; (iv) build consequential personal resources; (v) trigger upward spirals towards greater well-being in the future; and (vi) seed human flourishing. The theory also carries an important prescriptive message. People should cultivate positive emotions in their own lives and in the lives of those around them, not just because doing so makes them feel good in the moment, but also because doing so transforms people for the better and sets them on paths toward flourishing and healthy longevity. When positive emotions are in short supply, people get stuck. They lose their degrees of behavioral freedom and become painfully predictable. But when positive emotions are in ample supply, people take off. They become generative, creative, resilient, ripe with possibility and beautifully complex. The broaden-and-build theory conveys how positive emotions move people forward and lift them to the higher ground of optimal well-being.[9]

Integration is therefore at the heart of positive emotion and creates the foundation for resilience and well-being. Let's explore more deeply how integration manifests itself within the energy and information flow of an individual's own nervous system and between individuals within interpersonal relationships.

## NEURAL INTEGRATION

Within the brain itself, complex functions emerge from the coordination of neural activity in a range of circuits. Those regions that receive input and send output to widely distributed areas of the brain play an important role in neural integration. The limbic regions and associational circuits, especially

the prefrontal areas, serve such a coordinating function. From this neurobiological perspective, Tucker, Luu, and Pribram have stated that

> the theoretical challenge at the neural level is to go beyond labeling the func-
> tions of the frontal lobe to formulate the key neurophysiological mechanisms.
> These mechanisms link the operations of frontal cortex to the multiple sys-
> tems of the brain's control hierarchy, ranging from the control of arousal by
> brain-stem projection systems to the control of memory by reentrant corti-
> colimbic interactions. When sufficiently understood, these mechanisms must
> be found to regulate not only physiology of neural tissue, but the representa-
> tion and maintenance of the self.[10]

In this manner, neural integration is fundamental to self-organization,
and indeed to the brain's ability to create a sense of self. Tucker and colleagues
further suggest that integration within the brain may consist of at least three
forms, which focus on particular aspects of anatomic circuits: "vertical,"
"dorsal–ventral," and "lateral."[11] Vertical integration is the integration of
the "lower" functions of the brainstem and limbic regions with the "higher"
operations of the frontal neocortex, such
as cognitive and motor planning. In vertical integration, somewhat isolated processes at various layers of complexity or
"order" are coordinated into a functional
system. This vertical process is common throughout the brain and influences
such fundamental processes as memory and language formation.[12]

> Neural integration is fundamental
> to self-organization.

Dorsal–ventral integration focuses on the dual origins of the frontal cortex from the archicortical and paleocortical regions of the paralimbic cortex. As we've seen in Chapter 6, these differences begin in the embryo and
may stem from the asymmetry in what Trevarthen has called the "intrinsic
motive formation."[13] Each hemisphere has a dominant pathway: right with
dorsal and left with ventral. Each circuit or "stream" mediates differential
forms of motivational processes and motor control, and creates different representational processes on either side of the brain.[14] The finding of less hemispheric specialization in women may be proposed to be partly due to the
participation of both dorsal and ventral circuits in each hemisphere. Dorsal–
ventral integration would allow for less lateralization of the more complex
representational processes originating from each side of the brain.

Lateral integration is the coordination of functions of the circuits at a
similar level of complexity or order. Coordinating perceptual processes across
sensory modalities, such as bringing together vision with tactile and auditory
perceptions, to create a "whole picture" of an experience is an example of lateral integration. This integration may be mediated by associational neurons,
which link distinct systems. When lateral integration connects the complex

representational processes of one hemisphere to another, the term "bilateral" or "interhemispheric" integration can be used. The associational neurons that link various anatomically and functionally distinct regions on either side of the brain may be the means by which the coordination of interhemispheric information processing occurs. According to Trevarthen, the cerebral commissures (the corpus callosum and the anterior commissures) are "the only pathway through which the higher functions of perception and cognition, learning and voluntary motor coordination can be unified"; this is achieved through a sorting process, which he proposes "creates complementary sets of associative links between the cortical maps of various sensory and motor functions."[15] In this form of lateral integration, the isolated functions of each hemisphere can be coordinated into a functionally linked system.

The fact that the "greatest integration of sensory, motor, and evaluative information may occur in the primitive paralimbic cortex" has led Tucker and colleagues to suggest that these three forms of integration, each of which involves aspects of this region, may actually be interdependent.[16] For example, vertical integration is revealed in the capacity of the right hemisphere (especially the paralimbic orbitofrontal cortex) to have predominant control over certain "lower" functions, such as the regulation and representation of bodily function as mediated via the autonomic nervous system. Woltering and Lewis have presented a model that focuses on

> two types of emotion regulation—reactive and deliberate—and discusses the developmental trajectory of both types. We argue that the later-developing capacity for deliberate control builds on and coevolves with earlier-developing reactive control. . . . The focus is on specific neural "hubs," such as the anterior cingulate cortex and the orbitofrontal cortex, which serve as epicenters for the coupling of cortical and subcortical processes. We propose that an increasing coordination between brain regions during emotional situations subserves more effective and efficient regulation with development.[17]

In other words, the linkage of differentiated areas, or neural integration as exemplified in the activity of these middle prefrontal regions, is a fundamental part of self-regulation.

Lateral integration is revealed within REM sleep and encoding–retrieval processes, in which the left and right orbitofrontal cortices are involved in representational integration in dreams and the consolidation of memory. At a minimum, then, the orbitofrontal and other middle prefrontal areas (including the ventromedial, ventrolateral, and anterior cingulate cortices) coordinate vertical and possibly lateral integration.[18] (See Figure 4.1 in Chapter 4, as well as Figure 1.3 in Chapter 1.) The middle prefrontal region links the widely distributed areas of the cortex, limbic system (the amygdala and hippocampus), the brainstem, the body proper, and even the signals from other individuals' nervous systems in the form of empathic maps of other people. Future studies will need to explore further how these and other coordinating regions play a role in dorsal–ventral integration on one or both sides of the brain.[19]

Another illustration of how distinct regions of the brain may be coordinated into integrated circuits is in the connections of frontal cortex to the basal ganglia. As outlined by Steven Wise and colleagues, this integrated system functions to guide behavior by assessing a variety of inputs.[20] In their view, the basal ganglia mediate rule-guided behavior, whereas the frontal cortex provides alternatives that incorporate context-dependent processing. This can also be seen as an example of the integration of implicit encoding in the basal ganglia and explicit processing in the frontal cortex. This frontal cortex–basal ganglia system allows the individual to reject maladaptive rules that are no longer useful in the currently assessed situation. The integrated functioning of such a system has powerful implications for the acquisition and application of new behavioral responses.[21] This integration of "motor" areas (basal ganglia) with those thought of as responsible for more abstract "planning" (frontal lobes) may be an adaptive way our brains have evolved to integrate a wide array of systems.[22] This view is consistent with our earlier discussions of the prefrontal cortex, especially the orbitofrontal region, in its role of mediating response flexibility—the altering of responses based on unexpected or changing conditions.[23]

At an even more basic level of neurobiology, we can examine the notion of how neurons integrate their functioning within neural networks to produce neural net activation profiles. As we've seen, the brain learns from experience through the shaping of neuronal firing patterns that create these networks. van Ooyen and van Pelt have stated:

> As a result of these activity-dependent processes, a reciprocal influence exists between the formation of neuronal form and synaptic connectivity on the one hand, and neuronal and network activity on the other hand. A given network may generate activity patterns which modify the organization of the network, leading to altered activity patterns which further modify structural or functional characteristics, and so on . . . the realization is growing that electrical activity and neurotransmitters are not only involved in information coding, but also play an important role in shaping neuronal networks in which they operate.[24]

In this manner, basic neuronal connectivity creates representational abilities and also directly influences the nature of the network activity itself. What this means is that a process that links distinct circuits not only creates a new form of information processing, but also establishes a more complex, integrated network that influences its own capacities. Integrated systems, by virtue of their coordinated activities, establish their own characteristic features; the whole is greater than merely the sum of the individual parts. As we've seen, such neural integration becomes a central process that is directly related to self-regulation.[25]

The fundamental role of complexity has helped to clarify the development and functioning of neural networks and has pointed to the central role of "spatiotemporal integration."[26] Various levels of hierarchical systems—from sets of neurons to the interaction of complex circuits—involve space–time patterns of neuronal activity. What this suggests is that the brain is capable of representing, in the moment, patterns of activity in which direct influences from the past are encoded. As we've discussed, the organization of memory and the brain's function as an anticipation machine enable it to "represent the future." Such anticipatory mechanisms directly shape the ways in which linkages may be made across various processes and across time.

For example, the ways in which neural circuits anticipate experience may help us understand how the mind develops through a recursive set of interactions. As representational processes anticipate experience, they also seek particular forms of interactions to match their expectations. In this way, the "bias" of a system leads it to perceive, process, and act in a particular manner. The outcome of this bias is to reinforce the very features creating the system's bias. As development evolves, the circuits involved become more differentiated and more elaborately engrained in an integrated system that continues to support its own characteristics. These recursive and anticipatory features of development may be at the core of how the dorsal and ventral circuits influence the unfolding of the lateralization in hemispheric functioning. Infant studies suggest that traditional theories attempting to understand hemispheric lateralization and brain asymmetry may be looking at the problem from a limited end-product perspective. According to Trevarthen, a clearer understanding of the developmental origins of these different systems may be achieved by examining how the anticipation of encounters with the world influences each hemisphere in quite distinct ways. As Trevarthen explains:

> With a change of theory that recognizes the priority of intrinsic motor planning and prospective motor imagery in cognition, and that also takes into account the expression of emotional states related to anticipatory self-regulation and the subject's evaluation of the consequences of intended action, a different perspective on cerebral asymmetry of awareness and memory can be proposed, one that seeks the origins in cerebral activities that *anticipate* experience."[27]

This anticipation can be seen as emanating from a form of spatiotemporal integration: The mind creates complex representations as a process between perception (input) and action (output) in an effort to interact with an environment that changes across time and space. The value of such a representational process is that it allows the individual to anticipate the next moment in time, and in this way to act in a more adaptive manner, enhancing the chance for survival. Spatiotemporal integration may therefore be a fundamental feature of how the human mind has evolved.

## DEVELOPMENT AND INTEGRATIVE PROCESSES

How do integrative processes develop within the individual? What are the neural mechanisms that allow integration to occur? How do experiential and genetic factors transact in the development of integrative processes? One approach to answering these questions is to view the foundation of the mind as emanating from patterns in the flow of energy and information. As an emergent property of energy and information flow within the body and between people, the mind is a process that helps to self-organize these embodied and relational systems. The flow of this emergent self-organizational process, the mind, arises as patterns of engrained and novel interactions unfold across the lifespan. Because synaptic networks reflect prior experience, our lives are recursively reinforcing their own histories. For example, children's attachment to their parents evokes similar responses from their teachers.[28] Experience, as we've discussed repeatedly, activates neurons in such a manner that genes may become expressed and may produce alterations in neuronal connectivity. Information is transferred by the assembly of neural circuits into recruited clusters of activation that become functionally linked. This information transfer itself creates new representations and mental states. When new elements of informational processing are recruited into a new state of the system, this linkage of differentiated elements into a functional whole occurs and is the essence of integration. Such a flexible process, as we've seen, becomes disrupted in childhood trauma and in suboptimal attachment experiences. In contrast, typical development appears to move in the direction of more differentiated and linked states. How does this integration happen in the brain?

The capacity to link a widely distributed array of neural processes can be proposed to be mediated by neuronal fibers that serve to interconnect anatomically and functionally distributed regions of the brain. In this manner, differentiated information-processing modes, such as different sensory modalities, can become functionally linked.[29] This basic neuronal process may also help us to understand, for example, how highly engrained mental states, such as those of fear and shame, may become (or fail to become) integrated within the flow of the system's complex states. Synaptic patterns can evoke relational responses from others that reinforce these neural propensities. This is the "self-fulfilling" loop that gives us a sense of being "stuck" or "frozen" in unfulfilling ways of living. For example, we've seen that certain suboptimal attachment experiences produce multiple, incoherent working models of attachment and engrained, inflexible states of mind. These remain unintegrated across time within specialized and potentially dysfunctional self-states. We can propose that the creation of new neuronal linkages, then, allows the internal constraints of the brain's dynamical system to change. New interconnecting neuronal linkages may thus serve to integrate not only anatomically independent processes, but functionally isolated ones such as engrained mental states that have produced inflexibility. In the process of psychotherapy, the relationship with the therapist becomes a central factor in how to induce neural changes in these previously engrained synaptic networks.[30]

Central to this integration is emotion. As we've discussed earlier, emotion is inherently an integrative function that links internal processes and individuals together. This view reinforces the central role of emotion in self-regulation and in communication within interpersonal relationships. As the neurologist Antonio Damasio notes:

> Emotion is inherently an integrative function that links internal processes and individuals together.

> It would not be possible to discuss the integrative aspects of brain function without considering the operations that arise in large-scale neural systems; and it would be unreasonable not to single out emotion among the critical integrative components arising in that level. Yet, throughout the twentieth century, the integrated brain and mind have often been discussed with hardly any acknowledgment that emotion does exist, let alone that it is an important function and that understanding its neural underpinnings is of great advantage.[31]

Fortunately, great strides in examining the neurobiology and interpersonal nature of emotion have been made with the emergence of the subspecialty fields of affective and social neuroscience.[32]

Emotionally meaningful events can enable continued learning from experience throughout the lifespan. Such learning may be seen as, in effect, the ongoing development of the brain. Experience plays a primary role in stimulating new neuronal connections in both memory and developmental processes. Findings from neurobiology suggest that such development continues throughout the lifespan.[33] In particular, the neural circuitry facilitating integration may also continue to develop throughout life. Those neurons that serve to coordinate information from distributed regions may continue to develop—perhaps with genetic programming, with the inherent mechanisms of aging, and with specific forms of experience. For example, in studying the progressively increasing myelination across the lifespan in the hippocampal pathways that interconnect widely distributed regions, Francine Benes has indicated:

> Growth and development of regions in the human brain occur not only in childhood but also much later during adolescent and adult years. . . . Myelination represents one of the final stages in neuronal maturation where cells acquire a fatty lipid sheath around their axons, a change that increases the propagation of electrical signals from the neuronal cell body to terminal areas. . . . These axons might well play a role in the integration of emotional behaviors with cognitive processes, a putative function of the limbic cortex. . . . Therefore the functions influenced by this ongoing myelination may themselves "grow" and mature throughout adult life.[34]

In this manner, experiences and innate developmental processes may allow our neural capacity to integrate an array of processes throughout our lives. The mechanism of this differentiation of circuits, as we've discussed earlier, may involve a range of processes from the growth of axons into widely distributed regions of the brain, the establishment of new synaptic connections, and the increased conductance of nerve fibers via their increased myelination.[35] Recall that myelin increases the conduction speed down the axonal length by one hundred times and decreases the resting time between firings thirty-fold, making communication among myelinated neurons *three thousand times more effective*. These mechanisms may be at work in the dramatic maturation of the corpus callosum during the first decade of life, and perhaps, we can propose, in its ongoing development throughout life. Future studies may enable us to investigate how experience enhances or hinders the development of these integrating neural processes.[36]

The movement toward such integrating neural connections is consistent with complexity theory: Highly differentiated and functionally linked subsystems maximize the complexity achievable by a system. In this manner, it may be a natural developmental outcome for increasing levels of integration to occur across the lifespan.[37] One outcome of such a process for some individuals, we can imagine, might be the development of wisdom with age: The capacity to "see the forest for the trees" may emerge from an integrative capacity to focus on patterns over time and across situations, rather than on the details of particular events.[38] Disturbances in mental health, as we've discussed, may emanate from recursive processes that impair this natural movement toward integration. Fixed constraints to the system, either internal or external, may create an inflexible state for an individual. Typical development may thus continue to promote integration throughout life if it is unimpaired by elements of the individual's constitution, experiential history, or ongoing interpersonal relationships.

Internal processes and interpersonal relationships that entail subcomponent differentiation and intercomponent linkage can be proposed as those that promote healthy, ongoing development within and between individuals. Consider the musical analogy of a choir. At one extreme, each individual sings her own song, totally independently of the others. The ensuing cacophony occurs as a result of the lack of clustering of the individuals into a functional whole. There would be no cohesion, and the resultant sounds over time would be incoherent. Such a random set of isolated, though differentiated, interactions does little to move the system toward complexity. But at the other extreme, the exact matching of each singer's voice to those of the others produces an amplification of the mirrored sounds. Although the tune may be pleasing (and loud), it does little to maximize the complexity possible. If differentiated singers were to join together in a resonant integrational process, we might call that harmony. Neither independence nor mimicry creates complexity. When each singer has well-developed individual skills, integration allows them to contribute to a functional whole that has continuity and regularity on the one hand, and yet flexibility and spontaneity on the other. This is the vitality and fluidity of integrative harmony; it permits a FACES flow—flexible, adaptive, coherent, energized, and stable. As we've seen, such a blend allows for the movement toward maximal complexity within the individual mind and between minds. At the heart of such integration are emotion and the flow of energy and information through the system. Such a dynamic condition achieves stability as the system moves forward in time through the various states of activity. These reciprocal and cooperative processes may characterize the healthy ongoing development of the individual mind, dyadic relationships, and nurturing communities.[39] The blend of individual differentiation and interpersonal linkage allows each of us to move harmoniously forward in life, with our minds forever developing in a complex biological interdependence of our social and inner worlds.

## INTEGRATION OF MINDS

The concept of integration has also been applied to mental activity at a more macroscopic level, in both the intraindividual and interindividual domains. For example, several authors use the concept of "intraindividual" integration to refer to various ways in which developmental achievements and processes interrelate at one time or across the lifespan.[40] "Interindividual" integration focuses on the relationships between children and their caregivers and peers. From this psychological perspective, various layers of integration can be seen as interdependent, influencing one another in the moment and affecting the developmental trajectory of the child within a social world, as revealed in the extensive research findings from the field of attachment.[41]

Integration can also help us understand the notion of "selves" within a given individual. For some adults, their developmental path has led to a coherent set of interactions with the world—interactions that have enabled the emergence of various self-states, which perform their functions with relatively minimal conflict among themselves. Such individuals may live a comparatively carefree existence, without internal tumult or impairment in functioning. Part of the developmental challenge of typical adolescence, as identified by Susan Harter and her colleagues, is the resolution of potential conflicts among various adaptive "selves" defined by specific social relationship role contexts.[42] The teen years bring a significant change in metacognitive capacity, with the new ability to reflect on one's own existence in more complex and integrative ways than were possible at earlier stages of life. Adolescents become aware of conflictual role patterns in their early teens, but often only develop the capacity to resolve tensions about these roles in later adolescence. This lag time between the onset of awareness and the capacity for resolution may be a characteristic feature of typical adolescent development. As the need for various roles is accepted, and teenagers find ways to resolve potential conflicts within their experiences with peers and parents, an integration of selves across time and role relationships becomes possible. This is the essence of the integrative capacity to achieve coherence of the self.

Not all individuals are able to integrate multiple self-states into a coherent experience of the self. From early in development, the resolution of multiple models of attachment may be one of the determinants of later developmental outcome. Particular forms of self-states may have been constructed in relationship to different caregivers, resulting in potentially conflictual conditions. Within a given state, there may be cohesive functioning; across these self-states, however, spatiotemporal or "inter-state" integration may not be possible, given the inherent incompatibility of mental models, drives, and modes of emotion regulation. Experiences within relationships, models of such experiences, access to information, and the ways in which the mind comes to create a coherent perspective are important variables in determining emotional resilience or vulnerability. In other words, an integrative process across self-states may be essential to the acquisition of well-being.[43] The

> A "relational self" is a fundamental aspect of who we are.

capacity for such internal integration may be intimately related to inter-personal experience—derived initially from attachment relationships, and later shaped by individuals' ongoing involvement with parents, teachers, and peers. A "relational self" is a fundamental aspect of who we are.[44]

Culture can play a significant role in how the self develops within inter-personal relationships at home, at school, and in the community. Ethnic, racial, or religious background can serve as an organizing process for iden-tity as an adolescent emerges into the larger world.[45] How the adolescent comes to terms with identity may be related to how parents have integrated these processes into their own identity.[46] We all adapt to the many worlds in which we reside, with direct impacts on our sense of self.[47] Studies of autobiographical memory reveal that culture shapes how we remember our own lives and develop a narrative sense of self.[48] Facing the need to integrate multiple cultures into this sense of identity presents important developmen-tal challenges. This is particularly the case for those making transitions and living between two or more cultural worlds. As Chen, Benet-Martínez, and Bond have stated, "In the process of managing cultural environments and group loyalties, bilingual competence, and perceiving one's two cultural identities as integrated are important antecedents of beneficial psychological outcomes."[49]

Here we can see that "cultural integration" involves maintaining aspects of the self within varied cultural backgrounds, while also linking these some-times disparate ways of being. It also involves balancing an individual's inter-nal experiences with communication among individuals of different gen-erations from the various cultural backgrounds. *Integration requires a balance between differentiation and linkage.* So often there is a pressure to "blend in," which emphasizes becoming a part of the new and rejecting the old or vice versa, rather than to integrate, which requires respect for all the different worlds a person has come from and those in which the person now resides. Recent studies reveal that the meaning an adolescent derives from cultural identity, being a part of the family, and taking part in daily family responsi-bilities all influence the specificity of particular brain regions activated and the degree of stress reactivity in response to family expectation.[50] Making meaning in the face of cultural shifts in identity, then, can be seen as a part of cultural integration. As noted earlier in this book, achieving integration is more like making a fruit salad than making a smoothie, where the blended ingredients completely lose their original identity.

We can study various layers of integration, such as the coordination of elements of a given perceptual process into a hierarchy of functioning: sensory input, pattern analysis, and the creation of complex visual repre-sentations. We can also study the ways in which more widely distributed neural circuits interact to form a coherent pattern of increasingly complex processing, such as in the creation of multimodal representations that include perceptual and linguistic components. Such processes may involve the vertical, dorsal–ventral, and lateral aspects of integration discussed above. For example, the combination of linguistic and nonverbal prosodic elements of speech requires the bilateral integration of representational processes.[51] The brain is typically integrating information processing across widely distributed circuits at any given moment in time, or in a "synchronic" fashion. As Ciompi has suggested, emotion may be essential in such an integrative process at a given time ("synchronic"), as well as across time ("diachronic").[52] These aspects of integration may also play an important role in understanding the impact of culture on an individual's development. David, Florea, and Pop state:

> Cultural entities in the totality of their inner diversity demonstrate that the universal as a key concept of the contemporary world cannot be understood outside cultures as identity structures. Macro-history also implies "local history," [and] the universal at cultural level implies the particular not as simple mathematical sum but first and foremost as value and historical engagement. Current cultural unity can only exist through its structural and value diversity.[53]

Here again we see the power of the central concept of integration—the differentiation and linkage of elements of a system—to illuminate the nature of our collective human lives. The mind emerges as we live embedded in our social worlds and embodied in our neural structures. This is truly "the mind in context."[54]

What does integration at a given time or across time look like? We can propose the following possibilities. Synchronic integration involves the elements discussed in Chapter 5, which create a cohesive mental state. Various aspects of neural activity are clustered together within a functional state of mind as a part of vertical, dorsal–ventral, and lateral integration in a given moment in time. At another level, we can suggest that as an individual's states of mind flow across time, diachronic integration somehow links these together in a manner that facilitates flexible and adaptive functioning. This is spatiotemporal integration. Such cross-time integration serves as a mechanism of self-regulation, in that it serves to organize the flow of states. In Chapter 5, we have focused primarily on how complex systems can function as a cohesive state—a form of synchronic integration as we are defining it here. In this chapter, we are exploring ways in which the mind may create coherence across time through diachronic integration. As time itself flows, it is in fact difficult to distinguish between cohesion in the moment and coherence across time. In the physical world, when does a "moment" actually end? The complex system of the brain, however, has the capacity for abrupt shifts in state that more clearly define the neural edges of time. Though time itself may have no clear boundaries, these neural shifts give a functional reality to the temporal contrasts between states. In this manner, cohesion exists within a given state of mind as a form of synchronic integration. The recursive nature of systems establishes a continuity in a given self-state across time. As a given state changes, it goes through a phase transition involving the temporary disorganization and then reorganization of the system's state. In contrast to cohesion of a given self-state, coherence is created across states of mind as a form of diachronic integration. As we'll discuss, such abilities to create coherence can be proposed to be shaped in part by the individual's experiential history, which enables the acquisition of a core integrative process.

## ATTACHMENT AND INTEGRATION

Main, Hesse, and Goldwyn have suggested that the way adults can flexibly access information about childhood and reflect upon such information in a coherent manner determines their likelihood of raising securely attached children.[55] The abilities to reflect upon one's own childhood history, to conceptualize the mental states of one's parents, and to describe the impact of these experiences on personal development are the essential elements of coherent adult attachment narratives. Moreover, the capacity to reflect on the role of mental states in determining human behavior is associated with the capacity to provide sensitive and nurturing parenting.[56] Fonagy and colleagues have suggested that this reflective or mentalizing function is more than the capacity for introspection; it directly influences a self-organizational process within the individual.[57] This reflective function enables the parent to facilitate the self-organizational development of the child. The coherent organization of the mind depends upon an integrative process that enables such reflective processes to occur. Integrative coherence within the individual may depend upon interpersonal connections both early in development and later in life that cultivate emotional well-being—that is, "integrative health."

The coherence of one's own states of mind permits a form of relationship with others—especially one's own children, friends, or intimate partners—that fosters integration, reflective processes, and emotional well-being within the relationship and within the emerging minds of each person. In other words, internal integration allows for vital interpersonal connections that are themselves integrative.

> Internal integration allows for vital interpersonal connections that are themselves integrative.

Attachment studies suggest that coherence can be observed and measured within autobiographical narrative reflections. As Pearson and colleagues have stated, "congruity, unity and free-flowing connections" in such narratives are central features revealing what is thought to be "coherence of mind" in the AAI studies.[58] The intergenerational transmission of suboptimal parenting within insecure attachments is thought to be due to the persistence of incoherent adult stances toward attachment. Given the view that insecure attachment can be considered a risk factor for future difficulties,[59] understanding the nature of coherence becomes a pressing concern for parents and mental health professionals interested in early intervention and preventative measures.

What is incoherence of mind, and how can it be transformed into coherence? Incongruity, fragmentation, and restricted flow of information are the elements of such incoherence, as seen within the AAI narratives of individuals who are classified as dismissing, preoccupied, and unresolved/disoriented. Studies of those individuals who appear retrospectively to have had suboptimal attachment histories but receive "earned" secure/autonomous AAI classifications in the Main and Goldwyn system[60] reveal that their parenting, even under stressful conditions, is sensitive and nurturing.[61] Subsequent studies in which an infant's attachment status was identified as insecure, but now the individual as a young adult has an AAI classification as secure reveals a status sometimes called "prospective earned secure." These findings are points of active discussion in the field.[62] A general implication of these findings is that even with difficult past childhood experiences, the mind is capable of achieving an integrated perspective—one that is coherent and that permits parenting behavior to be sensitive and empathic. If integration is achieved, the trend toward transmission of insecure forms of attachment to the next generation can be prevented. Achieving coherence of mind thus becomes a central goal for creating emotional well-being in both oneself and one's offspring. As we'll see, such integration involves internal processes and their facilitation by interpersonal interactions.

Integration can be proposed to be a key process that influences the trajectory of developmental pathways toward resilience or toward vulnerability. For example, one factor in the adolescent onset of certain psychiatric disturbances, such as mood, eating, or identity disorders, may be the challenge of both social and neurological integration.[63] From the neural perspective, Fair and colleagues suggest:

> During development, both experience-dependent evoked activity and spontaneous waves of synchronized cortical activity are thought to support the formation and maintenance of neural networks. Such mechanisms may encourage tighter "integration" of some regions into networks over time

while "segregating" other sets of regions into separate networks. . . . We find that development of the proposed adult control networks involves both segregation (i.e., decreased short-range connections) and integration (i.e., increased long-range connections) of the brain regions that comprise them. Delay/disruption in the developmental processes of segregation and integration may play a role in disorders of control, such as autism, attention deficit hyperactivity disorder, and Tourette's syndrome.[64]

With regard to autism, for example, Rippon and colleagues present their "neuroscience model of neural integration or 'temporal binding.' We [have] proposed that autism is associated with abnormalities of information integration that [are] caused by a reduction in the connectivity between specialised local neural networks in the brain and possible overconnectivity within the isolated individual neural assemblies." These researchers suggest that the "'interactive specialisation' and the resultant stress on early and/or low-level deficits and their cascading effects on the developing brain" may explain the pervasive impact of these impediments to neural integration as the child grows.[65] Autism influences the quality of a child's relationships with family members, but experiences, such as the parent–child interactions, do not cause autism.[66] Here we see an example of how some genetic or toxic cause of impaired neural integration in the child's developing brain leads to impaired interpersonal integration within the social world in which the child lives.

Sometimes a child's experiences in the social world do in fact play a major role in creating challenges to the development of the child's brain and capacity for integration. Teicher and colleagues have demonstrated, for example, that exposure to verbal abuse by parents or by peers has a negative impact on the development of the corpus callosum, which integrates the left and right hemispheres.[67] The social world in which the child lives can offer relational experiences that shape how the self develops toward health. Within an individual's sense of self, social experiences influence the capacity to achieve integration across time. Those who are not fortunate enough to achieve a sense of coherence may live with adaptive selves whose goals are incompatible with each other; in such individuals, mental modules and the information they process create anxiety and conflict if shared across modalities. For these people, emotional imbalance may be due to the inability to integrate the self diachronically into a coherent whole. For example, an individual who has been humiliated repeatedly as a child may find rejection as an adolescent or adult extremely disorganizing. The self-state that needs affiliation and acceptance from others is in direct opposition to the self-state that needs to gain status and rise to a position of leadership in an organization; being in a position of authority inevitably involves evoking the displeasure of others. Such an individual may find her career hampered by such a conflict in needs.

Most people experience some degree of conflict between inner desires and outer realities. This may especially be true for those who are changing cultures, but the need for internal coherence and interpersonal belonging is a challenge for all adolescents, and perhaps for each of us across the lifespan. At times these desires for belonging are a part of fairly distinct states of mind, which can remain out of awareness for many individuals. Even without awareness, the mind may experience the emotional imbalance of such conflicts in the onset of depression, anxiety, uncontrolled rage, a feeling of meaninglessness and disconnection (as in a "false self"), loss of motivation, and interpersonal difficulties. Harter and coworkers' studies suggest that the more adolescents experience their roles as "false" and not "authentic," the more turmoil they feel.[68] Social contexts that force individuals to adapt via self-states that are not reflective of their own experiences, mental states, and needs may place these persons at higher risk of developing emotional disorders—of being vulnerable to "disintegration."

Attachment relationships may therefore serve as catalysts of risk or resilience, to the extent that they facilitate the flow of inauthentic versus authentic states within interactions with others. We can propose that *insecure attachments confer vulnerability because they fail to foster children's integrative self-organizational process.* Recall our basic proposal: Integrative communication cultivates the growth of integrative fibers in the brain. Secure attachment involves both the differentiation of child from parent and the empathic and attuned communication between the two. Suboptimal attachment, as we've seen, involves impediments to this differentiation and linkage. When such impairments have occurred, the child is left with a compromised regulatory system, because self-regulation depends upon neural integration. Development may begin in early childhood, when the basic regulatory circuits are first formed in an experience–dependent manner, but growth and development certainly do not end there. Later relationships with peers and teachers can also make a difference; interpersonal influences on the self-states that emerge to adapt to social contexts directly shape mental health. It seems clear that dyadic relationships beyond those with early caregivers may continue to influence the development of regulatory capacities.[69] Our regulatory capacities reflect the capacity for integration, in which we link prefrontal executive functions with the limbic, brainstem, and even visceral neural networks of the heart.[70] Our somatic and our social networks become linked within the neural integrative capacity of our embodied and relational brains. As Cicchetti

> Insecure attachments confer vulnerability because they fail to foster children's integrative self-organizational process.

and Rogosch have noted, resilience is not a trait or some fixed achievement, but is an emergent state function dependent upon self-organizational processes and continued interdependence within the social connections of families and cultures.[71]

*The capacity for self-integration, like the processes of the mind itself, is continually created by an interaction of internal neurophysiological processes and interpersonal relationships.* Resilience and emotional well-being are fundamental mental processes that emerge as the mind integrates the flow of energy and information across time and between minds.

As Ogawa and colleagues have paraphrased the work of Loevinger, "Integration is not a function of the self, it is what the self is."[72] They go on to state:

> Therefore, the failure to integrate salient experience represents profound distortion in the self system. When salient experience must be unnoticed, disallowed, unacknowledged, or forgotten, the result is incoherence in the self structure. Interconnections among experiences cannot be made, and the resulting gaps in personal history compromise both the complexity and the integrity of the self."[73]

# THE INTEGRATING SELF

## Creating Coherence

The integrating mind attempts to create a sense of coherence among multiple selves across time and across contexts. We have discussed in Chapter 5 how the inherent features of computation, complexity, and connectionism create a property of cohesion within a state of mind in a given slice of time. Self-states have a repeating pattern of cohesive activity, which lends a sense of historical continuity to their existence. If each of us existed as a continuous flow of states, this might be the end of the story. But as we've discussed, the complex systems of our minds are capable of abrupt transitions into markedly different states. These state transitions lack cohesion and continuity. How, then, does the mind achieve coherence across self-states? How can a four-dimensional sense of coherence be created with such discontinuous transitions across states?

The struggle to satisfy needs and desires within a complex social world is often filled with conflict. Examples can be found in many periods of life: a married adult's desire to explore his sexuality with other adults, but also to maintain affiliation with spouse and family; a young professional's struggle to balance her drive to achieve on a personal level with her need to be a part of a group process; an adolescent's need to have an identity as a member of his peer group, while at the same time seeking a sense of individuality and autonomy; a child's drive to master new situations and yet her desire to feel safe in a familiar environment. Each of these individuals can be seen as experiencing "conflictual needs," which are a part of the experience of segmented self-states. The properties we've seen in states of mind, the research on typical child and adolescent development, and the findings of cognitive neuroscience all suggest that in fact the usual functioning of the mind consists of many processes that can indeed function fairly autonomously. Just as the body is made up of its component parts, the mind as a whole system is made up of the activity of these multiple self-states.

At the transition between self-states, there may be a temporary disorganization or incohesion and discontinuity in the activity of the brain; however, once a new state of mind is instantiated, cohesion is reestablished. To understand this, let's review the way the mind functions as a self-organizational system.

Self-organization at the level of the mind must involve the integrative processing of multiple self-states across time and context. It is at the moments of transition that new self-organizational forms can be constructed. Indeed, integrating coherence of the mind is about state *shifts*. Congruity and unity emerge at the interface of how information and energy—the defining elements of the mind—flow across states. As Allan Schore has stated,

> the term "self-organization" can be imprecise and misleading, because first, despite the implications of the two words used to describe the process, self-organization occurs in interaction with another self—it is not monadic but dyadic. And second, the organization of brain systems does not involve a simple pattern of increments but rather large changes in organization. Development, the process of self-assembly, thus involves both progressive and regressive phenomena, and is best characterized as a sequence of processes of organization, disorganization, and reorganization.[74]

Integration is about how the mind creates a coherent self-assembly of information and energy flow across time and context. In this way, integration creates the subjective experience of self. When we view emotion as a fundamental process reflecting shifts in integration, we can see how the very experience of being alive entails being emotional. If our days become lifeless even before we die, integration has become fixed, change does not occur, and the internal sense of such rigidity is stagnation.

Some people can spend the vast majority of their time in cohesive, albeit relatively independent, self-states. If these states are not conflictual with one another—if the desires, beliefs, goals, and behaviors of one state are not in destructive competition with another—then what is the problem? Perhaps there is none. For these individuals, a coherent mind may be a natural developmental outcome of authentic nurturing relationships, supportive experiences with teachers in school, meaningful friendships, and identification with peer groups, which have all contributed to the development of a capacity for self-organization in a wide variety of contexts. *Integration establishes a sense of congruity and unity of the mind as it emerges within the flexible patterns of information and energy flow, within the embodied brain and in interaction with others. This is coherence.*

For other people, *conflicts among different needs, mental models, and self-states may lead to internal distress or external difficulties that create dysfunction. Such a conflict among self-states within an individual can create incoherence.* Incoherence may develop from insecure or conflictual attachments, difficulties in meeting school or job expectations, or significant trouble with finding companions in friendships or peer groups. Incoherence may be revealed in various ways, such as impairments in affect regulation, insecurity, unresolved trauma or loss, and dysfunctional social relationships. In a lifeless state, such people find themselves beached on the bank of rigidity. Other states of impaired integration fill them with chaos, a sense of dysregulation, and despair. Whether with professionals or in intimate relationships, an active approach to creating coherence may become necessary. This means bringing the flow of their lives back into the harmony of integration.

## The Adapting Mind: Disorganized Attachment as an Example of Impaired Integration

As noted in earlier chapters, the parents of children with disorganized attachments have provided frightened, frightening, or disorienting shifts in their own behavior. These experiences are conflictual for the children and lead to incoherent mental models.[75] Such a child may develop an internal mental model for each aspect of the parent's behavior. As mental models form the foundation for how we all perceive and make sense of the world, such conflictual models may create intense disruptions in this child's capacity for integration across these organizing processes of mind.[76] Abrupt shifts in parental state force the child to adapt with suddenly shifting states of his own. Such state shifts may occur if the nature of these experiences is profoundly incompatible with attachment, and/or if the child is neurobiologically capable of intense dissociative processes. With frequent experiences, the child can rapidly enter "altered states" to meet the interactive demands of the parent's sudden shifts in behavior. When such shifts are early, severe, and repeated, these states can become engrained in the child as self-states. The child both learns the processes of abrupt, dissociative state shifting and develops specific self-states that can be activated in response to specific external context cues. The result of these internal state shifts can be that the child may come to develop several forms of attachment with the parent: some avoidant, some ambivalent, some disorganized, and perhaps even some secure. These can be considered nonintegrated working models of attachment.

The quality of the relationship between the parent and child may thus vary significantly across repeated clusters of interactive experiences. Parent and child may enter various forms of "dyadic states" characterized by unique communication styles. A parent who disavows the existence of certain dyadic states (such as periods of terrifying a child), without later repairing such ruptured connections, will promote dissociative adaptations as a part of a disorganized attachment.[77] A parent with unresolved trauma or loss may enter trance-like states that are frightening to a child but are unrecognized and unacknowledged by the parent. Such state shifts lead to disconnections in attunement, which, if left unrepaired, can lead the child to have profoundly disturbing underlying feelings of shame and humiliation.[78]

Some individuals have experienced secure attachments with certain caregivers and disorganized ones with others. In such cases, isolation of the attuned dyadic states may maintain high functioning within self-systems that have reflective functioning, as well as having the capacity to integrate a coherent sense of self *across the self-states within that securely attached clustered system*. The AAI narratives of such persons may reveal an integrated coherence that on the surface appears to be highly functional. This is revealed in coherent stories about limited parts of the persons' lives. When certain psychosocial contexts, moments of stress, or less integrated subsystems emerge, then integration, reflective functioning, and narrative coherence may become impaired. In the narratives and lives of less well-functioning individuals, there may be a more generalized absence of any such reflective or integrative capacity, as a result of their more pervasive insecure attachment histories. These individuals may have had no developmental experience of interactive communication, which would have promoted such abilities. These individuals may have more difficulty utilizing internal or interpersonal resources, and thus have more marked impairments in their ability to cope with stress and to self-organize.

Giovanni Liotti has proposed that several different trajectories are possible in the setting of disorganized attachment.[79] If parental behavior becomes more predictable later in a child's life, even in the non-nurturing direction, then the child may minimize the conflict among the mental models of attachment developed in the context of the parent's abrupt and confusing shifts in behavior. In the case of a parent's becoming more predictable, then, the child may "settle" on one model or another. If the parent continues to exhibit disorienting behaviors, but these are not overly traumatizing, the child may develop the potential for future dissociation, especially under conditions of stress. A third pathway suggested by Liotti is that if the parent's behavior remains severely traumatizing and chronic, then the disorganized attachment may evolve into a dissociative disorder. At the extreme of this spectrum is dissociative identity disorder (formerly known as multiple personality disorder).

Elizabeth Carlson and colleagues, working with the Minnesota Longitudinal Study of Parents and Children, have provided longitudinal support for Liotti's proposal that children with disorganized attachments are predisposed to develop clinical symptoms of dissociation later in life.[80] There is also the controversial notion that dissociation itself may contribute to the vulnerability for developing clinical PTSD in those who later experience stressful events.[81] This idea, combined with Carlson's findings, suggests that disorganized attachment experiences early in life may perhaps lead to inadequate coping mechanisms and impaired interactive capacities. This vulnerability in turn makes these individuals less likely to be able to resolve trauma or grief, if such stressors are encountered later in life. In disorganized attachments, the core of the self remains fractured. As Ogawa and colleagues have stated:

> Children with disorganized attachments are predisposed to develop clinical symptoms of dissociation later in life.

> Self, in fact, refers to the integration and organization of diverse aspects of experience, and dissociation can be defined as the failure to integrate experience. . . . When experience is acknowledged and accepted, integration inevitably follows, because the self cannot help seeking meaning and coherence from experience. When experience is dissociated, however, integration is not possible, and to the extent that dissociation prevails, there is fragmentation of the self. A coherent, well-organized self depends on integration, and thus psychopathological dissociation represents a threat to optimal development of the self.[82]

For the child with disorganized attachment, in other words, relationship experiences have severely hampered the developmental acquisition of the capacity to achieve coherence. The segmentation of mental processes becomes an engrained process itself: dissociation.

What is dissociation? Numerous books have been written about the conceptualization, history, genesis, evaluation, psychopathology, and treatment of dissociative disorders. For the purposes of this chapter, let us look briefly at the self-organizational aspects of dissociative states of mind, and see how such states involve an impairment in the ability to achieve coherence of the self. I refer you to other sources for a more comprehensive review of this important area.[83]

Clinicians use the term "dissociation" to refer to a discontinuity in mental functioning that is a part of several disorders, such as panic disorder, borderline personality disorder, and PTSD. Dissociation includes the phenomena of depersonalization, derealization, and psychogenic amnesia. The term is also used to refer to a specific group of clinical disorders, including dissociative identity disorder, dissociative fugue, dissociative amnesia, and depersonalization disorder. In any of these latter conditions, there is a disruption in the integration of various processes, including memory, identity, perception, and consciousness.[84]

Clinical dissociation can be viewed as a dis-association in the usually integrative functioning of the mind. How does this happen? Mental functioning emanates from anatomically distinct and fairly autonomous circuits, each of which can be dis-associated from the function of the others. Studies of a drug called ketamine demonstrate that administering it to nondisordered participants leads to dissociative symptoms, such as depersonalization and derealization.[85] Subjects with prior histories of trauma experience the additional symptoms of terror and panic. Ketamine blocks the transmission of signals across the synapses of large neurons, which are especially plentiful in the associational regions of the cortex. One study demonstrated decreased blood flow in the middle prefrontal region, including the orbitofrontal and anterior cingulate regions, and these shifts were strongly correlated with dissociative symptoms.[86] This finding suggests that the dis-association of functions in dissociation may be mediated by a blockage in the integrative capacity of associational regions, which coordinate and balance an array of neural pathways.

The mind has layers of representational processes. These are created by various inputs from interactions with others and from more and more complex representational levels within the nervous system. Studies of brain function reveal that neural pathways have such layers of input, in which secondary and tertiary association areas link streams of neural activity into more and more complex networks of activation.[87] These processes in turn influence a widely distributed set of neural processes responsible for our emotional states, bodily response, reasoning, memory retrieval, and perceptual biases.

A pioneering neuroscientist, Francisco Varela, and his colleagues suggested the following in the summary of one of his last papers, titled "The Brainweb: Phase Synchronization and Large-Scale Integration":

> The emergence of a unified cognitive moment relies on the coordination of scattered mosaics of functionally specialized brain regions. Here we review the mechanisms of large-scale integration that counterbalance the distributed anatomical and functional organization of brain activity to enable the emergence of coherent behaviour and cognition. Although the mechanisms involved in large-scale integration are still largely unknown, we argue that the most plausible candidate is the formation of dynamic links mediated by synchrony over multiple frequency bands.[88]

Integration is at the heart of how our brains contribute to shape the moment-by-moment unfolding of experience in our subjective mental lives. When we embrace the view that the mind is not only embodied but also relational, we can then extend the concept of synchronization and integration to the notion of a "mindweb," which involves the synchronized firing and large-scale linkage of differentiated elements of multiple nodes of information and energy flow within our social networks. As Christakis and Fowler have revealed in their insightful research,[89] we are all interconnected to one another by three degrees of separation, such that a friend's friend's friend will be influenced by our own actions, for good or for bad. In our mindweb, we can sense that ripples of impact from our own intentions, carried out through kind and considerate empathic actions, could influence the overall synchronization and integration of the larger systems in which we globally live.

Within the embodied aspect of mind, it is illuminating to examine the areas that link widely separated neural circuits to one another to enable phase synchronization and large-scale functional integration. Naturally, the mirror neuron components of the resonance circuitry described in Chapter 4 play a large role. One aspect of this resonance circuitry is the middle prefrontal area. This region of the brain coordinates and balances a number of functions across time, and plays a crucial role in the integrative process.[90] As we've seen, these prefrontal areas link cortex, limbic area, brainstem, body, and even the social signals from other people together into one synchronized and integrated mindweb. Even the right and left prefrontal regions may coordinate their different functions with each other in an integrative fashion.[91] When injury occurs to this prefrontal region, various mental processes may thus be functionally isolated from one another, with these integrative circuits blocked.[92] As we've seen, these associational functions include body regulation, attuned communication, emotional balance, response flexibility, fear modulation, autonoetic consciousness (insight), empathy, morality, and intuition.[93] Isolation of these functions may be at the core of incoherence during dissociative experiences.

## OBSERVING INTEGRATION

### Coherence and Complexity

*We can propose that integration creates coherence by enabling the mind's flow of information and energy to achieve a balance in its movement toward maximizing complexity. This movement of the flow of states of mind can involve activity within an individual and with other people.* This balance means that the system moves between sameness and rigidity on the one hand, and novelty and chaos on the other. As we've seen, systems achieve stability as they flow between these extremes in their movement toward maximal complexity, like a choir singing in harmony. Within this optimal flow, processes are connected within a single mind and between minds. Integration involves the recruitment of internal and interpersonal processes into a mutually activating co-regulation. This is "resonance," the property of interacting systems that defines the influence of each on the other. We can thus look at resonance within both internal processes and interpersonal relationships to understand how the mind's movement toward integration brings about coherence.

Emotionally attuned and contingent communication between two individuals creates interpersonal resonance; each member of the dyad is influenced by the other. Within the brain, the neural process of "reentry" can help us to understand how distinct circuits can become involved in a resonating state.[94] Circuit $A$ sends signals to $B$, which in turn sends signals back to $A$, and so on. The reentrant activity of such a circuit links $A$ and $B$ as an integrated system at that moment. In this manner, $A$ and $B$ are part of a state-dependent process. In a different state, the activity of $A$ may have little influence on that of $B$. "Resonance" is a term that can thus be used to describe the nature of a system's contingent, reentrant, co-regulating influences on the interacting elements—whether these are clusters of neurons, circuits, systems, hemispheres, or entire brains and bodies (as in interpersonal communication). In resonance, the subcomponent parts become functionally linked in an integrated system.

Let's try to define the relationships among the terms "integration," "coherence," "cohesion," and "resonance." We've defined "integration" as the linkage of differentiated elements that creates coherence in the mind. "Coherence" is the state of the system in which many layers of neural functioning become activated and are flexibly linked to each other over time.[95] Complexity theory gives us some insight into why this linking process may occur: States of the system that maximize complexity achieve stability.[96] In this way, integration creates the experience of self changing over time. As the mind moves the system of energy and information flow in the body and in the social world toward complexity, it recruits various layers of processes into a cohesive state of mind. Cohesion is thus a state in which subcomponents become linked together at a given moment in time. As the mind emerges across time, cohesive states can become a part of a coherent flow. The linkages of subcomponents—whether in a given moment (cohesion) or across time (coherence)—are achieved by the process of integration. Integration recruits and connects differentiated subcomponent circuits into a larger functional system through a fundamental reentry process. The co-regulating, mutually influencing state of reentrant connections is

> Integration creates the experience of self changing over time.

called "resonance." In other words, *integration utilizes the resonance of different subsystems to achieve cohesive states and a coherent flow of states across time. Such a process creates a more complex, functionally linked system, which itself can become a subcomponent of even larger and more complex systems.*

Translating this often nonconscious process into words is quite a challenge. Within particular sensory modalities, for example, there may be a feeling of "connection" with the object in the focus of conscious attention. Looking at a flower can become a dynamic, consuming process in which the self and the flower lose their boundaries within conscious experience. The act of creation in many activities can feel as if some powerful flow of energy and information within the mind is occurring without intention and with a life of its own. Within interpersonal relationships, integration may be experienced as fullness of communication and spontaneity, in which the self is both fully present and lost within the flow of a vibrant, unpredictable, and yet reliable dyadic connection.

These experiences have the quality of "joining," in which the individual becomes a part of a process larger than a bodily defined, separate self. As integration occurs, the creation of coherence represents the flow of states of the system on the "fertile ground between order and chaos"[97]—a path of resonance with a balanced trajectory between rigidity and randomness. The particular "system" whose states are flowing may involve any level of functioning: localized circuits in the brain, larger neuronal systems, both hemispheres, or two or more people. The subjective experience of coherence will depend on the nature of the elements of the system activated in the resonance created by the integrative process.

Is there empirical support for the relationship between integration and the creation of such joining experiences? One possible source of corroboration may come from the studies of "optimal experiences" by Mihaly Csikszentmihalyi.[98] In these investigations, participants who had the experience of "flow"—a process in which one creatively loses oneself in an activity—often seemed to have well-developed skills at becoming highly focused and fully immersed in an activity, such as athletics, playing music, or writing. Csikszentmihalyi has suggested that such flow experiences involve an individual's moving between the boundaries of boredom on the one hand and anxiety on the other. We can propose that these experiences maximize the complexity of an individual's states in their movement between rigidity/order (boredom) and randomness/chaos (anxiety). We can also suggest that such experiences actually become self-reinforcing, as they facilitate the development of integrative processes within the individual that enhance the capacity for joining in a variety of contexts. The capacity for such a joining process may be revealed in an individual's immersion within an activity ("flow"), as well as within the collaborative communication of interpersonal relationships. This possibility is supported by Csikszentmihalyi's finding that individuals who experienced flow tended to have a combination of highly specialized individual skills and a capacity for being socially integrated with others. Future studies may be helpful in exploring the possible ways in which the capacities for joining within activities and within interpersonal relationships are related to each other as well as to the development of integrative processes, and perhaps emotional well-being, across the lifespan.

## The Narrative Process

What other evidence is available to help us more fully understand the integrative process and to further support the proposal that it plays an important role in our lives? There are several sources of data. The first we will examine is the integrative function of narratives. Studies of child development reveal that by the third year of life, a "narrative" function emerges in children and allows them to create stories about the events they encounter during their lives.[99] These narratives are sequential descriptions of people and events that condense numerous experiences into generalizing and contrasting stories. New experiences are compared to old ones. Similarities are noted in creating generalized rules, and differences are highlighted as memorable exceptions to these rules. The stories are about making sense of events and the mental experiences of the characters. Filled with the elements of the characters' internal experience in the context of interactions with others in the world, these stories appear to be functioning to create a sense of coherent comprehension of the individual in the world across time.

Is this related to a drive to create coherence among the disparate aspects of one's own mind? We could argue that it is, but this is not necessarily the case. Narratives may at times selectively focus on the minds of others and on external contexts, not on one's own internal experience. Children begin as biographers and emerge into autobiographers. As Dennie Wolf has discussed, a child begins to develop an "authorial self" by two years of age. In her view, "authorship is the ability to act independent[ly] of the impinging facts of a situation." Such a process requires the ability to "uncouple" various versions of experience, as well as the "emergence of explicit forms of representation to mark the nature of and movement among the stances of the self."[100] This view is based on the notion that the child can adopt different perspectives on or versions of the experience of self. As Wolf states, "Our most immediate definition of self is that of a coherent and distinctive center: a bodily container, an anchor point for our sense of agency, a single source for our emotions (no matter how chaotic), or a kind of volume where the chapters of a very personal history accumulate."[101] As the child experiences different domains of self-experience (or "self-states," as we have defined them), the authorial self is challenged to incorporate these different "versions of the self" into an autobiographical narrative process. The development of such a personal process, as we've seen in other domains, is extremely dependent upon social experience.[102]

The narrative process in this way attempts to make sense of the world and of one's own mind and its various states. In some individuals, however, one sees narratives that reflect upon a particular self-state without creating a more global coherence of the mind as a whole. The narrative may be cohesive in its logical consistencies, but incoherent in its lack

> The narrative process is thus a fundamental building block of an integrative mode.

of flexibility across time and states. The narrative process is thus a fundamental building block of an integrative mode, but insufficient by itself to create coherence across self-states through time. Let's look at three other sources of data that can help us explore the nature of integration and its potential relationship to the narrative process.

## Hidden Observers

A second source of information regarding the integrative process consists of studies of nondisordered participants in hypnotic or trance-like states. In this condition, the vast majority of the population appears to have a third-party observing capacity, which has been called a "hidden observer," "observing ego," "internal self-helper," or "inner guide."[103] The hidden observer reveals itself under hypnosis or guided imagery as a form of mental output that makes comments about the person: "Dan is working too much; he should slow down and relax more," or "Her need to get this project done is interfering with her ability to exercise. She should stop being so busy with the project." This function reveals the mind's capacity for processing mindsight, representing states of mind, and processing the context of an experience over time. Comments such as these, made under the hypnotic condition of focused internal concentration, are intended to *alter the functioning* of the individual as a whole. This appears to be not just an observing function (information representation), but also an effort to use this information to change other aspects of behavior (processing the information and causing further effects). We can therefore view the hidden observer as an integrative attempt of the mind to create a sense of coherence across its own states through time and contexts.

Does the hidden observer exist beyond the conditions of hypnosis? Several sources of information suggest that it does. First of all, as we've just seen, children develop the capacity at an early age to narrate their own lives from multiple perspectives, including the third-person, observer perspective.

Second, studies of memory reveal that people have the capacity for observer recollections in which they recall themselves from a distant perspective, seeing themselves in a scene from the past as if they were watching themselves from afar.[104] Furthermore, clinical studies of patients with a variety of disorders reveal an internal process that comments on ongoing experience. In patients with dissociative disorders, an "internal self-helper" that attempts to coordinate some of the disparate activities of the mind is quite a common self-state.[105] Individuals with depression may experience an "internal voice" that is demeaning and pessimistic, and that further entrenches the negative, depressed mood.

What does the hidden observer tell us about interpersonal experience? In examining the relationship between hypnosis and developmental processes, Brian Vandenberg states, first, that hypnosis reveals how "social exchange and intrapsychic functioning interpenetrate, that self and other, cognitive and social, individual and culture are intimately enmeshed"; second, that it suggests that "thought and experience are not always continuous, seamless, autonomous, and internal but involve discontinuities, dislocations, and alterations that are structured by contextual factors"; and, third, that hypnotic states reflect "the childhood experience of lability of grounding, and of 'receiving speech' from an authoritative other who provides stability in an uncertain world."[106] Communication with a parent, in other words, can enable a child to achieve a sense of coherence in the face of confusing shifts in the internal and external worlds. Could it be that children's early relationship experiences with contingent communication and reflective dialogue facilitate the development of an "internal voice" that addresses the self from a third-person perspective and helps integrate a sense of coherence? Could this form of thought be the internalization of interpersonal dialogue, as Lev Vygotsky has suggested?[107] Some of the features of mindfulness traits (touched on in Chapter 1) are the capacities for self-observation, emotional equilibrium, and awareness of events as they are happening, along with the abilities to suspend judgments and to name the inner experiences of the mind. Interestingly, some executive functions have been found to be associated with mentalization ability and with relational experiences with parents.[108] If parental sensitivity and mentalization are associated with the development of executive functions[109]—and preliminary studies do suggest that mindfulness traits and a parent's own security of attachment are correlated[110]—then one can see how each of these internal and interpersonal functions may share the common mechanism of integration. Future studies examining the relationships among parent–child attachment, executive function, discourse, narrative, and even the hidden observer will help further elucidate the developmental origin of these integrative processes.

## Hemispheric Laterality

A third source of information supporting the existence of an integrative mode of processing consists of research on the specialized functions of the brain's two hemispheres. The following findings (many of which have been reviewed earlier) have been consistently obtained in investigations ranging from studies of "split-brain" patients to studies involving brain function imaging. When information is presented to only the left hemisphere, verbal output reflects an effort to create a story or make sense of what it sees or hears. Michael Gazzaniga and colleagues have called this the "interpreter" function of the left hemisphere.[111] For the isolated left hemisphere, these words are confabulations—made-up stories that fit with the data, but are unrelated to the gist or context of the situation. In these studies, the left hemisphere appears to lack the contextual representations of the right hemisphere, but nevertheless creates a story to explain the limited information at its disposal. The left hemisphere uses syllogistic reasoning, stating major and minor premises and deducing logical conclusions from a limited set of data in an attempt to clarify cause–effect relationships. For example, if a subject with an isolated left hemisphere is asked about a picture showing a boy and his father, the left hemisphere will take the details of the scene and create a fabricated explanation of what the two people are doing. Surrounding features, such as the fact that the other parts of the picture reveal a baseball game, or the facial expressions of the pair, are ignored. These contextual elements do not appear to be perceived by the left hemisphere, or at least they are ignored when it comes to explaining what the scene is about. The left hemisphere's interpreter function seems to be driven primarily by a need to reason about cause–effect relationships. It seems uninterested in establishing some coordinated or coherent view of "truth" or in understanding the internal mental intention of other people.[112] Some authors have suggested that the left hemisphere may be primarily responsible for the creation of distorted and "false" memories of past experiences.[113]

In contrast to the left, the right hemisphere appears to be able to make sense of the essential meaning of what it is able to perceive: Contextual information is perceived and processed, and the gist of a situation is sized up and understood. The right hemisphere does not use syllogistic logic to deduce conclusions about cause–effect relationships, but rather represents information about the environment. Such information includes the relationships of various components of experience, including elements of mental processes and spatial relationships. Since the right hemisphere is predominantly non-verbal, the output of its processing must be expressed in non-word-based ways, such as drawing a picture or pointing to a pictorial set of options to make its output known to the external world.

As discussed at length in prior chapters, these hemispheric differences have embryological origins and reflect a dominance of processing in the dorsal or ventral circuits on each side of the brain. Numerous studies support the view that the capacity for mindsight is right-hemisphere-dominant. The registration and regulation of bodily state, the perception and expression of nonverbal signals of affective state, the coordination of social and emotional input with the appraisal centers of the brain, and the retrieval of autobiographical memory all appear to be predominantly mediated by the right hemisphere. Because the input from the body is registered primarily in the right cortical regions, such as the right anterior insula and right anterior cingulate, the right hemisphere is more directly influenced by interoceptive data. These somatic inputs, "wisdom of the body," shape our emotional state and have primary access to right hemisphere consciousness. We become aware of our nonrational world by way of nonworded right-hemisphere representational processing. The capacity to represent states of mind within the mind is probably mediated within the right hemisphere's domains of processing. We have thus proposed that reflective function, which permits mentalizing, is likely to be mediated primarily by the right hemisphere.

> The capacity for mindsight is right-hemisphere-dominant.

These laterality studies suggest several relevant aspects of the mind's functioning. The left hemisphere tries to create explanations for the information it receives, but it lacks the ability to process the context of this information, and so its conclusions are based on selected details without relational meaning. The left hemisphere's interpreter deduces an explanation that is superficially logical, but is often without contextual substance if this hemisphere is acting in isolation from information from the right hemisphere. The right hemisphere processes the overall gist of a scene and creates a context-rich representational "understanding." The right hemisphere specializes in the ability to perceive the mental states of others and to represent others' minds. Although it may not use syllogistic reasoning to interpret and deduce cause–effect relationships, it has a reflective understanding of the social world of other minds.[114]

## Making Sense of Minds

An important implication of the three sets of studies reviewed to this point is that people are constantly trying to "make sense" of what they experience. On one level, making sense means trying to understand cause–effect relationships—what is happening and why it happened. Why does the mind try to do this? (Even the asking of this question reflects the human mind's need to make sense of things, including the mind itself!) A straightforward answer comes from the reverse-engineering approach of evolutionary thinking: Individuals whose brains were able to understand cause–effect relationships were more likely to survive and to pass on their genetic material. Why? Because if the mind can perceive the events of the world, remember them, extract cause–effect relationships (understanding, making sense), and use these processes to influence the outcome of future behavior in the world, then it will be more likely to survive. As we have noted throughout this book, the brain functions as an anticipation machine; it takes data from the perceived world and prepares itself for the next event. Individuals whose brains were good at anticipating did better than those whose brains merely lived in the here-and-now. For instance, it was easier to avoid a lion if people figured out that a growl (cause) could indicate the presence of a lion who would eat them (effect). Such is the basis for learning. Such is the basis for making sense of the world.

Making sense of the social world of minds is a bit more complicated, but it involves the same basic problem of cause–effect relationships. What does the scowl of another person "mean"? How do the subtle and rapid signals, both verbal and nonverbal, from other people reveal what is happening and what may happen next? Knowing whom to trust and whom to be wary of is essential in negotiating one's way through the human world of social interactions. The states of mind of others—their intentions, beliefs, attitudes, and emotions—predispose an individual to behave in a certain way. *The ability to anticipate the behavior of others is dependent upon the ability to understand other minds.*

Functioning in a complex social network enhances people's capacity to survive as individuals, reproduce, and create a group of like-minded individuals who share such a capacity. This can be seen as a form of interindividual integration. Shared mentalizing abilities permit the group to function as a cohesive system composed of linked individuals. This allows for a "group state" to be achieved, which can facilitate the development of a highly effective problem-solving system to meet challenges in a world filled with competition. Being a member of such a group confers a sense of safety, security, and stability on an individual. This is the way we participate in the larger mindweb, which enables energy and information to emerge within the interactions of many interconnected individuals. The Internet reveals how such a web of human minds can function as an interconnected whole with its own emergent properties.

When we examine our individual lives across developmental time, a number of studies suggest complex relationships among early attachment history, experiences with teachers, relationships with friends, and social competence in peer groups.[115] One of these studies has shown, for example, that peer acceptance and leadership abilities are associated with a history of secure attachments.[116] Relationships, both early and later in life, clearly make a difference as our lives evolve. Overall, these findings support the notion that an individual continues to develop in interaction with an evolving set of internal processes as well as social experiences within interpersonal and group relationships.

Through the life course, the individual mind attempts to create a coherent internal, interpersonal, and group experience. Such an integrative process places the system of the individual mind within the context of complex social forces, which directly shape the life course in often unpredictable ways. As Glenn Elder has described:

> Life course theory and research alert us to this real world, a world in which lives are lived and where people work out paths of development as best they can. It tells us how lives are socially organized in biological and historical time, and how the resulting social pattern affects the way we think, feel and act.[117]

Our minds are in this manner continually processing both internal and social experiences as we develop through time.

Natural selection has enabled our minds to evolve mindsight capacities. Being able to navigate our way through an intense social world requires the ability to make sense of other minds. Communicating the more elaborate and intricate learned aspects of this mentalizing knowledge to others allows the benefits of one individual's wisdom and experience to be shared with others in the group. This knowledge is transmitted from one individual to others in the group by means of storytelling. *Making sense of other minds is the essential stuff of narratives.* This means that the mentalizing representations of the right hemisphere may need to be integrated with the interpreting ones of the left in both the expression and reception of such information. What can stories tell us about such an integrative process?

## AN INTERPERSONAL NEUROBIOLOGY VIEW OF STORIES

### Narrative and Neural Integration

Narrative may have originated as a fundamental part of social discourse. Recall that stories are created within a social context between human minds. The process of narrative is thus inherently social. The contents of stories are human lives and mental experiences. Describing an IPNB view of stories may be helpful in elucidating the fundamental processes involved in how narrative facilitates the integration of coherence within the mind. Let's first review some aspects of the neural integration involved in stories.

The hippocampus is considered a "cognitive mapper": It gives the brain a sense of the self in space and in time, regulates the order of perceptual categorizations, and links mental representations to emotional appraisal centers.[118] These are multiple layers of integration.

A number of authors propose that the associational areas of the neocortex, such as the prefrontal regions (including the orbitofrontal cortex) that link various widely distributed representational processes together, are fundamental to narrative and form dynamic global maps or complex representations in order to establish a sensorimotor integration of the self across space and time.[119] This capacity allows for the anticipation of and planning for future events. This is autonoetic consciousness. Such a spatiotemporal integrating process is proposed to be fundamental to the narrative mode of cognition. This mapping process may be at the heart of autobiographical narrative and the way the mind attempts to achieve a sense of coherence among its various states: trying to make sense of the self in the past, the present and the anticipated future. We can propose that the capacity of the mind to create such a global map of the self across time and various contexts—to have autonoetic consciousness—is an essential feature of integration that may continue to develop throughout life.

Narrative can also be viewed as requiring both right- and left-hemisphere modes of processing information. The right brain's perceptually rich, analogic, context-dependent, autonoetic, mentalizing representations create much of the imagery and many of the themes of the narrative process. The logical, linear, "making sense" interpretations of these representations and the communication of narrative details stem from the left hemisphere's interpretive and linguistic processing of representations. On each side of the brain, these processes may reflect a vertical integration of various representational processes. As the dorsal tract processes (dominant in the right hemisphere) interconnect with those of the ventral tract (dominant in the left hemisphere), dorsal–ventral integration begins to occur. Within these forms of integration, processes on the right begin to be integrated with those on the left. We can propose the following bilateral integration process for narratives: The left hemisphere's drive to understand cause–effect relationships is a primary motivation of the narrative process. Coherent narratives, however, require participation of both the interpreting left hemisphere and the mentalizing right hemisphere. *Coherent narratives are created through interhemispheric integration.*

Integration that recruits multiple layers of circuits may create the most complex states as it links various forms of representation throughout the brain (and between brains). Vertical, dorsal–ventral, lateral, interhemispheric, and spatiotemporal forms of integration are all present within the narrative process. The "drive to make sense of the mind," drawing on these

> Coherent narratives are created through interhemispheric integration.

multidimensional layers of integration, may in part be seen as a way the brain achieves a more stable (complex) connection among its various representational processes. The left hemisphere's effort to find cause–effect relationships draws upon the right hemisphere's retrieval of autobiographical and mentalizing representations. Such multilayered integration may exist independently of narration. In other words, the mind may be internally driven to link these layers of representational processes as a function of achieving coherence within the mind itself. Such internal coherence may be revealed within the middle prefrontal cortex's capacity for response flexibility and may reflect the integration of a range of prefrontally mediated processes. As we attempt to communicate a shareable set of representations within autobiographical stories, we must use the linguistic translations and interpretations of the left hemisphere in order to express the narrative of our lives. Such a communication process lets us see for ourselves, and share with others, the fundamental way in which our minds come to integrate experience.

As we've discussed in Chapter 2, Endel Tulving and colleagues have postulated a dual role for the frontal lobes on each side of the brain. In their "hemispheric encoding–retrieval asymmetry" hypothesis, the left hemisphere is seen as the primary mediator of autobiographical encoding, whereas the right is responsible for retrieval—and recent studies suggest that this is independent of the type of input, verbal or nonverbal.[120] Autonoetic consciousness gives us the ability to perform "mental time travel," in which we can represent the self in the past, present, and future.[121] These studies suggest that the ability to make sense of the past and the capacity to create our future are intimately interwoven. We have also discussed the possibility that the consolidation of memory into permanent storage may require REM sleep and dreaming, and thus may depend on the synchronous activation of both hemispheres. We have proposed that this bilateral activation of the brain may permit a rhythmic process in which right frontal activation retrieves autobiographical representations from more posterior regions of the right brain. The transfer of this information to the left prefrontal regions may then allow reencoding to occur. In essence, this may be the encoding of the newly assembled representations created from retrieved memory. Items in long-term (nonpermanent) storage in this way may be retrieved (right side) and encoded (left side) in a process that integrates information from recent and more distant past experiences, as well as from imagination, current perception, and random activations. As Winson and others have suggested, the electrical activity and neuroendocrine milieu of the REM stage of sleep may allow for the consolidation of memory via the induction of the long-term potentiation of synaptic connections.[122] This bilateral encoding–retrieval process may facilitate the creation of new and strengthened associational links. This process may also reveal how memory retrieval acts as a "memory modifier" in this setting of bilateral activation, permitting recent recollections of the day's experiences to be synthesized with prior elements of memory within a constructive and thematic narrative process.

In this proposal, interhemispheric integration is essential for memory consolidation. Dreaming, REM sleep, and cortical consolidation become the integrating processes that mediate autobiographical narrative. Blockage of these integrating processes may be seen as the core of unresolved trauma and may be revealed as one form of incoherence in autobiographical narratives. Autonoetic consciousness may thus be impaired as the ability to integrate representations of the self across past, present, and future is disrupted in lack of resolution. This proposal regarding narrative, consolidation, and bilateral integration is a hypothesis in need of validation. As Milner, Squire, and Kandel have noted, we are still far from understanding the exact mechanisms behind the consolidation process.[123] Future research will need to clarify exactly how this consolidation process occurs.

The ways in which interpersonal experience shapes both implicit memory and explicit memory directly affect our life stories. Narratives, though they draw on flexibly accessible explicit memory, are also influenced by the more reflective retrieval of implicit recollections. Our dreams and stories may contain implicit aspects of our lives even without our awareness of their origins in the past. In fact, storytelling may be a primary way in which we can linguistically communicate to others—as well as to ourselves—the sometimes hidden contents of our implicitly remembering minds. Stories make available perspectives on the emotional themes of our implicit memory that may otherwise be consciously unavailable to us as remnants of prior experiences. This may be one reason why journal writing and intimate communication with others, which are so often narrative processes, have such powerful organizing effects on the mind: They allow us to modulate our emotions and make sense of the world. Integration, as observed in coherent narratives, directly shapes self-regulation.

## Narrative and Interpersonal Integration

The narrative process also enables a form of interpersonal integration. The external expression of narrative through storytelling is inherently influenced by listeners' expectations. In this way, early attachment experiences have a direct effect on how children learn to narrate their lives and perhaps to develop autonoetic consciousness. Patterns of collaborative communication allow children to develop what Trevarthen has called "narratives of cooperative awareness."[124] As parents reflect with their securely attached children on the mental states that create their shared subjective experience, they are joining with them in an important co-constructive process of understanding how the mind functions. The inherent feature of secure attachment—contingent, collaborative communication—is also a fundamental component in how interpersonal relationships facilitate internal integration in a child. We can propose that a parent's engaging in what we have called "reflective dialogue" (focusing on the central importance of mental states in human behavior and their manifestations as feelings, perceptions, intentions, goals, beliefs, and desires) is also central to both secure attachment and the integrative process of co-construction of narratives. Social competence and a sense of autonomy, mastery, and self-determination are aspects of resilience that secure attachment fosters.[125] We can propose that integration also becomes a developmental capacity within the foundation of nurturing and reflective early relationships.

Secure attachment facilitates integration in the developing child by allowing for different forms of interpersonal resonance to occur. Left-hemisphere-to-left-hemisphere resonance takes the form of verbal communication within a linear, logical mode of discourse. Right-hemisphere-to-right-hemisphere resonance involves the nonverbal components of communication, such as tone of voice, gestures, and facial expressions. *In the co-construction of stories, parent and child enter into a dyadic form of bilateral resonance: Each person enters a state of interhemispheric integration, which is facilitated by interpersonal communication.* In this manner, secure attachment involves an intimate dance of resonant processes involving left-to-left, right-to-right, and bilateral-to-bilateral communication. This highly complex form of collaborative communication allows the dyad to move into highly resonant states, and also enables the child's mind to develop its own capacity for integration. Such a capacity may be at the heart of self-regulation. In essence, integrative communication initiates the activity and reinforces the connections within integrative neural circuits. Integrative communication cultivates neural integration.

> In the co-construction of stories, parent and child enter into a dyadic form of bilateral resonance.

With insecure attachments, such contingent, resonant communication often does not occur and neural integration is compromised. For example, the avoidantly attached child's and dismissing adult's experience can be understood in part as dominated by a primarily left-hemisphere form of communication. These interactions may stem from the parent's tendency to access primarily the nonmentalizing representations of a dominant left-hemisphere interpreter. In fact, studies of the correspondence between affective expression (right hemisphere) and verbal communication (left hemisphere) reveal such a dis-association in these dyads.[126] The capacity to blend the nonverbal/prosodic elements of dialogue with those of semantic/linguistic meaning requires the harmonious collaboration between the hemispheres.[127] As Sroufe has noted, "shared emotion is the fabric of social relationships" and "provides the rhythm or punctuation in human interaction and communication."[128] Thus avoidant attachment reveals an emotional impairment in the ability of two minds to communicate fully.[129] Resonance and the capacity to integrate experience in a complex and interhemispheric way are significantly restricted. This absence of shared emotion produces a severe restriction in the level of interpersonal connection that parent and child are able to achieve. Such a condition reflects the central role emotion plays as an integrating process, both within the mind and between minds.

Within an individual, bilateral integration may occur in creative processes of many forms. My clinical work with insecurely attached individuals who experience a transformation in their "state of mind with respect to attachment" within psychotherapy or other emotionally involving relationships suggests that their new experience of interpersonal connection allows them to achieve new levels of mental coherence.[130] This new capacity for integration—both interpersonal and internal—may create a sense of vitality and a release of creative energy and ideas, leading to an invigorating sense of personal expression. Such spontaneous and energized processes can give rise to participation in various activities, such as painting, music, dance, poetry, creative writing, or sculpture. It can also yield a deeper sense of creativity and appreciation within the "everyday" experience of life: communication with others, walks down the street, new appreciation of the richness of perceptions, feelings of being connected to the flow of the moment. As noted in earlier discussions, secure attachment and mindfulness traits have been shown to correlate with each other.[131] This finding suggests that secure attachment, mindfulness, and even mental well-being all share neural integration as a common fundamental mechanism. Life becomes a process, not merely a product. This experience of creativity may in part be derived from the way in which activated elements in one modality freely recruit those in another. This is truly how integration broadens and builds connections in our lives. Much of this is nonconscious, but the new resonance among processes can give rise to an awareness of the activated flow of an emerging, coherent mind. Many people find this sense of vitality, intensity, and clarity to be quite exhilarating.

The integrating experience of resonance also gives rise to a sense of spontaneity and creativity when it occurs between two people. Such vibrant connections between minds can be seen within various kinds of emotional relationships, such as those of romantic partners, friends, colleagues, teachers and students, therapists and patients, and parents and children. Two people become companions on a mutually created journey through time. Interpersonal integration can be seen in spontaneous, resonant communication that flows freely and is balanced between continuity, familiarity, and predictability on one side and flexibility, novelty, and uncertainty on the other. Neither partner of a dyad is fully predictable, yet each is quite familiar. Each one's differences are honored and encouraged, while compassionate communication connects each to the other. The collaborative communication between the two is not merely a reflective mirror, but a reciprocal, contingent process that moves the pair into vibrant states neither alone could achieve. The resultant evolving process creates a sense of the emerging complexity and coherence of integrating minds.

Integration is a central organizing principle for how the human mind develops across the lifespan. It can inform the way we approach child rearing in education and in families,[132] in psychotherapy,[133] and in our understanding of contemplation.[134] Learning to be flexible and fully present in our lives, and being kind and compassionate to others and to ourselves, are the ultimate outcomes of living an integrated life.

## REFLECTIONS: INTEGRATING MINDS

As the mind emerges within the flow of self-states, it creates coherence across these states by a process we have defined as "integration." Integration allows the mind to experience the mutual co-regulation of energy flow and information processing, which permits adaptive, coordinated functioning. Incoherence derives from the inflexible, maladaptive, and restricted flow of energy and information within the mind across time. Interpersonal processes can facilitate integration by altering the restrictive ways in which the mind may have come to organize itself.

Creating coherence is a lifetime project. Integration is a process, not a final accomplishment. This process perhaps is best seen as a form of "resonance," defined as the mutually influencing interactions between two or more relatively independent and differentiated entities. This resonance allows two systems to amplify and co-regulate each other's activity. In the case of one mind, integration allows for the spontaneous flow of energy and information within the whole brain and body. This spontaneity does not mean random activation, but the flexible influence of layers of processes upon each other. By contrast, insecure attachment patterns produce incoherence. Individuals' adaptations to suboptimal parenting experiences place marked restrictions on their capacity for resonance—within their own minds and with other minds.

Autobiographical narratives can reveal integration or incoherence. A coherent narrative reveals a blending of left- and right-hemisphere processes. The interpreting left hemisphere is driven to weave a tale of what it knows. When access to the right hemisphere's representational processes is limited, such a tale is incoherent. When the mentalizing, primary emotional, somatosensory, and autobiographical processes of the right hemisphere can be drawn upon, the left brain is able to "make sense" by integrating a coherent life story. Bilateral integration promotes coherent narratives.

The multilayered resonance of contingently communicating dyadic states allows each individual to acquire new integrative capacities. Two people connect across space by means of the flow of energy and information from both sides of each brain. This flow is contained within patterns of communication. As seen in attachment relationships, the development of the mind depends upon the basics of contingent, collaborative communication. Acquiring the capacity for integrating coherence comes from dyadic communication. Emotional attunement, reflective dialogue, co-construction of narrative, memory talk, and the interactive repair of disruptions in connection are all fundamental elements of secure attachment and of effective growth enhancing interpersonal relationships.

Connections between minds therefore involve a dyadic form of resonance in which energy and information are free to flow across two brains. When such a process is in full activation, the vital feeling of connection is exhilarating. When interpersonal communication is "fully engaged"— when the joining of minds is in full force—there is an overwhelming sense of immediacy, clarity, and authenticity. It is in these heightened moments of engagement, these dyadic states of resonance, that one can appreciate the power of relationships to nurture and to heal the mind.

# Epilogue
## A Framework for Cultivating Integration

A s we come to the end of our journey into the developing mind, I want to
make some brief suggestions about ways of applying the approach to integration described in this book. When a person, dyad, family, group, organization, or community experiences chaos and/or rigidity, then we know that
integration is impaired.[1] The key to moving the system toward well-being is
to identify which elements are not differentiated and/or linked. This search-
and-integrate process is helped by categorizing a set of "domains of integration" that can be the focus of the effort to bring health to a system.

The following nine domains are important areas for energy and information to flow in an integrated way to create well-being, as described in various ways within this book's nine chapters. These domains are also areas in
which integration can be blocked. They provide a reasonable way to describe
the terrain of differentiation and linkage. The nine domains are integration
of consciousness, bilateral integration, vertical integration, memory integra-
tion, narrative integration, state integration, interpersonal integration, temporal integration, and transpirational integration. Together, they represent
one way to begin to apply IPNB and its integration framework to your daily
life in a practical and, I hope, useful way.

In each of these domains, we can ask the following general questions.
What aspects of this domain can be segregated functionally, temporally, or
spatially so that differentiation is possible? How can this domain's subcomponents be differentiated, or their differences cultivated and refined? Once
they are differentiated, how do they become linked? Is the linkage severely
restricted, limiting integration? Is the linkage accompanied by long-lasting
dissolution of the differentiation, so that subcomponents lose their authentic, unique specializations? Linkage naturally entails "phase synchronization" so that resonance is achieved in the moment, but remember once again

that achieving integration is more like making a fruit salad than making a smoothie: Individual components do not become lost in the blender. Heterogeneous functioning imbues integration with a sense of harmony, rather than the sameness of a homogeneous mixture.

## THE NINE DOMAINS OF INTEGRATION

### Integration of Consciousness

What can be differentiated within consciousness? As we have explored in Chapter 1, the subjective experience of awareness (the quality of knowing) and the object of awareness (that which is known) are separable elements of our conscious experience. Furthermore, the various objects of awareness can be differentiated from one another—the five senses from sight to touch; the sixth sense of the interior of the body; the "seventh sense" of mental activities; and our "eighth sense" of our interconnections with others and the world. When these aspects of consciousness are not differentiated, the experience of being aware can have a blurry quality, like an out-of-focus photo. The resulting image lacks depth, clarity, and stability. What we see is blurred in the focus of our attention. We may also view the object of attention as the totality of our identity when we do not distinguish awareness from that object of which we are aware. An intense emotion becomes who we are, not what we are feeling temporarily at that moment in time.

A practical approach to cultivating the integration of consciousness is the "Wheel of Awareness" practice—a form of focusing attention in an integrative, mindful way, as discussed in Chapter 7. In this metaphor for the mind, the hub represents awareness, and the points on the rim of the wheel represent that which we can be aware of—from sights and sounds to our sense of the body, our thoughts and feelings, and even our sense of connections to others. These are the elements of consciousness that can be differentiated from one another, and then linked. A metaphoric spoke can be sent systematically from the hub to any point on the rim. This integrative practice has been found to be quite useful with a wide range of people, including elementary school children. It is designed to be an integration-of-consciousness practice, but it also meets all the criteria for being a mindfulness practice: It cultivates curiosity, observation, acceptance, and a loving stance toward the self and others.

### Bilateral Integration

As we've seen, the left and right hemispheres are quite distinct from one another. The two hemispheres have "intrinsic factors" from life *in utero* that differentiate the two sides. As we have explored in Chapter 6, impediments to differentiation can be present from innate causes (e.g., autism and nonverbal learning disabilities) or from experiential causes (e.g., suboptimal attachment). Impaired differentiation means that linkage is not possible, given that one needs to link elements that are distinct from one another. In autism, for example, there may be a premature closure of the early period of differentiation; as a result, the brain is actually larger, but its various areas are not uniquely specialized.[2] In avoidant attachment, the hypothesis is that the left hemisphere is excessively differentiated and the right is underdifferentiated. Interventions would then be created to promote differentiation first, and then to cultivate linkages.

Linkage of the left and right hemispheres happens naturally in most people, so that we can say the brain generally works as an integrated whole. But for some, this does not occur. We can see impaired bilateral integration with incoherent narratives, with dysfunctional interpersonal interactions, and with blocked access to an internal awareness of emotions and bodily sensations. A systematic program can be created to promote the collaborative work of each of these ways of knowing and being in the world, left and right.[3] The key in the overall approach to integration is to remember that the linkage of differentiated parts is a natural drive of a system to organize itself as it maximizes complexity. For bilateral integration, what this often means is discovering the fundamental process that is preventing each way of knowing from being equally valued; it may be a response to an event, the avoidance of a feeling, or a belief. With this new awareness, cooperation across the corpus callosum can then be achieved. Remember this: Openness to the body's sensation and the accompanying wash of emotion is a nonrational, often ambiguous experience that can create a sense of vulnerability. These right-sided subjective sensations may feel quite fragile in the face of the more rational, logic-based, and language-defined left. Vulnerability is a sign of strength, however. Protecting the sometimes timid right in the face of the sometimes overly certain (and dogmatic) left is important in promoting bilateral integration. At other times and for other people, an excessively flooding right hemisphere needs the clear and rational soothing of the more somatically distant left hemisphere. Neither side is better than the other. The key to living a creative and fulfilling life is collaboration, not obliteration. Integration across the hemispheres entails respecting differences while cultivating collaborative connections between these two important but distinct ways of knowing.

## Vertical Integration

If consciousness arises from the complex assemblies of neural firing in temporary phase synchronizations that involve a range of neural processes, especially in the cortex, then vertical integration entails the awareness of subcortical input. Literally, this means focusing conscious attention on the data from the body proper, the brainstem, and the limbic regions. Because these areas are anatomically "lower" than the cortex, we call this "vertical integration." Differentiation along this axis is usually well established, given that *in utero* growth of the fetal nervous system occurs from bottom to top, and then from back to front. Recall that the nervous system has extensive innervation throughout the whole of the body—reaching to our muscles and bones, and distributed throughout our hollow organs, giving us the visceral input of the heart, lungs, and intestines. All of this "wisdom of the body" comes up the vagal nerve and up Lamina I in the spinal cord; makes stopovers in the brainstem and limbic/hypothalamic regulatory areas; and emerges into the middle prefrontal cortical regions of the anterior cingulate and insula, primarily on the right side of the brain. I am using the word "brain" here to mean the brain in the skull, or "head brain." It is reasonable to call the intestinal input the "gut brain" and the heart's input the "heart brain." The "brain" is an embodied brain. Vertical integration makes this reality a part of conscious experience.

A simple exercise can offer others a direct experience of vertical integration—or the lack of it. Say "no" firmly seven times, and then follow that with a gentler "yes" seven times. "No" often elicits the reactive brainstem states of fight–flight–freeze. "Yes" activates the state of openness and social engagement, involving limbic and prefrontal modulation of the state of reactivity to one of receptivity. These bodily felt sensations of being reactive versus being receptive are a part of interoception—literally, the perception of the interior, which is what enables us to cultivate vertical integration. Often when someone has difficulty with interoception, there are important causes; going gently into this terrain is helpful. The window of tolerance for being aware of bodily states can be quite narrow if early attachment experiences were not supportive or if someone is innately sensitive or has intense responses. We live in our bodies, but sometimes we treat the body more like a transportation vehicle for the head than like a sanctuary of peace and pleasure, clarity and intuition.

## Memory Integration

In Chapter 2, we have explored the layers of memory as they move from initial encoding in implicit forms of perception, bodily sensation, emotion, and behavioral response into the assembled puzzle pieces of explicit factual and autobiographical memory storage. As a child grows, he develops the important, socially shaped capacity to have a sense of self across time. This is embedded in implicit circuitry, and then is integrated by the hippocampus into explicit memory. Sometimes this process is blocked, as in trauma. When differentiated implicit memory remains in pure form, it can be seen as the flooding of emotion and images, automatic and sometimes rigidly dysfunctional behavioral habits, and intrusive bodily sensations. Implicit memory also involves mental models based on prior experiences that filter our perceptions. One important aspect of implicit memory is that it can be retrieved and influence our conscious experience without our knowing that something from the past is having an impact on our lives.

Memory integration is the linkage of differentiated implicit memory into the explicit forms of factual and autobiographical memory with which we can exercise intention and choice. This makes our lives more flexible. Memory integration can make the difference between PTSD, with its impairments, and posttraumatic growth. Understanding memory integration helps bring clarity and resolution to overwhelming past events.

## Narrative Integration

We humans are a storytelling species—one that "knows we know" (*Homo sapiens sapiens*). For at least forty thousand years (since the days of our early cave paintings), we have been making sense of our world by bringing the inside out, sharing what we see through our eyes with others. Narrative development is rich with examples of how our interpersonal relationships shape not only what and how we remember, but also how we learn to put words together to tell our experiences to others in story form. A story is the linear telling of a sequence of events, and so naturally narrative integration involves the left hemisphere's linguistic, logical, linear drive to explain the cause–effect relationships of things in life. But autobiographical storage and the ability to understand our mental lives are predominantly right-sided affairs, suggesting that to tell a coherent story of our lives, we need collaboration between these two differentiated, lateralized ways of seeing and being in the world.

Narrative integration is the way we harness the power of the left and the storage of the right to make sense of our lived experience. The emergence of coherent narratives thus arises from bilateral integration and from intra-hemisphere integration. Sometimes a coherent narrative can seem to have "appeared out of nowhere"—for example, as a person comes to resolution of some troubling event. James Pennebaker and colleagues have shown that the mere act of writing in a journal (as compared to dancing or drawing as an expression of a difficult past experience), even if never shown to anyone else, can have profound positive effects on bodily and mental well-being.[4] Narrative integration is about making sense of our lives, and the research is clear that it makes sense to make sense.

## State Integration

We've seen throughout our journey, and especially in Chapter 5, that the emergent mind arises from the interaction of neural and relational processes. Within our families, or with particular friends, we can become more likely to act in certain ways. We should choose our life partners and our friends wisely, as they will profoundly influence not just what we do and talk about, but actually who we will be. We are relational creatures, and the "self" is created in part within relationships. But our state of being in the moment—the self-state that arises—is also shaped by the synaptic shadows that reflect the ways we have adapted to our past experiences; by how those experiences have affected us directly; and also by innately determined neural development processes, such as genes, epigenetic controls, and toxic exposures. In other words, neural connections are shaped by both experience and by constitution to create personality. "Personality" can be described as the proclivity to travel down certain developmental pathways that directly shape self-regulation and our emotional lives.

How can one state of being, or state of mind, be differentiated from another? If I am in need of solitude, do I give myself permission to have time alone? Or is my gregarious state dominant, and do I thus feel guilty about saying "no" to offers for social events? Recognizing and then respecting the differing and often conflictual needs of distinct self-states is a part of "inter-state" integration. This can entail cultivating coherent functioning within a given state. So I give myself permission to learn to sail, and I cultivate a guilt-free (or minimally guilty) state of pleasure with time on the water, wind in my face, and tiller in my hand. This is a part of "intra-state" integration. Living a rich and full life entails at least these two aspects of differentiating (inter-state and intra-state) and then linking the many selves that define who we are. We also have an "interpersonal state," which involves the next domain of integration.

## Interpersonal Integration

Moving from "me" to "we" involves the differentiation of a personal, individual self and then the linkage of this self to another. A balanced relationship is an integrated entity. Often people come for clinical help with relational difficulties; they find their connections with others filled with chaos or rigidity. Fighting, emotional outbursts, and impulsive and sometimes destructive behaviors can dominate a relationship. For others, or at other times, a stagnant quality of predictability and boredom fill the relational landscape. In either case, integration is impaired. When one searches for the impediments to differentiation and/or linkage, they are often found in both members of the relationship.

The synaptic side of relational conflict can be revealed with the narrative window that the AAI offers. If this is being explored with a couple, then often we see how the partners get lost in familiar places; in other words, they have self-fulfilling prophecies that arise to reinforce the very conditions that these persons had as children. Interpersonal integration involves the honoring and relishing of differences while cultivating compassionate connections with others. One of the challenges of making interpersonal integrative changes is that people can fear being engulfed by another's needs, or having their own needs for closeness, once acknowledged, go unmet. The retreat into isolation can sometimes feel more controllable than being flooded with a sense of needing another person for comfort and connection.

As we've discussed, for some the feeling of shame is subterranean, beneath the radar of awareness, and yet it dominates the relational world. With shame, people can have a buried belief of the self as defective, unworthy of connection, "damaged goods." When people learn both conceptually and viscerally that shame has its developmental roots in impaired attachment, the path is opened to heal that early relational wound. It may have been a person's way of preserving her sanity to think that she as a child was the defective one, rather than seeing her parents as the ones in trouble. The young child would have been paralyzed by terror of death if she believed that her parents were not able to be protective. Such reflections are the gateway to letting shame be understood and released. With such internal changes, the opportunity for interpersonal integration is made available; people can feel whole as they remain differentiated and yet deeply and intimately linked to others.

## Temporal Integration

As we journey through life connecting with others, we also live within the homes of our bodies, which travel across the course of a lifespan with us. Not only do we have bodily selves, but we have cortices that are able to make maps of all sorts of things, including maps of time. These dogs sitting by my side as I write do not have the cortical architecture (we think) to make a map of time. When the sun rises, they know I'll feed them soon, and they are excited. Each meal is like the first time they've eaten. Yet we humans often compare what is happening now with what occurred before. We may know that today is unique, but we also know that we cannot be certain of anything that life may bring. We may long for certainty, but we know that we cannot predict or control the outcome of things. We also know, because of our time-mapping cortical columns, that nothing lasts forever. Everything is transient. We all must die. My dogs are probably blessed with not having to worry about all of this.

Temporal integration is the way we differentiate our longings for certainty, permanence, and immortality from—and link them with—the reality of life's uncertainty, transience, and mortality. When people deny one or the other side of this temporal slate, rigidity or chaos can ensue. A dear friend recently had a cancer successfully removed, yet she became profoundly depressed. At fifty years of age, she told me, she had never thought she'd have to face becoming ill or dying. She actually is not that unusual, as many people deny death and live as if this will never befall them. Her depression, even in the face of her full recovery from the surgery, is an example of a rigidity that comes from impaired temporal integration. These existential issues are a theme of our common humanity and a fundamental part of the world's major religions. Learning to embrace our longing for certainty and constancy in the face of life's realities is the essence of embracing temporal integration at the heart of our human lives.

## Transpirational Integration

In my work as a psychotherapist over the past twenty-five years, I have found that using this model of integration has been a powerful way to reconceptualize human development. As people I worked with in therapy dove deeply into the eight domains just discussed, they would come to a common shift in their lives. This signaled the need to conceptualize a ninth domain of integration.

Transpirational integration signifies "breathing across" the other domains of integration—a kind of "integration of integration." This form of integration involves a person's sense of coming to feel connected to a larger whole. The "larger" here refers to a sense of belonging to something bigger than merely a bodily defined sense of self (as in vertical integration), or even to friends and family, as in interpersonal integration. Transpirational integration has the feeling that joining with others to give back to the world is as natural as taking care of oneself. For example, people may find themselves with a deep drive to help with cleaning up the local environment, reducing hunger in the community, or working to reduce child slavery or trafficking of young women. Even when the outcome of their efforts may not be known for decades, people may still feel the drive to become part of something larger than themselves—something that will make this home we share, our planet Earth, a better place for years ahead.

## INTEGRATION AND THE "SELF"

The word "self" can be misleading. For some, "self" is a personalized identity defined by the body. "I" feed "myself" dinner, meaning that this body
is eating food. But when we experience the integration of consciousness,
such as in doing the Wheel of Awareness practice, we come to distinguish
the experience of knowing (the wheel's hub) from that which is known (the
wheel's rim).[5] Many come to sense the infinite possibility of awareness contained within the differentiated inner hub. This awareness often gives rise
to a sense of knowing that the body, a point on the rim, is only one of many
ways to define what "the self" actually is. Defining the self as a singular noun
is limiting. A broader view is that a self is a part of a much larger interconnected whole: the self can be seen as a "plural verb." When we reflect on the
notion of mind as an emergent process of energy and information flow in our
bodies and in our relationships, we come to sense that our personal experience is a "node" in which energy and information flows through us, connects us to other nodes of flow, and makes us a part of a larger "mindweb" of
interconnected individuals now, and across time. Within that interconnected
whole rests the many ways we can experience our "selves" in the world.

Science reveals our deeply social and neurally embodied minds. When
we embrace this perspective, we can see how health emerges from the integration of our interpersonal and bodily selves. Studies of happiness, health,
and wisdom each reveal that positive attributes are associated with helping
others and giving back to the world. We achieve a deep sense of meaning and
accomplishment when we are devoted to something beyond our personal,
individual concerns. Integration creates health and expands our sense of who
we are in life, connecting us to others and a wider sense of ourselves. Being
compassionate to others, and to ourselves, is a natural outcome of the healthy
development of the mind. Kindness and compassion are integration made
visible. If we take on the challenge of integration across its many domains,
we may just be able to make a meaningful difference in the lives of people
here now, and for future generations to come.

# Glossary

**Action potential:** The process of the neuron in which charged particles, or ions, flow in and out of the membrane to create the equivalent of an electric flow down the long axonal length of the neuron.

**Affect:** The way an internal emotional state is externally revealed. Also called "affective expression."

**Affect regulation:** The mechanisms by which emotion and its expression are modulated.

**Alignment:** The process by which the internal state of one person is altered to reflect the internal state of another individual.

**Amygdala:** Part of the centrally located limbic regions of the brain. This almond-shaped cluster of neurons is involved in the appraisal of meaning, the processing of social signals, and the activation of emotion. Along with the orbitofrontal cortex and anterior cingulate, it plays a crucial role in coordinating perceptions with memory and behavior.

**Anterior cingulate cortex:** A curved structure at the top of the limbic area/bottom of the prefrontal region that coordinates a number of processes, including the focus of attention, the registration of bodily states (such as pain), and the social representation of interactions (such as rejection).

**Anterior insula:** The frontmost part of the **insula** (see below). It serves as a ventrolateral prefrontal region that transfers information in a vertical fashion between the cortex and the subcortical regions, including the limbic areas and the body proper.

**Apoptosis:** The diminution or pruning of synaptic connections in the absence of stimulating experience. Also called **parcellation**.

**Appraisal–arousal:** The second phase of an emotional response, following initial orientation and preceding the creation of categorical emotion.

**Attention:** The process that regulates the flow of information. Attention can be within awareness as "focal attention," or it can be outside of awareness as "nonfocal attention."

**Attractor states:** Reinforced patterns or activated states of mind that are fairly stable in specific conditions or contexts. These states "attract" particular neuron firing patterns that then reinforce their own creation. Attractor states constitute a way that a system organizes itself and achieves stability in the moment.

**Autonoesis/autonoetic consciousness:** Self-knowing awareness, associated with episodic and autobiographical memory and connected to "mental time travel"— the linkage of past, present, and anticipated future.

**Autonomic nervous system:** A system extending from the head down into the body; it regulates heart rate, respiration, and other bodily functions. Sometimes abbreviated as "ANS." A basic view of the ANS is that it consists of two branches, a sympathetic branch (the "accelerator") and a parasympathetic branch (the "brakes"). See **sympathetic nervous system** and **parasympathetic nervous system**.

**Awareness:** The mental experience of consciousness. Awareness involves a sense of knowing and often includes that which is known.

**Axon:** A long portion of a neuron, which extends from the cell body out to make synaptic connections with other neurons.

**Basal ganglia:** A set or cluster of neurons beneath the outer cortex, thought to mediate rule-guided behavior.

**Brain:** Here viewed as the extended nervous system distributed throughout the entire body and intimately interwoven with the physiology of the body as a whole. It is the embodied neural *mechanism* that shapes the flow of energy and information.

**Brainstem:** A lower brain structure, deep within the skull. It mediates states of arousal and alertness, and regulates the physiological state of the body (temperature, respiration, heart rate). It also houses the clusters of neurons that activate the fight–flight–freeze survival reactions.

**Categorical affects:** The external expressions of categorical emotions.

**Categorical emotions:** The third stage of an emotional response; they involve differentiation of initial orientation and appraisal–arousal. Sadness, anger, fear, surprise, and joy are examples of categorical emotions. See also **primary emotions** and **emotions**.

**Cell membrane:** The protein–lipid layer surrounding the cell. For the nervous system, the cell membrane functions to transfer electrochemical energy flow in the form of an action potential (ions flowing in and out of neuron through the membrane) and chemical release via neurotransmitters at the far end of the axon.

**Central nervous system:** The components of the nervous system, such as the skull-enclosed part of the brain, that connect with the peripheral nervous system (which is spread throughout the body). Sometimes abbreviated as "CNS."

**Cerebellum:** A portion of the brain at the back of the skull that plays an important role in integrating bodily information with emotional and cognitive processing.

**Circuit:** A set of interconnected neurons that are linked by genetics and experience to carry out specific functions, such as perception or action.

**Coherence:** The fluid and adaptive flow of integrated elements across time. Coherence is created across states of mind as a form of diachronic (across-time) integration.

**Cohesion:** The quality of elements sticking together. Cohesion exists within a given state of mind as a form of synchronic (in-the-moment) integration. Cohesive states of mind can be highly functional and responsive to the environment, but if they are excessively rigid and not flexible across time, they can lead to dysfunctional reactions.

**Conceptual (or categorical) representations:** Prelinguistic representations that symbolizes the mind's creation of ideas, such as notions about the mind itself. They have no direct correlates in the external, three-dimensional world and so are abstract—for example, freedom or compassion.

**Consciousness:** The subjective experience of being aware. It has two dimensions: access to information, and the phenomenal or subjective personal quality of an experience. See also **awareness**.

**Consilience:** The discovery of common findings from independent disciplines. The term was popularized by E. O. Wilson in 1998. Consilience is the intellectual approach to the field of IPNB.

**Constraints:** Factors that are modified by complex systems in order to balance continuity and flexibility. Constraints are internal (e.g., synaptic strengths) and external (e.g., interpersonal relationships). Constraints form the context that shapes the mind.

**Contingent communication:** A way in which the signals of one person are (1) perceived, (2) made sense of, and (3) responded to in a timely and effective manner. They are based on affect attunement and sensitivity to another's nonverbal signals.

**Corpus callosum:** The connecting fibers that link the left and the right hemispheres of the brain.

**Cortex:** See **neocortex**.

**Cortical consolidation:** The process by which encoded memories are integrated into cortical representations for long-term storage and are then free from dependence on the hippocampus for retrieval. It may be a fundamental outcome of dreaming and sleep.

**Corticosteroids/cortisol:** Sometimes known as the "stress hormone," cortisol is released during stress to alter metabolism in an adaptive manner.

**Default mode of the brain:** The resting state of brain function that is present when an individual is given no task to perform.

**Dendrites:** The receiving ends of neurons.

**Dorsal:** A term referring to the back of something, as opposed to the ventral side. See **ventral**.

**Dorsal dive:** The activation of the dorsal branch of the primitive vagal nerve, in which blood pressure and heart rate both drop when a sense of helplessness arises and a flaccid freeze or feigned death response is engaged. It can lead to fainting.

**Ecphoric sensation:** A feeling that a recalled memory is accurate, whether or not it is. Ecphoric sensations give the signal that something is coming from the past. *Déjà vu* may be an example of a neurologically activated ecphoric sensation in the absence of accurate recall.

**Ecphory:** The process of reactivating explicit memory when there is a match between retrieval cue and memory representation.

**Elaborative appraisals:** Brain processes that assess whether a stimulus is "good" or "bad," and that determine whether an organism should move toward or away from the stimulus.

**Emergence/emergent property:** A process arising from the interactions of a complex system's basic parts. Emergence makes the whole greater than the sum of its parts.

**Emotions:** Changes in the state of integration. Within the brain, an emotion links various systems together to form a state of mind. It also serves to connect one mind to another. Emotional processing prepares the brain and the rest of the body for action, to "evoke motion." See also **primary emotions** and **categorical emotions**.

**Emotion regulation:** See **affect regulation**.

**Encoding:** The process by which neural activation during experience alters synaptic strengths.

**Energy:** A term from physics that means the capacity to do something. Energy comes in various forms, such as kinetic, thermal, nuclear, electrical, and chemical. The nervous system functions by way of the flow of electrochemical energy.

**Engram:** The initial impact of an experience on the brain; the encoding of a new memory.

**Epigenesis:** The process in which experience alters the regulation of gene expression by way of changing the various molecules (histones and methyl groups) on the chromosome.

**Episodic memory:** The encoding, storage, and retrieval of a sense of self as experienced in one specific episode of time.

**Experience-dependent:** The form of neural growth in which novel experience induces the activation of genes to create the proteins that result in new synapse formation or synapse strengthening.

**Experience-expectant:** The form of neural growth in which synapses grow on the basis of genetic information, and the maintenance of these synapses relies upon the exposure of the organism to "expected" stimuli, such as light, sound, or caregiving. Lack of such stimuli leads to the loss of these genetically established connections.

**Explicit memory:** The layer of memory that during recall is coupled with an internal sensation of remembering. There are two forms: **semantic memory** (factual) and **episodic memory** (with repeated episodes being called "autobiographical"). The encoding or deposition of explicit memory requires focal, conscious attention. Without focal attention, or with excessive stress hormone (cortisol) release, items are not encoded explicitly but are encoded in implicit form.

**Frontal lobes:** The lobes at the front of the cerebral cortex; they make linkages among widely distributed processes fundamental to higher thinking and planning.

**Gene expression:** The process by which information on the chromosome, a gene, is transcribed into RNA and then translated into proteins so that changes in anatomic structure can be created. For the nervous system, gene expression leads to synaptic growth. Epigenetic factors regulate gene expression.

**Glial cells:** Fundamental cells of the nervous system, numbering in the trillions; they are generally smaller than neurons and carry out a number of functions. They support neurons through myelin production and regulating blood flow.

**Hippocampus:** Located in the central part of the brain, this seahorse-shaped structure is a part of the medial temporal lobe limbic area. The hippocampus plays a central role in flexible forms of memory, in the recall of facts and autobiographical details. It gives the brain a sense of the self in space and in time, regulates the order of perceptual categorizations, and links mental representations to emotional appraisal centers.

**Hypothalamic–pituitary–adrenocortical (HPA) axis:** A system that responds to stress and its function over time, which can be adversely affected by trauma.

**Hypothalamus:** Located in the lower region of the brain, near the pituitary, this structure is responsible for physiological homeostasis as a master hormone regulator.

**Implicit memory:** Involves parts of the brain that do not require conscious, focal attention during encoding or retrieval. Perceptions, emotions, bodily sensations, and behavioral response patterns are all examples of implicit layers of processing.

Mental models (schema or generalizations of repeated experiences) and priming (getting ready to respond) are basic components. Implicit memory in its unintegrated form lacks a sense that something is being recalled from the past.

**Information:** Patterns of energy that have symbolic meaning. Information is also an active process, in that it gives rise to further processing in cascades of associations and linked meanings that emerge over time.

**Insula:** A structure in the middle prefrontal cortex that links bodily processes to higher cortical areas. Information from the body streams up the spinal cord's Lamina I and reaches to the brainstem and then the insula. First the dorsal and then the right anterior part of the insula seem to be involved in the process of **interoception** (see below). Its direct link to other middle prefrontal areas, such as the anterior cingulate, by way of spindle cells has been associated with forms of self-awareness.

**Integration:** In general, the linkage of differentiated elements. The mind's process of linking differentiated parts (distinct modes of information processing) into a functional whole is postulated to be the fundamental mechanism of health. Without integration, chaos, rigidity, or both ensue. Integration is both a process and a structural dimension, and can be examined, for example, in the functional and anatomic studies of the nervous system.

**Internal working model:** A mental model derived from experiences. Repeated interaction with an attachment figure shapes a child's mental models and expectations for future interactions. These working models are open to change throughout the lifespan.

**Interoception:** The ability to know what we are feeling—to become aware of internal bodily states and affective arousal. This awareness seems to involve action of the right anterior insula in the prefrontal cortex and is correlated with the capacity for empathy for the feelings of others.

**Interpersonal neurobiology (IPNB):** A consilient field that embraces all branches of science, as it seeks the common, universal findings across independent ways of knowing in order to expand our understanding of the mind and well-being.

**Lateral prefrontal cortex:** Also known as the "dorsolateral prefrontal cortex," this region is thought to be a primary center for focal, conscious attention as it links to activities in other regions of the brain.

**Limbic regions:** Located in the central part of the brain called the medial temporal lobe, these areas include the amygdala and hippocampus; they coordinate input from the higher cortical regions, with streams of input from the lower brainstem and the body proper. Limbic structures permit integration of a wide range of mental processes, such as appraisal of meaning, processing of social signals, and the activation of emotion. The limbic area evolved during our mammalian evolution and is thought to be essential for attachment.

**Long-term potentiation:** A way in which the firing of neurons strengthens their synaptic connections to one another and increases the probability that the pattern will be repeated. Sometimes abbreviated as "LTP." This is one process by which experience leads to structural changes in the linkages among neurons during the encoding of events into long-term memory.

**Memory:** The way past events affect future function; the probability that a particular neural network pattern will be activated in the future. See also **implicit memory** and **explicit memory**.

**Mentalization:** The ability to understand other people's minds; a form of **metacognition** (see below). It is also related to theory of mind, mind-mindedness, mind perception, psychological-mindedness, reflective function, and aspects of **mindsight**.

**Metacognition:** A form of "thinking about thinking" that starts developing in the early years of life. It includes learning that there is a distinction between actual reality and the appearance of reality ("the appearance–reality distinction"); that feelings influence thinking and behavior (part of "emotional intelligence"); that what you believe and perceive and what I believe or perceive may both have validity but be different ("representational diversity"); and that what we believe at this moment may change in the future ("representational change").

**Middle prefrontal cortex:** A portion of the cerebral cortex consisting of medial, ventral, orbitofrontal, and anterior cingulate cortices. The neural circuits in this interconnected set of regions function to integrate the processing of social information, autobiographical consciousness, the evaluation of meaning, the activation of arousal, bodily response, and higher cognitive processing. Nine middle prefrontal functions are body regulation, attuned communication, emotional balance, fear modulation, flexibility of response, insight, empathy, morality, and intuition. These are the outcomes of mindfulness meditation practice and (the first eight) of secure attachment relationships.

**Mind:** A process that includes at least three fundamental aspects: (1) personal, subjective experience; (2) awareness; and (3) a regulatory function that is an emergent, self-organizing process of the extended nervous system and relationships. A core aspect of mind is defined as an embodied and relational process that *regulates* the flow of energy and information.

**Mindful awareness:** Awareness of present-moment experience, with intention and purpose, without grasping at judgments. It includes having an open stance toward oneself and others, emotional equanimity, and the ability to describe the inner world of the mind.

**Mindsight:** The ability to see the internal world of self and others, not just to observe behavior. It is the way we not only sense but also shape energy and information flow within the triangle of mind, brain, and relationships and move that flow toward integration.

**Mindsight maps:** Creating representations of the mind within the mind. Three such mindsight maps are of "me" (insight), "you" (empathy), and "we" (a sense of belonging to a larger whole).

**Modality:** An organizational functional process of the brain that links similar representation modules into a mode, such as those involving visual perception to form the visual mode. Modes or modalities can themselves be coordinated to form a "system"—in this case example, a system of cross-modality perception linking vision with hearing.

**Module:** A set of neural circuits carrying a certain type of (usually localized) information and using a similar form of neural signal or code. Modules can be linked together to form a mode; modes come together to form a system.

**Mood:** The general tone of emotions across time. A bias in the system toward certain categorical emotions. Mood shapes the interpretation of perceptual processing and gives a "slant" to thinking, self-reflection, and recollections.

**Myelin:** The fatty sheath created by glial cells that forms insulation around the long axonal lengths of neurons, so that the speed of neuronal firing is increased one hundred times and the resting or refractory period is decreased by thirty times. As a result of practice, myelin thus increases the effective communication among interconnected neurons by three thousand times, creating the enhanced functioning necessary for skill building.

**Neocortex:** Also known as the **cortex** (or "cerebral cortex"), this is the outer layer of the cerebral hemispheres. It consists of highly folded layers, usually about six cells deep, filled with "cortical columns" of highly linked neuronal clusters. Their communication with other columnar areas allows more and more complex functions to emerge. The neocortex mediates information-processing functions, such as perception, thinking, and reasoning.

**Neural integration:** Linkage of differentiated neurons within the brain. It results in optimal self-regulation with balance and coordination of disparate regions into a functional whole.

**Neural net profile:** The recruitment of various activated neuronal circuits into a localized memory representation or, more globally, into a state of mind.

**Neural network:** A set of interconnected neurons.

**Neural pathways:** A term used to denote the functional linkage of neural circuits.

**Neurobiology:** The study of how neurons work and how the nervous system functions.

**Neuron:** A basic type of cell in the nervous system. It is consists of a cell body, receiving ends called **dendrites**, and a long **axon** that reaches out to other neurons at a synaptic linkage.

**Neuroplasticity:** The overall process by which brain connections are changed by experience, including the way we pay attention.

**Noesis:** A way of knowing that can include semantic knowledge as well as nonconceptual knowing; it is the sense we have of knowing about the world and about ourselves.

**Orbitofrontal cortex:** A part of the prefrontal cortex just behind the eyes. This important region is molded by relational experience and interacts with other aspects of the middle prefrontal cortex in shaping attachment and self-awareness.

**Parallel distributed processing:** The ability of a system such as the spider-web-like brain to process different types of stimuli simultaneously across different neural networks in a rapid and highly complex manner. Sometimes abbreviated as "PDP." PDP processors, animate or inanimate, can learn from experience.

**Parasympathetic nervous system:** One of two branches of the **autonomic nervous system**. The parasympathetic branch is inhibitory and de-arousing, producing, for example, decreases in heart rate, respiration, and alertness. See also **sympathetic nervous system**.

**Parcellation:** The pruning of synaptic connections. Also called **apoptosis**.

**Perceptual representations:** Constructed bits of information created from the synthesis of present sensory experience with past memory and generalizations contained in experientially derived mental models. These representations are the essence of top-down processing, in that what we perceive is shaped by our past experiences.

**Polyvagal theory:** A theory posited by Steven Porges. According to this theory, humans have a reactive state of fight–flight–freeze and a more receptive state that activates the "social engagement system" and makes the individual open to interacting with others. "Neuroception" is the process posited by this theory, which suggests that we are continually evaluating the context of a situation for its inherent threats to survival.

**Prefrontal cortex:** Central to the processes of creating meaning and emotion and of enabling a flexibility of response, it sits at the interface between lower regions (brainstem and limbic areas) receiving input from the body and higher regions (the cortex) involved in integrating information. It includes the dorsolateral prefrontal cortex; ventral areas such as the insula; and medial structures such as the orbitofrontal cortex, the ventromedial prefrontal cortex, and, in some frameworks, the anterior cingulate cortex.

**Presymbolic representation:** A neural net profile of activation from sensory input that is as close to the input as possible, with a minimum of top-down influences from prior experience. See **sensory representation**.

**Primary emotions:** The shifts in brain state that result from the initial orientation and elaborated appraisal and arousal processes. Primary emotions are the beginning of how the mind creates meaning. They are not to be confused with categorical, or basic, emotions. See also **emotions** and **categorical emotions**.

**Recruitment:** A process that temporarily links distinct, differentiated elements into a functional whole. Emotions recruit distributed neuronal clusters to fire together into a cohesive state in the moment.

**Recursive:** The quality by which processes feed back on themselves to reinforce their own patterns of activation.

**Reentry:** A process by which positive feedback loops reinforce the initial patterns of activity, as in neural firing in the brain or in communication patterns within relationships. Reentry recursively stabilizes a neuronal firing pattern in that moment and allows the processing to become a part of conscious experience.

**Reflective function:** The ability of one person to perceive and reflect upon the mental world of the self and of other. The ability to create representations of the mind of oneself or another.

**Remembering:** The construction of a new neural net profile with features of the old engram and elements of memory from other experiences, as well as influences from the present state of mind.

**Representations:** Patterns of neural firing that serve as mental symbols. Different types of representation are processed in different parts of the brain. This term can be used for "neural representations" (neural net profiles that symbolize something) or for "mental representations" (the subjective experience of knowing something).

**Resonance:** The mutual influence of interacting systems on each other; it allows two or more entities to become a part of one functional whole.

**Resonance circuits:** Interconnected neural regions, including mirror neurons, that enable a person to tune in to others and align her internal states with others. The resonance circuits include the insula, which brings information down from the cortex to the limbic areas, the brainstem, and the body proper; then these lower inputs arise through the spinal cord to reach to the anterior insula and then to other areas of the middle prefrontal cortex, where mindsight maps of "me," "you," and "we" are constructed.

**Response flexibility:** The ability to respond flexibly and creatively to new or changing conditions instead of responding automatically and reflexively. Mediated by the middle prefrontal cortex, it allows the individual to pause and put a space between impulse and action.

**Retrieval:** The process of reactivating a neural firing pattern similar to, but never identical with, the engram first encoded for an experience.

**Semantic memory:** A form of explicit memory dealing with facts.

**Sensory representation:** The mental experience or neural firing pattern that contains information symbolizing sensations from the outside world, the body, and the brain itself.

**Somatic maps:** Representations in the brain of the physiological state of the rest of the body. A secondary somatic map is formed by the anterior insula from primary maps in the dorsal insula and allows us not only to be aware of the body's signals, but to pause and reflect on the body's input (interoception) and then do something intentionally to modify it.

**State of mind:** An overall way that mental processes, such as emotions, thought patterns, memories, and behavioral planning, are brought together into a functional and cohesive whole. A state of mind is shaped by the total pattern of activations in the brain at a particular moment. It coordinates activity in the moment, and it creates a pattern of brain activation that can become more likely in the future. States of mind allow the brain to achieve cohesion in functioning.

**State-dependent:** The process by which the context—internal and external—influences the functioning of a particular process.

**Sympathetic nervous system:** One of two branches of the **autonomic nervous system**. The sympathetic system excites and arouses, producing, for example, increases in heart rate, respiration, sweating, and states of alertness. See also **parasympathetic nervous system**.

**Subcortical:** A term referring to neural regions below the cortex, including the limbic areas and the brainstem in the skull portion of the nervous system, and sometimes also the neural processing of regions in the body proper.

**Synapse:** The linkage between two neurons. The synapse is often a small space between the end of one neuron's axons and the dendrites or cell body of another neuron; neurons communicate with each other through this space via the release of neurotransmitters from the presynaptic neuron and their reception by the receptors embedded in the membrane of the postsynaptic neuron.

**Thalamus:** A structure that sits atop the brainstem. It serves as a gateway for incoming sensory information and has extensive connections to other brain regions, including the neocortex. Activity of the thalamocortical circuit may be a central process for the mediation of conscious experience.

**Ventral:** Refers to the "belly side" of something, as opposed to the dorsal side. See **dorsal**.

**Vitality affects:** The external expression of primary emotional states.

**Working memory:** Holding something in the "front of the mind" for a brief period of time, so that the item can be the focus of attention, sorted, and altered for further information processing.

# Notes

**Preface to the First Edition**

1. Kandel (1998).
2. Stoller (1985, p. x).


**Chapter 1**

1. Wilson (1998); Slingerland and Collard (2011).
2. *Webster's New World College Dictionary* (1997, p. 1085).
3. Choudhury and Slaby (2012).
4. Meaney (2010).
5. Doidge (2007).
6. Doty (2007); Schmidt-Hellerau (2002); Shulman (2001).
7. Gazzaniga (2004).
8. Luijk et al. (2010); Meaney (2010).
9. Siegel (2010a).
10. American Psychiatric Association (2000).
11. Kandel et al. (2000).
12. Green et al. (1998, p. 427).
13. Doidge (2007).
14. Porges (2011).
15. Llinas (2002).
16. Damasio (1994/2005); Edelman (1993).
17. Zhang and Meaney (2010).
18. Teicher (2010); Teicher et al. (2004, 2006).
19. Zhang and Raichle (2010).
20. Kandel et al. (2000).
21. Achard et al. (2005).
22. Teicher (2002).
23. McGowan et al. (2009).
24. De Bellis (2005); Rees (2010).
25. Meaney (2010); Sweatt (2009); Ogren and Lombroso (2008).
26. Brown et al. (2003).

27. Szyf et al. (2010); Meaney (2010).
28. Doidge (2007).
29. Siegel (2010a).
30. Wiesel and Hubel (1963).
31. Bowlby (1969, 1988b).
32. Schick et al. (2007).
33. Kornfield (2008); Guastello et al. (2009); Howe and Lewis (2005); Lewis (2005a).
34. Zhou et al. (2006).
35. Zhou et al. (2006).
36. Kauffman (1996); Guastello et al. (2009).
37. Teicher (2010); Teicher et al. (2004/2006).
38. Zhang and Raichle (2010).
39. Bookheimer et al. (2000); Damasio (2000); Fosha et al. (2009).
40. Halpern et al. (2005); McGilchrist (2009).
41. Kagan and Snidman (2004).
42. Perry (2002); Sroufe and Siegel (2011).
43. Worthman et al. (2010).
44. Ridley (2003).
45. Doidge (2007); Begley (2007).
46. Yagmurlu and Altan (2009).
47. Howe and Lewis (2005).
48. Meaney (2010); Lewis (2005a, 2005b); Lanius et al. (2011).
49. Triandis and Suh (2002).
50. Someya et al. (2000); Eliot (2010).
51. Eliot (2010).
52. Isles and Wilkinson (2008).
53. Caspi et al. (2003); Kilpatrick et al. (2007); Munafo et al. (2009); Risch et al. (2009); Caspers et al. (2009).
54. McGowan et al. (2009); Karr, Morse, and Wiley (2012).
55. Guastello et al. (2009).
56. Holsboer (2001); Joëls et al. (2004).
57. Gross (2002).
58. McGowan et al. (2009).
59. Kagan and Fox (2006); Kagan and Snidman (2004).
60. Bradley et al. (2001); Pettit et al. (2001).
61. Rakel et al. (2009).
62. Ainsworth et al. (1978); see also Fonagy and Target (2005); Slade et al. (2005).
63. Schore (2001, 2003a, 2003b); Tronick (2007).
64. Meinz and Main (2011).
65. Fonagy and Target (2005).
66. Schore (2001, 2003a, 2003b); Tronick (2007).
67. Cozolino (2008).
68. Siegel (2010a, 2010b).
69. Siegel (2010a, 2010b); Siegel and Hartzell (2003); Siegel and Bryson (2011).
70. Guastello et al. (2009).
71. Chalmers (2007).
72. Edelman and Tononi (2000a); Merker (2007).
73. Merker (2007); Crick and Koch (2003); Edelman and Tononi (2000b).
74. Crick and Koch (2003); Derakhshan (2010).

75. Doidge (2007); Pascual-Leone et al. (2005).
76. Haggard (2008).
77. Koch and Preuschoff (2007).
78. Siegel (2010b).
79. Wallace (2010).
80. Freud (1895/1966).
81. Koch and Tsuchiya (2007).
82. Rakel et al. (2009).
83. Cortina and Liotti (2010); Trevarthen and Reddy (2006); Tronick (2007).
84. Daprati et al. (2010); Merker (2007).
85. Eisenberger and Lieberman (2004).
86. Keller (1903/2010).
87. Vygotsky (1934/1986, p. 41).
88. Posner and Rothbart (1998).
89. Anderson (2002).
90. Perner and Dienes (2003); Ferrari et al. (2001); Zelazo et al. (2007); Rakison (2007); Zelazo (2004).
91. *New Oxford American Dictionary* (2005); Princeton University (2010).
92. Saxe (2006).
93. Perner and Dienes (2003).
94. Trevarthen (2009a).
95. Perner and Dienes (2003).
96. Stern (1985).
97. Rakison (2007); Immordino-Yang (2011).
98. Kabat-Zinn (2005).
99. Siegel (2007a).
100. Brown and Ryan (2003); Davidson and Begley (2012).
101. Baer et al. (2006).
102. Urry et al. (2004).
103. Krasner et al. (2009).
104. Jacobs et al. (2011).
105. Kabat-Zinn (2005).
106. DiNoble (2009).
107. Siegel (2007a).

## Chapter 2

1. Kandel (2006).
2. Schacter et al. (2007).
3. Matyushkin (2007).
4. Tang et al. (2010); McClelland et al. (2002); Bowers (2009).
5. Kandel (2001); Barnes and Finnerty (2010).
6. Minshew and Williams (2007); Hughes (2007).
7. Bowers (2009).
8. Barnes and Finnerty (2010); Bailey and Kandel (2009); Abraham and Robins (2005); Tang et al. (2010).
9. LeBaron et al. (2008); Rosenzweig et al. (2002).
10. Milner et al. (1998, p. 463).
11. LeDoux (2003a).

12. Shatz (1992); see also Tsien (2000) and Cooper (2005).
13. Hebb (1949, pp. 69–70).
14. Freud (1888), cited in Amacher (1965); see also Doidge (2007).
15. Mechelli et al. (2004); Ganis et al. (2009).
16. Peters et al. (2009).
17. Babiloni et al. (2006); Chiu et al. (2006); Hoscheidt et al. (2010).
18. Mendelsohn et al. (2010); Raposo et al. (2009).
19. Govindarajan et al. (2006); Schafe et al. (2005).
20. Nelson and Fivush (2004).
21. Hoscheidt et al. (2010).
22. Easton and Eacott (2009); Voss and Paller (2007, 2008); Squire (2004); Paller and Wagner (2002); Paller et al. (2009).
23. Brainerd and Reyna (2004).
24. Gonsalves and Paller (2002).
25. Gerhardstein and West (2003); Repacholi and Meltzoff (2007); Hayne (2004).
26. Voss and Paller (2008); Thomson et al. (2010).
27. Salomons et al. (2004); Barnes and Finnerty (2010); Gallace and Spence (2009).
28. Bahrick and Hollich (2008); Bahrick (2004).
29. Johnson-Laird (1983).
30. Hampe and Grady (2005); Schacter et al. (2007).
31. Bayen et al. (2007).
32. Pinker (2005).
33. Zhang and Meaney (2010).
34. Belsky and Fearon (2008).
35. Fonagy et al. (2002, 2007).
36. Perry et al. (1995).
37. Carver and Cluver (2009); Newcombe et al. (2007); Marsh et al. (2008).
38. Johnson (2001).
39. Levita and Muzzio (2010).
40. Paller et al. (2009, p. 196).
41. Christakis and Fowler (2009).
42. Fivush and Nelson (2004).
43. Bauer (2006).
44. Bauer (2006); Bauer et al. (2010).
45. Howard et al. (2007); Vandekerckhove (2009); Wheeler (2000).
46. Tulving (2005); Oddo et al. (2010).
47. Nelson and Fivush (2004); Nelson (2003a).
48. Nelson (2003a, p. 3).
49. Nelson (2003a, pp. 3–4).
50. Reese and Newcombe (2007).
51. Fivush and Nelson (2006, p. 235).
52. Fivush (2011).
53. Jack et al. (2009, p. 496).
54. Fivush (2011, p. 559).
55. Ballesteros et al. (2006); Wiltgen et al. (2004); Chun and Turk-Browne (2007).
56. Baddeley (2003); Buchsbaum and D'Esposito (2009).
57. Ehlis et al. (2008); Wendelken et al. (2008).
58. Buchsbaum and D'Esposito (2009, p. 255).
59. Ranganath et al. (2005); Khader et al. (2007); Ruchkin et al. (2003).
60. Baddeley (2010); Öztekin et al. (2010).

61. Paller and Voss (2004).
62. Wiltgen et al. (2004); Hayashi et al. (2004).
63. Born (2010); Diekelmann et al. (2009).
64. Vertes and Eastman (2003); J. M. Siegel (2001).
65. Wiltgen et al. (2004).
66. Wiltgen et al. (2004).
67. Vandekerckhove (2009); Wheeler (2000); Neath (2010); Zion-Golumbic et al. (2010); Ryan et al. (2008); Burianova et al. (2010).
68. Svoboda et al. (2006, p. 2189).
69. Zion-Golumbic (2010); Ryan et al. (2008); Burianova et al. (2010); Svoboda et al. (2006); Addis et al. (2004).
70. Addis et al. (2004); Markowitsch (2003).
71. Addis et al. (2004); Ryan et al. (2008); Markowitsch (2003).
72. Markowitsch (2003); Oddo et al. (2010).
73. Natsoulas (2003); Mitchell et al. (2005); Tulving (2005).
74. Ramus et al. (2007); Schnell et al. (2007); Tsukiura and Cabeza (2008).
75. Lyons et al. (2002); Hane and Fox (2006); Minagawa-Kawai et al. (2009); Noriuchi et al. (2008).
76. Rempel-Clower (2007); Whittle et al. (2009).
77. Schore (2010); Kalin et al. (2007); Schwartz et al. (2010).
78. Willis et al. (2010); Beer (2007); McDonald (2007).
79. Sutton (2010).
80. Polyn et al. (2009); Steinvorth et al. (2005).
81. Markowitsch et al. (2003).
82. Storm et al. (2005).
83. Squire et al. (2007).
84. Freud (1895/1966); see Christianson and Lindholm (1998).
85. Wang (2008a); Howe (2003, 2004).
86. Bauer (2008); Hayne (2004).
87. Hudson and Mayhew (2009).
88. Bauer et al. (2010).
89. Bauer (2007).
90. Thompson and Madigan (2007).
91. Bauer et al. (2010).
92. Thompson and Madigan (2007); Bauer et al. (2010).
93. Morrison and Conway (2010).
94. Hayne and Simcock (2009).
95. Reese and Newcombe (2007).
96. Bergen (2009).
97. Bauer et al. (1998, p. 677).
98. Oliver and Plomin (2007).
99. Strayer and Roberts (2004); Saarni (2007).
100. Nisbett and Miyamoto (2005).
101. Morris et al. (2007).
102. Lyons et al. (2002).
103. Nelson and Carver (1998, pp. 798–799); see also Howe et al. (2009); Wang et al. (2007).
104. Levine et al. (2009).
105. de Quervain et al. (2007); Kensinger (2004).
106. Elzinga et al. (2005, p. 211).

107. Clarke and Butler (2008).
108. Turk-Browne et al. (2006); Degonda et al. (2005); de Quervain et al. (2009); Clarke and Butler (2008); Chun and Turk-Browne (2007); Elzinga et al. (2005).
109. van Stegeren et al. (2010).
110. LaBar and Cabeza (2006).
111. McGaugh (1992, pp. 261–262).
112. Cicchetti and Curtis (2006); Barco et al. (2008); Sweatt (2004); Doidge (2007); Kandel (2001).
113. Doidge (2007); Weinberger (2008).
114. McLin et al. (2002).
115. Doidge (2007).
116. Post et al. (1998, p. 849); see also Fitzgerald et al. (2006).
117. de Quervain et al. (2009).
118. McEwen (2008); Lupien et al. (2004).
119. Wang et al. (2010); Frodi (2010); Shin et al. (2006).
120. Siegel (1995a, 1996, 2001b); Sigman and Siegel (1992); Elzinga and Bremner (2002); Rodrigues et al. (2009); Roozendaal et al. (2007); Phelps (2004).
121. Bower and Sivers (1998, p. 631).
122. Lupien et al. (2004); Kim and Diamond (2002); Elzinga and Bremner (2002); Packard and Cahill (2001).
123. Clarke and Butler (2008).
124. Amir et al. (2010).
125. Lensvelt-Mulders et al. (2008); Marmar et al. (2006); Briere et al. (2005); van der Velden and Wittman (2008); Wittmann et al. (2006).
126. Wang et al. (2010); Frodi et al. (2010); Shin et al. (2006).
127. Heim et al. (2008).
128. Heim et al. (2008); Talbot et al. (2009).
129. McGaugh et al. (2006); Wiltgen et al. (2004).
130. Sterpenich et al. (2009); Diekelmann et al. (2009).
131. Tulving et al. (1994); Wheeler et al. (1997).
132. Babiloni et al. (2006); Habib et al. (2003).
133. Spaniola et al. (2009).
134. Kinsbourne (1972).
135. O'Neill et al. (2010); Diekelmann and Born (2010); Axmacher et al. (2009).
136. Axmacher et al. (2009).
137. Gaensbauer and Jordan (2009); Dalgleish et al. (2008).
138. Schore (2009a).
139. Teicher et al. (2004); Jackowski et al. (2009); Karl et al. (2006).
140. Spaniola et al. (2009); Eustache and Desgranges (2008).
141. Bremner (2007); Shin et al. (2006).
142. Jackowski et al. (2009); Teicher et al. (2006).
143. Elzinga et al. (2005); Amir et al. (2010).
144. de Quervain et al. (2009); Rauch et al. (2006); Liberzon and Sripada (2007).
145. Brewin (2007); McNally and Geraerts (2009).
146. Karpinski and Scullin (2009).
147. Loftus (2006); Geraerts et al. (2008).
148. Cicchetti and Toth (1998).
149. Fivush (1998, p. 713).
150. Christianson and Lindholm (1998, pp. 774, 776).
151. Henry (2009); Fox and Hoelscher (2010).

152. Lynch and Cicchetti (1998, p. 744).
153. Teicher (2010).
154. Lynch and Cicchetti (1998, pp. 756–757).
155. Bremner and Narayan (1998, p. 881–882).
156. Hauser et al. (2007); McAdams (2001).
157. Bruner (2003); Nelson (2006); Bauer et al. (2010).
158. Anderson-Fye (2010).
159. Wang (2006).
160. Fivush et al. (2010).
161. Wang (2006, p. 1804).
162. Vygotsky (1934/1986).
163. Hammack (2008); McLean et al. (2007); Conway and Pleydell-Pearce (2000).
164. Conway et al. (2005, pp. 337–338); see also Wang (2001, 2004); Wang and Brockmeier (2002).
165. Markus and Kitayama (1991).
166. Conway et al. (2005, p. 747); see also Conway et al. (2002); Wang and Conway (2004).
167. Bruner (2003); McAdams (2001).
168. Nelson (2006).
169. Mar (2004); Colle et al. (2007); Gal et al. (2009).
170. Riessman (2003).
171. Mar (2004); Pasupathi et al. (2007).
172. Reed (1994, p. 278).

## Chapter 3

1. Main (1999); Simpson and Belsky (2008).
2. Hofer (2006).
3. Ainsworth (1988).
4. Siegel and Hartzell (2003).
5. Bowlby (1969, 1988a).
6. Main et al. (2005); Cicchetti et al. (1995); Sroufe et al. (2005).
7. Main (1996).
8. Main et al. (2005).
9. Greenberg et al. (2001).
10. Weinfield et al. (2008); Margalit (2004).
11. Weinfield et al. (2008, p. 90).
12. Gillath et al. (2006); Edelstein and Gillath (2008).
13. Cassidy and Shaver (2008); Mikulincer and Shaver (2007); Hazan et al. (2006); Roisman et al. (2007a, 2008).
14. Trevarthen (1993).
15. Trevarthen (1993).
16. Stern (1985); Haft and Slade (1989).
17. Ainsworth (1988); Tronick (2007).
18. Fosha et al. (2009); Ferber (2008).
19. Schore (2001).
20. Schore (2000).
21. Tronick (2007).
22. Stern (1985); Sroufe et al. (2005).

23. Bowlby (1988b); see also Ainsworth (1993).
24. Bowlby (1988a).
25. Schore (1994).
26. Bretherton and Munholland (2008).
27. Main (1995).
28. Belsky and Fearon (2008).
29. van IJzendoorn et al. (2006).
30. Hrdy (2009).
31. Main (1999).
32. Ainsworth et al. (1978).
33. Ainsworth et al. (1978).
34. Main and Solomon (1986).
35. Main et al. (2003); Solomon and George (2008); Hesse (1999a).
36. Sroufe et al. (2005); Jimerson et al. (2000).
37. Simpson and Belsky (2008); Dozier and Rutter (2008); Dozier et al. (2001); Steele et al. (2008).
38. Dozier et al. (2001); Dozier and Rutter (2008).
39. Bowlby (1988a).
40. Cicchetti et al. (2006).
41. Sroufe et al. (2005); Waters et al. (2000); Main et al. (2005); Grossman et al. (2005).
42. Siegel (2001a); Hofer (2006).
43. Hesse et al. (2010); Ainsworth (1988).
44. Ainsworth et al. (1978).
45. van IJzendoorn and Bakermans-Kranenburg (2008).
46. Main et al. (2005).
47. Main et al. (2005).
48. Main et al. (2005).
49. Hesse and Main (2006); Main et al. (2005).
50. Main et al. (2005); van IJzendoorn and Bakermans-Kranenburg (2006).
51. Vaughn et al. (2008); Moriceau and Sullivan (2005); Bokhorst et al. (2003).
52. van IJzendoorn and Bakermans-Kranenburg (2006).
53. McGowan et al. (2009).
54. Polan and Hofer (2008); Gervai (2009).
55. Lickliter (2008).
56. Bokhorst et al. (2003, p. 1769).
57. Cyr et al. (2010).
58. Madigan et al. (2006).
59. Schore (2003a, 2003b); Tronick (2007); Cozolino (2006).
60. Main and Hesse (1990).
61. Liotti (1992); Main and Morgan (1996).
62. Main et al. (1985).
63. George et al. (1996).
64. George et al. (1996); Steele and Steele (2008).
65. Steele and Steele (2008); Hesse (2008); Bakermans-Kranenburg and van IJzendoorn (2009).
66. Brennan (1998); Roisman et al. (2007b, 2008).
67. Steele and Steele (2008); Main et al. (2005).
68. Hesse (1999b); de Haas et al. (1994).
69. Hesse (2008).

70. Waters et al. (2000); Weinfield et al. (2008); Sroufe et al. (2005); Main et al. (2005).
71. Bokhorst et al. (2003); Dozier et al. (2001); Dozier et al. (2008); Steele et al. (2003).
72. Siegel (2010a, 2010b); see also Steele and Steele (2008).
73. Hesse (2008); Main et al. (2005).
74. Sagi et al. (1994); Bakermans-Kranenburg and van IJzendoorn (1993).
75. Madigan et al. (2006).
76. Fonagy and Target (2005); Grienenberger et al. Slade (2005); Oppenheim and Koren-Karie (2002), Oppenheim et al. (2004); van IJzendoorn et al. (2006); Bernier and Dozier (2003); Goldberg et al. (2003); Lyons-Ruth et al. (2005); Berlin et al. (2008).
77. Siegel and Hartzell (2003).
78. Meinz and Main (2011).
79. Bakermans-Kranenburg and van IJzendoorn (2008).
80. Ellis et al. (2011).
81. Main et al. (2005).
82. Main et al. (2003).
83. Steele and Steele (2008); Main et al. (2005).
84. Main et al. (2005).
85. Main et al. (2005).
86. Hesse (1996).
87. Grice (1975).
88. Main and Goldwyn (1998, p. 46).
89. Main and Goldwyn (1998).
90. Hesse and Main (2000); Hesse et al. (2003); Hesse (2008).
91. Gloger-Tippelt et al. (2002).
92. Gloger-Tippelt et al. (2002).
93. Slade et al. (2005); Steele and Steele (2008); van IJzendoorn and Bakermans-Kranenburg (2008); Hesse (2008).
94. Main et al. (2005); Hughes et al. (2006).
95. Main et al. (2005).
96. van IJzendoorn et al. (2008); Barone (2003).
97. Main et al. (2005); Vaughn et al. (2008); Sroufe et al. (2005).
98. Weinfield et al. (2004).
99. Sroufe et al. (2005); Main et al. (2005).
100. Vaughn et al. (2008); Belsky and Fearon (2008); Mangelsdorf et al. (2000).
101. Wade and Kendler (2000).
102. Bokhorst et al. (2003); Dozier and Rutter (2008); Stovall-McClough and Dozier (2004).
103. van IJzendoorn et al. (2006).
104. van IJzendoorn et al. (2006).
105. Hazan et al. (2006).
106. Ainsworth (1988, p. 1).
107. Main et al. (2005).
108. Ammaniti et al. (2000).
109. Main (1995); Benoit et al. (1992); Crowell et al. (1992); Greenberg et al. (1997).
110. See, e.g., Cassidy and Shaver (2008).
111. Dozier and Rutter (2008); Schore (2001); Hofer (2006).
112. Wallis and Steele (2001); Riggs and Jacobvitz (2002); Patrick et al. (1994); Kobak et al. (1991); Fonagy et al. (2008).

113. Sroufe et al. (2005); Bateman and Fonagy (2008); Muris et al. (2004); DeKlyen and Greenberg (2008).
114. DeKlyen and Greenberg (2008).
115. MacDonald et al. (2008, p. 493); see also Schore (2002); Hesse et al. (2003); van der Kolk (2003).
116. Noll-Hussong et al. (2010); Trickett et al. (2010); Swain et al. (2007); Dozier et al. (2006); Solomon and Siegel (2003); Fearon et al. (2010).
117. Berlin et al. (2008); Cicchetti et al. (2006); Fonagy et al. (2008).
118. Main (1995).
119. Rentesi et al. (2010, p. 7).
120. Llorente et al. (2010b); Lovic (2010).
121. Choy and van den Buuse (2007); Llorente et al. (2010a).
122. Polan and Hofer (2008); Rentesi et al. (2010).
123. Chen et al. (2010).
124. Brodsky and Lombroso (1998, pp. 2, 3).
125. Doidge (2007); Greenberg (2010).
126. Teicher and Andersen (2009); Andersen et al. (2008).
127. Glaser et al. (2006, p. 229).
128. Schore (1997, p. 618).
129. Schore (1996).
130. Worthman et al. (2010).
131. Doidge (2007).
132. MacDonald et al. (2008); Schore (2002); Palaszynski and Nemeroff (2009).
133. Berlin et al. (2008); Main et al. (2005).
134. Dozier et al. (2008); Green and Goldwyn (2002); Brown and Wright (2003).
135. DeKlyen and Greenberg (2008); Dozier and Rutter (2008).
136. Warren et al. (2000); Sroufe et al. (2005).
137. Renken et al. (1989).
138. Carlson (1998).
139. Madigan et al. (2007); see also Zajac and Kobak (2009); van IJzendoorn and Bakermans-Kranenburg (2006); Meins et al. (2001); Moran et al. (2008).
140. Madigan et al. (2006.); van IJzendoorn and Bakermans-Kranenburg (2008).
141. Berlin et al. (2008); Meloy (2003); van IJzendoorn and Bakermans-Kranenburg (2006).
142. Main et al. (2005); Schore and Schore (2008).
143. Main (1995, p. 451).
144. Schore (2000).
145. Ainsworth et al. (1978); see also de Wolff and van IJzendoorn (1997).
146. Fonagy and Target (2005); Slade et al. (2005); Bowlby (1988a).
147. Fonagy and Target (2005).
148. Fonagy and Target (2005); Legerstee et al. (2007); Markova and Legerstee (2006).
149. Tronick (2007, 2009).
150. Tronick (2007); Fosha et al. (2009).
151. Schore (2003a, 2003b).
152. Tronick (2009); Palombo et al. (2009).
153. Ainsworth (1988); Hazan et al. (2006).
154. Peterson et al. (2006).
155. Main et al. (2003).
156. Hesse (1996).

157. Siegel and Hartzel (2003); Hesse et al. (2003); Hesse (2008); Wallin (2007).
158. Fonagy and Target (2005); Allen et al. (2008).
159. Main (1995).
160. Main et al. (2003, 2005); Roisman et al. (2002).
161. Pearson et al. (1994); Benoit (2009); Roisman et al. (2002).
162. Pearson et al. (1994); Benoit (2009); Roisman et al. (2002).
163. Roisman et al. (2002, 2007a); Hesse (2008); Conradi and de Jonge (2009); Pearson et al. (1994).
164. Pearson et al. (1994); Conradi and de Jonge (2009); Roisman et al. (2002).
165. Main et al. (2005).
166. Fox and Hane (2008); Hill–Soderlund et al. (2008).
167. Ainsworth et al. (1978).
168. Main et al. (2005).
169. Solomon and George (2008); George and West (2003).
170. Fonagy and Target (2005); Main et al. (2005).
171. Main et al. (2003).
172. Bowlby (1969).
173. Hill–Soderlund et al. (2008).
174. Allen et al. (2008); Fonagy and Target (2005); Fonagy (2001).
175. Edelstein and Gillath (2008); Haggerty et al. (2010).
176. Edelstein and Gillath (2008); Haggerty et al. (2010); Courage and Howe (2010).
177. Sroufe et al. (2010).
178. Sroufe et al. (2005).
179. Siegel (2010a); Murray et al. (2007).
180. Tyron and McKay (2009).
181. Schacter (1996); Rubin (1986); Burt (2008).
182. Wheeler et al. (1997).
183. Wheeler et al. (1997); Kinsbourne (1972).
184. M. Main and E. Hesse (personal communication, 1999).
185. Behrens et al. (2011, p. 1003).
186. LaBar and Cabeza (2006); Schmidt and Saari (2007).
187. Sergerie et al. (2006); Paz et al. (2006).
188. Thomsen and Berntsen (2008).
189. Main (1996).
190. Ainsworth et al. (1978).
191. Main (1995).
192. Sroufe et al. (2005); Siegel (2004).
193. Aitken and Trevarthen (1997).
194. Stern (1985).
195. Main (1991); Bowlby (1973).
196. Main (1991).
197. Main et al. (2003).
198. Main and Goldwyn (1998).
199. Hesse et al. (2003); Siegel (2004).
200. Johns and Mewhort (2009); Huber et al. (2008).
201. Lang et al. (2001).
202. Hesse (1996); see also Bretherton and Munholland (2008).
203. Coan (2008); Schore (2001).
204. Main et al. (2003).
205. Solomon and George (2008).

206. Liotti (1992); Main and Hesse (1990).
207. Main and Hesse (1990); see also Lyons-Ruth and Jacobvitz (2008).
208. Main (1995); Hesse (1999b); see also Lyons-Ruth and Jacobvitz (2008).
209. Lyons-Ruth and Jacobvitz (2008); Cyr et al. (2010); Main et al. (2005).
210. Lyons-Ruth and Jacobvitz (2008); Main et al. (2005).
211. Putnam and Carlson (1998).
212. Main et al. (2005).
213. Sroufe et al. (2005); Zilberstein and Messer (2010).
214. Atkinson and Goldberg (2004); Fosha (2003).
215. Toth et al. (2009).
216. Main et al. (2005).
217. Siegel (2001b).
218. Hesse and Main (2000); Hesse and Main (2006); see also Abrams et al. (2006);
     Madigan et al. (2006).
219. Madigan et al. (2006).
220. Main et al. (2005); Hesse (2008).
221. Main et al. (2003).
222. Siegel (2001b, 2010a).
223. Moran et al. (2005); Moran et al. (2008).
224. Hesse and van IJzendoorn (1998).
225. Riggs et al. (2007).
226. Walker (2007).
227. Hesse and Main (1999).
228. MacDonald et al. (2008); Madigan et al. (2007).
229. Madigan et al. (2006).
230. Hesse (1996).
231. Siegel (1996a, 1996b).
232. Main and Hesse (1990); Hesse and Main (2000).
233. Jacobvitz et al. (2006); Madigan et al. (2006).
234. Abrams et al. (2006).
235. Keller et al. (2006).
236. Siegel (1996a).
237. Perry et al. (1995).
238. Lyons-Ruth and Jacobvitz (2008).
239. Yehuda and McFarlane (1995).
240. Lyons-Ruth and Jacobvitz (2008).
241. Schore (2001); Meaney (2010); Teicher et al. (2003).

## Chapter 4

1. Carlson (2007).
2. Frederick (2009).
3. Walden and Kim (2005); Nichols et al. (2010).
4. Fosha et al. (2009).
5. Davidson et al. (2003b).
6. Hariman and Lucaites (2008).
7. Panksepp (1998); Borod (2000).
8. LeDoux (1996); Brothers (1997).
9. Pessoa (2008); Davidson et al. (2003c).

10. Lewis et al. (2008).
11. Davidson et al. (2003c); Kober et al. (2008).
12. Stemmler (2003).
13. van Kleef et al. (2010).
14. Bar (2009).
15. Panksepp (2009).
16. Porges (2009).
17. Dodge (1991, p. 159).
18. Sroufe (1996, p. 15).
19. Siegel (2009a).
20. Pessoa (2008, p. 148).
21. Bradley (2008); Carlson (2007).
22. Ellsworth and Scherer (2003); Bradley (2008).
23. Ellsworth and Scherer (2003); Davidson et al. (2003a); Balcani and Mazza (2009).
24. Ellsworth and Scherer (2003).
25. Bradley (2008, p. 1).
26. Newman and Lorenz (2003).
27. Sroufe (1996).
28. Davidson et al. (2003a).
29. Siegel (2010a).
30. Derryberry and Reed (2003); Kagan (2003).
31. Rubin et al. (2009).
32. Matsumoto et al. (2009).
33. Kagan (2010).
34. Ellsworth and Scherer (2003); Barrett et al. (2009); Davidson et al. (2003b).
35. Ekman and Lama (2009); Levenson (2003).
36. Barrett (2006, p. 20).
37. Damasio et al. (2003).
38. Ellsworth and Scherer (2003).
39. Damasio et al. (2003).
40. Roberson et al. (2007).
41. Sauter et al. (2009).
42. van Bakel and Riksen-Walraven (2008); Haley and Stransbury (2003).
43. Leppänen (2006); Venn et al. (2006); Milders et al. (2010); Phillips et al. (2003).
44. George et al. (1997).
45. Johnson et al. (2000); Harkess and Tucker (2000).
46. Trevarthen (2009a); Behrens et al. (2007).
47. van Bakel and Riksen-Walraven (2008); Haley and Stansbury (2003).
48. Damasio et al. (2000).
49. Schore (1998); LeDoux (1996).
50. Rolls and Grabenhorst (2008).
51. Wataru et al. (2004).
52. Mesquita et al. (2010).
53. Siegel (2007a).
54. Schmitz and Johnson (2006); Craig (2010); Critchley et al. (2004).
55. Craig (2002); Davidson et al. (2003a).
56. Rolls and Grabenhorst (2008); Bechara et al. (2000).
57. Critchley (2005).
58. Berridge (2003).

59. Carlson (2007); Rolls and Grabenhorst (2008); Bechara et al. (2000).
60. Davis (1992); Lieberman et al. (2005); LeDoux (2003b).
61. Dębiec and LeDoux (2009).
62. Porges (2011).
63. Carlson (2007); van IJzendoorn et al. (2010).
64. Velmans (2009).
65. Sinnet et al. (2009); Miller and Cohen (2001); Ochsner and Schacter (2003).
66. Tanji and Hoshi (2008).
67. Llinas (2008).
68. Crick (1994); Llinas (1990).
69. Grossberg (1999); Raffone and Pantani (2010).
70. Edelman and Tononi (2000a, 2000b).
71. Miller and Cohen (2001).
72. Kringelbach (2005); Fuster (2008); Mayer et al. (2000).
73. Craig (2009).
74. Craig (2009).
75. James (1884); Panksepp (1982); Panksepp and Biven (2012); Davidson and Begley (2012).
76. Ellsworth and Scherer (2003).
77. Poldrack et al. (2008); Roozendaal et al. (2009).
78. Haxby et al. (2002).
79. Forgas (2008).
80. Diamond (2006); Posner et al. (2005); Pollak (2005).
81. Gallese et al. (1996).
82. Mukamel et al. (2010).
83. Carr et al. (2003).
84. Mukamel et al. (2010).
85. Meltzoff et al. (2009); Shimada and Hiraki (2006).
86. Mukamel et al. (2010, p. 750).
87. Berridge (2003).
88. Siegel (2007a).
89. Siegel (2007a); Ochsner and Schacter (2003).
90. Happaney et al. (2004); Ochsner and Schacter (2003); Perlman and Pelphrey (2010); Davidson et al. (2003a).
91. Siegel (2010a); Decety and Michalska (2010).
92. Happaney et al. (2004).
93. Ochsner and Schacter (2003).
94. Cheng et al. (2010); Jackson et al. (2006); Siegel (2007a).
95. Janig (2003).
96. Hardan (2006); Girgis et al. (2007).
97. Perlman and Pelphrey (2010).
98. Nobre et al. (1999, p. 12).
99. Siegel (2007a); Ghahremani et al. (2010).
100. Mesulam (1998, p. 1013).
101. Main (1991, 1995, 1996, 2000).
102. Hesse (1996).
103. Schore (2005).
104. Happaney et al. (2004).
105. Carlson (2007); Ochsner and Schacter (2003).
106. Kühn et al. (2010); Stemmler (2003); Mori and Mori (2009).

107. Kringelbach (2005); Critchley (2005, 2009); McGilchrist (2009).
108. Blakeslee and Blakeslee (2007).
109. Critchley (2005).
110. Rose and Rudolph (2006).
111. Rose and Rudolph (2006).
112. Taylor et al. (2000, 2002).
113. Sowell (2011).
114. Iacoboni (2009a, 2009b).
115. Green and Phillips (2004); Bloch (2008).
116. Carlson (2007).
117. Trevarthen (2009a).
118. Mehrabian (2008); Reilly and Seibert (2003).
119. Carlson (2007); Damasio et al. (2003).
120. Schore (2003b; 2009b).
121. Springer and Deutsch (1993); Nass and Koch (1991).
122. Krohne (2003); Rotenber (2004).
123. Krohne (2003); Davidson and Begley (2012).
124. Ross et al. (2007).
125. Damasio et al. (2003).
126. Fox (1994); Davidson and Begley (2012).
127. McManis et al. (2002).
128. Diego et al. (2006); Field and Diego (2008).
129. Levitin (2006).
130. Alossa and Castelli (2009).
131. Pessoa (2008).
132. Buckner and Carroll (2006); Lebreton et al. (2008); McGilchrist (2009).
133. McGilchrist (2009).
134. Schore (2009b).
135. Lewis (1995); Fox (1994).
136. Ross et al. (2007).
137. Schore (2009b); Cozolino (2006); Badenoch (2011).
138. Mcquaid et al. (2007).
139. Baer et al. (2006).
140. DiNoble (2009).
141. Cresswell et al. (2007).
142. Gross and Thompson (2007).
143. Sroufe (1996, p. 159).
144. Calkins (1994).

# Chapter 5

1. Plaut and McClelland (2010); Szu-Han and Morris (2010); Rogers and McClelland (2008); Tse et al. (2007); McClelland and Rogers (2003); Raffone and Van Leeuwen (2001).
2. Thagard (2002).
3. Eggermont (2005); Globerson et al. (2009); Brenner et al. (2000); Jacobs et al. (2009); Bell (2007); Furber et al. (2007).
4. Anders et al. (2008).
5. Voss and Paller (2007, 2009).

6. Perry (2002); Baccus and Horowitz (2005); Horowitz (2001).
7. Fuster (2006, 2009).
8. Kawasaki et al. (2005); Erk et al. (2006); Longe et al. (2009); Ochsner et al. (2009).
9. Beer et al. (2006).
10. van der Kolk et al. (2005); van der Kolk and Courtois (2005); Bluhm et al. (2009).
11. Livneh and Parker (2005); Vallacher et al. (2002); Witherington (2007).
12. McClelland et al. (2002); McClelland Rogers (2003); Boldrini et al. (1998).
13. Kröger (2007); Neme and Mireles (2008); Cicchetti and Rogosch (1997b).
14. Kauffman (1996); Lewis and Granic (2000); Cicchetti and Rogosch (1997a); Kroger (2007); Fonagy and Target (2007).
15. Guastello et al. (2009).
16. Guastello et al. (2009); Sulis and Trofimova (2001); Ward (2002).
17. Doebeli (1993).
18. Pinker (2005); Sherwood et al. (2008); Frankenhuis and Ploeger (2007); Goldsmith (2009); Buller (2009).
19. Bowers (2009); Plaut and McClelland (2010); Botvinick and Plaut (2009).
20. McClelland and Rumelhart (1986).
21. Plaut and McClelland (2010); Bowers (2009); Sporns (2010).
22. Mercado (2008); Gilson et al. (2009).
23. Rimol et al. (2010).
24. Sherwood et al. (2008); Riegler (2008).
25. Holtmaat and Svoboda (2009); Trachtenberg et al. (2002).
26. Robertson and Combs (1995).
27. Boldrini et al. (1998, p. 25).
28. Globus and Arpaia (1993).
29. Thelen and Smith (1994); see Dawson-Tunik et al. (2004).
30. Shatz (1990); personal communication October 15, 2011.
31. Post and Weiss (1997, p. 911; emphasis added).
32. Fogel et al. (2002); Anderson (2002).
33. American Psychiatric Association (2000).
34. Sporns (2010).
35. Cicchetti and Rogosch (2009).
36. Zhang and Raichle (2010); Raichle (2010); Raichle and Snyder (2007); Fox and Greicius (2010).
37. Chepenik et al. (2010).
38. Bluhm et al. (2009).
39. Teicher (2000, 2002); Teicher et al. (2002, 2003, 2004); Andersen and Teicher (2004).
40. Guastello et al. (2009); Fogel et al. (1997); Globus and Arpaia (1993); Chamberlain (1995); Jackson (1991); March and Mulle (1998).
41. Fairfax (2008); Simon et al. (2010); Ursu and Carter (2009).
42. Coan (2010).
43. Garcia-Toroa and Aguirre (2007); Normann et al. (2007).
44. Ammaniti and Trentini (2009).
45. Shmueli-Goetz et al. (2008); Fonagy et al. (2007); Fonagy and Target (2005).
46. Eisenberger et al. (2007).
47. Cohan et al. (2006); Eisenberger et al. (2011).
48. Fonagy et al. (2003); Hesse and Main (2000, 2006).

49. Friedman et al. (2010); Ritter et al. (2007); Crown et al. (2002); Beebe et al. (2005).
50. Lewis et al. (2006); Howe and Lewis (2005); Lewis (2005b); Lamm and Lewis (2010).
51. Woltering and Lewis (2009, p. 160).
52. Fogel (2000a, 2000b); Hsu and Fogel (2003).
53. Schore (1997, p. 600); see also Schore (2009a).
54. Shinbrot et al. (1993).
55. Lewis (2005b, p. 272).
56. Boldrini et al. (1998, p. 25).
57. Lewis (2005b, p. 272; emphasis in original).
58. Ridout et al. (2009); Guyer et al. (2007); Surguladze et al. (2004); Gollan et al. (2008).
59. Hofer (1990, p. 74).
60. Harter (2012); Harter (1988); Harter et al. (1997).
61. Harter et al. (1997); Pfeifer et al. (2009).
62. Pfeifer et al. (2009).
63. Sroufe (1996).
64. Kim and Cicchetti (2010); Alink et al. (2009); Kim et al. (2009).
65. Harter et al. (1997).
66. Harter et al. (1997).
67. Harter (2012).
68. Walsh et al. (2010); van IJzendoorn et al. (2010).
69. Belsky et al. (2007); Bakermans-Kranenburg and van IJzendoorn (2007, 2011); Bakermans-Kranenburg et al. (2008); Ellis et al. (2011).
70. Tronick (2007).
71. Cicchetti and Rogosch (1997b).
72. McGowan et al. (2009).
73. Siegel (2007a).
74. O'Donohue (1997, pp. 101, 118).
75. Chamberlain (1995); Howe and Lewis (2005).

## Chapter 6

1. Liu et al. (2010); Perani et al. (2010); Halpern et al. (2005).
2. Morris et al. (2006).
3. Jermakowicz and Casagrande (2007).
4. deCharms and Zador (2000).
5. Doidge (2007).
6. Pinker (1999); for an opposing view, see Fodor (2000).
7. Sahin et al. (2009).
8. Barsalou et al. (2003); van Dantzig et al. (2008).
9. Farb et al. (2007); Siegel (2007a, 2007b, 2010b).
10. Mesquita et al. (2010).
11. Uddin et al. (2007); Iacoboni (2008); Craig (2010).
12. Edelman (1993).
13. Edelman and Tononi (2000a).
14. Edelman and Tononi (2000b, p. 144; emphasis in original).
15. Edelman and Tononi (2000a).

16. Wheeler et al. (1997); see also Lemmon and Moore (2001); Quoidbach et al. (2008); Piolino et al. (2009).
17. Vandekerckhove (2009); Lemmon and Moore (2001).
18. Buckner (1996); see also Ferbinteanu et al. (2006); Kircher and David (2003).
19. Nisbett and Miyamoto (2005); see *http://cbd.ucla.edu* for more information.
20. Trevarthen (1990b, p. 357); see also Fonagy et al. (2007); Trevarthen (2005a).
21. Trevarthen (2001, 2009a).
22. Trevarthen (1996, p. 583).
23. McGilchrist (2009); Halpern et al. (2005).
24. Trevarthen (1996, 2005a, 2009b); McGilchrist (2009); Hugdahl and Davidson (2003).
25. McGilchrist (2009); Hugdahl and Westerhausen (2010).
26. Tucker et al. (1995, pp. 233–234); see also Scherf et al. (2007).
27. Tucker et al. (1995, p. 222).
28. Tucker et al. (1995, p. 223); see also Tang (2003).
29. McGilchrist (2009); Hugdahl and Westerhausen (2010).
30. Springer and Deutsch (1993); McGilchrist (2009).
31. McGilchrist (2009); Hugdahl and Davidson (2003); Hugdahl and Westerhausen (2010).
32. Toga and Thompson (2003).
33. Buck and VanLear (2002).
34. Ornstein et al. (1979); Buck and VanLear (2002).
35. Stroganova et al. (2004).
36. Hugdahl and Westerhausen (2010); Yoshida et al. (2007); Evert and Emen (2003).
37. Gazzaniga (2004); Leclercq (2002).
38. Gazzaniga (1996).
39. Sato and Aoki (2006); Gainotti (2005).
40. Damasio (2001); Adolphs and Damasio (2000).
41. Indersmitten and Gur (2003); Heilman et al. (2000); Porges (2011).
42. Eckert et al. (2009); Vanderhasselt et al. (2007).
43. Craig (2002).
44. Ustinova et al. (2001); Schore (2003b); Wager et al. (2008).
45. Kimura et al. (2004); Sato and Aoki (2006); Tapiero and Fillon (2007).
46. Balconi and Lucchiari (2008).
47. Alfano and Cimino (2008); Hofman (2009); Tondowski et al. (2007); Smith and Bulman-Fleming (2004, 2005, 2006); Balconi and Lucchiari (2008).
48. Smith and Bulman-Fleming (2005); Schultheiss et al. (2009).
49. Alfano and Cimino (2008, p. 219; emphasis in original).
50. Harmon-Jones et al. (2010); Hane et al. (2008); Maxwell and Davidson (2007); Balconi and Mazza (2009).
51. Harmon-Jones et al. (2010, p. 61).
52. Urry et al. (2004).
53. Ross et al. (1994).
54. Ross et al. (2007).
55. Keenan et al. (2001).
56. Ross et al. (2007).
57. Narumoto et al. (2001); Sim and Martinez (2005).
58. Goel et al. (2004); Fournier et al. (2008); Mason and Macrae (2004); Carrington and Bailey (2008).

59. Ashman et al. (2008); Forbes et al. (2006); Allen and Kline (2004); Jones et al. (2004).
60. Ashman et al. (2008); Field et al. (2005).
61. Jones et al. (2004).
62. Newman et al. (2002).
63. Newman et al. (2002).
64. Schick et al. (2007).
65. Thatcher et al. (1987); Chiron et al. (1997).
66. Teicher et al. (2006).
67. Teicher et al. (2006).
68. Thatcher (2007).
69. DeOliveira et al. (2005); Moran et al. (2008).
70. Fonagy et al. (2007).
71. Carrington and Bailey (2008).
72. Carrington and Bailey (2008).
73. Fonagy et al. (2007); Gergely and Unoka (2008).
74. Aitken and Trevarthen (1997, pp. 653–654).
75. Brazelton and Greenspan (2002); see also Dunn (2003).
76. Aitken and Trevarthen (1997, pp. 655, 664).
77. Ritter et al. (2007).
78. Rueckert and Naybar (2008); Amunts et al. (2007); Tranel et al. (2005).
79. Tranel et al. (2005).
80. Sowell (2011).
81. Chura et al. (2010); Bourne and Gray (2009); Cohen-Bendahan et al. (2004).
82. Worthman et al. (2010).
83. Szyf et al. (2010); Meaney (2010).
84. Cela-Conde et al. (2009); Godard and Flori (2010).
85. Kaiser et al. (2007); Sommer et al. (2004).
86. Coney (2002).
87. Levy (1969); see also Ecuyer-Dab and Robert (2004).
88. Kaiser et al. (2007); Sommer et al. (2004).
89. Levy (1969).
90. Rogers (2000); Csermely (2004).
91. Thatcher (2007).
92. Cramer and Riley (2008); Dancause et al. (2005); Desmurget et al. (2007); Duffau (2006).
93. Begley (2007); Doidge (2007).
94. Hall and Lifshitz (2010); Thompson et al. (2009); Mizelle (2008).
95. Seung et al. (2005); Altenmüller (2001); Levitin (2006).
96. Levitin (2006).
97. Hubel (1967).
98. Spencer (2004).
99. Stanislawa (2000); Chisholm (2000).
100. Begley (2007); Doidge (2007); Kempermann et al. (2002).
101. Zhang and Raichle (2010).
102. Hall and Lifshitz (2010); Thompson et al. (2009); Doidge (2007).
103. Zhang and Raichle (2010).
104. Siegel (2010a).
105. Post and Weiss (1997, p. 925).
106. Siegel (2010a).

107. Kagan and Fox (2006); Goldsmith et al. (2000); Davidson and Begley (2012).
108. Schmidt (1999); Spere et al. (2005).
109. Shulman et al. (2010).
110. Miller and Coll (2007); Findlay and Coplan (2008); Kagan and Snidman (2004).
111. Levy (1969).
112. Bloom and Hynd (2005); McGilchrist (2009).
113. Engle and Smith (2010); Evans and Federmeier (2009); Slotnick and Moo (2006).
114. Schacter (1996, p. 141).
115. Goldberg and Costa (1981).
116. Edwards (1999).
117. McGilchrist (2009); Stark et al. (2008).
118. Stark et al. (2008); Sporns (2010).
119. Decety and Chaminade (2003); Shamay-Tsoory et al. (2003); Ritblatt (2000).
120. Thatcher (2007).
121. Gopnik and Meltzoff (2006).
122. Fonagy and Target (1997, pp. 690–691).
123. Wasserstein and Stefanatos (2000); Lindner and Rosén (2006).
124. Baron-Cohen (2008); see also Shanker and Stieben (2009); Uddin et al. (2008).
125. Dapretto et al. (2005).
126. Uddin et al. (2008).
127. Siegel (2010a, 2010b).
128. Fonagy and Target (1997); see also Lemche et al. (2007).
129. Fonagy and Target (1997).
130. Behrens et al. (2011).
131. M. Main, personal communication (January 1999).
132. Hesse (1999b).
133. Siegel (2010a).

## Chapter 7

1. Ciompi (1991).
2. Sroufe (1996).
3. Hofer (1994).
4. Calkins and Hill (2007); Gross and Thompson (2007); Panksepp (2001); Tronick (2007).
5. Feldman (2007); Reck et al. (2004).
6. Sroufe (1996).
7. Schore (2003a).
8. Damasio (1998, p. 84).
9. Schore (2003b); Fosha et al. (2009).
10. Fonagy et al. (2002); Gross and Thompson (2007); Baumeister and Vohs (2004).
11. Cole and Deater-Deckard (2009); Beauregard et al. (2006); Austin et al. (2007); Etkin and Wager (2007).
12. American Psychiatric Association (2000).
13. Zhang and Raichle (2010); Raichle (2010); Raichle and Snyder (2007).
14. Phillips et al. (2008); Dickstein et al. (2008); Post et al. (2001).
15. Miklowitz et al. (2009).

16. Siegel (2007a, 2007b).
17. Sroufe et al. (2005).
18. Cole et al. (2009b); Johnson et al. (2003); Waller and Scheidt (2006).
19. Goleman (2006); Siegel (2010a).
20. Saxena et al. (2009); Siegel (2010b).
21. Gross (2007); Schore (2003a, 2003b); Fosha et al. (2009); Davidson and Begley (2012).
22. Kagan and Snidman (2004, 2007); Lengua and Kovacs (2005); Coplan et al. (2007); Miller et al. (2010); Suveg et al. (2010).
23. Heinicke et al. (2006); Sroufe et al. (2005, 2010); Sroufe and Siegel (2011).
24. Gross (2007); Schore (2003a, 2003b); Fosha et al. (2009); Lewis (2005b).
25. Aftanasa and Golosheykina (2005); Lutz et al. (2008); Waugh et al. (2010).
26. Dawson et al. (2008).
27. Ashman et al. (2008); Tronick and Reck (2009); Field and Diego (2008); Diego et al. (2006).
28. Stern (1985); Field (1994); Atzil et al. (2011); Barret et al. (2011).
29. Fonagy et al. (2007); Tronick (2004).
30. Schore (2001); Strathearn (2011); Atzil et al. (2011).
31. Schore (2003b).
32. Wig et al. (2009).
33. King et al. (2001); Heim et al. (2000, 2002); de Kloet et al. (2006).
34. McGowan et al. (2009).
35. Teicher (2000, 2002, 2010); Andersen et al. (2008).
36. Kim and Jung (2006); Myers and Davis (2007); LeDoux (2003b).
37. Sroufe (1996).
38. Camras (1992); see also Campos et al. (2004).
39. Malatesta-Magai (1991); see also Cole et al. (2009a); Cunningham et al. (2009).
40. Zahn-Waxler (2010); Brand and Klimes-Dougan (2010).
41. Cole et al. (2003); Raval et al. (2007); Anolli et al. (2008); Soto et al. (2005).
42. Vygotsky (1934/1986).
43. Eid and Diener (2009).
44. Lewis et al. (2008).
45. Northoff and Bermpohl (2004).
46. Wager et al. (2008, p. 1048).
47. Wager et al. (2008, p. 1037).
48. Goleman (2006).
49. Porges (2011); Siegel (2007a); Fossati et al. (2003); D'Argembeau et al. (2007); Mano et al. (2011); Schmitz and Johnson (2006).
50. Cole et al. (2003); Winsler (2009).
51. Hassin et al. (2005); Velmans (2009); Mudrik et al. (2011); Van Opstal et al. (2011).
52. Kabat-Zinn (2005); Siegel (2007a, 2007b).
53. Hanna et al. (2011); Paulson et al. (2011); Voorhoeve et al. (2011); Knobe and Nichols (2008); Slingerland and Collard (2011); and see Lau et al. (2004).
54. Edelman (2000); Sporns et al. (2000); Sporns and Tononi (2007); Block (2007); Velik (2009).
55. Nobre et al. (2007); Taylor et al. (2007); Alvarez and Emory (2006); Koechlin and Summerfield (2007); Melloni et al. (2007); Mayer et al. (2011); Obhi et al. (2011).

56. Nobre et al. (1999, p. 12); see also O'Doherty (2007); Bechara et al. (2000); Rolls (2004).
57. Siegel (2010a, 2010b, 2012).
58. Zelazo (2004).
59. Cole et al. (2009a); Sodian and Frith (2008).
60. Hansen and Markman (2005); Bialystock and Senman (2004); Courtin and Merlot (2004).
61. Lang et al. (2001); Voss et al. (2008).
62. Oatley (2007); Tulving (2005).
63. Malatesta-Magai (1991); McDowell and Parke (2000); Chiao et al. (2008); see also Ekman (2009).
64. Raval et al. (2007).
65. Masuda et al. (2008).
66. Craig (2002); Critchley et al. (2004); Critchley (2004).
67. Masuda et al. (2008).
68. Nisbett and Miyamoto (2005).
69. Harter (2012).
70. Chen et al. (2006).
71. Milders et al. (2010); Wager et al. (2008).
72. Kagan and Snidman (2004).
73. Davidson and Begley (2012).
74. Davidson and Begley (2012, p. xii).
75. Goldberg (1990).
76. Davidson and Begley (2012, p. xiv).
77. Begley (2007); Doidge (2007).
78. Davidson and Begley (2012, p. xvii).
79. Berkovich-Ohana et al. (2011); Davanger et al. (2010); Ives-Deliperi et al. (2010); Jang et al. (2011); Jha et al. (2007); Kilpatrick et al. (2011); Lazar et al. (2005); Manna et al. (2010).
80. Siegel (2010a, 2011b, 2012).

## Chapter 8

1. Sporns (2010); Fox et al. (2005); Lewis (2005b).
2. Rizzolatti et al. (2001, 2006); Gallese (2005); Iacoboni et al. (2005).
3. Iacoboni (2008).
4. Siegel (2007a).
5. Hofer (2006).
6. Ferber et al. (2007); Ferber and Makhoul (2004).
7. McCraty et al. (1998).
8. Cicchetti and Rogosch (2009); Knitzer and Raver (2002); Greenberg et al. (1993); Kochanska and Aksan (2004); Sroufe et al. (2005); Sroufe and Siegel (2011); Karr-Morse and Wiley (2012).
9. Sroufe et al. (2005).
10. Sroufe and Siegel (2011).
11. Schore (2009a, 2009b).
12. Brodal (2010).
13. Panksepp (1998, 2009, 2010); Panksepp and Biven (2012).

14. Schore (2003b); Gilbert and Andrews (1998); Trevarthen and Aitken (2001, 2003); Tangney and Dearing (2002); Rogoff (2003); Sander (1964); Stern (1985); Trevarthen (2005b, 2005c); Trevarthen et al. (2006); Nathanson (2009).
15. Sroufe (1996).
16. Schore (2003a, 2003b).
17. Schore (2003a, 2003b); see also Bruce (2006); Rutter (2005).
18. Trumbull (2008).
19. Zhong et al. (2008); Mei et al. (2008).
20. Behrens et al. (2007); van IJzendoorn et al. (2006); Bakermans-Kranenburg and van IJzendoorn (2009).
21. Banks et al. (2007); Schore and Schore (2008).
22. Legerstee et al. (2007).
23. Field (1985); Schore (1994).
24. Tronick (2007).
25. Siegel and Hartzell (2003).
26. Farber and Siegel (2011).
27. Schore (2003a, 2003b).
28. Minagawa-Kawai et al. (2009); Bartels and Zeki (2004).
29. Rolls and Grabenhorst (2008).
30. Panksepp (1998, 2009); Panksepp and Biven (2012).
31. Daniels et al. (2011).
32. Panksepp (2010, pp. 485–486; capital letters in original; brackets added).
33. Dunbar (2003); Norman et al. (2009); Burish et al. (2004); Barton (1996).
34. Porges (2009, 2011).
35. Porges (2011).
36. Iacoboni and Dapretto (2006); Dapretto et al. (2005).
37. Scott-Van Zeeland et al. (2010).
38. Wana et al. (2010); see also Purvis et al. (2007); Hughes (2012).
39. Main et al. (2005); Hesse (2008); Bakermans-Kranenburg and van IJzendoorn (2009).
40. Swain et al. (2007); van IJzendoorn et al. (2008); Bakermans-Kranenburg and van IJzendoorn (2008).
41. Ellis et al. (2011).
42. Sroufe and Siegel (2011).
43. Laible and Panfile (2009).
44. Sroufe et al. (2005); Strathearn (2011).
45. Sroufe et al. (2005); Cassidy and Shaver (2008); Atzil et al. (2011).
46. Hesse et al. (2003); Porges (2011).
47. Blakemore and Choudhury (2006); Doidge (2007); Erraji et al. (2005); Davidson and Begley (2012).
48. Northoff and Bermpohl (2004); Siegel (2007a).
49. Andersen and Teicher (2004, 2008a, 2008b); Andersen et al. (2008); Teicher et al. (2004, 2009); van Harmelin et al. (2010); McGreenery et al. (2006).
50. Noll and Shenk (2010); Andersen and Teicher (2008a); Stoltenborgh et al. (2011); Purvis et al. (2007).
51. Fonagy et al. (2002); Allen et al. (2008).
52. Siegel (2010a, 2010b).
53. Walden (1991).
54. See Siegel (2010a) for a more in-depth exploration and case examples.

55. Sroufe et al. (2005); Liotti (2007).
56. Main and Goldwyn (1998).
57. Siegel (2010b).
58. Edwards (1999).
59. Edwards (1999).
60. Dutra et al. (2009); MacDonald et al. (2008).
61. van IJzendoorn et al. (2010).
62. Tedeschi and Calhoun (2004); Haidt (2006); see also Curtis and Cicchetti (2003).
63. Hesse and Main (2006).
64. Main et al. (2008); Siegel (2001a, 2010a); Neimeyer and Levitt (2001); Mackenzie (2009); Klein and Boats (2010); Hesse (2008).
65. Nader (2006).
66. Calhoun and Tedeschi (2006); Nader (2006).
67. Hesse (2008).
68. Vicentic et al. (2006); Khoury et al. (2006).
69. Bowlby (1980).
70. Siegel (2010a, 2010b).

# Chapter 9

1. Lewis (2005b); Varela et al. (2001); Velik (2010); Tucker et al. (2000).
2. Siegel (2010a, 2010b).
3. Siegel (2012); Siegel and Bryson (2011).
4. Sporns (2010, p. 54; emphasis in original).
5. Fredrickson (2004, p. 1367).
6. Wooley et al. (2010).
7. Fredrickson (2004, p. 1372).
8. Zhang and Raichle (2010).
9. Fredrickson (2004, p. 1375).
10. Tucker et al. (1995, p. 214).
11. Tucker (2007).
12. Tucker et al. (2000, 2008).
13. Trevarthen (2005c, 2009b); see also Cowley (2008).
14. Stephan et al. (2007); Knyazeva et al. (2009).
15. Trevarthen (1990b, p. 49); see also Trevarthen (2007).
16. Tucker et al. (1995, p. 218); see also Tucker (2002).
17. Woltering and Lewis (2009, p. 160).
18. Tucker and Luu (2006); Tucker et al. (2008).
19. Rosa et al. (2009); Stephan et al. (2007); Saur et al. (2008).
20. Wise et al. (1996).
21. Hikosaka and Isoda (2010); Cameron et al. (2009).
22. Genovesio et al. (2005); Levy and Dubois (2006); Nambu (2008).
23. Ragozzino (2007); Kim and Ragozzino (2005); Genovesio et al. (2005).
24. van Ooyen and van Pelt (1994, pp. 245–246).
25. Woltering and Lewis (2009).
26. Guo et al. (2007); Pillow et al. (2008); Huk and Shadlen (2005).
27. Trevarthen (1996, pp. 571–572; emphasis in original).
28. Sroufe et al. (2005); Sroufe and Siegel (2011).

29. Budinger et al. (2006); Yu and Ballard (2004); Fuster (2006).
30. Siegel (2010a, 2010b).
31. Damasio (1998, p. 83).
32. Cacioppo et al. (2006); Davidson (2003); Izard (2010); Davidson and Begley (2012).
33. Doidge (2007); Craik and Bialystok (2006); Lindenberger (2001); Cozolino (2006); Sohur et al. (2006).
34. Benes (1998, p. 1489).
35. Coyle (2009); Markham and Greenough (2004); Wallace et al. (2010).
36. Deak et al. (2007).
37. Casey et al. (2005); Tucker-Drob (2009).
38. Cozolino (2008).
39. Guastello et al. (2009).
40. Amiot et al. (2007).
41. Cassidy and Shaver (2008).
42. Harter (2012).
43. Showers and Zeigler-Hill (2007).
44. Chen et al. (2006).
45. Hill et al. (2007).
46. Mann (2004); Kiang and Harter (2008).
47. LeVine (2010); Haberstadt and Lozada (2011).
48. Wang (2008b).
49. Chen et al. (2008, p. 803).
50. Fuligni (2011).
51. Van Lancker Sidtis et al. (2006); Kelly et al. (2010).
52. Ciompi (1991); see also Posner et al. (2005); Sutton (2006).
53. David et al. (2010, p. 1158).
54. Mesquita et al. (2010).
55. Main et al. (2008).
56. Meinz and Main (2011).
57. Fonagy et al. (2007).
58. Pearson et al. (1994, p. 360).
59. Brumariu and Kerns (2008); Sroufe et al. (2005).
60. Main and Goldwyn (1998).
61. Brumariu and Kerns (2008); Sroufe et al. (2005).
62. Roisman et al. (2002, 2007a); Hesse (2008).
63. Berkman et al. (2000); Zhang and Raichle (2010).
64. Fair et al. (2007, p. 13507).
65. Rippon et al. (2007, p. 164).
66. Frith (2004).
67. Teicher et al. (2010); Teicher (2007).
68. Harter (2012); Kiang and Harter (2008).
69. Sroufe et al. (2005); Feeney and VanVleet (2010); Laurent and Powers (2007); Cassidy and Shaver (2010).
70. Thayer et al. (2009).
71. Cicchetti and Rogosch (1997b); see also Flores et al. (2005).
72. Ogawa et al. (1997, p. 871), paraphrasing Loevinger (1976).
73. Ogawa et al. (1997, pp. 871–872).
74. Schore (1997, p. 607).

75. Lyons-Ruth and Jacobvitz (2008); Hesse and Main (2000); Bernier and Meins (2008); Fearon et al. (2010).
76. Harter and Leary (2003).
77. Sroufe et al. (2005); Judd (2005).
78. Fosha et al. (2009); Hane and Fox (2006); Harrist and Waugh (2002); Meins et al. (2001); Nicolosi (2009).
79. Liotti (1992).
80. Carlson (1998); Sroufe et al. (2005).
81. Bryant (2007); Bronner et al. (2009); Simeon et al. (2006).
82. Ogawa et al. (1997, p. 856).
83. Dell and O'Neil (2009); Dutra et al. (2009); Siegel (1995b, 1996a, 1996b).
84. American Psychiatric Association (2000).
85. Curran and Morgan (2000); Schönenberg et al. (2008).
86. Deakin et al. (2008).
87. Sporns et al. (2004); Ciaramelli and di Pellegrino (2011).
88. Varela et al. (2001, p. 229).
89. Christakis and Fowler (2009).
90. Siegel (2007a); Ciaramelli and di Pellegrino (2011); Oliviera-Souza et al. (2011).
91. Goel et al. (2007).
92. Siegel (2010a).
93. Siegel (2007a).
94. Tucker et al. (2008).
95. Thagard (2002).
96. Guastello et al. (2009); Sporns (2010).
97. A quote from the bulletin board of the First Presbyterian Church Preschool, Los Angeles.
98. Csikszentmihalyi (1990/2008).
99. Nelson (2003b, 2006).
100. Wolf (1990, p. 185).
101. Wolf (1990, p. 183).
102. Fivush and Nelson (2004); Hammack (2008); McLean et al. (2007); Rueda et al. (2005); Zelazo et al. (2008); see also Starmans and Bloom (2011); Hanna (2011); Izenberg (2011).
103. Hilgard (1977).
104. Piolino et al. (2007); Crawley and French (2005).
105. Dell and O'Neil (2009).
106. Vandenberg (1998, pp. 265–266).
107. Vygotsky (1934/1986).
108. Hughes and Ensor (2005); Chasiotis et al. (2006).
109. Bernier et al. (2010).
110. DiNoble (2009).
111. Gazzaniga et al. (1996); see also Leclercq (2002).
112. Ortigue et al. (2009).
113. Abe et al. (2008).
114. McGilchrist (2009).
115. Sroufe et al. (2005); Dwyer et al. (2010); Benson et al. (2006).
116. Sroufe et al. (2005).
117. Elder (1998, p. 9).
118. Iaria et al. (2007); McNaughton et al. (2006).

119. Herzog et al. (2006); Douglas and Marton (2007); Galetto et al. (2011); Keane and Verfaellie (2011); Sanford and Emmott (2012); Wallentin et al. (2011).
120. Tulving et al. (1994); Gagnon et al. (2010); Habib et al. (2003); Babiloni et al. (2006).
121. Quoidbach et al. (2008); Buckner and Carroll (2007).
122. Winson (1993); Anton et al. (2009); Ravassard et al. (2009); Stickgold and Walker (2007).
123. Milner et al. (1998); see also Wiltgen et al. (2004).
124. Trevarthen (1990a, 1993).
125. Alink et al. (2009); Cicchetti and Rogosch (2009); Moller et al. (2008); Teicher et al. (2006).
126. Beebe and Lachman (1994).
127. Ross (1996); Ethofer et al. (2005).
128. Sroufe (1996, p. 17).
129. Strathearn (2011).
130. Siegel (2010a, 2010b).
131. DiNoble (2009).
132. Siegel and Bryson (2011); Siegel and Hartzell (2003).
133. Siegel (2010a, 2010b).
134. Siegel (2007a, 2007b, 2010b).

## Epilogue

1. Siegel and Bryson (2011); Siegel and Hartzell (2003); Zuckerman et al. (2005); Siegel (2006, 2009b, 2010a, 2010b), Siegel and Pierce-McCall (2009), Epstein et al. (2009); Badenoch (2011).
2. Frith (2004).
3. Siegel (2010a).
4. Ramirez-Esparza and Pennebaker (2006).
5. Siegel (2010b, 2012).

# References

Abe, N., Okuda, J., Suzuki, M., Sasaki, H., Matsuda, T., Mori, E., et al. (2008). Neural correlates of true memory, false memory, and deception. *Cerebral Cortex, 18*(12), 2811–2819.

Abraham, W., & Robins, A. (2005). Memory retention: The synaptic stability versus plasticity dilemma. *Trends in Neurosciences, 28*(2), 73–78.

Abrams, K. Y., Rifkin, A., & Hesse, E. (2006). Examining the role of parental frightened/frightening subtypes in predicting disorganized attachment within a brief observational procedure. *Development and Psychopathology, 18*(2), 345–361.

Achard, S., Bullmore, E., Salvador, R., Suckling, J., & Whitcher, B. (2005). A resilient, low-frequency, small-world human brain functional network with highly connected association cortical hubs. *Journal of Neuroscience, 26*(1), 63–72.

Addis, D., Moscovitch, M., Crawley, A., & McAndrews, M. (2004). Recollective qualities modulate hippocampal activation during autobiographical memory retrieval. *Hippocampus, 14*(6), 752–762.

Adolphs, R., & Damasio, A. (2000). Neurobiology of emotion at a systems level. In J. Borod (Ed.), *The neuropsychology of emotion* (pp. 194–213). New York: Oxford University Press.

Aftanasa, L., & Golosheykina, S. (2005). Impact of regular meditation practice on EEG activity at rest and during evoked negative emotions. *International Journal of Neuroscience, 115*(6), 893–909.

Ainsworth, M. D. S. (1988, January). *On security.* Paper presented at a meeting of attachment experts in Stony Brook, NY. Ovid Database.

Ainsworth, M. D. S. (1993). Attachments and other affectional bonds across the life cycle. In C. M. Parkes, J. Stevenson-Hinde, & P. Marris (Eds.), *Attachment across the life cycle* (pp. 33–51). New York: Routledge.

Ainsworth, M. D. S., Blehar, M. C., Waters, E., & Wall, S. (1978). *Patterns of attachment: A psychological study of the Strange Situation.* Hillsdale, NJ: Erlbaum.

Aitken, K. J., & Trevarthen, C. (1997). Self–other organization in human psychological development. *Development and Psychopathology, 9,* 653–678.

Alfano, K. M., & Cimino, C. R. (2008). Alteration of expected hemispheric asymmetries: Valence and arousal effects in neuropsychological models of emotion. *Brain and Cognition, 66*(3), 213–220.

Alink, L. R. A., Cicchetti, D., Kim, J., & Rogosch, F. A. (2009). Mediating and moderating processes in the relation between maltreatment and psychopathology: Mother–child relationship quality and emotion regulation. *Journal of Abnormal Child Psychology, 37*(6), 831–843.

Allen, J. G., Fonagy, P., & Bateman, A. W. (2008). *Mentalizing in clinical practice.* Arlington, VA: American Psychiatric Publishing.

Allen, J. J. B., & Kline, J. P. (2004). Frontal EEG asymmetry, emotion, and psychopathology: The first, and the next 25 years. *Biological Psychology, 67*(1–2), 1–5.

Alossa, N., & Castelli, L. (2009). Amusia and musical functioning. *European Neurology, 61,* 269–277.

Altenmüller, E. O. (2001). How many music centers are in the brain? *Annals of the New York Academy of Sciences, 930,* 273–280.

Alvarez, J. A., & Emory, E. (2006). Executive function and the frontal lobes: A meta-analytic review. *Neuropsychology Review, 16*(1), 17–42.

Amacher, P. (1965). Freud's neurological education and its influence on psychoanalytic theory. *Psychological Issues, 4*(4), 5–93.

American Psychiatric Association. (2000). *Diagnostic and statistical manual of mental disorders* (4th ed., text rev.). Washington, DC: Author.

Amiot, C. E., de la Sablonniere, R., Terry, D. J., & Smith, J. R. (2007). Integration of social identities in the self: Toward a cognitive-developmental model. *Personality and Social Psychology Review, 11*(4), 364–388.

Amir, N., Leiner, A. S., & Bomyea, J. (2010). Implicit memory and posttraumatic stress symptoms. *Cognitive Therapy and Research, 34*(1), 49–58.

Ammaniti, M., & Trentini, C. (2009). How new knowledge about parenting reveals the neurobiological implications of intersubjectivity: A conceptual synthesis of recent research. *Psychoanalytic Dialogues, 19*(5), 537–555.

Ammaniti, M., van IJzendoorn, M. H., Speranza, A., & Tambelli, R. (2000). Internal working models of attachment during late childhood and early adolescence: An exploration of stability and change. *Attachment and Human Development, 2*(3), 328–346.

Amunts, K., Armstrong, E., Malikovic, A., Hömke, L., Mohlberg, H., Schleicher, A., et al. (2007). Gender-specific left–right asymmetries in human visual cortex. *Journal of Neuroscience, 27*(6), 1356–1364.

Anders, J. R., Fincham, J. M., & Stocco, A. (2008). A central circuit of the mind. *Trends in Cognitive Sciences, 12*(4), 136–143.

Andersen, S. L., & Teicher, M. H. (2004). Delayed effects of early stress on hippocampal development. *Neuropsychopharmacology, 29*(11), 1988–1993.

Andersen, S. L., & Teicher, M. H. (2008a). Desperately driven and no brakes: Developmental stress exposure and subsequent risk for substance abuse. *Neuroscience and Biobehavioral Reviews, 33*(4), 516–524.

Andersen, S. L., & Teicher, M. H. (2008b). Stress, sensitive periods and maturational events in adolescent depression. *Trends in Neurosciences, 31*(4), 183–191.

Andersen, S. L., Tomoda, A., Vincow, E. S., Valente, E., Polcari, A., & Teicher, M. H. (2008). Preliminary evidence for sensitive periods in the effect of childhood sexual abuse on regional brain development. *Journal of Neuropsychiatry and Clinical Neurosciences, 20*(3), 292–301.

Anderson, P. (2002). Assessment and development of executive function (EF) during childhood. *Child Neuropsychology, 8*(2), 71–82.

Anderson-Fye, E. (2010). Ethnographic case study: Maria—Cultural change and posttraumatic stress in the life of a Belizean adolescent girl. In C. M. Worthman, P. M. Plotsky, D. S. Schecher, & C. A. Cummings (Eds.), *Formative experiences: The interaction of caregiving, culture, and developmental psychobiology* (pp. 331–343). New York: Cambridge University Press.

Anolli, L., Wang, L., Mantovani, F., & De Toni, A. (2008). The voice of emotion in Chinese and Italian young adults. *Journal of Cross-Cultural Psychology, 39*(5), 565–598.

Anton, S. J., Seibt, J., Dumoulin, M., Jha, S. K., Steinmetz, N., Coleman, T., et al. (2009). Mechanisms of sleep-dependent consolidation of cortical plasticity. *Neuron, 61*(3), 454–466.

Ashman, S. B., Dawson, G., & Panagiotides, H. (2008). Trajectories of maternal depression over 7 years: Relations with child psychophysiology and behavior and role of contextual risks. *Development and Psychopathology, 20,* 55–77.

Atkinson, L., & Goldberg, S. (2004). *Attachment issues in psychopathology and intervention.* Mahwah, NJ: Erlbaum.

Atzil, S., Hendler, T., & Feldman, R. (2011). Specifying the neurobiological basis of human attachment: Brain, hormones, and behavior in synchronous and intrusive mothers. *Neuropsychopharmacology, 36,* 2603–2615.

Austin, M. A., Riniolo, T. C., & Porges, S. W. (2007). Borderline personality disorder and emotion regulation: Insights from the polyvagal theory. *Brain and Cognition, 65*(1), 69–76.

Axmacher, N., Draguhn, A., Elger, C., & Fell, J. (2009). Memory processes during sleep: Beyond the standard consolidation theory. *Cellular and Molecular Life Sciences, 66*(14), 2285–2297.

Babiloni, C., Vecchio, F., Cappa, S., Pasqualetti, P., Rossi, S., Miniussi, C., et al. (2006). Functional frontoparietal connectivity during encoding and retrieval processes follows HERA model: A high-resolution study. *Brain Research Bulletin, 68*(4), 203–212.

Baccus, J., & Horowitz, M. J. (2005). Role-relationship models: Addressing maladaptive interpersonal patterns and emotional distress. In M. W. Baldwin (Ed.), *Interpersonal cognition* (pp. 334–358). New York: Guilford Press.

Baddeley, A. (2003). Working memory: Looking back and looking forward. *Nature Reviews Neuroscience, 4*(10), 829–839.

Baddeley, A. (2010). Long-term and working memory: How do they interact? In L. Backman & L. Nyberg (Eds.), *Memory, aging and the brain: A festschrift in honour of Lars-Göran Nilsson* (pp. 7–23). New York: Psychology Press.

Badenoch, B. (2011). *The brain-savvy therapist's workbook.* New York: Norton.

Baer, R. A., Smith, G. T., Hopkins, J., Krietemeyer, J., & Toney, L. (2006). Using self-report assessment methods to explore facets of mindfulness. *Assessment, 13*(1), 27–45.

Bahrick, L. E. (2004). The development of perception in a multimodal environment. In G. Bremner & A. Salter (Eds.), *Theories of infant development* (pp. 90–120). Malden, MA: Blackwell.

Bahrick, L. E., & Hollich, G. (2008). Intermodal perception. In M. Haith & J. B. Benson (Eds.), *Encyclopedia of infant and early childhood development* (Vol. 2, pp. 164–176). Oxford: Academic Press.

Bailey, C., & Kandel, E. (2009). Synaptic and cellular basis of learning. In G. G. Bernsten & J. T. Cacioppo (Eds.), *Handbook of neuroscience for the behavioral sciences* (Vol. 1, pp. 528–551). Hoboken, NJ: Wiley.

Bakermans-Kranenburg, M. J., & van IJzendoorn, M. H. (1993). A psychometric study of the Adult Attachment Interview: Reliability and discriminant validity. *Developmental Psychology, 29,* 870–879.

Bakermans-Kranenburg, M. J., & van IJzendoorn, M. H. (2007). Genetic vulnerability or differential susceptibility in child development: The case of attachment. *Journal of Child Psychology and Psychiatry, 48*(12), 1160–1173.

Bakermans-Kranenburg, M. J., & van IJzendoorn, M. H. (2008). Oxytocin receptor (OXTR) and serotonin transporter (5-HTT) genes associated with observed parenting. *Social Cognitive and Affective Neuroscience, 3,* 128–134.

Bakermans-Kranenburg, M. J., & van IJzendoorn, M. H. (2009). The first 10,000 Adult Attachment Interviews: Distributions of adult attachment representations in clinical and non-clinical groups. *Attachment and Human Development, 11*(3), 223–263.

Bakermans-Kranenburg, M. J., & van IJzendoorn, M. H. (2011). Differential susceptibility to rearing environment depending on dopamine-related genes: New evidence and a meta-analysis. *Development and Psychopathology, 23*(1), 39–52.

Bakermans-Kranenburg, M. J., van IJzendoorn, M. H., Pijlman, F. T. A., Mesman, J., & Juffer, F. (2008). Experimental evidence for differential susceptibility: Dopamine D4 receptor polymorphism (DRD4 VNTR) moderates intervention effects on toddlers' externalizing behavior in a randomized controlled trial. *Developmental Psychology, 44*(1), 293–300.

Balconi, M., & Lucchiari, C. (2008). Consciousness and arousal effects on emotional face processing as revealed by brain oscillations: A gamma band analysis. *International Journal of Psychophysiology, 67*(1), 41–46.

Balconi, M., & Mazza, G. (2009). Brain oscillations and BIS/BAS (behavioral inhibition/activation system) effects on processing masked emotional cues: ERS/ERD and coherence measures of alpha band. *International Journal of Psychophysiology, 74*(2), 158–165.

Ballesteros, S., Reales, J., García, E., & Carrasco, M. (2006). Selective attention affects implicit and explicit memory for familiar pictures at different delay conditions. *Psicothema, 18*(1), 88–99.

Banks, S. J., Eddy, K. T., Angstadt, M., Nathan, P. J., & Phan, K. L. (2007). Amygdala–frontal connectivity during emotion regulation. *Social Cognitive and Affective Neuroscience, 2*(4), 303–312.

Bar, M. (2009). A cognitive neuroscience hypothesis of mood and depression. *Trends in Cognitive Sciences, 13*(11), 456–463.

Barco, A., Jancic, D., & Kandel, E. (2008). CREB-dependent transcription and synaptic plasticity. In S. S. Dudek (Ed.), *Transcriptional regulation by neuronal activity: To the nucleus and back* (pp. 127–154). New York: Springer.

Barnes, S., & Finnerty, G. (2010). Sensory experience and cortical rewiring. *The Neuroscientist, 16*(2), 186–198.

Baron-Cohen, S. (2008). Theories of the autistic mind. *The Psychologist, 21*(2), 112–116.

Barone, L. (2003). Developmental protective and risks factors in borderline personality disorder: A study using the Adult Attachment Interview. *Attachment and Human Development, 5*(1), 64–77.

Barrett, L. F. (2006). Solving the emotion paradox: Categorization and the experience of emotion. *Personality and Social Psychology Review, 10*(1), 20–46.

Barrett, L. F., Gendron, M., & Huang, Y.-M. (2009). Do discrete emotions exist? *Philosophical Psychology, 22*(4), 427–437.

Barrett, J., Wonch, K. E., Gonzalez, A., Ali, N., Steiner, M., Hall, G. B., et al. (2011). Maternal affect and quality of parenting experiences are related to amygdala response to infant faces. *Social Neuroscience, 1–17.*

Barsalou, L. W., Simmons, W. K., Barbey, A. K., & Wilson, C. D. (2003). Grounding conceptual knowledge in modality-specific systems. *Trends in Cognitive Sciences, 7*(2), 84–91.

Bartels, A., & Zeki, S. (2004). The neural correlates of maternal and romantic love. *NeuroImage, 21*(3), 1155–1166.

Barton, R. A. (1996). Neocortex size and behavioural ecology in primates. *Biological Sciences, 263*(1367), 173–177.

Bateman, A., & Fonagy, P. (2008). Mentalization-based treatment and borderline personality disorder. In J. F. Clarkin, P. Fonagy, & G. O. Gabbard (Eds.), *Psychodynamic psychotherapy for personality disorders: A clinical handbook* (pp. 187–208). Arlington, VA: American Psychiatric Publishing.

Bauer, P. J. (2006). Constructing a past in infancy: A neuro-developmental account. *Trends in Cognitive Sciences, 10*(4), 175–181.

Bauer, P. J. (2007). *Remembering the times of our lives: Memory in infancy and beyond.* Mahwah, NJ: Erlbaum.

Bauer, P. J. (2008). Amnesia, infantile. In M. M. Haith & J. B. Benson (Eds.), *Encyclopedia of infant and early childhood development* (pp. 51–62). Boston: Elsevier/Academic Press.

Bauer, P. J., Kroupina, M. G., Schwade, J. A., Dropik, P. L., & Saeger Wewerka, S. (1998). If memory serves, will language?: Later verbal accessibility of early memories. *Development and Psychopathology, 10,* 655–680.

Bauer, P. J., San Souci, P., & Pathman, T. (2010). Infant memory. *Wiley Interdisciplinary Reviews: Cognitive Science, 1*(2), 267–277.

Baumeister, R., & Vohs, K. D. (Eds.). (2004). *Handbook of self-regulation: Research, theory, and applications.* New York: Guilford Press.

Bayen, U., Smith, R., McDaniel, M., & Einstein, G. (2007). *Prospective memory: An overview and synthesis of an emerging field.* Thousand Oaks, CA: Sage.

Beauregard, M., Paquette, V., & Lèvesque, J. (2006). Dysfunction in the neural circuitry of emotional self-regulation in major depressive disorder. *NeuroReport, 17*(8), 843–846.

Bechara, A., Damasio, H., & Damasio, A. R. (2000). Emotion, decision making and the orbitofrontal cortex. *Cerebral Cortex, 10*(3), 295–307.

Beebe, B., Jaffe, J., & Lachmann, F. (2005). A dyadic systems view of communication. In J. S. Auerbach, K. N. Levy, & C. E. Schaffer (Eds.), *Relatedness, self-definition and mental representation* (pp. 23–42). New York: Routledge.

Beebe, B., & Lachman, F. M. (1994). Representation and internalization in infancy: Three principles of salience. *Psychoanalytic Psychology, 11,* 127–166.

Beer, J. (2007). The importance of emotion–social cognition interactions for social functioning: Insights from orbitofrontal cortex. In E. Harmon-Jones & P. Winkielman (Eds.), *Social neuroscience: Integrating biological and psychological explanations of social behavior* (pp. 15–30). New York: Guilford Press.

Beer, J., John, O., Scabini, D., & Knight, R. (2006). Orbitofrontal cortex and social behavior: Integrating self-monitoring and emotion–cognition interactions. *Journal of Cognitive Neuroscience, 18*(6), 871–879.

Begley, S. (2007). *Train your mind, change your brain: How a new science reveals our extraordinary potential to transform ourselves.* New York: Ballantine Books.

Behrens, K. Y., Gribneau-Bahm, N., Li, Y., & O'Boyle, M. W. (2011). Electroencephalographic responses to photographs: A case study of three women with distinct Adult Attachment Interview classifications. *Psychological Reports, 108*(3), 993–1010.

Behrens, K. Y., Hesse, E., & Main, M. (2007). Mothers' attachment status as determined by the Adult Attachment Interview predicts their 6-year-olds' reunion responses: A study conducted in Japan. *Developmental Psychology, 43*(6), 1553–1567.

Bell, A. (2007). Towards a cross-level theory of neural learning. *AIP Conference Proceedings, 954*(1), 56–73.

Belsky, J., Bakermans-Kranenburg, M. J., & van IJzendoorn, M. H. (2007). For better and for worse: Differential susceptibility to environmental influences. *Current Directions in Psychological Science, 16*(6), 300–304.

Belsky, J., & Fearon, R. M. P. (2008). Precursors of attachment security. In J. Cassidy & P. R. Shaver (Eds.), *Handbook of attachment: Theory, research, and clinical applications* (2nd ed., pp. 295–316). New York: Guilford Press.

Benes, F. M. (1998). Human brain growth spans decades. *American Journal of Psychiatry, 155*(11), 1489.

Benoit, D. (2009). Efficacy of attachment-based interventions. In R. E. Tremblay, R. G.

Barr, & R. DeV. Peters (Eds.), *Encyclopedia on Early Childhood Development* (pp. 1–6). Montréal, Quebec: Centre of Excellence for Early Childhood Development.

Benoit, D., Zeanah, C. H., Boucher, C., & Minde, K. K. (1992). Sleep disorders in early childhood: Association with insecure maternal attachment. *Journal of the American Academy of Child and Adolescent Psychiatry, 31*, 86–93.

Benson, M. J., McWey, L. M., & Ross, J. J. (2006). Parental attachment and peer relations in adolescence: A meta-analysis. *Research in Human Development, 3*(1), 33–43.

Bergen, P. (2009). The effects of mother training in emotion-rich, elaborative reminiscing on children's shared recall and emotion knowledge. *Journal of Cognition and Development, 10*(3), 162–187.

Berkman, L. F., Glass, T., Brissette, I., & Seeman, T. E. (2000). From social integration to health: Durkheim in the new millennium. *Social Science and Medicine, 51*(6), 843–857.

Berkovich-Ohana, A., Glicksohn, J., & Goldstein, A. (2012). Mindfulness-induced changes in gamma band activity—Implications for the default mode network, self-reference and attention. *Clinical Neurophysiology.*

Berlin, L. J., Zeanah, C. H., & Lieberman, A. F. (2008). Prevention and intervention programs for supporting early attachment security. In J. Cassidy & P. R. Shaver (Eds.), *Handbook of attachment: Theory, research, and clinical applications* (2nd ed., pp. 745–761). New York: Guilford Press.

Bernier, A., Carlson, S. M., & Whipple, N. (2010). From external regulation to self-regulation: Early parenting precursors of young children's executive functioning. *Child Development, 81*(1), 326–339.

Bernier, A., & Dozier, M. (2003). Bridging the attachment transmission gap: The role of maternal mind-mindedness. *International Journal of Behavioral Development, 27*, 355–365.

Bernier, A., & Meins, E. (2008). A threshold approach to understanding the origins of attachment disorganization. *Developmental Psychology, 44*, 969–982.

Berridge, K. C. (2003). Comparing the emotional brains of humans and other animals. In R. J. Davidson, K. R. Scherer, & H. H. Goldsmith (Eds.), *Handbook of affective sciences* (pp. 25–51). New York: Oxford University Press.

Bialystock, E., & Senman, S. (2004). Executive processes in appearance–reality tasks: The role of inhibition of attention and symbolic representation. *Child Development, 75*(2), 562–579.

Blakemore, S.-J., & Choudhury, S. (2006). Development of the adolescent brain: Implications for executive function and social cognition. *Journal of Child Psychology and Psychiatry, 47*(3–4), 296–312.

Blakeslee, S., & Blakeslee, M. (2007). *The body has a mind of its own: How body maps in your brain help you do (almost) everything better.* New York: Random House.

Bloch, M. (2008). Truth and sight: Generalizing without universalizing. *Journal of the Royal Anthropological Institute, 14*, S2–S32.

Block, N. (2007). Consciousness, accessibility, and the mesh between psychology and neuroscience. *Behavioral and Brain Sciences, 30*(5–6), 481–499.

Bloom, J. S., & Hynd, G. W. (2005). The role of the corpus callosum in interhemispheric transfer of information: Excitation or inhibition? *Neuropsychology Review, 15*(2), 59–71.

Bluhm, R., Williamson, P., Osuch, E., Frewen, P., Stevens, T., Boksman, K., et al. (2009). Alterations in default network connectivity in posttraumatic stress disorder related to early-life trauma. *Journal of Psychiatry and Neuroscience, 34*(3), 187–194.

Bokhorst, C. L., Bakermans-Kranenburg, M. J., Fearon, R. M., van IJzendoorn, M. H., Fonagy, P., & Schuengel, C. (2003). The importance of shared environment in mother–infant attachment security: A behavioral genetic study. *Journal of Personality Disorders, 74*(6), 1769–1782.

Boldrini, M., Placidi, G. P. A., & Marazziti, D. (1998). Applications of chaos theories to psychiatry: A review and future perspectives. *International Journal of Neuropsychiatric Medicine, 3*, 22–29.

Bookheimer, S. Y., Hariri, A. R., & Mazziotta, J. C. (2000). Modulating emotional responses: Effects of a neocortical network on the limbic system. *NeuroReport, 11*(1), 43–48.

Born, J. (2010). Slow-wave sleep and the consolidation of long-term memory. *World Journal of Biological Psychiatry, 11*(1), 16–21.

Borod, J. C. (2000). *The neuropsychology of emotion.* New York: Oxford University Press.

Botvinick, M., & Plaut, D. (2009). Empirical and computational support for context-dependent representations of serial order: Reply to Bowers, Damian, and Davis (2009). *Psychological Review, 116*(4), 998–1002.

Bourne, V. J. J., & Gray, D. L. (2009). Hormone exposure and functional lateralisation: Examining the contributions of prenatal and later life hormonal exposure. *Psychoneuroendocrinology, 34*(8), 1214–1221.

Bower, G. H., & Sivers, H. (1998). Cognitive impact of traumatic events. *Development and Psychopathology, 10*, 625–654.

Bowers, J. (2009). On the biological plausibility of grandmother cells: Implications for neural network theories in psychology and neuroscience. *Psychological Review, 116*(1), 220–251.

Bowlby, J. (1969). *Attachment and loss: Vol. 1. Attachment.* New York: Basic Books.

Bowlby, J. (1973). *Attachment and loss: Vol. 2. Separation and anger.* New York: Basic Books.

Bowlby, J. (1980). *Attachment and loss: Vol. 3. Loss: Sadness and depression.* New York: Basic Books.

Bowlby, J. (1988a). *A secure base: Parent–child attachment and healthy human development.* New York: Basic Books.

Bowlby, J. (1988b). Attachment and loss: Retrospect and prospect. *American Journal of Orthopsychiatry, 52*(4), 664–678.

Bradley, M. M. (2008). Natural selective attention: Orienting and emotion. *Psychophysiology, 46*(1), 1–11.

Bradley, R. H., Corwyn, R. F., Burchinal, M., McAdoo, H. P., & Coll, C. G. (2001). The home environments of children in the United States: Part II. Relations with behavioral development through age thirteen. *Child Development, 72*(6), 1868–1886.

Brainerd, C., & Reyna, V. (2004). Fuzzy-trace theory and memory development. *Developmental Review, 24*(4), 396–439.

Brand, A. E., & Klimes-Dougan, B. (2010). Emotion socialization in adolescence: The roles of mothers and fathers. *New Directions for Child and Adolescent Development, 2010*(128), 85–100.

Brazelton, T. B., & Greenspan, S. I. (2002). *The irreducible needs of children: What every child must have to grow, learn, and flourish.* Cambridge, MA: Perseus.

Bremner, J. D. (2007). Neuroimaging in posttraumatic stress disorder and other stress-related disorders. *Neuroimaging Clinics of North America, 17*(4), 523–538.

Bremner, J. D., & Narayan, M. (1998). The effects of stress on memory and the hippocampus throughout the life cycle: Implications for childhood development and aging. *Development and Psychopathology, 10*, 871–888.

Brennan, K. A., Clark, C. L., & Shaver, P. R. (1998). Self-report measurement of adult attachment: An integrative overview. In J. A. Simpson & W. S. Rholes (Eds.), *Attachment theory and close relationships* (pp. 46–76). New York: Guilford Press.

Brenner, N., Strong, S., Koberle, R., Bialek, W., & Van Steveninck, R. (2000). Synergy in a neural code. *Neural Computation, 12*(7), 1531–1552.

Bretherton, I., & Munholland, K. A. (2008). Internal working models in attachment relationships: Elaborating a central construct in attachment theory. In J. Cassidy & P. R. Shaver (Eds.), *Handbook of attachment: Theory, research, and clinical applications* (2nd ed., pp. 102–130). New York: Guilford Press.

Brewin, C. (2007). Remembering and forgetting. In M. J. Friedman, T. M. Terence, & P. A. Resick (Eds.), *Handbook of PTSD: Science and practice* (pp. 116–134). New York: Guilford Press.

Briere, J., Scott, C., & Weathers, F. (2005). Peritraumatic and persistent dissociation in the presumed etiology of PTSD. *American Journal of Psychiatry, 162*, 2295–2301.

Brodal, P. (2010). *The central nervous system: Structure and function.* New York: Oxford University Press.

Brodsky, M., & Lombroso, P. J. (1998). Molecular mechanisms of developmental disorders. *Development and Psychopathology, 10*, 1–20.

Bronner, M. B., Kayser, A., Knoester, H., Bos, A. P., Last, B. F., & Grootenhuis, M. A. (2009). A pilot study on peritraumatic dissociation and coping styles as risk factors for posttraumatic stress, anxiety and depression in parents after their child's unexpected admission to a pediatric intensive care unit. *Child and Adolescent Psychiatry and Mental Health, 3*, 33.

Brothers, L. (1997). *Friday's footprint: How society shapes the human mind.* New York: Oxford University Press.

Brown, J., Cooper-Kuhn, C. M., Gage, F. H., Kempermann, G., Kuhn, H. G., van Praag, H., et al. (2003). Enriched environment and physical activity stimulate hippocampal but not olfactory bulb neurogenesis. *European Journal of Neuroscience, 17*(10), 2042–2046.

Brown, K. W., & Ryan, R. M. (2003). The benefits of being present: Mindfulness and its role in psychological well-being. *Journal of Personality and Social Psychology, 84*(4), 822–848.

Brown, L. S., & Wright, J. (2003). The relationship between attachment strategies and psychopathology in adolescence. *Psychology and Psychotherapy: Theory, Research, and Practice, 76*(4), 351–367.

Bruce, D. P. (2006). Applying principles of neurodevelopment to clinical work with maltreated and traumatized children. In N. B. Webb (Ed.), *Working with traumatized youth in child welfare* (pp. 27–52). New York: Guilford Press.

Brumariu, L. E., & Kerns, K. A. (2008). Mother–child attachment and social anxiety symptoms in middle childhood. *Journal of Applied Developmental Psychology, 29*(5), 393–402.

Bruner, J. S. (2003). *Making stories: Law, literature, life.* Cambridge, MA: Harvard University Press.

Bryant, R. (2007). Does dissociation further our understanding of PTSD? *Journal of Anxiety Disorders, 21*(2), 183–191.

Buchsbaum, B. R., & D'Esposito, M. (2009). Is there anything special about working memory? In F. Roesler, C. Ranganath, B. Roder, & R. H. Kluwe (Eds.), *Neuroimaging of human memory: Linking cognitive processes to neural systems* (pp. 255–261). New York: Oxford University Press.

Buck, R., & VanLear, C. A. (2002). Verbal and nonverbal communication: Distinguishing symbolic, spontaneous, and pseudo-spontaneous nonverbal behavior. *Journal of Communication, 52*(3), 522–541.

Buckner, R. L. (1996). Beyond HERA: Contributions of specific prefrontal brain areas to long-term memory retrieval. *Psychonomic Bulletin, 3*, 149–158.

Buckner, R. L., & Carroll, D. C. (2006). Self-projection and the brain. *Trends in Cognitive Sciences, 11*(2), 49–57.

Budinger, E., Heil, P., Hess, A., & Scheich, H. (2006). Multisensory processing via early cortical stages: Connections of the primary auditory cortical field with other sensory systems. *Neuroscience, 143*(4), 1065–1083.

Buller, D. (2009, January). Four fallacies of pop evolutionary psychology. *Scientific American,* pp. 74–81.

Burianova, H., McIntosh, A., & Grady, C. (2010). A common functional brain network for autobiographical, episodic, and semantic memory retrieval. *NeuroImage, 49*(1), 865–874.

Burish, M. J., Kueh, H. Y., & Wang, S.S.-H. (2004). Brain architecture and social complexity in modern and ancient birds. *Brain, Behavior and Evolution, 63,* 107–124.

Burt, C. D. (2008). Time, language, and autobiographical memory. *Language Learning, 58*(S1), 123–141.

Cacioppo, J. T., Visser, P. S., & Pickett, C. L. (2006). *Social neuroscience: People thinking about thinking people.* Cambridge, MA: MIT Press.

Calhoun, L. G., & Tedeschi, R. G. (2006). *The handbook of posttraumatic growth: Research and practice.* Mahwah, NJ: Erlbaum.

Calkins, S. D. (1994). Origins and outcomes of individual differences in emotion regulation. In N. A. Fox (Ed.), The development of emotion regulation: Biological and behavioral considerations. *Monographs of the Society for Research in Child Development, 59*(2–3, Serial No. 240), 53–72.

Calkins, S. D., & Hill, A. (2007). Caregiver influences on emerging emotion regulation: Biological and environmental transactions in early development. In J. J. Gross (Ed.), *Handbook of emotion regulation* (pp. 229–248). New York: Guilford Press.

Cameron, I. G. M., Coe, B. C., Watanabe, M., Stroman, P. W., & Munoz, D. P. (2009). Role of the basal ganglia in switching a planned response. *European Journal of Neuroscience, 29*(12), 2413–2425.

Campos, J. J., Frankel, C. B., & Camras, L. A. (2004). On the nature of emotion regulation. *Child Development, 75*(2), 377–394.

Camras, L. A. (1992). Expressive development and basic emotions. *Cognition and Emotion, 3,* 269–283.

Carlson, E. A. (1998). A prospective longitudinal study of disorganized and psychiatric relapse: A meta-analysis. *Archives of General Psychiatry, 55,* 547–552.

Carlson, N. R. (2007). *Physiology of behavior* (9th ed.). Boston: Pearson Education.

Carr, L., Iacoboni, M., Dubeau, M. C., Maziotta, J. C., & Lenzi, L. G. (2003). Neural mechanisms of empathy in humans; A relay from neural systems for imitation to limbic areas. *Proceedings of the National Academy of Sciences USA, 100,* 5497–5502.

Carrington, S. J., & Bailey, A. J. (2008). Are there theory of mind regions in the brain?: A review of the neuroimaging literature. *Human Brain Mapping, 30*(8), 2313–2335.

Carver, L., & Cluver, A. (2009). Stress effects on the brain system underlying explicit memory. In J. A. Quas & R. Fivush (Eds.), *Emotion and memory in development: Biological, cognitive, and social considerations* (pp. 278–312). New York: Oxford University Press.

Casey, B. J., Tottenham, N., Liston, C., & Durston, S. (2005). Imaging the developing brain: What have we learned about cognitive development? *Trends in Cognitive Sciences, 9*(3), 104–110.

Caspers, K. M., Paradiso, S., Yucuis, R., Troutman, B., Arndt, S., & Philibert, R. (2009). Association between the serotonin transporter promoter polymorphism (5-HTTLPR) and adult unresolved attachment. *Developmental Psychology, 45*(1), 64–76.

Caspi, A., Sugden, K., Moffitt, T. E., Taylor, A., Craig, I. W., Harrington, H., et al. (2003).

Influence of life stress on depression: Moderation by a polymorphism in the 5-HTT gene. *Science, 301*(5631), 386–389.

Cassidy, J., & Shaver, P. R. (Eds.). (2008). *Handbook of attachment: Theory, research, and clinical applications* (2nd ed.). New York: Guilford Press.

Cela-Conde, C. J. J., Ayala, F. J., Munar, E., Maestú, F., Nadal, M., Capó, M. A., et al. (2009). From the cover: Sex-related similarities and differences in the neural correlates of beauty. *Proceedings of the National Academy of Sciences USA, 106*(10), 3847–3852.

Chalmers, D. (2007). The hard problem of consciousness. In. M. Valmans & S. Schneider (Eds.), *The Blackwell companion to consciousness* (pp. 223–235). New York: Blackwell.

Chamberlain, L. (1995). Strange attractors in patterns of family interaction. In R. Robertson & A. Combs (Eds.), *Chaos theory in psychology and the life sciences* (pp. 267–273). Mahwah, NJ: Erlbaum.

Chasiotis, A., Kiessling, F., Hofer, J., & Campos, D. (2006). Theory of mind and inhibitory control in three cultures: Conflict inhibition predicts false belief understanding in Germany, Costa Rica and Cameroon. *International Journal of Behavioral Development, 30*, 249–260.

Chen, J., Yamahachi, H., & Gilbert, C. D. (2010). Experience-dependent gene expression in adult visual cortex. *Cerebral Cortex, 20*(3), 650–660.

Chen, S., Boucher, H. C., & Tapias, M. P. (2006). The relational self revealed: Integrative conceptualization and implications for interpersonal life. *Psychological Bulletin, 132*(2), 151–179.

Chen, S. X., Benet-Martínez, V., & Bond, M. H. (2008). Bicultural identity, bilingualism, and psychological adjustment in multicultural societies: Immigration-based and globalization-based acculturation. *Journal of Personality, 76*(4), 803–838.

Cheng, Y., Chen, C., Lin, C. P., Chou, K. H., & Decety, J. (2010). Love hurts: An fMRI study. *NeuroImage, 51*(2), 923–929.

Chepenik, L. G., Raffo, M., Hampson, M., Lacadie, C., Wang, F., Jones, M. M., et al. (2010). Functional connectivity between ventral prefrontal cortex and amygdala at low frequency in the resting state in bipolar disorder. *Psychiatry Research: Neuroimaging, 182*, 207–210.

Chiao, J. Y., Iidaka, T., Gordon, H. L., Nogawa, J., Bar, M., Aminoff, E., et al. (2008). Cultural specificity in amygdala response to fear faces. *Journal of Cognitive Neuroscience, 20*(12), 2167–2174.

Chiron, C., Jambaque, I., Nabbot, R., Lounes, R., Syrota, A., & Dulac, O. (1997). The right brain is dominant in human infants. *Brain, 120*, 1057–1065.

Chisholm, K. (2000). Attachment in children adopted from Romanian orphanages: Two case studies. In P. M. Crittenden & A. H. Claussen (Eds.), *The organization of attachment relationships: Maturation, culture, and context* (pp. 171–189). New York: Cambridge University Press.

Chiu, C., Schmithorst, V., Brown, R., Holland, S., & Dunn, S. (2006). Making memories: A cross-sectional investigation of episodic memory encoding in childhood using fMRI. *Developmental Neuropsychology, 29*(2), 321–340.

Choudhury, S., & Slaby, J. (2012). *Critical neuroscience: A handbook of the social and cultural contexts*. West Sussex, UK: Wiley-Blackwell.

Choy, K., & van den Buuse, M. (2007). Attenuated disruption of prepulse inhibition by dopaminergic stimulation after maternal deprivation and adolescent corticosterone treatment in rats. *European Neuropsychopharmacology, 18*(1), 1–13.

Christakis, N. A., & Fowler, J. H. (2009). *Connected: The surprising power of our social networks and how they shape our lives*. New York: Little, Brown.

Christianson, S. A., & Lindholm, T. (1998). The fate of traumatic memories in childhood and adulthood. *Development and Psychopathology, 10*, 761–780.

Chun, M., & Turk-Browne, N. (2007). Interactions between attention and memory. *Current Opinion in Neurobiology, 17*(2), 177–184.

Chura, L. R. R., Lombardo, M. V., Ashwin, E., Auyeung, B., Chakrabarti, B., Bullmore, E. T., et al. (2010). Organizational effects of fetal testosterone on human corpus callosum size and asymmetry. *Psychoneuroendocrinology, 35*(1), 122–132.

Ciaramelli, E., & di Pelligrino, G. (2011). Ventromedial prefrontal cortex and the future of morality. *Emotion Review, 3*(3), 308–309.

Cicchetti, D., Ackerman, B. P., & Izard, C. (1995). Emotions and emotion regulation in developmental psychopathology. *Development and Psychopathology, 7*, 1–10.

Cicchetti, D., & Curtis, W. J. (2006). The developing brain and neural plasticity: Implications for normality, psychopathology, and resilience. In D. Cicchetti & D. J. Cohen (Eds.), *Developmental psychopathology: Developmental neuroscience, second edition* (Vol. 2, pp. 1–64). Hoboken, NJ: Wiley.

Cicchetti, D., & Lynch, M. (1993). Toward an ecological/transactional model of community violence and child maltreatment: Consequences for children's development. *Psychiatry, 53*, 96–118.

Cicchetti, D., & Rogosch, F. A. (Eds.). (1997a). Self-organization [Special issue]. *Development and Psychopathology, 9*(4).

Cicchetti, D., & Rogosch, F. A. (1997b). The role of self-organization in the promotion of resilience in maltreated children. *Development and Psychopathology, 9*, 797–816.

Cicchetti, D., & Rogosch, F. A. (2009). Adaptive coping under conditions of extreme stress: Multilevel influences on the determinants of resilience in maltreated children. *New Directions for Child and Adolescent Development, 2009*(124), 47–59.

Cicchetti, D., Rogosch, F. A., & Toth, S. L. (2006). Fostering secure attachment in infants in maltreating families through preventive interventions. *Development and Psychopathology, 18*(3), 623–649.

Cicchetti, D., & Toth, S. (Eds.). (1998). Risk, trauma, and memory [Special issue]. *Development and Psychopathology, 10*(4).

Ciompi, L. (1991). Affects as central organising and integrating factors: A new psychosocial/biological model of the psyche. *British Journal of Psychiatry, 159*, 97–105.

Clarke, A. J., & Butler, L. T. (2008). Dissociating word stem completion and cued recall as a function of divided attention at retrieval. *Memory, 16*(1), 763–772.

Coan, J. A. (2008). Toward a neuroscience of attachment. In J. Cassidy & P. R. Shaver (Eds.), *Handbook of attachment: Theory, research, and clinical applications* (2nd ed., pp. 241–268). New York: Guilford Press.

Coan, J. A. (2010). Emergent ghosts of the emotion machine. *Emotion Review, 2*(3), 274–285.

Coan, J. A., Schaefer, H. S., & Davidson, R. J. (2006). Lending a hand: Social regulation of the neural response to threat. *Psychological Science, 17*(12), 1032–1039.

Cohen-Bendahan, C. C., Buitelaar, J. K., van Goozen, S. H. M., & Cohen-Kettenis, P. T. (2004). Prenatal exposure to testosterone and functional cerebral lateralization: A study in same-sex and opposite-sex twin girls. *Psychoneuroendocrinology, 29*(7), 911–916.

Cole, P. M., Bruschi, C. J., & Tamang, B. L. (2003). Cultural differences in children's emotional reactions to difficult situations. *Child Development, 73*(3), 983–996.

Cole, P. M., & Deater-Deckard, K. (2009). Emotion regulation, risk, and psychopathology. *Journal of Child Psychology and Psychiatry, 50*(11), 1327–1330.

Cole, P. M., Dennis, T. A., Smith-Simon, K.E., & Cohen, L. H. (2009a). Preschoolers' emotion regulation strategy understanding: Relations with emotion socialization and child self-regulation. *Social Development, 18*(2), 324–352.

Cole, P. M., Llera, S. J., & Pemberton, C. K. (2009b). Emotional instability, poor emotional awareness, and the development of borderline personality. *Development and Psychopathology, 21*(4), 1293–1310.

Colle, L., Baron, S.-C., Wheelwright, S., & van Der Lely, H. K. J. (2007). Narrative discourse in adults with high-functioning autism or Asperger syndrome. *Journal of Autism and Developmental Disorders, 38*(1), 28–40.

Coney, J. (2002). Lateral asymmetry in phonological processing: Relating behavioral measures to neuroimaged structures. *Brain and Language, 80*(3), 355–365.

Conradi, H. J., & de Jonge, P. (2009). Recurrent depression and the role of adult attachment: A prospective and a retrospective study. *Journal of Affective Disorders, 116*(1), 93–99.

Conway, M. A., & Pleydell-Pearce, C. W. (2000). The construction of autobiographical memories in the self memory system. *Psychological Review, 107*, 261–288.

Conway, M. A., Pleydell-Pearce, C. W., Whitecross, S., & Sharpe, H. (2002). Brain imaging autobiographical memory. In B. H. Ross (Ed.), *The psychology of learning and motivation: Advances in research and theory* (Vol. 41, pp. 229–264). San Diego, CA: Academic Press.

Conway, M. A., Wang, Q., Hanyu, K., & Haque, S. (2005). A cross-cultural investigation of autobiographical memory: On the universality and cultural variation of the reminiscence bump. *Journal of Cross-Cultural Psychology, 36*(6), 739–749.

Cooper, S. J. (2005). Donald O. Hebb's synapse and learning rule: A history and commentary. *Neuroscience and Biobehavioral Reviews, 28*(8), 851–874.

Coplan, R. J., Arbeau, K. A., & Armer, M. (2007). Don't fret, be supportive!: Maternal characteristics linking child shyness to psychosocial and school adjustment in kindergarten. *Journal of Abnormal Child Psychology, 36*(3), 359–371.

Cortina, M., & Liotti, G. (2010). The intersubjective and cooperative origins of consciousness: An evolutionary-developmental approach. *Journal of the American Academy of Psychoanalysis and Dynamic Psychiatry, 38*(2), 291–314.

Courage, M. L., & Howe, M. L. (2010). Autobiographical memory: Individual differences and developmental course. In A. Gruszka, G. Matthews, & B. Szymura (Eds.), *Handbook of individual differences in cognition: Attention, memory, and executive control* (pp. 403–417). New York: Springer.

Courtin, C., & Merlot, A.-M. (2004). Metacognitive development of deaf children: Lessons from the appearance–reality and false belief tasks. *Developmental Science, 8*(1), 16–25.

Cowley, S. J. (2008). The codes of language: Turtles all the way up? In M. Barbieri (Ed.), *Biosemiotics, vol. 1, part 4, The codes of life* (pp. 319–345). The Dordrecht, Netherlands: Springer.

Coyle, D. (2009). *The talent code.* New York: Bantam/Random House.

Cozolino, L. (2006). *The neuroscience of human relationships: Attachment and the developing social brain.* New York: Norton.

Cozolino, L. (2008). *The healthy aging brain: Sustaining attachment, attaining wisdom.* New York: Norton.

Craig, A. D. (2002). How do you feel? Interoception: The sense of the physiological condition of the body. *Nature Reviews Neuroscience, 2*(8), 655–666.

Craig, A. D. (2009). How do you feel—now?: The anterior insula and human awareness. *Nature Reviews Neuroscience, 10*, 59–70.

Craig, A. D. (2010). The sentient self. *Brain Structure and Function, 214*(5–6), 1863–2661.

Craik, F. I. M., & Bialystok, E. (2006). Cognition through the lifespan: Mechanisms of change. *Trends in Cognitive Sciences, 10*(3), 131–138.

Cramer, S. C., & Riley, J. D. (2008). Neuroplasticity and brain repair after stroke. *Current Opinion in Neurology, 21*, 76–82.

Crawley, S., & French, C. (2005). Field and observer viewpoint in remember–know memories of personal childhood events. *Memory, 13*(7), 673–681.

Cresswell, J. D., Eisenberger, N. I., & Lieberman, M. D. (2007). *Neurobehavioral correlates of mindfulness during social exclusion*. Unpublished manuscript, University of California, Los Angeles.

Crick, F. (1994). *The astonishing hypothesis*. New York: Scribner.

Crick, F., & Koch, C. (2003). A framework for consciousness. *Nature Neuroscience*, 119–126.

Critchley, H. D. (2004). The human cortex responds to an interoceptive challenge. *Proceedings of the National Academy of Sciences USA, 101*(17), 6333–6334.

Critchley, H. D. (2005). Neural mechanisms of autonomic, affective, and cognitive integration. *Journal of Computational Neurology, 493*(1), 154–166.

Critchley, H. D. (2009). Psychophysiology of neural, cognitive, and affective integration: fMRI and autonomic indicants. *International Journal of Psychophysiology, 73*(2), 88–94.

Critchley, H. D., Wiens, S., Rotshtein, P., Ohman, A., & Dolan, R. J. (2004). Neural systems supporting interoceptive awareness. *Nature Neuroscience, 7*(2), 189–195.

Crowell, J. A., O'Connor, E., Wollmers, G., Sprafkin, J., & Rao, U. (1992). Mothers' conceptualizations of parent–child relationships: Relation to mother–child interaction and child behavior problems. *Development and Psychopathology, 3*, 431–444.

Crown, C. L., Feldstein, S., Jasnow, M. D., Beebe, B., & Jaffe, J. (2002). The cross-modal coordination of interpersonal timing: Six-week-olds infants' gaze with adults' vocal behavior. *Journal of Psycholinguistic Research, 31*(1), 1–23.

Csermely, D. (2004). Lateralisation in birds of prey: Adaptive and phylogenetic considerations. *Behavioural Process, 67*(3), 511–520.

Csikszentmihalyi, M. (2008). *Flow: The psychology of optimal experience*. New York: Harper Perennial Modern Classics. (Original work published 1990)

Cunningham, J. N., Kliewer, W., & Garner, P. W. (2009). Emotion socialization, child emotion understanding and regulation, and adjustment in urban African American families: Differential associations across child gender. *Development and Psychopathology, 21*(1), 261–283.

Curran, H. V., & Morgan, C. (2000). Cognitive, dissociative and psychotogenic effects of ketamine in recreational users on the night of drug use and 3 days later. *Addiction, 95*(4), 575–590.

Curtis, W. J., & Cicchetti, D. (2003): Moving research on resilience into the 21st century: Theoretical and methodological considerations in examining the biological contributors to resilience. *Development and Psychopathology, 15*, 773–810.

Cyr, C., Euser, E. M., Bakermans-Kranenburg, M. J., & van IJzendoorn, M. H. (2010). Attachment security and disorganization in maltreating and high-risk families: A series of meta-analyses. *Development and Psychopathology, 22*(1), 87–108.

Dalgleish, T., Hauer, B., & Kuyken, W. (2008). The mental regulation of autobiographical recollection in the aftermath of trauma. *Current Directions in Psychological Science, 17*(4), 259–263.

Damasio, A. R. (1998). Emotion in the perspective of an integrated nervous system. *Brain Research Reviews, 26*, 83–86.

Damasio, A. R. (2000). *The feeling of what happens: Body and emotion in the making of consciousness*. Orlando, FL: Harcourt Brace.

Damasio, A. R. (2001). Emotion and the human brain. *Annals of the New York Academy of Sciences, 935*, 101–106.

Damasio, A. R. (2005). *Descartes' error: Emotion, reason, and the human brain*. New York: Penguin. (Original work published 1994)

Damasio, A. R., Adolphs, R., & Damasio, H. (2003). The contributions of the lesion method to the functional neuroanatomy of emotion. In R. J. Davidson, K. R. Scherer, & H. H. Goldsmith (Eds.), *Handbook of affective sciences* (pp. 66–92). New York: Oxford University Press.

Damasio, A. R., Grabowski, T. J., Bechara, A., Damasio, H., Ponto, L. L. B., Parvizi, J., et al. (2000). Subcortical and cortical brain activity during the feeling of self-generated emotions. *Nature Neuroscience, 3*, 1049–1056.

Dancause, N., Barbay, S., Frost, S. B., Plautz, E. J., Chen, D., Zoubina, E. V., et al. (2005). Extensive cortical rewiring after brain injury. *Journal of Neuroscience, 25*(44), 10167–10179.

Daniels, D., Baker, L., Daniels, D., Killen, J., & Siegel, D. J. (2011). *Patterns of developmental pathways (PDP): How temperament and attachment intertwine in the creation of adult personality.* Manuscript submitted for publication.

Daprati, E., Sirigu, A., & Nico, D. (2010). Body and movement: Consciousness in the parietal lobes. *Neuropsychologia, 48*(3), 756–762.

Dapretto, M., Davies, M. S., Pfeifer, J. H., Scott, A. A., Sigman, M., Bookheimer, S. Y., et al. (2005). Understanding emotions in others: Mirror neuron dysfunction in children with autism spectrum disorders. *Nature Neuroscience, 9*, 28–30.

D'Argembeau, A., Ruby, P., Collette, F., Degueldre, C., Balteau, E., Luxen, A., et al. (2007). Distinct regions of the medial prefrontal cortex are associated with self-referential processing and perspective taking. *Journal of Cognitive Neuroscience, 19*(6), 935–944.

Davanger, S., Ellingsen, O., Holen, A., & Hugdahl, K. (2010). Meditation-specific prefrontal cortical activation during acem meditation: An fMRI study. *Perceptual and Motor Skills, 111*(1), 291–306.

David, D., Florea, C., & Pop, A. (2010). Culture-process and phenomenon, synchronic and diachronic, particular and universal. *Procedia—Social and Behavioral Sciences, 2*(2), 1158–1163.

Davidson, R. J. (2003). Affective neuroscience and psychophysiology: Toward a synthesis. *Psychophysiology, 40*(5), 655–665.

Davidson, R. J., & Begley, S. (2012). *The emotional life of your brain: How its unique patterns affect the way you think, feel, and live—and how you can change them.* New York: Penguin.

Davidson, R. J., Pizzagalli, D., Nitschke, J. B., & Kalin, N. (2003a). Parsing the subcomponents of emotion and disorders of emotion: Perspectives from affective neuroscience. In R. J. Davidson, K. R. Scherer, & H. H. Goldsmith (Eds.), *Handbook of affective sciences* (pp. 8–24). New York: Oxford University Press.

Davidson, R. J., Scherer, K. R., & Goldsmith, H. H. (Eds.). (2003b). *Handbook of affective sciences.* New York: Oxford University Press.

Davidson, R. J., Scherer, K. R., & Goldsmith H. H. (2003c). Introduction: Neuroscience. In R. J. Davidson, K. R. Scherer, & H. H. Goldsmith (Eds.), *Handbook of affective sciences* (pp. 3–7). New York: Oxford University Press.

Davis, M. (1992). The role of the amygdala in fear and anxiety. *Annual Review of Neuroscience, 15*, 353–375.

Dawson, G., Klinger, L. G., Panagiotides, H., Hill, D., & Spieker, S. (2008). Frontal lobe activity and affective behavior of infants of mothers with depressive symptoms. *Child Development, 63*(3), 725–737.

Dawson-Tunik, T., Fischer, K., & Stein, Z. (2004). Do stages belong at the center of developmental theory?: A commentary on Piaget's stages. *New Ideas in Psychology, 22*(3), 255–263.

Deak, G. O., Bartlett, M. S., & Jebara, T. (2007). New trends in cognitive science: Integrative approaches to learning and development. *Neurocomputing, 70*(13–15), 2139–2147.

Deakin, J. F. W., Lees, J., McKie, S., Hallak, J. E. C., Williams, S. R., & Dursun, S. M. (2008). Glutamate and the neural basis of the subjective effects of ketamine. *Archives of General Psychiatry, 65*(2), 154–164.

De Bellis, M. D. (2005). The psychobiology of neglect. *Child Maltreatment, 10*(2), 150–172.

Dębiec, J., & LeDoux, J. E. (2009). The amygdala and the neural pathways of fear. In P. J. Shiromani, T. M. Keane, & J. E. LeDoux (Ed.), *Post-traumatic stress disorder: Basic science and clinical practice* (pp. 23–38). Totowa, NJ: Humana Press.

Decety, J., & Chaminade, T. (2003). When the self represents the other: A new cognitive neuroscience view on psychological identification. *Consciousness and Cognition, 12*(4), 577–596.

Decety, J., & Michalska, K. J. (2010) Neurodevelopmental changes in the circuits underlying empathy and sympathy from childhood to adulthood. *Developmental Science, 13*(6), 886–899.

deCharms, R. C., & Zador, A. (2000). Neural representation and the cortical code. *Annual Review of Neuroscience, 23*(1), 613–647.

Degonda, N., Mondadori, C. R. A., Bosshardt, S., Schmidt, C. F., Boesiger, P., Nitsch, R. M., et al. (2005). Implicit associative learning engages the hippocampus and interacts with explicit associative learning. *Neuron, 46*(3), 505–520.

de Haas, M., Bakermans-Kranenburg, M., & van IJzendoorn, M. H. (1994). The Adult Attachment Interview and questionnaires for attachment style, temperament and memories of parental behavior. *Journal of Genetic Psychology, 155*, 471–486.

DeKlyen, M., & Greenberg, M. T. (2008). Attachment and psychopathology in childhood. In J. Cassidy & P. R. Shaver (Eds.), *Handbook of attachment: Theory, research, and clinical applications* (2nd ed., pp. 637–665). New York: Guilford Press.

de Kloet, E. R., Joels, M., & Holsboer, F. (2006). Stress and the brain: From adaptation to disease. *Nature Reviews Neuroscience, 6*, 463–475.

Dell, P. F., & O'Neil, J. A. (Eds.). (2009). *Dissociation and the dissociative disorders: DSM-V and beyond*. New York: Routledge.

DeOliveira, C. A. A., Moran, G., & Peterson, D. (2005). Understanding the link between maternal adult attachment classifications and thoughts and feelings about emotions. *Attachment and Human Development, 7*(2), 153–170.

de Quervain, D. J., Aerni, A., Schelling, G., & Roozendaal, B. (2009). Glucocorticoids and the regulation of memory in health and disease. *Frontiers in Neuroendocrinology, 30*(3), 358–370.

de Quervain, D. J., Kolassa, I.-T., Ert, V., Onyut, P. L., Neuner, F., Elbert, T., et al. (2007). A deletion variant of the 2b-adrenoceptor is related to emotional memory in Europeans and Africans. *Nature Neuroscience, 10*, 1137–1139.

Derakhshan, I. (2010). It is all quiet in the minor hemisphere: An investigation into the laterality of consciousness, attention and vision in the human brain. *Biomedicine International, 1*(1), 3–15.

Derryberry, D., & Reed, M. (2003). Information processing approaches to individual differences in emotional reactivity. In R. J. Davidson, K. R. Scherer, & H. H. Goldsmith (Eds.), *Handbook of affective sciences* (pp. 681–697). New York: Oxford University Press.

Desmurget, M., Bonnetblanc, F., & Duffau, H. (2007). Contrasting acute and slow growing lesions: A new door to brain plasticity. *Brain, 130*(4), 898–914.

de Wolff, M. S., & van IJzendoorn, M. H. (1997). Sensitivity and attachment: A metaanalysis of parental antecedents of infant attachment. *Child Development, 68, 571–591.*

Diamond, A. (2006). Interrelated and interdependent. *Developmental Science, 10*(1), 152–158.

Dickstein, D., Brazel, A., Goldberg, L., & Hunt, J. (2008). Affect regulation in pediatric bipolar disorder. *Child and Adolescent Psychiatric Clinics of North America, 18*(2), 405–420.

Diego, M. A., Field, T., Jones, N. A., & Hernandez-Reif, M. (2006). Withdrawn and intrusive maternal interaction style and infant frontal EEG asymmetry shifts in infants of depressed and non-depressed mothers. *Infant Behavior and Development, 29*(2), 220–229.

Diekelmann, S., & Born, J. (2010). The memory function of sleep. *Nature Reviews Neuroscience, 11*, 114–126.

Diekelmann, S., Wilhelm, I., & Born, J. (2009). The whats and whens of sleep-dependent memory consolidation. *Sleep Medicine Reviews, 13*(5), 309–321.

DiNoble, A. (2009). *Examining the relationship between adult attachment style and mindfulness traits.* Unpublished doctoral dissertation, California Graduate Institute of the Chicago School of Professional Psychology.

Dodge, K. A. (1991). Emotion and social information processing. In J. Garber & K. A. Dodge (Eds.), *The development of emotion regulation and dysregulation* (pp. 159–181). Cambridge, UK: Cambridge University Press.

Dodge, K. A. (1993). Social-cognitive mechanisms in the development of conduct disorder and depression. *Annual Review of Psychology, 44*, 559–584.

Doebeli, M. (1993). The evolutionary advantage of controlled chaos. *Proceedings of the Royal Society of London: Series B. Biological Sciences, 254*, 281–285.

Doidge, N. (2007). *The brain that changes itself: Stories of personal triumph from the frontiers of brain science.* New York: Penguin.

Doty, R. W. (2007). Alkmaion's discovery that brain creates mind: A revolution in human knowledge comparable to that of Copernicus and of Darwin. *Neuroscience, 147*(3), 561–568.

Douglas, R. J., & Martin, K. A. C. (2007). Mapping the matrix: The ways of neocortex. *Neuron, 56*, 226–236.

Dozier, M., Manni, M., Gordon, K. M., Peloso, E., Gunnar, M. A., Stovall-McClough, K., et al. (2006). Foster children's diurnal production of cortisol: An exploratory study. *Child Maltreatment, 11*(2), 189–197.

Dozier, M., & Rutter, M. (2008). Challenges to the development of attachment relationships faced by young children in foster and adoptive care. In J. Cassidy & P. R. Shaver (Eds.), *Handbook of attachment: Theory, research, and clinical applications* (2nd ed., pp. 698–717). New York: Guilford Press.

Dozier, M., Stovall, K. C., Albus, K. E., & Bates, B. (2001). Attachment for infants in foster care: The role of caregiver state of mind. *Child Development, 72*, 1467–1477.

Dozier, M., Stovall-McClough, C., & Albus, K. E. (2008). Attachment and psychopathology in adulthood. In J. Cassidy & P. R. Shaver (Eds.), *Handbook of attachment: Theory, research, and clinical applications* (2nd ed., pp. 718–744). New York: Guilford Press.

Duffau, H. (2006). Brain plasticity: From pathophysiological mechanisms to therapeutic applications. *Journal of Clinical Neuroscience, 13*(9), 885–897.

Dunbar, R. (2003). The social brain: Mind, language, and society in evolutionary perspective. *Annual Review of Anthropology, 32*, 163–181.

Dunn, J. (2003). Emotional development in early childhood: A social relationship perspective. In R. J. Davidson, K. R. Scherer, & H. H. Goldsmith (Eds.), *Handbook of affective sciences* (pp. 332–346). New York: Oxford University Press.

Dutra, L., Ilaria, B., Siegel, D. J., & Lyons-Ruth, K. (2009). The relational context of dissociative phenonmena. In P. F. Dell & J. A. O'Neil (Eds.), *Dissociation and the dissociative disorders: DSM-V and beyond* (pp. 83–92). New York: Routledge.

Dwyer, K. M., Fredstrom, B. K., Rubin, K. H., Booth-LaForce, C., Rose-Krasnor, L., & Burgess, K. B. (2010). Attachment, social information processing, and friendship quality of early adolescent girls and boys. *Journal of Social and Personal Relationships, 27*(1), 91–116.

Easton, A., & Eacott, M. (2009). Recollection of episodic memory within the medial temporal lobe: Behavioural dissociations from other types of memory. *Behavioural Brain Research, 215*(2), 310–317.

Eckert, M. A., Menon, V., Walczak, A., Ahlstrom, J., Denslow, S., Horwitz, A., et al. (2009). At the heart of the ventral attention system: The right anterior insula. *Human Brain Mapping, 30*(8), 2530–2541.

Ecuyer-Dab, I., & Robert, M. (2004). Have sex differences in spatial ability evolved from male competition for mating and female concern for survival? *Cognition, 91*(3), 221–257.

Edelman, G. M. (1993). *Bright air, brilliant fire: On the matter of the mind.* New York: Basic Books.

Edelman, G. M., & Tononi, G. (2000a). *A universe of consciousness: How matter becomes imagination.* New York: Basic Books.

Edelman, G. M., & Tononi, G. (2000b). Reentry and the dynamic core: Neural correlates of conscious experience. In T. Mezinger (Ed.), *Neural correlates of consciousness: Empirical and conceptual questions* (pp. 139–151). Cambridge, MA: MIT Press.

Edelstein, R. S., & Gillath, O. (2008). Avoiding interference: Adult attachment and emotional processing biases. *Personality and Social Psychology Bulletin, 34*(2), 171–181.

Edwards, B. (1999). *The new drawing on the right side of the brain.* New York: Penguin Putnam.

Eggermont, J. (2005). Correlated neural activity: Epiphenomenon or part of the neural code? In R. Konig, P. Heil, E. Budinger, & H. Scheich (Eds.), *The auditory cortex: A synthesis of human and animal research* (pp. 255–273). Hove, UK: Psychology Press.

Ehlis, A., Bähne, C., Jacob, C., Herrmann, M., & Fallgatter, A. (2008). Reduced lateral prefrontal activation in adult patients with attention-deficit/hyperactivity disorder (ADHD) during a working memory task: A functional near-infrared spectroscopy (fNIRS) study. *Journal of Psychiatric Research, 42*(13), 1060–1067.

Eid, M., & Diener, E. (2009). Norms for experiencing emotions in different cultures: Inter- and intranational differences. In E. Diener (Ed.), *Culture and well-being: The collected works of Ed Diener* (pp. 169–202). New York: Springer.

Eisenberger, N. I., & Lieberman, M. D. (2004). Why rejection hurts: A common neural alarm system for physical and social pain. *Trends in Cognitive Sciences, 8*(7), 294–300.

Eisenberger, N. I., Master, S. L., Inagaki, T. K., Taylor, S. E., Shirinyan, D., Lieberman, M. D., et al. (2011). Attachment figures activate a safety signal-related neural region and reduce pain experience. *PNAS, 108*(28), 11721–11726.

Eisenberger, N. I., Taylor, S. E., Gable, S. L., Hilmert, C. J., & Lieberman, M. D. (2007). Neural pathways link social support to attenuated neuroendocrine stress responses. *NeuroImage, 35*(4), 1601–1612.

Ekman, P. (2009). *Telling lies: Clues to deceit in the marketplace, politics, and marriage* (4th ed.). New York: Norton.

Ekman, P., & Lama, D. (2009). *Emotional awareness: Overcoming the obstacles to psychological balance.* New York: Holt Paperbacks.

Elder, G. H. (1998). The life course as developmental theory. *Child Development, 69,* 1–12.

Eliot, L. (2010, May). The truth about boys and girls. *Scientific American Mind,* pp. 22–29.

Ellis, B. J., Boyce, W. T., Belsky, J., Bakermans-Kranenburg, M. J., & van IJzendoorn, M. H. (2011). Differential susceptibility to the environment: An evolutionary-neurodevelopment theory. *Development and Psychopathology, 23,* 7–28.

Ellsworth, P. C., & Scherer K. R. (2003). Appraisal processes in emotion. In R. J. Davidson, K. R. Scherer, & H. H. Goldsmith (Eds.), *Handbook of affective sciences* (pp. 572–595). New York: Oxford University Press.

Elzinga, B. M., Bakker, A., & Bremner, J. D. (2005). Stress-induced cortisol elevations are associated with impaired delayed, but not immediate recall. *Psychiatry Research, 134*(3), 211–223.

Elzinga, B. M., & Bremner, J. D. (2002). Are the neural substrates of memory the final common pathway in posttraumatic stress disorder (PTSD)? *Journal of Affective Disorders, 70*(1), 1–17.

Engle, J. A. A., & Smith, M. L. (2010). Attention and material-specific memory in children with lateralized epilepsy. *Neuropsychologia, 48*(1), 38–42.

Epstein, R. M., Siegel, D. J., & Silberman, J. (2009). Self-monitoring in clinical practice: A challenge for medical educators. *Journal of Continuing Education in the Health Professions, 28*(1), 5–13.

Erk, S., Abler, B., & Walter, H. (2006). Cognitive modulation of emotion anticipation. *European Journal of Neuroscience, 24*(4), 1227–1236.

Erraji, L.-B., Underwood, M. D., Arango, V., Galfalvy, H., Pavlidis, P., Smyrniotopoulos, P., et al. (2005). Molecular aging in human prefrontal cortex is selective and continuous throughout adult life. *Biological Psychiatry, 57*(5), 549–558.

Ethofer, T., Anders, S., Erb, M., Herbert, C., Weithoff, S., Kissler, J., et al. (2005). Cerebral pathways in processing of affective prosody: A dynamic causal modeling study. *NeuroImage, 30*(2), 580–587.

Etkin, A., & Wager, T. D. (2007). Functional neuroimaging of anxiety: A meta-analysis of emotional processing in PTSD, social anxiety disorder, and specific phobia. *American Journal of Psychiatry, 164*, 1476–1488.

Eustache, F., & Desgranges, B. (2008). MNESIS: Towards the integration of current multisystem models of memory. *Neuropsychology Review, 18*(1), 53–69.

Evans, K. M., & Federmeier, K. D. (2009). Left and right memory revisited: Electrophysiological investigations of hemispheric asymmetries at retrieval. *Neuropsychologia, 47*(2), 303–313.

Evert, D. D., & Emen, M. (2003). Hemispheric asymmetries for global and local processing as a function of stimulus exposure duration. *Brain and Cognition, 51*(1), 115–142.

Fair, D. A., Dosenbach, N. U. F., Church, J. A., Cohen, A. L., Brahmbhatt, S., Miezin, F. M., et al. (2007). Development of distinct control networks through segregation and integration. *Proceedings of the National Academy of Sciences USA, 104*(33), 13507–13512.

Fairfax, H. (2008). The use of mindfulness in obsessive compulsive disorder: Suggestions for its application and integration in existing treatment. *Clinical Psychology and Psychotherapy, 15*(1), 53–59.

Farb, N. A. S., Segal, Z. V., Mayberg, H., Bean, J., McKeon, D., Fatima, Z., et al. (2007). Attending to the present: Mindfulness meditation reveals distinct neural modes of self-reference. *Social Cognitive and Affective Neuroscience, 2*(4), 313–322.

Farber, H. R., & Siegel, D. J. (2011). Parental presence: An interpersonal neurobiology approach to healthy relationships between adults and their parents. In S. M. Dunham, S. B. Dermer, & J. Carlson (Eds.), *Poisonous parenting: Toxic relationships between parents and their adult children* (pp. 49–62). New York: Routledge.

Fearon, P., Bakermans-Kranenburg, M. J., van IJzendoorn, M. H., Lapsley, A., & Roisman, G. I. (2010). The significance of insecure attachment and disorganization in the development of children's externalizing behavior: A meta-analytic study. *Child Development, 81*(2), 435–456.

Feeney, B. C., & VanVleet, M. (2010). Growing through attachment: The interplay of attachment and exploration in adulthood. *Journal of Social and Personal Relationships, 72*(2), 226–234.

Feldman, R. (2007). Parent–infant synchrony: Biological foundations and developmental outcomes. *Current Directions in Psychological Science, 16*(6), 340–345.

Ferber, S. G. (2008). The concept of coregulation between neurobehavioral subsystems: The logic interplay between excitatory and inhibitory ends. *Behavioral and Brain Sciences, 31*, 337–338.

Ferber, S. G., Feldman, R., & Makhoul, I. R. (2007). The development of maternal touch across the first year of life. *Early Human Development, 84*(6), 363–370.

Ferber, S. G., & Makhoul, I. R. (2004). The effect of skin-to-skin contact (kangaroo care) shortly after birth on the neurobehavioral responses of the term newborn: A randomized, controlled trial. *Pediatrics, 113*(4), 858–865.

Ferbinteanu, J., Kennedy, P. J., & Shapiro, M. L. (2006). Episodic memory: From brain to mind. *Hippocampus, 16*(9), 691–703.

Ferrari, M., Pinard, A., & Runions, K. (2001). Piaget's framework for a scientific study of consciousness. *Human Development, 44*, 195–213.

Field, T. (1985). Attachment as psychobiological attunement: Being on the same wavelength. In M. Reite & T. Field (Eds.), *The psychobiology of attachment and separation* (pp. 415–454). Orlando, FL: Academic Press.

Field, T. (1994). The effects of mother's physical and emotional unavailability on emotion regulation. In N. A. Fox (Ed.), The development of emotion regulation: Biological and behavioral considerations. *Monographs of the Society for Research in Child Development, 59*(2–3, Serial No. 240), 208–227.

Field, T., & Diego, M. (2008). Maternal depression effects on infant frontal EEG asymmetry. *International Journal of Neuroscience, 118*(8), 1081–1108.

Field, T., Hernandez-Reif, M., & Diego, M. (2006). Intrusive and withdrawn depressed mothers and their infants. *Developmental Review, 26*(1), 15–30.

Field, T., Hernandez-Reif, M., Vera, Y., Gil, K., Diego, M., Bendell, D., et al. (2005). Anxiety and anger effects on depressed mother–infant spontaneous and imitative interactions. *Infant Behavior and Development, 28*(1), 1–9.

Findlay, L., & Coplan, R. J. (2008). Come out and play: Shyness in childhood and the benefits of organized sports participation. *Canadian Journal of Behavioural Science, 40*(3), 153–161.

Fitzgerald, D. A., Angstadt, M., Jelsone, L. M., Nathan, P. J., & Phan, K. L. (2006). Beyond threat: Amygdala reactivity across multiple expressions of facial affect. *NeuroImage, 30*(4), 1441–1448.

Fivush, R. (1998). Children's recollections of traumatic and nontraumatic events. *Development and Psychopathology, 10*, 699–716.

Fivush, R. (2011). The development of autobiographical memory. *Annual Review of Psychology, 62*, 559–582.

Fivush, R., Bohanek, J. G., & Marin, K. (2010). Patterns of family narrative co-construction in relation to adolescent identity and well-being. In K. C. McLean & M. Pasupathi (Eds.), *Narrative development in adolescence* (pp. 45–63). New York: Springer

Fivush, R., & Nelson, K. (2004). Culture and language in the emergence of autobiographical memory. *Psychological Science, 15*(9), 573–577.

Fivush, R., & Nelson, K. (2006). Parent–child reminiscing locates the self in the past. *British Journal of Developmental Psychology, 24*(1), 235–251.

Flores, E., Rogosch, F. A., & Cicchetti, D. (2005). Predictors of resilience in maltreated and nonmaltreated Latino children. *Developmental Psychology, 41*(2), 338–351.

Fodor, J. (2000). *The mind doesn't work that way.* Cambridge, MA: MIT Press.

Fogel, A. (2000a). Systems, attachment, and relationships. *Human Development, 43*(6), 314–320.

Fogel, A. (2000b). Developmental pathways in close relationships. *Child Development, 71*(5), 1150–1151.

Fogel, A., de Koeyer, I., Secrist, C., & Nagy, R. (2002). Dynamic systems theory places the scientist in the system. *Behavioral and Brain Sciences, 25*(5), 623.

Fogel, A., Lyra, M. C. D. P., & Valsiner, J. (Eds.). (1997). *Dynamics and indeterminism in developmental and social processes*. Mahwah, NJ: Erlbaum.

Fonagy, P. (2001). *Attachment theory and psychoanalysis*. New York: Other Press.

Fonagy, P., Gergely, G., Jurist, E., & Target, M. (2002). *Affect regulation, mentalization, and the development of the self*. London: Karnac Books.

Fonagy, P., Gergely, G., & Target, M. (2007). The parent–infant dyad and the construction of the subjective self. *Journal of Child Psychology and Psychiatry, 48*(3–4), 288–328.

Fonagy, P., Luyten, P., Bateman, A., Gergely, G., Strathearn, L., Target, M., et al. (2008). Attachment and personality pathology. In J. F. Clarkin, P. Fonagy, & G. O. Gabbard (Eds.), *Psychodynamic psychotherapy for personality disorders: A clinical handbook* (pp. 37–88). Arlington, VA: American Psychiatric Publishing.

Fonagy, P., & Target, M. (1997). Attachment and reflective function: Their role in self-organization. *Development and Psychopathology, 9*, 679–700.

Fonagy, P., & Target, M. (2005). Bridging the transmission gap: An end to an important mystery of attachment research? *Attachment and Human Development, 7*(3), 333–343.

Fonagy, P., Target, M., Gergely, G., Allen, J., & Bateman, A. (2003). The developmental roots of borderline personality disorder in early attachment relationships: A theory and some evidence. *Psychoanalytic Inquiry, 23*(3), 412–459.

Forbes, E. E. E., Shaw, D. S., Fox, N. A., Cohn, J. F., Silk, J. S., & Kovacs, M. (2006). Maternal depression, child frontal asymmetry, and child affective behavior as factors in child behavior problems. *Journal of Child Psychology and Psychiatry, 47*(1), 79–87.

Forgas, J. (2008). Affect and cognition. *Perspectives on Psychological Science, 3*(2), 94–101.

Fosha, D. (2003). Dyadic regulation and experiential work with emotion and relatedness in trauma and disorganized attachment. In M. F. Solomon & D. J. Siegel (Eds.), *Healing trauma: Attachment, mind, body and brain* (pp. 221–282). New York: Norton.

Fosha, D., Siegel, D. J., & Solomon, M. F. (Eds.). (2009). *The healing power of emotion: Affective neuroscience, development and clinical practice*. New York: Norton.

Fossati, P., Hevenor, S. J., Graham, S. J., Grady, C., Keightley, M. L., Craik, F., et al. (2003). In search of the emotional self: An fMRI study using positive and negative emotional words. *American Journal of Psychiatry, 160*(11), 1938–1945.

Fournier, N., Calverley, K. L., Wagner, J. P., Poock, J. L., & Crossley, M. (2008). Impaired social cognition 30 years after hemispherectomy for intractable epilepsy: The importance of the right hemisphere in complex social functioning. *Epilepsy and Behavior, 12*(3), 460–471.

Fox, M. D., & Greicius, M. (2010). Clinical applications of resting state functional connectivity. *Frontiers in Systems Neuroscience, 4*, 19.

Fox, M. D., Snyder, A. Z., Vincent, J. L., Corbetta, M., Van Essen, D. C., & Raichle, M. E. (2005). The human brain is intrinsically organized into dynamic, anticorrelated functional networks. *Proceedings of the National Academy of Sciences USA, 102*(27), 9673–9678.

Fox, N. A. (Ed.). (1994). The development of emotion regulation: Biological and behavioral considerations. *Monographs of the Society for Research in Child Development, 59*(2–3, Serial No. 240).

Fox, N. A., & Hane, A. A. (2008). Studying the biology of human attachment. In J. Cassidy & P. R. Shaver (Eds.), *Handbook of attachment: Theory, research, and clinical application* (2nd ed., pp. 217–240). New York: Guilford Press.

Fox, S., & Hoelscher, K. (2010). *The political economy of social violence: Theory and evidence from a cross-country study* (Crisis States Working Paper No. 72, Series 2). London: London Schools of Economics.

Frankenhuis, W., & Ploeger, A. (2007). Evolutionary psychology versus Fodor: Arguments for and against the massive modularity hypothesis. *Philosophical Psychology, 20*(6), 687–710.

Frederick, R. J. (2009). *Living like you mean it: Use the wisdom and power of your emotions to get the life you really want.* San Francisco: Jossey-Bass.

Fredrickson, B. (2004). The broaden-and-build theory of positive emotion. *Philosophical Transactions of the Royal Society of London: Series B. Biological Sciences, 359,* 1367–1377.

Freud, S. (1966). Project for a scientific psychology. In J. Strachey (Ed. & Trans.), *The standard edition of the complete psychological works of Sigmund Freud* (Vol. 1, pp. 281–397). London: Hogarth Press. (Original work published 1895)

Friedman, D., Beebe, B., Jaffe, J., Ross, D., & Triggs, S. (2010). Microanalysis of 4-month infant vocal affect qualities and maternal postpartum depression. *Clinical Social Work Journal, 38*(1), 8–16.

Frith, U. (2004). *Autism: Mind and brain.* Oxford, UK: Oxford University Press.

Frodi, T., Reinhold, E., Koutsouleris, N., Reiser, M., & Meisenzahl, E. M. (2010). Interaction of childhood stress with hippocampus and prefrontal cortex volume reduction in major depression. *Journal of Psychiatric Research, 44*(13), 799–807.

Fuligni, A. (2011, January 27). *Social identity and the motivation and well being of adolescents.* Oral presentation at the UCLA Center for Culture, Brain, and Development Winter Seminar, UCLA.

Furber, S. B., Brown, G., Bose, J., Cumpstey, J. M., Marshall, P., & Shapiro, J. L. (2007). Sparse distributed memory using rank-order neural codes. *IEEE Transactions on Neural Networks, 18*(3), 648–659.

Fuster, J. M. (2006). The cognit: A network model of cortical representation. *International Journal of Psychophysiology, 60*(2), 125–132.

Fuster, J. M. (2008). *The prefrontal cortex* (4th ed.). Burlington, MA: Elsevier/Academic Press.

Fuster, J. M. (2009). Cortex and memory: Emergence of a new paradigm. *Journal of Cognitive Neuroscience, 21*(11), 2047–2072.

Gaensbauer, T. J., & Jordan, L. (2009). Psychoanalytic perspectives on early trauma: Interviews with thirty analysts who treated an adult victim of a circumscribed trauma in early childhood. *Journal of the American Psychoanalytic Association, 57*(4), 947–977.

Gagnon, G., Blanchet, S., Grondin, S., & Schneider, C. (2010). Paired-pulse transcranial magnetic stimulation over the dorsolateral prefrontal cortex interferes with episodic encoding and retrieval for both verbal and non-verbal materials. *Brain Research, 1344,* 148–158.

Gainotti, G. (2005). Emotions, unconscious processes, and the right hemisphere. *Neuro-Psychoanalysis, 7*(1), 71–81.

Gal, E., Bauminger, N., Goren-Bar, D., Pianesi, F., Stock, O., Zancanaro, M., et al. (2009). Enhancing social communication of children with high-functioning autism through a co-located interface. *AI and Society, 24*(1), 75–84.

Gallace, A., & Spence, C. (2009). The cognitive and neural correlates of tactile memory. *Psychological Bulletin, 135*(3), 380–406.

Gallese, V. (2005). Embodied simulation: From neurons to phenomenal experience. *Phenomenology and the Cognitive Sciences, 4,* 23–48.

Gallese, V., Fadiga, L., Fogassi, L., & Rizzolati, G. (1996). Action recognition in the premotor cortex. *Brain: A Journal of Neurology, 119*(2), 593–609.

Ganis, G., Thompson, W., & Kosslyn, S. (2009). Visual mental imagery: More than 'seeing with the mind's eye.' In J. R. Brockmole (Ed.), *The visual world in memory* (pp. 215–249). New York: Psychology Press.

Garcia, M.-T., & Aguirre, I. (2007). Biopsychosocial model in depression revisited. *Medical Hypotheses, 68*(3), 683–691.

Gazzaniga, M. S. (1996). *Cognitive neuroscience and the future of psychiatry*. Plenary address to the American Association of Directors of Psychiatric Residency Training, San Francisco.

Gazzaniga, M. S. (Ed.). (2004). *The cognitive neurosciences III*. Cambridge, MA: MIT Press.

Gazzaniga, M. S., Eliassen, J. C., Nisenson, L., Wessinger, C. M., & Baynes, K. B. (1996). Collaboration between the hemispheres of a callosotomy patient: Emerging right hemisphere speech and the left brain interpreter. *Brain, 119*, 1255–1262.

Genovesio, A., Brasted, P. J., Mitz, A. R., & Wise, S. P. (2005). Prefrontal cortex activity related to abstract response strategies. *Neuron, 47*(2), 307–320.

George, C., Kaplan, N., & Main, M. (1996). *An Adult Attachment Interview: Interview protocol* (3rd ed.). Unpublished manuscript, University of California at Berkeley.

George, C., & West, M. (2003). The Adult Attachment Projective: Measuring individual differences in attachment security using projective methodology. In M. J. Hilsenroth, D. L. Segal, & M. Hersen (Eds.), *Comprehensive handbook of psychological assessment* (Vol. 2, pp. 431–448). Hoboken, NJ: Wiley.

George, M. S., Ketter, T. A., Parekh, P. I., Gill, D. S., Marangell, L., Pazzaglia, P. J., et al. (1997). Depressed subjects have decreased rCBF activation during facial emotion recognition. *International Journal of Neuropsychiatric Medicine, 2*, 45–55.

Geraerts, E., Bernstein, D. M., Merckelbach, H., Linders, C., Raymaekers, L., & Loftus, E. F. (2008). Lasting false beliefs and their behavioral consequences. *Psychological Science, 19*(8), 749–753.

Gergely, G., & Unoka, Z. (2008). Attachment, affect-regulation, and mentalization: The developmental origins of the representational affective self. In C. Sharp, P. Fonagy, & I. Goodyer (Eds.), *Social cognition and developmental psychopathology* (p. 305–342). New York: Oxford University Press.

Gerhardstein, P., & West, R. (2003). Relation between perceptual input and infant memory. In J. W. Fagen & H. Hayne (Eds.), *Progress in infancy research* (Vol. 3, pp. 121–158). Mahwah, NJ: Erlbaum.

Gervai, J. (2009). Environmental and genetic influences on early attachment. *Child and Adolescent Psychiatry and Mental Health, 3*, 25.

Ghahremani, D. G., Monterosso, J., Jentsch, J. D., Bilder, R. M., & Poldrack, R. A. (2010). Neural components underlying behavioral flexibility in human reversal learning. *Cerebral Cortex, 20*(8), 1843–1852.

Gilbert, P., & Andrews, B. (Eds.). (1998). *Shame: Interpersonal behavior, psychopathology, and culture*. New York: Oxford University Press.

Gillath, O., Mikiulincer, M. P., Fitzsimons, G. M., Shaver, P. R., Schachner, D. A., & Bargh, J. A. (2006). Automatic activation of attachment-related goals. *Development and Psychopathology, 32*(10), 1375–1388.

Gilson, M., Thomas, D. A., Burkitt, A. N., Grayden, D. B., & Van Hemmen, J. (2009). Interplay between spike-timing-dependent plasticity and neuronal correlations gives rise to network structure. *BMC Neuroscience, 10*(1), 101–102.

Girgis, R. R., Minshew, N. J., Melhem, N. M., Nutche, J. J., Keshavan, M. S., & Hardan, A. Y. (2007). Volumetric alterations of the orbitofrontal cortex in autism. *Progress in Neuro-Psychopharmacology and Biological Psychiatry, 31*(1) 41–45.

Glaser, J., van Os, J., Portegijs, P. M., & Myin-Germeys, I. (2006). Childhood trauma and emotional reactivity to daily life stress in adult frequent attenders of general practitioners. *Journal of Psychosomatic Research, 61*(2), 229–236.

Globerson, A., Stark, E., Vaadia, E., & Tishby, N. (2009). The minimum information principle and its application to neural code analysis. *Proceedings of the National Academy of Sciences USA, 106*(9), 3490–3495.

Globus, G., & Arpaia, J. P. (1993). Psychiatry and the new dynamics. *Biological Psychiatry, 35,* 352–364.

Gloger-Tippelt, G., Gomile, B., Koenig, L., & Vetter, J. (2002). Attachment representations in 6-year-olds: Related longitudinally to the quality of attachment in infancy and mothers' attachment representations. *Attachment and Human Development, 4*(3), 318–339.

Godard, O., & Flori, N. (2010) Sex differences in face processing: Are women less lateralized and faster than men? *Brain and Cognition, 73*(3), 167–175.

Goel, V., Shuren, J., Sheesley, L., & Grafman, J. (2004). Asymmetrical involvement of frontal lobes in social reasoning. *Brain, 127*(4), 783–790.

Goel, V., Tierney, M., Sheesley, L., Bartolo, A., Vartanian, O., & Grafman, J. (2007). Hemispheric specialization in human prefrontal cortex for resolving certain and uncertain inferences. *Cerebral Cortex, 17*(10), 2245–2250.

Goldberg, E., & Costa, L. D. (1981). Hemispheric differences in the acquisition and use of descriptive systems. *Brain and Language, 14,* 144–173.

Goldberg, L. R. (1990). An alternative "description of personality": The big-five factor structure. *Journal of Personality and Social Psychology, 59*(6), 1216–1229.

Goldberg, S., Benoit, D., Blokland, K., & Madigan, S. (2003). Atypical maternal behavior, maternal representations and infant disorganized attachment. *Development and Psychopathology, 15,* 239–257.

Goldsmith, H. H., Lemery, K. S., Aksan, N., & Buss, K. A. (2000). Temperamental substrates of personality. In V. J. Molfese, D. L. Molfese, & R. R. McCrae (Eds.), *Temperament and personality development across the life span* (pp. 1–32). Mahwah, NJ: Erlbaum.

Goldsmith, T. (2009). How scandalous is knowledge of evolutionary psychology? *Society, 46*(4), 341–346.

Goleman, D. (2006). *Emotional intelligence: Why it can matter more than IQ* (10th anniversary ed.). New York: Bantam/Random House.

Gollan, J., Pane, H., McCloskey, M., & Coccaro, E. (2008). Identifying differences in biased affective information processing in major depression. *Psychiatry Research, 159*(1–2), 18–24.

Gonsalves, B., & Paller, K. A. (2002). Mistaken memories: Remembering events that never happened. *The Neuroscientist, 8*(5), 391–395.

Gopnik, A., & Meltzoff, A. N. (2006). Minds, bodies, and persons: Young children's understanding of the self and others as reflected in imitation and theory of mind research. In S. T. Parker, R. W. Mitchell, & M. L. Boccia (Eds.), *Self-awareness in animals and humans: Developmental perspectives* (pp. 166–1186). Cambridge, UK: Cambridge University Press.

Govindarajan, A., Kelleher, R., & Tonegawa, S. (2006). A clustered plasticity model of long-term memory engrams. *Nature Reviews Neuroscience, 7*(7), 575–583.

Green, J., & Goldwyn, R. (2002). Attachment disorganisation and psychopathology: New findings in attachment research and their potential implications for developmental psychopathology in childhood. *Journal of Child Psychology and Psychiatry, 43*(7), 835–846.

Green, M. J., & Phillips, M. L. (2004). Social threat perception and the evolution of paranoia. *Neuroscience and Biobehavioral Reviews, 23*(3), 338–342.

Green, T., Neinemann, S. F., & Gusella, J. F. (1998). Molecular neurobiology and genetics: Investigation of neural function and dysfunction. *Neuron, 20,* 427–444.

Greenberg, M. E. (2010). Signaling networks that control synapse development and cognitive function. In Harvey Society (Ed.), *The Harvey lectures* (Series 102, pp. 73–102). Hoboken, NJ: Wiley.

Greenberg, M. T., DeKlyen, M., Speltz, M. L., & Endriga, M. C. (1997). The role of attachment processes in externalizing psychopathology in young children. In L. Atkinson & K. J. Zucker (Eds.), *Attachment and psychopathology* (pp. 196–222). New York: Guilford Press.

Greenberg, M. T., Speltz, M. L., & DeKlyen, M. (1993). The role of attachment in the early development of disruptive behavior problems. *Development and Psychopathology, 5*, 191–213.

Greenberg, M. T., Speltz, M. L., DeKlyen, M., & Jones, K. (2001). Correlates of clinic referral for early conduct problems: Variable and person-oriented approaches. *Development and Psychopathology, 13*(2), 255–276.

Grice, H. P. (1975). Logic and conversation. In P. Cole & J. L. Moran (Eds.), *Syntax and semantics III: Speech acts* (pp. 41–58). New York: Academic Press.

Grienenberger, J., Kelly, K., & Slade, A. (2005). Maternal reflective functioning, mother–infant affective communication, and infant attachment: Exploring the link between mental states of observed caregiving behavior in the intergenerational transmission of attachment. *Attachment and Human Development, 7*, 299–311.

Gross, J. J. (2002). Emotion regulation: Affective, cognitive, and social consequences. *Psychophysiology, 29*, 281–291.

Gross, J. J. (Ed.). (2007). *Handbook of emotion regulation.* New York: Guilford Press.

Gross, J. J., & Thompson, R. A. (2007). Emotion regulation: Conceptual foundations. In J. J. Gross (Ed.), *Handbook of emotion regulation* (pp. 3–26). New York: Guilford Press.

Grossberg, S. (1999). The link between brain learning, Attention, and Consciousness. *Consciousness and Cognition, 8*(1), 1–44.

Grossman, K. E., Grossman, K., & Waters, E. (Eds.). (2005). *Attachment from infancy to adulthood: The major longitudinal studies.* New York: Guilford Press.

Guastello, S. J., Koopmans, M., & Pincus, D. (Eds.). (2009). *Chaos and complexity in psychology: The theory of nonlinear dynamical systems.* Cambridge, UK: Cambridge University Press.

Guo, K., Robertson, R. G., Pulgarin, M., Nevado, A., Panzeri, S., Thiele, A., et al. (2007). Spatio-temporal prediction and inference by V1 neurons. *European Journal of Neuroscience, 26*(4), 1045–1054.

Guyer, A., McClure, E., Adler, A., Brotman, M., Rich, B., Kimes, A., et al. (2007). Specificity of facial expression labeling deficits in childhood psychopathology. *Journal of Child Psychology and Psychiatry, 48*(9), 863–871.

Haberstadt, A. G., & Lozada, F. T. (2011). Emotion development in infancy through the lens of culture. *Emotion Review, 3*(2), 158–168.

Habib, R., Nyberg, L., & Tulving, E. (2003). Hemispheric asymmetries of memory: The HERA model revisited. *Trends in Cognitive Sciences, 7*(6), 241–245.

Haft, W. L., & Slade, A. (1989). Affect attunement and maternal attachment: A pilot study. *Infant Mental Health Journal, 10*, 157–172.

Haggard, P. (2008). Human volition: Toward a neuroscience of will. *Nature Neuroscience, 9*, 934–946.

Haggerty, G. D., Siegfert, C. J., & Weinberger, J. (2010). Examining the relationship between current attachment status and freely recalled autobiographical memories of childhood. *Psychoanalytic Psychology, 27*, 27–41.

Haidt, J. (2006). *The happiness hypothesis.* New York: Basic Books.

Haley, D. W., & Stansbury, K. (2003). Infant stress and parent responsiveness: Regulation of physiology. *Child Development, 74*(5), 1534–1546.

Hall, K. D. D., & Lifshitz, J. (2010). Diffuse traumatic brain injury initially attenuates and later expands activation of the rat somatosensory whisker circuit concomitant with neuroplastic responses. *Brain Research, 1323*, 161.

Halpern, M. E., Güntürkün, O., Hopkins, W. D., & Rogers, L. J. (2005). Lateralization of the vertebrate brain: Taking the side of model systems. *Journal of Neuroscience, 25*(45), 10351–10357.

Hammack, P. L. (2008). Narrative and the cultural psychology of identity. *Personality and Social Psychology Review, 12*(3), 222–247.

Hampe, B., & Grady, J. E. (Eds.). (2005). *From perception to meaning: Image schemas in cognitive linguistics.* Berlin: de Gruyter.

Hane, A. A., & Fox, N. A. (2006). Ordinary variations in maternal caregiving influence human infants' stress reactivity. *Psychological Science, 17*(6), 550–556.

Hane, A. A., Fox, N. A., Henderson, H. A., & Marshall, P. J. (2008). Behavioral reactivity and approach–withdrawal bias in infancy. *Developmental Psychology, 44*(5), 1491–1496.

Hanna, R. (2011). What is the self? *Annals of the New York Academy of Sciences, 1234*(1), 121–123.

Hanna, R., Izenberg, G., Martin, R., Wiley, N., & Seigel, J. (2011). Me, myself, and I: The rise of the modern self. *Annals of the New York Academy of Sciences, 1234*(1), 108–120.

Hansen, M. B., & Markman, E. M. (2005). Appearance questions can be misleading: A discourse-based account of the appearance–reality problem. *Cognitive Psychology, 50*(3), 233–263.

Happaney, K., Zelaso, P. D., & Stuss, D. T. (2004). Development of orbitofrontal function: Current themes and future directions. *Brain and Cognition, 55*(1), 1–10.

Hardan, A. Y. (2006). Magnetic resonance imaging study of the orbitofrontal cortex in autism. *Journal of Child Neurology, 21*(10), 866–861.

Hariman, R., & Lucaites, J. L. (2008). Visual tropes and late-modern emotion in U.S. public culture. *Poroi, 5*(2), 47–93.

Harkess, K. L., & Tucker, D. M. (2000). Motivation of neural plasticity: Neural mechanisms in the self-organization of depression. In M. D. Lewis & I. Granic (Eds.), *Emotion, development, and self-organization: Dynamic systems approaches to emotional development* (pp. 186–208). Cambridge, UK: Cambridge University Press.

Harmon-Jones, E., Peterson, C. K., & Harmon-Jones, C. (2010). Anger, motivation, and asymmetrical frontal cortical activations. In M. Potegal, G. Stemmler, & C. Spielberger (Eds.), *International handbook of anger: Constituent and concomitant biological, psychological, and social processes* (pp. 61–78). New York: Springer Science & Business Media.

Harrist, A. W., & Waugh, R. M. (2002). Dyadic synchrony: Its structure and function in children's development. *Developmental Review, 22*, 555–592.

Harter, S. (1988). Developmental processes in the construction of the self. In T. D. Yawkey & J. E. Johnson (Eds.), *Integrative processes and socialization: Early to middle childhood* (pp. 45–78). Hillsdale, NJ: Erlbaum.

Harter, S. (2012). *The construction of the self: Developmental and sociocultural foundations* (2nd ed.). New York: Guilford Press.

Harter, S., Bresnick, S., Bouchey, H. A., & Whitsell, N. R. (1997). The development of multiple role-related selves during adolescence. *Development and Psychopathology, 9*, 835–854.

Harter, S., & Leary, M. R. (2003). The development of self-representations during childhood and adolescence. In M. R. Leary (Ed.), *Handbook of self and identity* (pp. 610–642). New York: Guilford Press.

Hassin, R. R., Uleman, J. S., & Baragh, J. A. (2005). *The new unconscious.* New York: Oxford University Press.

Hauser, S. T., Golden, E., & Allen, J. P. (2007). Narrative in the study of resilience. *Psychoanalytic Study of the Child, 61*, 205–227.

Haxby, J. V., Hoffman, E. A., & Gobbini, M. I. (2002). Human neural systems for face recognition and social communication. *Biological Psychiatry, 51*(1), 59–67.

Hayashi, M. L., Choi, S., Rao, B. S. S., Jung, H., & Lee, H. (2004). Altered cortical synaptic morphology and impaired memory consolidation in forebrain-specific dominant negative PAK transgenic mice. *Neuron, 42*(5), 773–787.

Hayne, H. (2004). Infant memory development: Implications for childhood amnesia. *Developmental Review, 24*(1), 33–73.

Hayne, H., & Simcock, G. (2009). Memory development in toddlers. In M. L. Courage & N. Cowan (Eds.), *The development of memory in infancy and childhood* (pp. 43–68). New York: Psychology Press.

Hazan, C., Campa, M., & Gur-Yaish, N. (2006). What is adult attachment? In M. Mikulincer & G. S. Goodman (Eds.), *Dynamics of romantic love: Attachment, caregiving, and sex* (pp. 47–101). New York: Guilford Press.

Hebb, D. O. (1949). *The organization of behavior: A neuropsychological theory.* New York: Wiley.

Heilman, K. M., Blonder, L. X., Bowers, D., & Crucian, G. P. (2000). Neurological disorders and emotional dysfunction. In J. Borod (Ed.), *The neuropsychology of emotion* (pp. 367–412). New York: Oxford University Press.

Heim, C., Newport, D. J., Heit, S., Graham, Y. P., Wilcox, M., Bonsall, R., et al. (2000). Pituitary–adrenal and autonomic responses to stress in women after sexual and physical abuse in childhood. *Journal of the American Medical Association, 284*(5), 592–597.

Heim, C., Newport, D. J., Mletzko, T., Miller, A. H., & Nemeroff, C. B. (2008). The link between childhood trauma and depression: Insights from HPA axis studies in humans. *Psychoneuroendocrinology, 33*(6), 693–710.

Heim, C., Newport, D. J., Wagner, D., Wilcox, M. M., Miller, A. H., & Nemeroff, C. B. (2002). The role of early adverse experience and adulthood stress in the prediction of neuroendocrine stress reactivity in women: A multiple regression analysis. *Depression and Anxiety, 25*(3), 117–125.

Heinicke, C. M., Goorsky, M., Levine, M., Ponce, V., Ruth, G., Silverman, M., et al. (2006). Pre- and postnatal antecedents of a home-visiting intervention and family developmental outcome. *Infant Mental Health Journal, 27*(1), 91–119.

Henry, S. (2009). School violence beyond Columbine: A complex problem in need of an interdisciplinary analysis. *American Behavioral Scientist, 52*(9), 1246–1265.

Herzog, A., Kube, K., de Lima, A. D., Michaelis, B., & Voigt, T. (2006, April). *Connection strategies in neocortical networks.* Paper presented at the European Symposium on Artificial Neural Networks, Bruges, Belgium.

Hesse, E. (1996). Discourse, memory and the Adult Attachment Interview: A note with emphasis on the emerging cannot classify category. *Infant Mental Health Journal, 17,* 4–11.

Hesse, E. (1999a). *Unclassifiable and disorganized responses in the Adult Attachment Interview and in the infant strange situation procedure: Theoretical proposals and empirical findings.* Unpublished doctoral dissertation, Leiden University, Leiden, The Netherlands.

Hesse, E. (1999b). The Adult Attachment Interview: Historical and current perspectives. In J. Cassidy & P. R. Shaver (Eds.), *Handbook of attachment: Theory, research, and clinical applications* (pp. 395–433). New York: Guilford Press.

Hesse, E. (2008). The Adult Attachment Interview: Protocol, method of analysis, and empirical studies. In J. Cassidy & P. R. Shaver (Eds.), *Handbook of attachment: Theory, research, and clinical applications* (2nd ed., pp. 552–598). New York: Guilford Press.

Hesse, E., & Main, M. (1999). Unresolved/disorganized responses to trauma in non-maltreating parents: Previously unexamined risk factor for offspring. *Psychoanalytic Inquiry, 19,* 4–11.

Hesse, E., & Main, M. (2000). Disorganized infant, child, and adult attachment: Collapse in behavioral and attentional strategies. *Journal of the American Psychoanalytic Association, 48*(4), 1097–1127.

Hesse, E., & Main, M. (2006). Frightened, threatening, and dissociative parental behavior in low-risk samples: Description, discussion, and interpretations. *Development and Psychopathology, 18*(2), 309–343.

Hesse, E., Main, M., Abrams, K. Y., & Rifkin, A. (2003). Unresolved states regarding loss or abuse can have "second-generation" effects: Organization, role inversion, and frightening ideation in the offspring of traumatized, non-maltreating parents. In M. F. Solomon & D. J. Siegel (Eds.), *Healing trauma: Attachment, mind, body, and brain* (pp. 57–106). New York: Norton.

Hesse, E., Main, M., & Siegel, D. J. (2010, December). *Interpersonal neurobiology and the clinical applications of the Adult Attachment Interview.* Paper presented at the UCLA-Lifespan Learning Conference, Los Angeles.

Hesse, E., & van IJzendoorn, M. H. (1998). Parental loss of close family members and propensities towards absorption in offspring. *Developmental Science, 1*, 299–305.

Hikosaka, O., & Isoda, M. (2010). Switching from automatic to controlled behavior: Cortico-basal ganglia mechanisms. *Trends in Cognitive Sciences, 14*(4), 154–161.

Hilgard, E. R. (1977). *Divided consciousness: Multiple controls in human thought and action.* New York: Wiley.

Hill, N. B., Bromell, L. Tyson, D. F., & Flint, R. (2007). Developmental commentary: Ecological perspectives on parental influences during adolescence. *Journal of Clinical Child and Adolescent Psychology, 36*(3), 367–377.

Hill-Soderlund, A. L., Mills-Koonce, W. R., Propper, C., Calkins, S. D., Granger, D. A., Moore, G. A., et al. (2008). Parasympathetic and sympathetic responses to the Strange Situation in infants and mothers from avoidant and securely attached dyads. *Developmental Psychobiology, 50*(4), 361–376.

Hofer, M. (1990). Early symbiotic processes: Hard evidence from a soft place. In R. A. Glick & S. Bone (Eds.), *Pleasure beyond the pleasure principle* (pp. 55–78). New Haven, CT: Yale University Press.

Hofer, M. A. (1994). Hidden regulators in attachment, separation, and loss. In N. A. Fox (Ed.), The development of emotion regulation: Biological and behavioral considerations. *Monographs of the Society for Research in Child Development, 59*(2–3, Serial No. 240), 192–207.

Hofer, M. A. (2006). Psychobiological roots of early attachment. *Current Directions of Psychological Science, 15*(2), 84–88.

Hofman, D. (2009). The frontal laterality of emotion: A historical overview. *Netherlands Journal of Psychology, 64*(3), 112–118.

Holsboer, F. (2001). Stress, hypercortisolism and corticosteroid receptors in depression: Implications for therapy. *Journal of Affective Disorders, 62*(1), 77–91.

Holtmaat, A., & Svoboda, K. (2009). Experience-dependent structural synaptic plasticity in the mammalian brain. *Nature Reviews Neuroscience, 10*(9), 647–658.

Horowitz, M. J. (2001). Configurational analysis of the self: A states-of-mind approach. In M. J. Christopher (Ed.), *Self-relations in the psychotherapy process* (pp. 67–86). Washington, DC: American Psychological Association.

Hoscheidt, S., Nadel, L., Payne, J., & Ryan, L. (2010). Hippocampal activation during retrieval of spatial context from episodic and semantic memory. *Behavioural Brain Research, 212*(2), 121–132.

Howard, M., Jing, B., Addis, K., & Kahana, M. (2007). Semantic structure and episodic memory. In T. K. Landauer, D. S. McNamara, S. Dennis, & W. Kintsch (Eds.), *Handbook of latent semantic analysis* (pp. 121–141). Mahwah, NJ: Erlbaum.

Howe, M. L. (2003). When autobiographical memory begins. *Developmental Review, 23*(4), 471–494.

Howe, M. L. (2004). Early memory, early self, and the emergence of autobiographical memory. In D. R. Beike, J. M. Lampinen, & D. A. Behrend (Eds.), *The self and memory* (pp. 45–74). New York: Psychology Press.

Howe, M. L., Courage, M. L., & Rooksby, M. (2009). The genesis and development of autobiographical memory. In M. Courage & N. Cowan (Eds.), *The development of memory in infancy and childhood* (pp. 177–187). New York: Psychology Press.

Howe, M. L., & Lewis, M. (2005). The importance of dynamic systems approaches for understanding development. *Developmental Review, 25*(3–4), 247–251.

Hrdy, S. B. (2009). *Mothers and others: The evolutionary origins of mutual understanding.* Cambridge, MA: Belknap Press of Harvard University Press.

Hsu, H., & Fogel, A. (2003). Social regulatory effects of infant nondistress vocalization on maternal behavior. *Developmental Psychology, 39*(6), 976–991.

Hubel, D. H. (1967). Effects of distortion of sensory input on the visual cortex and the influence of the environment. *Physiologist, 10*, 17–45.

Huber, D. E., Clark, T. F., Curran, T., & Winkielman, P. (2008). Effects of repetition priming on recognition memory: Testing a perceptual fluency—disfluency model. *Journal of Experimental Psychology: Learning, Memory, and Cognition, 34*(6), 1305–1324.

Hudson, J., & Mayhew, E. M. Y. (2009). The development of memory for recurring events. In M. L. Courage & N. Cowan (Eds.), *The development of memory in infancy and childhood* (pp. 69–92). New York: Psychology Press.

Hugdahl, K., & Davidson, R. J. (Eds.). (2003). *The asymmetrical brain.* Cambridge, MA: MIT Press.

Hugdahl, K., & Westerhausen, R. (Eds.). (2010). *The two halves of the brain: Information processing in the cerebral hemispheres.* Cambridge, MA: MIT Press.

Hughes, C., & Ensor, R. (2005). Executive function and theory of mind in 2 year-olds: A family affair? *Developmental Neuropsychology, 28*, 645–668.

Hughes, D. A. (2007). *Attachment-focused family therapy.* New York: Norton.

Hughes, J. (2007). Autism: The first firm finding = underconnectivity? *Epilepsy and Behavior, 11*(1), 20–24.

Hughes, P., Turton, P., McGauley, G., & Fonagy, P. (2006). Factors that predict infant disorganization in mothers classified as U in pregnancy. *Attachment and Human Development, 8*(2), 113–122.

Huk, A. C., & Shadlen, M. N. (2005). Neural activity in macaque parietal cortex reflects temporal integration of visual motion signals during perceptual decision making. *Journal of Neuroscience, 25*(45), 10420–10436.

Iacoboni, M. (2008). *Mirroring people.* New York: Picador.

Iacoboni, M. (2009a). Imitation, empathy, and mirror neurons. *Annual Review of Psychology, 60*, 653–670.

Iacoboni, M. (2009b). Neurobiology of imitation. *Current Opinion in Neurobiology, 19*(6), 661–665.

Iacoboni, M., & Dapretto, M. (2006). The mirror neuron system and the consequences of its dysfunction. *Nature Reviews Neuroscience, 7*, 942–951.

Iacoboni, M., Molnar-Szakacs, I., Gallese, V., Buccino, G., Mazziotta, J. C., & Rizzolatti, G. (2005). Grasping the intentions of others with one's own mirror neuron system. *PLOS Biology, 3*(3), e79.

Iaria, G., Chen, J., Guariglia, C., Ptito, A., & Petrides, M. (2007). Retrosplenial and hippocampal brain regions in human navigation: Complementary functional contributions to the formation and use of cognitive maps. *European Journal of Neuroscience, 25*(3), 890–899.

Immordino-Yang, M. H. (2011). Me, my "self" and you: Neuropsychological relations between emotion, self-awareness, and morality. *Emotion Review, 3*(3), 313–315.

Indersmitten, T., & Gur, R. C. (2003). Emotion processing in chimeric faces: Hemispheric asymmetries in expression and recognition of emotions. *Journal of Neuroscience, 23*(9), 3820–3825.

Isles, A. R., & Wilkinson, L. S. (2008). Epigenetics: What is it and why is it important to mental disease? *British Medical Bulletin, 85*(1), 35–45.

Ives-Deliperi, V. L., Solms, M., & Meintjes, E. M. (2010). The neural substrates of mindfulness: An fMRI investigation. *Social Neuroscience, 6*(3), 231–242.

Izenberg, G. (2011). The modern notion of self has reached its ultimate conclusion. *Annals of the New York Academy of Sciences, 1234*(1), 124–126.

Izard, C. (2010). The many meanings/aspects of emotion: Definitions, functions, activation and regulation. *Emotion Review, 2*(4), 363–370.

Jack, F., MacDonald, S., Reese, E., & Hayne, H. (2009). Maternal reminiscing style during early childhood predicts the age of adolescents' earliest memories. *Child Development, 80*(2), 496–505.

Jackowski, A. P., de Araujo, C. M., de Lacerda, A. L. T., Mari, J. D. J., & Kaufman, J. (2009). Neurostructural imaging findings in children with post-traumatic stress disorder: Brief review. *Psychiatry and Clinical Neurosciences, 63*(1), 1–8.

Jackson, E. A. (1991). Controls of dynamic flows with attractors. *Physical Review A, 44,* 4389–4853.

Jackson, P. L., Brunet, E., Meltzoff, A. N., & Decety, J. (2006). Empathy examined through the neural mechanisms involved in imagining how I feel versus how you feel pain. *Neuropsychologia, 44*(5), 752–761.

Jacobs, A., Fridman, G., Douglas, R., Alam, N., Latham, P., Prusky, G., et al. (2009). Ruling out and ruling in neural codes. *Proceedings of the National Academy of Sciences USA, 106*(14), 5936–5941.

Jacobs, T. L., Epel, E. S., Lin, J., Blackburn, E. H., Wolkowitz, O. M., Bridwell, D. A., et al. (2011). Intensive meditation training, immune cell telomerase activity, and psychological mediators. *Psychoneuroendocrinology, 36*(5), 664–681.

Jacobvitz, D., Leon, K., & Hazen, N. (2006). Does expectant mothers' unresolved trauma predict frightened/frightening maternal behavior?: Risk and protective factors. *Development and Psychopathology, 18*(2), 363–379.

James, W. (1884). What is an emotion? *Mind, 9, 188–205.*

James, W. (1890). *The principles of psychology.* New York: Holt.

Jang, J. H., Jung, W. H., Kang, D. H., Byun, M. S., Kwon, S. J., Choi, C. H., et al. (2011). Increased default mode network connectivity associated with meditation. *Neuroscience Letters, 487*(3), 358–362.

Janig, W. (2003). The autonomic nervous system and its coordination by the brain. In R. J. Davidson, K. R. Scherer, & H. H. Goldsmith (Eds.), *Handbook of affective sciences* (pp. 135–186). New York: Oxford University Press.

Jermakowicz, W. J., & Casagrande, V. A. (2007). Neural networks a century after Cajal. *Brain Research Reviews, 55*(2), 264.

Jha, A. P., Krompinger, J., & Baime, M. J. (2007). Mindfulness training modifies subsystems of attention. *Cognitive, Affective, and Behavioral Neuroscience, 7*(2), 109–119.

Jimerson, S., Egeland, B., Sroufe, L., & Carlson, B. (2000). A prospective longitudinal study of high school dropouts examining multiple predictors across development. *Journal of School Psychology, 38*(6), 529–549.

Joëls, M., Karst, H., Alfarez, D., Heine, V. M., Qin, Y., van Riel, E., et al. (2004). Effects of chronic stress on structure and cell function in rat hippocampus and hypothalamus. *Informa Healthcare, 7*(4), 221–231.

Johns, E. E., & Mewhort, D. J. K. (2009). Test sequence priming in recognition memory. *Journal of Experimental Psychology: Learning, Memory, and Cognition, 35*(5), 1162–1174.

Johnson, M. H. (2001). Functional brain development in humans. *Nature Reviews Neuroscience, 2*, 472–483.

Johnson, P. A., Hurley, R. A., Benkelfat, C., Herpertz, S. C., & Taber, K. H. (2003). Understanding emotion regulation in borderline personality disorder: Contributions of neuroimaging. *Journal of Neuropsychiatry and Clinical Neurosciences, 15*, 397–402.

Johnson, S. L., Hayes, A. M., Field, T. M., Schneiderman, N., & McCabe, P. M. (Eds.). (2000). *Stress, coping, and depression*. Mahwah, NJ: Erlbaum.

Johnson-Laird, P. N. (1983). *Mental models: Towards a cognitive science of language, inference, and consciousness*. Cambridge, MA: Harvard University Press.

Jones, N. A., McFall, B. A., & Diego, M. A. (2004). Patterns of brain electrical activity in infants of depressed mothers who breastfeed and bottle feed: The mediating role of infant temperament. *Biological Psychology, 67*(1–2), 103–124.

Judd, P. H. (2005). Neurocognitive impairment as a moderator in the development of borderline personality disorder. *Development and Psychopathology, 17*, 1173–1196.

Kabat-Zinn, J. (2005). *Coming to our senses: Healing ourselves and the world through mindfulness*. New York: Hyperion.

Kagan, J. (2003). Behavioral inhibition as a temperamental category. In R. J. Davidson, K. R. Scherer, & H. H. Goldsmith (Eds.), *Handbook of affective sciences* (pp. 320–331). New York: Oxford University Press.

Kagan, J. (2010). *The temperamental thread: How genes, culture, time and luck make us who we are*. New York: Dana Press.

Kagan, J., & Fox, N. A. (2006). Biology, culture, and temperamental biases. In W. Damon & R. M. Lerner (Series Eds.) & N. Eisenberg (Vol. Ed.), *Handbook of child psychology: Vol. 3. Social, emotional, and personality development* (6th ed., pp. 167–225). Hoboken, NJ: Wiley.

Kagan, J., & Snidman, N. (2004). *The long shadow of temperament*. Cambridge, MA: Harvard University Press.

Kagan, J., & Snidman, N. (2007). Temperament and biology. In D. Coch, K. W. Fischer, & G. Dawson (Eds.), *Human behavior, learning, and the developing brain: Atypical development* (pp. 219–246). New York: Guilford Press.

Kaiser, A., Kuenzli, E., Zappatore, D., & Nitsch, C. (2007). On females' lateral and males' bilateral activation during language production: A fMRI study. *International Journal of Psychophysiology, 63*(2), 192–198.

Kalin, N., Shelton, S., & Davidson, R. (2007). Role of the primate orbitofrontal cortex in mediating anxious temperament. *Biological Psychiatry, 62*(10), 1134–1139.

Kandel, E. R. (1998). A new intellectual framework for psychiatry. *American Journal of Psychiatry, 155*, 457–469.

Kandel, E. R. (2001). The molecular biology of memory storage: A dialogue between genes and synapses. *Science, 294*(5544), 1030–1038.

Kandel, E. R. (2006). *In search of memory: The emergence of a new science of mind*. New York: Norton.

Kandel, E. R., Schwartz, J. H., & Jessell, T. M. (2000). *Principles of neural science* (4th ed.). New York: McGraw-Hill.

Karl, A., Schaefer, M., Malta, L. S., Dörfel, D., Rohleder, N., & Werner, A. (2006). A meta-analysis of structural brain abnormalities in PTSD. *Neuroscience and Biobehavioral Reviews, 30*(7), 1004–1031.

Karpinski, A. C., & Scullin, M. H. (2009). Suggestibility under pressure: Theory of mind, executive function, and suggestibility in preschoolers. *Journal of Applied Developmental Psychology, 30*(6), 749–763.

Karr-Morse, R., & Wiley, M. S. (2012). *Scared sick: The role of childhood trauma in adult disease.* New York: Basic Books.

Kauffman, S. (1996). *At home in the universe: Self-organization and complexity.* Oxford, UK: Oxford University Press.

Kawasaki, H., Adolphs, R., Oya, H., Kovach, C., Damasio, H., Kaufman, O., et al. (2005). Analysis of single-unit responses to emotional scenes in human ventromedial prefrontal cortex. *Journal of Cognitive Neuroscience, 17*(10), 1509–1518.

Keenan, J. P., Nelson, A., O'Connor, M., & Pascual-Leone, A. (2001). Self-recognition and the right hemisphere. *Nature, 409*(6818), 305.

Keller, A., Lhewa, D., Rosenfeld, B., Sachs, E., & Aladjem, A. (2006). Traumatic experiences and psychological distress in an urban refugee population seeking treatment services. *Journal of Nervous and Mental Disease, 194*(3), 188–194.

Keller, H. (2010). *The story of my life.* New York: Signet Classics. (Original work published 1903)

Kelly, S. D., Creigh, P., & Bartolotti, J. (2010). Integrating speech and iconic gestures in a Stroop-like task: Evidence for automatic processing. *Journal of Cognitive Neuroscience, 22*(4), 683–694.

Kempermann, G., Gast, D., & Gage, F. H. (2002). Neuroplasticity in old age: Sustained fivefold induction of hippocampal neurogenesis by long-term environmental enrichment. *Annals of Neurology, 52*(2), 135–143.

Kensinger, E. A. (2004). Remembering emotional experiences: The contribution of valence and arousal. *Reviews in Neuroscience, 15*(4), 241–253.

Khader, P., Ranganath, C., Seemüller, A., & Rösler, F. (2007). Working memory maintenance contributes to long-term memory formation: Evidence from slow event-related brain potentials. *Cognitive, Affective, and Behavioral Neuroscience, 7*(3), 212–224.

Khoury, A. E., Gruber, S. H. M., Mørk, A., & Mathé, A. A. (2006). Adult life behavioral consequences of early maternal separation are alleviated by escitalopram treatment in a rat model of depression. *Progress in Neuro-Psychopharmacology and Biological Psychiatry, 30*(3), 535–540.

Kiang, L., & Harter, S. (2008). Do pieces of the self-puzzle fit?: Integrated/fragmented selves in biculturally-identified Chinese Americans. *Journal of Research in Personality, 42*(6), 1657–1662.

Kilpatrick, D. G., Koenen, K. C., Ruggiero, K. J., Acierno, R., Galea, S., Resnick, H. S., et al. (2007). The serotonin transporter genotype and social support and moderation of posttraumatic stress disorder and depression in hurricane-exposed adults. *American Journal of Psychiatry, 164*(11), 1693–1699.

Kilpatrick, L. A., Suyenobu, B. Y., Smith, S. R., Bueller, J. A., Goodman, T., Creswell, J. D., et al. (2011). Impact of mindfulness-based stress reduction training on intrinsic brain connectivity. *NeuroImage, 56*(1), 290–298.

Kim, J., & Cicchetti, D. (2010). Longitudinal pathways linking child maltreatment, emotion regulation, peer relations, and psychopathology. *Journal of Child Psychology and Psychiatry, 51*(6), 706–716.

Kim, J., Cicchetti, D., Rogosch, F. A., & Manly, J. T. (2009). Child maltreatment and trajectories of personality and behavioral functioning: Implications for the development of personality disorder. *Development and Psychopathology, 21*(3), 889–912.

Kim, J., & Ragozzino, M. E. (2005). The involvement of the orbitofrontal cortex in learning under changing task contingencies. *Neurobiology of Learning and Memory, 83*(2), 125–133.

Kim, J. J., & Diamond, D. M. (2002). The stressed hippocampus, synaptic plasticity and lost memories. *Nature Reviews Neuroscience, 3*, 453–462.

Kim, J. J., & Jung, M. W. (2006). Neural circuits and mechanisms involved in Pavlovian fear conditioning: A critical review. *Neuroscience and Biobehavioral Reviews, 30*(2), 188–202.

Kimura, Y., Yoshino, A., Takahashi, Y., & Nomura, S. (2004). Interhemispheric difference in emotional response without awareness. *Physiology and Behavior, 82*(4), 727–731.

King, J. A., Mandansky, D., King, S., Fletcher, K. E., & Brewer, J. (2001). Early sexual abuse and low cortisol. *Psychiatry and Clinical Neurosciences, 55*(1), 71–74.

Kinsbourne, M. (1972). Eye and head turning indicates cerebral lateralization. *Science, 176*, 539–541.

Kircher, T., & David, A. (Eds.). (2003). *The self in neuroscience and psychiatry.* Cambridge, UK: Cambridge University Press.

Klein, K., & Boats, A. (2010). Coherence and narrative structure in personal accounts of stressful experiences. *Journal of Social and Clinical Psychology, 29*(3), 256–280.

Knitzer, J., & Raver, C. C. (2002). *Ready to enter: What research tells policymakers about strategies to promote social and emotional school readiness among three- and four-year-old children* (Promoting the Emotional Well-Being of Children and Families Policy Paper No. 3). New York: National Center for Children in Poverty, Columbia University Mailman School of Public Health.

Knobe, J., & Nichols, S. (2008). *Experimental philosophy.* New York: Oxford University Press.

Knyazeva, M. G., Fornari, E., & Meuli, R. (2009). Interhemispheric integration at different spatial scales: The evidence from EEG coherence and fMRI. *Journal of Neurophysiology, 96*(1), 259–275.

Kobak, R. R., Sudler, N., & Gamble, W. (1991). Attachment and depressive symptoms during adolescence: A developmental pathways analysis. *Development and Psychopathology, 3*(4), 461–474.

Kober, H., Barrett, L. F., Joseph, J., Bliss-Moreau, E., Lindquist, K., & Wager, T. D. (2008). Functional grouping and cortical–subcortical interactions in emotion: A meta-analysis of neuroimaging studies. *NeuroImage, 42*(2), 998–1031.

Koch, C., & Preuschoff, K. (2007). Betting the house on consciousness. *Nature Neuroscience, 10*, 140–141.

Koch, C., & Tsuchiya, N. (2007). Attention and consciousness: Two distinct brain processes. *Trends in Cognitive Sciences, 11*(1), 16–22.

Kochanska, G., & Aksan, N. (2004). Development of mutual responsiveness between parents and their young children. *Child Development, 75*(6), 1657–1676.

Koechlin, E., & Summerfield, C. (2007). An information theoretical approach to prefrontal executive function. *Trends in Cognitive Sciences, 11*(6), 229–235.

Kornfield, J. (2008). *The wise heart: A guide to the universal teachings of Buddhist psychology.* New York: Bantam.

Krasner, M. S., Epstein, R. M., Beckman, H., Suchman, A. L., Chapman, B., Mooney, C. J., et al. (2009). Association of an educational program in mindful communication without burnout, empathy, and attitudes among primary care physicians. *Journal of the American Medical Association, 302*, 1284–1293.

Kringelbach, M. (2005). The human orbitofrontal cortex: Linking reward to hedonic experience. *Nature Reviews Neuroscience, 6*, 691–702.

Kröger, H. (2007). Biological and physical principles in self-organization of brain. *AIP Conference Proceedings, 905*(1), 168–174.

Krohne, H. W. (2003). Individual differences in emotional reactions and coping. In R. J. Davidson, K. R. Scherer, & H. H. Goldsmith (Eds.), *Handbook of affective sciences* (pp. 698–725). New York: Oxford University Press.

Kühn, S., Müller, B. C., van der Leij, A., Dijksterhuis, A., Brass, M., & van Baaren, R. B.

(2010). Neural correlates of emotional synchrony. *Social Cognitive and Affective Neuroscience, 6*(3), 368–374.

LaBar, K. S., & Cabeza, R. (2006). Cognitive neuroscience of emotional memory. *Nature Reviews Neuroscience, 7*, 54–64.

Laible, D., & Panfile, T. (2009). Mother–child reminiscing in the context of secure attachment relationships. In J. Quas & R. Fivush (Eds.), *Emotion and memory in development: Biological, cognitive, and social considerations* (pp. 166–195). New York: Oxford University Press.

Lamm, C., & Lewis, M. (2010). Developmental change in the neurophysiological correlates of self-regulation in high- and low-emotion conditions. *Developmental Neuropsychology, 35*(2), 156–176.

Lang, A. J., Craske, M. G., Brown, M., & Ghaneian, A. (2001). Fear-related state dependent memory. *Cognition and Emotion, 15*(5), 695–703.

Lanius, R. A., Bluhm, R. L., & Frewen, P. A. (2011). How understanding the neurobiology of complex PTSD can inform clinical practice: A social cognitive and affective neuroscience approach. *Acta Psychiatrica Scandinavica, 124*(5), 331–348.

Lau, H., Rogers, D., Haggard, P., & Passingham, R. E. (2004). Attention to intention. *Science, 303*(5661), 1208–1210.

Laurent, H., & Powers, S. (2007). Emotion regulation in emerging adult couples: Temperament, attachment, and HPA response to conflict. *Biological Psychology, 76*(1–2), 61–71.

Lazar, S. W., Kerr, C. E., Wasserman, R. H., Gray, J. R., Greve, D. N., Treadway, M. T., et al. (2005). Meditation experience is associated with increased cortical thickness. *NeuroReport, 16*(17), 1893–1897.

LeBaron, R., Hernandez, R., Navarro, M., Orfila, J., Curry, L., & Martinez, J. (2008). Focal adhesion-like processes underlie induction of long-term potentiation in the Schaffer collateral–CA1 region of the hippocampus. In R. D. Fields (Ed.), *Beyond the synapse: Cell–cell signaling in synaptic plasticity* (pp. 160–168). New York: Cambridge University Press.

Lebreton, M., Barnes, A., Miettunen, J., Peltonen, L., Ridler, K., Veijola, J., et al. (2008). The brain structural disposition to social interaction. *European Journal of Neuroscience, 29*, 2247–2252.

Leclercq, M. (2002). Theoretical aspects of the main components and functions of attention. In M. Leclercq & P. Zimmerman (Eds.), *Applied neuropsychology of attention* (pp. 3–55). London: Psychology Press.

LeDoux, J. E. (1996). *The emotional brain: The mysterious underpinning of emotional life.* New York: Simon & Schuster.

LeDoux, J. E. (2003a). *Synaptic self: How our brains become who we are.* New York: Penguin.

LeDoux, J. E. (2003b). The emotional brain, fear, and the amygdala. *Cellular and Molecular Neurobiology, 23*(4–5), 727–738.

Legerstee, M., Markova, G., & Fisher, T. (2007). The role of maternal affect attunement in dyadic and triadic communication. *Infant Behavior and Development, 30*(2), 296–306.

Lemche, E., Kreppner, J. M., Joraschky, P., & Klann-Delius, G. (2007). Attachment organization and the early development of internal state language: A longitudinal perspective. *International Journal of Behavioral Development, 31*(3), 252–262.

Lemmon, K., & Moore, C. (2001). Binding the self in time. In C. Moore, K. Lemmon, & K. Skene (Eds.), *The self in time: Developmental perspectives* (pp. 163–180). Mahwah, NJ: Psychology Press.

Lengua, L. J., & Kovacs, E. A. (2005). Bidirectional associations between temperament and parenting and the prediction of adjustment problems in middle childhood. *Journal of Applied Developmental Psychology, 26*(1), 21–38.

Lensvelt-Mulders, G., van der Hart, O., van Ochten, J. M., van Son, M. J. M., Steele, K., & Breeman, L. (2008). Relations among peritraumatic dissociation and posttraumatic stress: A meta-analysis. *Clinical Psychology Review, 28*(7), 1138–1151.

Leppänen, J. M. (2006). Emotional information processing in mood disorders: A review of behavioral and neuroimaging findings. *Current Opinion in Psychiatry, 19,* 34–39.

Levenson, R. W. (2003). Autonomic specificity and emotion. In R. J. Davidson, K. R. Scherer, & H. H. Goldsmith (Eds.), *Handbook of affective sciences* (pp. 212–224). New York: Oxford University Press.

Levine, L. J., Lench, H. C., & Safer, M. A. (2009). Functions of remembering and misremembering emotion. *Applied Cognitive Psychology, 23*(8), 1059–1075.

LeVine, R. A. (2010). Plasticity and variation: Cultural influences on parenting and early child development within and across populations. In C. M. Worthman, P. M. Plotsky, D. S. Schecher, & C. A. Cummings (Eds.), *Formative experiences: The interaction of caregiving, culture, and developmental psychobiology* (pp. 9–11). New York: Cambridge University Press.

Levita, L., & Muzzio, I. (2010). Role of the hippocampus in goal-oriented tasks requiring retrieval of spatial versus non-spatial information. *Neurobiology of Learning and Memory, 93*(4), 581–588.

Levitin, D. J. (2006). *This is your brain on music: The science of a human obsession.* New York: Dutton.

Levy, J. (1969). Possible basis for the evolution of the human brain. *Nature, 224,* 614–615.

Levy, R., & Dubois, B. (2006). Apathy and the functional anatomy of the prefrontal cortex–basal ganglia circuits. *Cerebral Cortex, 16*(7), 916–928.

Lewis, M., Haviland-Jones, J. M., & Barrett, L. F. (Eds.). (2008). *Handbook of emotions* (3rd ed.). New York: Guilford Press.

Lewis, M. D. (1995). Cognition–emotion feedback and the self-organization of developmental paths. *Human Development, 38,* 71–102.

Lewis, M. D. (2005a). Bridging emotion theory and neural biology through dynamic systems modeling. *Behavioral and Brain Sciences, 28*(2), 169–194.

Lewis, M. D. (2005b). Self-organizing individual differences in brain development. *Developmental Review, 25*(3–4), 252–277.

Lewis, M. D., Lamm, C., Segalowitz, S., Stieben, J., & Zelazo, P. (2006). Neurophysiological correlates of emotion regulation in children and adolescents. *Journal of Cognitive Neuroscience, 18*(3), 430–443.

Liberzon, I., & Sripada, C. S. (2007). The functional neuroanatomy of PTSD: A critical review. *Progress in Brain Research, 167,* 151–169.

Lickliter, R. (2008). The growth of developmental thought: Implications for a new evolutionary psychology. *New Ideas in Psychology, 26*(3), 359–369.

Lieberman, M. D., Hariri, A., Jarcho, J. M., Eisenberger, N. I., & Bookheimer, S. Y. (2005). An fMRI investigation of race-related amygdala activity in African-American and Caucasian-American individuals. *Nature Neuroscience, 8*(6), 720–722.

Lindenberger, U. (2001). Lifespan theories of cognitive development. In N. J. Smelser & P. B. Baltes (Eds.), *International encyclopedia of the social and behavioral sciences* (pp. 8848–8854). Amsterdam: Elsevier.

Lindner, J. L. L., & Rosén, L. A. (2006). Decoding of emotion through facial expression, prosody and verbal content in children and adolescents with Asperger's syndrome. *Journal of Autism and Developmental Disorders, 36*(6), 769–777.

Liotti, G. (1992). Disorganized/disoriented attachment in etiology of dissociative disorders. *Dissociation, 5,* 196–204.

Liotti, G. (2007). Internal working models of attachment in the therapeutic relationship.

In P. Gilbert & R. L. Leahy (Eds.), *The therapeutic relationship in the cognitive behavioral psychotherapies* (pp. 143–162). New York: Routledge.

Liu, Y, Balériaux, D., Kavec, M., Metens, T., Absil, J., Denolin, V., et al. (2010). Structural asymmetries in motor and language networks in a population of healthy preterm neonates at term equivalent age: A diffusion tensor imaging and probabilistic tractography study. *NeuroImage, 51*(2), 783–788.

Livneh, H., & Parker, R. (2005). Psychological adaptation to disability: Perspectives from chaos and complexity theory. *Rehabilitation Counseling Bulletin, 49*(1), 17–28.

Llinas, R. R. (1990). Intrinsic electrical properties of mammalian neurons and CNS function. *Fidia Research Foundation Neuroscience Award Lectures, 4,* 175–194.

Llinas, R. R. (2002). *I of the vortex: From neurons to self.* Cambridge, MA: MIT Press.

Llinas, R. R. (2008). Of self and self-awareness: The basic neuronal circuit in human consciousness and the generation of self. *Journal of Consciousness Studies, 15*(9), 64–74.

Llorente, R., Llorente-Berzal, A., Petrosino, S., Marco, E., Guaza, C., & Prada, C. (2010a). Gender-dependent cellular and biochemical effects of maternal deprivation on the hippocampus of neonatal rats: A possible role for the endocannabinoid system. *Developmental Neurobiology, 68*(11), 1334–1347.

Llorente, R., O'Shea, E., Gutierrez-Lopez, M., Llorente-Berzal, A., Colado, M. I., & Viveros, M. (2010b). Sex-dependent maternal deprivation effects on brain monoamine content in adolescent rats. *Neuroscience Letters, 479*(2), 112–117.

Loevinger, J. (1976). *Ego development.* San Francisco: Jossey-Bass.

Loftus, E. F. (2006). Recovered memories. *Annual Review of Clinical Psychology, 2,* 469–498.

Longe, O., Senior, C., & Rippon, G. (2009). The lateral and ventromedial prefrontal cortex work as a dynamic integrated system: Evidence from fMRI connectivity analysis. *Journal of Cognitive Neuroscience, 21*(1), 141–154.

Lovic, V. (2010). *The effects of maternal deprivation, through artificial rearing, on impulsiveness in rats.* Unpublished doctoral thesis, University of Toronto.

Luijk, M. P., Saridjan, N., Tharner, A., van IJzendoorn, M. H., Bakermans-Kranenburg, M. J., Jaddoe, V. W., et al. (2010). Attachment, depression, and cortisol: Deviant patterns in insecure-resistant and disorganized infants. *Developmental Psychobiology, 52*(5), 441–452.

Lupien, S. J., Fiocco, A., Wan, N., Maheu, F., Lord, C., Scramek, T., et al. (2004). Stress hormones and human memory function across the lifespan. *Psychoneuroendocrinology, 30*(3), 225–242.

Lutz, A., Slagter, H. A., Dunne, J. D., & Davidson, R. J. (2008). Attention regulation and monitoring in meditation. *Trends in Cognitive Sciences, 12*(4), 163–169.

Lynch, M., & Cicchetti, D. (1998). Trauma, mental representation, and the organization of memory for mother-referent material. *Development and Psychopathology, 10,* 739–760.

Lyons, D. M., Afarian, H., Schatzberg, A. F., Sawyer-Glover, A., & Moseley, M. E. (2002). Experience-dependent asymmetric variation in primate prefrontal morphology. *Behavioural Brain Research, 136,* 51–59.

Lyons-Ruth, K., & Jacobvitz, D. (2008). Attachment disorganization: Genetic factors, parenting contexts, and developmental transformation from infancy to adulthood. In J. Cassidy & P. R. Shaver (Eds.), *Handbook of attachment: Theory, research, and clinical applications* (2nd ed., pp. 666–697). New York: Guilford Press.

Lyons-Ruth, K., Yellin, C., Melnick, S., & Atwood, G. (2005). Expanding the concept of unresolved mental states: Hostile/helpless states of mind on the Adult Attachment Interview are associated with disrupted mother–infant communication and infant disorganization. *Development and Psychopathology, 17,* 1–23.

MacDonald, H. Z., Beeghly, M., Grant-Knight, W., Augustyn, M., Woods, R. W., Cabral, H., et al. (2008). Longitudinal association between infant disorganized attachment and childhood posttraumatic stress symptoms. *Development and Psychopathology, 20*(2), 493–508.

Mackenzie, C. (2009). Personal identity, narrative integration, and embodiment. In S. Campbell, L. Meynell, & S. Sherwin (Eds.), *Embodiment and agency* (pp. 100–125). University Park: Pennsylvania State University Press.

Madigan, S., Bakermans-Kranenburg, M. J., van IJzendoorn, M. H., Moran, G., Pederson, D. R., & Benoit, D. (2006). Unresolved states of mind, anomalous parental behavior, and disorganized attachment: A review and meta-analysis of a transmission gap. *Attachment and Human Development, 8*(2), 89–111.

Madigan, S., Moran, G., Schuengel, C., Pederson, D. R., & Otten, R. (2007). Unresolved maternal attachment representations, disrupted maternal behavior and disorganized attachment in infancy: Links to toddler behavior problems. *Journal of Child Psychology and Psychiatry, 48*(10), 1042–1050.

Main, M. (1991). Metacognitive knowledge, metacognitive monitoring, and singular (coherent) versus multiple (incoherent) models of attachment: Findings and directions for future research. In C. M. Parkes, J. Stevenson-Hinde, & P. Marris (Eds.), *Attachment across the life cycle* (pp. 127–159). London: Routledge.

Main, M. (1995). Attachment: Overview, with implications for clinical work. In S. Goldberg, R. Muir, & J. Kerr (Eds.), *Attachment theory: Social, developmental, and clinical perspectives* (pp. 407–474). Hillsdale, NJ: Analytic Press.

Main, M. (1996). Introduction to the special section on attachment and psychopathology: 2. Overview of the field of attachment. *Journal of Consulting and Clinical Psychology, 64*, 237–243.

Main, M. (1999). Mary D. Salter Ainsworth: Tribute and portrait. *Psychoanalytic Inquiry, 19*(5), 682–736.

Main, M. (2000). The organized categories of infant, child, and adult attachment: Flexible vs. inflexible attention under attachment-related stress. *Journal of the American Psychoanalytic Association, 48*, 1055–1095.

Main, M., & Goldwyn, R. (1984). *Adult attachment scoring and classification system.* Unpublished manuscript, University of California at Berkeley.

Main, M., & Goldwyn, R. (1998). *Adult attachment scoring and classification systems* (Version 6.3). Unpublished manuscript, University of California at Berkeley.

Main, M., Goldwyn, R., & Hesse, E. (2003). *Adult attachment scoring and classification system.* Unpublished manuscript, University of California, Berkeley.

Main, M., & Hesse, E. (1990). Parents' unresolved traumatic experiences are related to infant disorganized status: Is frightened and/or frightening parental behavior the linking mechanism? In M. T. Greenberg, D. Cicchetti, & E. M. Cummings (Eds.), *Attachment in the preschool years: Theory, research, and intervention* (pp. 161–182). Chicago: University of Chicago Press.

Main, M., Hesse, E., & Goldwyn, R. (2008). Studying difference in language usage in recounting attachment history: An introduction to the AAI. In H. Steele & M. Steele (Eds.), *Clinical applications of the Adult Attachment Interview* (pp. 31–68). New York: Guilford Press.

Main, M., Hesse, E., & Kaplan, N. (2005). Predictability of attachment behavior and representational processes at 1, 6, and 19 years of age: The Berkeley longitudinal study. In K. E. Grossmann, K. Grossman, & E. Waters (Eds.), *Attachment from infancy to adulthood: The major longitudinal studies* (pp. 245–304). New York: Guilford Press.

Main, M., Kaplan, N., & Cassidy, J. (1985). Security in infancy, childhood, and adulthood:

A move to the level of representation. In I. Bretherton & E. Waters (Eds.), Growing points of attachment theory and research. *Monographs of the Society for Research in Child Development, 50*(2–3, Serial No. 209), 66–104.

Main, M., & Morgan, H. (1996). Disorganization and disorientation in infant Strange Situation behavior: Phenotypic resemblance to dissociative states. In L. K. Michelson & W. J. Ray (Eds.), *Handbook of dissociation: Theoretical, empirical, and clinical perspectives* (pp. 107–138). New York: Plenum Press.

Main, M., & Solomon, J. (1986). Discovery of an insecure-disorganized/disoriented attachment pattern. In T. B. Brazelton & M. Yogman (Eds.), *Affective development in infancy* (pp. 95–124). Norwood, NJ: Ablex.

Main, M., & Solomon, J. (1990). Procedures for identifying infants as disorganized/disoriented during the Ainsworth Strange Situation. In M. T. Greenberg, D. Cicchetti, & E. M. Cummings (Eds.), *Attachment in the preschool years: Theory, research, and intervention* (pp. 121–160). Chicago: University of Chicago Press.

Malatesta-Magai, C. (1991). Development of emotion expression during infancy: General course and patterns of individual difference. In J. Garber & K. A. Dodge (Eds.), *The development of emotion regulation and dysregulation* (pp. 49–68). Cambridge, UK: Cambridge University Press.

Mangelsdorf, S. C., McHale, J. L., Diener, M., Goldstein, L. H., & Lehn, L. (2000). Infant attachment: Contributions of infant temperament and maternal characteristics. *Infant Behavior and Development, 23*(2), 175–196.

Mann, M. A. (2004). Immigrant parents and their emigrant adolescents: The tension of inner and outer worlds. *American Journal of Psychoanalysis, 64*(2), 143–153.

Manna, A., Raffone, A., Perrucci, M. G., Nardo, D., Ferretti, A., Tartaro, A., et al. (2010). Neural correlates of focused attention and cognitive monitoring in meditation. *Brain Research Bulletin, 82*(1–2), 46–56.

Mano, Y., Sugiura, M., Tsukiura, T., Chiao, J. Y., Yomogida, Y., Jeong, H., et al. (2011). The representation of social interaction in episodic memory: A functional MRI study. *NeuroImage, 57*(3), 1234–1242.

Mar, R. A. (2004). The neuropsychology of narrative: Story comprehension, story production and their interrelation. *Neuropsychologia, 42*(10), 1414–1434.

March, J. S., & Mulle, K. (1998). *OCD in children and adolescents: A cognitive-behavioral treatment manual.* New York: Guilford Press.

Margalit, M. (2004). Second-generation research on resilience: Social-emotional aspects of children with learning disabilities. *Learning Disabilities Research and Practice, 19*(1), 45–48.

Marini, A., Galetto, V., Zampieri, E., Vorano, L., Zettin, M., & Carlomagno, S. (2011). Narrative language in traumatic brain injury. *Neuropsychologia, 49*(10), 2904–2910.

Markham, J. A., & Greenough, W. T. (2004). Experience-driven brain plasticity: Beyond the synapse. *Neuron Glia Biology, 1*(4), 351–363.

Markova, G., & Legerstee, M. (2006). Contingency, imitation, and affect sharing: Foundations of infants' social awareness. *Developmental Psychology, 42*(1), 132–141.

Markowitsch, H. (2003). Autonoetic consciousness. In T. Kircher & A. David (Eds.), *The self in neuroscience and psychiatry* (pp. 180–196). New York: Cambridge University Press.

Markowitsch, H., Vandekerckhove, M. P. V., Lanfermann, H., & Russ, M. O. (2003). Engagement of lateral and medial prefrontal areas in the ecphory of sad and happy autobiographical memories. *Cortex, 39*(4), 643–665.

Markus, H. R., & Kitayama, S. (1991). Culture and the self: Implications for cognition, motion, and motivation. *Psychological Review, 98*(2), 224–253.

Marmar, C. R., McCaslin, S. E., Metzler, T. J., Best, S., Weiss, D. S., Fagan, J., et al. (2006).

Predictors of posttraumatic stress in police and other first responders. *Annals of the New York Academy of Sciences, 1071*, 1–18.

Marsh, R., Gerber, A. J., & Peterson, B. S. (2008). Neuroimaging studies of normal brain development and their relevance for understanding childhood neuropsychiatric disorders, *Journal of the American Academy of Child and Adolescent Psychiatry, 47*(11), 1233–1251.

Mason, M. F., & Macrae, C. N. (2004). Categorizing and individuating others: The neural substrates of person perception. *Journal of Cognitive Neuroscience, 16*(10), 1785–1795.

Masuda, T., Ellsworth, P. C., Mesquita, B., Leu, J., Tanida, S., & Van de Veerdonk, E. (2008). Placing the face in context: Cultural differences in the perception of facial emotion. *Journal of Personality and Social Psychology, 94*(3), 365–381.

Matsumoto, D., Willingham B., & Olide, A. (2009). Sequential dynamics of culturally moderated facial expressions of emotion. *Psychological Science, 20*(10), 1269–1274.

Matyushkin, D. (2007). The possible neurophysiological basis of the inner self. *Human Physiology, 33*(6), 701–709.

Maxwell, J. S. S., & Davidson, R. J. (2007). Emotion as motion: Asymmetries in approach and avoidant actions. *Psychological Science, 18*(12), 1113–1119.

Mayer, A. R., Teshiba, T. M., Franco, A. R., Ling, J., Shane, M. S., Stephen, J. M., et al. (2011). Modeling conflict and error in the medial frontal cortex. *Human Brain Mapping* [Epub ahead of print].

Mayer, E. A., Naliboff, B., & Munakata, J. (2000). The evolving neurobiology of gut feelings. *Progress in Brain Research, 122*, 195–206.

McAdams, D. P. (2001). The psychology of life stories. *Review of General Psychology, 5*(2), 100–122.

McClelland, J. L., McNaughton, B., & O'Reilly, R. (2002). Why there are complementary learning systems in the hippocampus and neocortex: Insights from the successes and failures of connectionist models of learning and memory. *Psychological Review, 102*(3), 419–457.

McClelland, J. L., & Rogers, T. (2003). The parallel distributed processing approach to semantic cognition. *Nature Reviews Neuroscience, 4*(4), 310–322.

McClelland, J. L., & Rumelhart, D. E. (Eds.). (1986). *Parallel distributed processing: Explorations in the microstructure of cognition* (Vols. 1 and 2). Cambridge, MA: MIT Press.

McCraty, R., Atkinson, M., Tomasion, D., & Tiller, W. A. (1998). The electricity of touch: Detection and measurement of cardiac energy exchange between people. In K. H. Pribram & J. King (Eds.), *Brain and values: Is a biological science of values possible?* (pp. 359–379). Hillsdale, NJ: Erlbaum.

McDonald, S. (2007). The social, emotional and cultural life of the orbitofrontal cortex. *Brain Impairment, 8*(1), 41–51.

McDowell, D. J., & Parke, R. D. (2000). Differential knowledge of display rules for positive and negative emotions: Influences from parents, influences on peers. *Social Development, 9*(4), 415–432.

McEwen, B. S. (2008). Central effects of stress hormones in health and disease: Understanding the protective and damaging effects of stress and stress mediators. *European Journal of Pharmacology, 583*(2–3), 174–185.

McGaugh, J. L. (1992). Affect, neuromodulatory systems, and memory storage. In S. A. Christianson (Ed.), *Handbook of emotion and memory* (pp. 245–268). Hillsdale, NJ: Erlbaum.

McGaugh, J. L., Roozendaal, B., & Okuda, S. (2006). Role of stress hormones and the amygdala in creating lasting memories. In N. Kato, M. Kawata, & R. K. Pitman (Eds.), *PTSD: Brain mechanisms and clinical implications* (pp. 89–103). Tokyo: Springer-Verlag.

McGilchrist, I. (2009). *The master and his emissary: The divided brain and the making of the Western world.* New Haven, CT: Yale University Press.

McGowan, P. O., Sasaki, A., D'Alessio, A. C., Dymov, S., Labonté, B., Szyf, M., et al. (2009). Epigenetic regulation of the glucocorticoid receptor in human brain associates with childhood abuse. *Nature Neuroscience, 12,* 342–348.

McGreenery, C. E., Polcari, A., Samson, J. A., & Teicher, M. H. (2006). Sticks, stones, and hurtful words: Relative effects of various forms of childhood maltreatment. *American Journal of Psychiatry, 163,* 993–1000.

McLean, K. C., Pasupathi, M., & Pals, J. L. (2007). Selves creating stories creating selves: A process model of self-development. *Personality and Social Psychology Review, 11*(3), 262–278.

McLin, D. E., Miasnikov, A. A., & Weinberger, N. M. (2002). Induction of behavioral associative memory by stimulation of the nucleus basalis. *Proceedings of the National Academy of Sciences USA, 99*(6), 4002–4007.

McManis, M. H., Kagan, J., Snidman, N. C., & Woodward, S. A. (2002). EEG asymmetry, power, and temperament in children. *Developmental Psychobiology, 41*(2), 169–177.

McNally, R. J., & Geraerts, E. (2009). A new solution to the recovered memory debate. *Perspectives on Psychological Science, 4*(2), 126–134.

McNaughton, B. L., Battaglia, F. P., Jensen, O., Moser, E. I., & Moser, M. (2006). Path integration and neural basis of the 'cognitive map.' *Nature Reviews Neuroscience, 7,* 663–678.

Mcquaid, N., Bigelow, A. E., McLaughlin, J., & Maclean, K. (2008). Maternal mental state language and preschool children's attachment security: Relation to children's mental state language and expressions of emotional understanding. *Social Development, 17*(1), 61–83.

Meaney, M. J. (2010). Epigenetics and the biological definition of gene × environment interactions. *Child Development, 81*(1), 41–79.

Mechelli, A., Price, C., Friston, K., & Ishai, A. (2004). Where bottom-up meets top-down: Neuronal interactions during perception and imagery. *Cerebral Cortex, 14*(11), 1256–1265.

Mehrabian, A. (2008). Communication without words. In C. D. Mortensen (Ed.), *Communication theory* (2nd ed., pp. 193–200). New Brunswick, NJ: Transaction.

Mei, T., Zhiyan, W., Mingyi, Q., Jun, G., & Lili, Z. (2008). Transferred shame in the cultures of interdependent-self and independent self. *Journal of Cognition and Culture, 8*(1–2), 163–178.

Meins, E., Fernyhough, C., Fradley, E., & Tuckey, M. (2001). Rethinking maternal sensitivity: Mothers' comments on infants' mental processes predict security of attachment at 12 months. *Journal of Child Psychology and Psychiatry, 42*(5), 637–648.

Meinz, P., & Main, M. (2011, April 3). *The evolution of Mary Ainsworth's understanding of attachment: Changes in her conceptualization of security and its precursors* Poster presented at the biennial meeting of the Society for Research in Child Development, Montréal.

Melloni, L., Molina, C., Pena, M., Torres, D., Singer, W., & Rodriguez, E. (2007). Synchronization of neural activity across cortical areas correlates with conscious perception. *Journal of Neuroscience, 27*(11), 2858–2865.

Meloy, J. R. (2003). Pathologies of attachment, violence, and criminality. In A. M. Goldstein & I. B. Weiner (Eds.), *Handbook of psychology: Vol. 11. Forensic psychology* (pp. 509–526). New York: Wiley.

Meltzoff, A. N., Kuhl, P. K. Movellan, J., & Sejnowski, T. J. (2009). Foundations for a new science of learning. *Science, 325*(5938), 284–288.

Mendelsohn, A., Furman, O., & Dudai, Y. (2010). Signatures of memory: Brain coactivations during retrieval distinguish correct from incorrect recollection. *Frontiers in Behavioral Neuroscience, 4,* 18.

Mercado, E., III. (2008). Neural and cognitive plasticity: From maps to minds. *Psychological Bulletin, 134*(1), 109–137.

Merker, B. (2007). Consciousness without a cerebral cortex: A challenge for neuroscience and medicine. *Behavioral and Brain Sciences, 30* (1), 63–81.

Mesquita, B., Barrett, L. F., & Smith, E. R. (Eds.). (2010). *The mind in context.* New York: Guilford Press.

Mesulam, M. M. (1998). Review article: From sensation to cognition. *Brain, 121,* 1013–1052.

Miklowitz, D. J., Alatiq, Y., Goodwin, G. M., Geddes, J. R., Fennell, V., Dimidjian, S., et al. (2009). A pilot study of mindfulness-based cognitive therapy for bipolar disorder. *International Journal of Cognitive Therapy, 2*(4), 373–382.

Mikulincer, M., & Shaver, P. R. (2007). *Attachment in adulthood: Structure, dynamics, and change.* New York: Guilford Press.

Milders, M., Bell, S., Platt, J., Serrano, R., & Runcie, O. (2010). Stable expression recognition abnormalities in unipolar depression. *Psychiatry Research, 179*(1), 38–42.

Miller, E. K., & Cohen, J. D. (2001). An integrative theory of prefrontal cortex function. *Annual Review of Neuroscience, 24,* 167–202.

Miller, S. R., & Coll, E. (2007). From social withdrawal to social confidence: Evidence for possible pathways. *Current Psychological Research and Reviews, 26*(2), 86–101.

Miller, S. R., Tserakhava, V., & Miller, C. J. (2010). "My child is shy and has no friends: What does parenting have to do with it?" *Journal of Youth and Adolescence, 40*(4), 442–452.

Milner, B., Squire L. R., & Kandel, E. R. (1998). Cognitive neuroscience and the study of memory. *Neuron, 20,* 445–468.

Minagawa-Kawai, Y., Matsuoka, S., Dan, I., Naoi, N., Nakamura, K., & Kojima, S. (2009). Prefrontal activation associated with social attachment: Facial-emotion recognition in mothers and infants. *Cerebral Cortex, 19*(2), 284–292.

Minshew, N., & Williams, D. (2007). The new neurobiology of autism: Cortex, connectivity, and neuronal organization. *Archives of Neurology, 64*(7), 945–950.

Mitchell, J. P., Banagi, M. R., & Macrae, C. N. (2005). The link between social cognition and self-referential thought in the medial prefrontal cortex. *Journal of Cognitive Neuroscience, 17,* 1306–1315.

Mizelle, J. C. (2008). Modulation of cortical activity by visual and proprioceptive sensory demand in knee movement. *Dissertation Abstracts International, 69*(6b), 3433B.

Moller, A. C., Elliot, A. J., E., & Friedman, R. (2008). When competence and love are at stake: Achievement goals and perceived closeness to parents in an achievement context. *Journal of Research in Personality, 42,* 1386–1391.

Moran, G., Bailey, H. N., Gleason, K., DeOliveira, C. A., & Peterson, D. R. (2008). Exploring the mind behind unresolved attachment: Lessons from and for attachment-based interventions with infants and their traumatized mothers. In H. Steele & M. Steele (Eds.), *Clinical applications of the Adult Attachment Interview* (pp. 371–398). New York: Guilford Press.

Moran, G., Pederson, D. R., & Krupka, A. (2005). Maternal unresolved attachment status impedes the effectiveness of interventions with adolescent mothers. *Infant Mental Health Journal, 26*(3), 231–249.

Mori, K., & Mori, H. (2009). Another test of the passive facial feedback hypothesis: When your face smiles, you feel happy. *Perceptual and Motor Skills, 109*(1), 76–78.

Moriceau, S., & Sullivan, R. M. (2005). Neurobiology of infant attachment. *Developmental Psychobiology, 47*(3), 230–242.

Morris, A. S., Silk, J. S., Steinberg, L., Myers, S. S., & Robinson, L. R. (2007). The role of the family context in the development of emotion regulation. *Social Development, 16*(2), 361–388.

Morris, R., Tarassenko, L., & Kenward, M. (2006). *Cognitive systems: Information processing meets brain science.* London: Elsevier/Academic Press.

Morrison, C. A., & Conway, M. A. (2010). First words and first memories. *Cognition, 116*(1), 23–32.

Mudrik, L., Breska, A., Lamy, D., & Deouell, L. Y. (2011). Integration without awareness: Expanding the limits of unconscious processing. *Psychological Science, 22*(6), 764–770.

Mukamel, R., Ekstrom, A. D., Kaplan, J., Iacoboni, M., & Fried, I. (2010). Single-neuron responses in humans during execution and observation of actions. *Current Biology, 20*(8), 750–756.

Munafo, M. R., Durrant, C., Lewis, G., & Flint, J. (2009). Gene × environment interaction at the serotonin transporter locus. *Biological Psychiatry, 65*(3), 211–219.

Muris, P., Meesters, C., Morren, M., & Moorman, L. (2004). Anger and hostility in adolescents: Relationships with self-reported attachment style and perceived parental rearing styles. *Journal of Psychosomatic Research, 57*(3), 257–264.

Murray, E. A., O'Doherty, J. P., & Schoenbaum, G. (2007). What we know and do not know about the functions of the orbitofrontal cortex after 20 years of cross-species studies. *Journal of Neuroscience, 27*(31), 8166–8169.

Myers, K. M., & Davis, M. (2007). Mechanisms of fear extinction. *Molecular Psychiatry, 12*, 120–150.

Nader, K. O. (2006). Childhood trauma: The deeper wound. In J. P. Wilson (Ed.), *The posttraumatic self: Restoring meaning and wholeness to personality* (pp. 117–156). New York: Routledge.

Nambu, A. (2008). Seven problems on the basal ganglia. *Current Opinion in Neurobiology, 18*(6), 595–604.

Narumoto, J., Okada, T., Sadato, N., Fukui, K., & Yonekura, Y. (2001). Attention to emotion modulates fMRI activity in human right superior temporal sulcus. *Cognitive Brain Research, 12*(2), 225–231.

Nass, R., & Koch, D. (1991). Innate specialization for emotion: Temperament differences in children with left versus right brain damage. In N. Amir, I. Rapin, & D. Branski (Eds.), *Pediatric neurology: Vol. 1. Behavior and cognition of the child with brain dysfunction* (pp. 1–17). Basel: Karger.

Nathanson, D. L. (2009). *Shame and pride: Affect, sex, and the birth of the self.* New York: Norton.

Natsoulas, T. (2003). What is this autonoetic consciousness? *Journal of Mind and Behavior, 24*(2), 229–254.

Neath, I. (2010). Evidence for similar principles in episodic and semantic memory: The presidential serial position function. *Memory and Cognition, 38*(5), 659–666.

Neimeyer, R. A., & Levitt, H. (2001). Coping and coherence: A narrative perspective on resilience. In C. R. Snyder (Ed.), *Coping with stress: Effective people and processes* (pp. 47–67). New York: Oxford University Press.

Nelson, C. A., & Carver, L. J. (1998). The effects of stress and trauma on brain and memory: A view from developmental cognitive neuroscience. *Development and Psychopathology, 10*, 793–810.

Nelson, K. (2003a). Narrative and self, myth and memory: Emergence of the cultural self. In

R. Fivush & C. A. Haden (Eds.), *Autobiographical memory and the construction of a narrative self: Developmental and cultural perspectives* (pp. 3–28). Mahwah, NJ: Erlbaum.

Nelson, K. (2003b). Self and social functions: Individual autobiographical memory and collective narrative. *Memory, 11*(2), 125–136.

Nelson, K. (2006). *Narratives from the crib.* Cambridge, MA: Harvard University Press.

Nelson, K., & Fivush, R. (2004). The emergence of autobiographical memory: A social cultural developmental theory. *Psychological Review, 111*(2), 486–511.

Neme, A., & Mireles, V. (2008). Self-organizing maps with refractory periods. *AIP Conference Proceedings, 1060*(1), 19–25.

*New Oxford American Dictionary* (2nd ed.). (2005). New York: Oxford University Press.

Newcombe, N. S., Lloyd, M. E., & Ratliff, K. R. (2007). Development of episodic and autobiographical memory: A cognitive neuroscience perspective. *Advances in Child Development and Behavior, 35*, 37–85.

Newman, A. J. J., Bavelier, D., Corina, D., Jezzard, P., & Neville, H. J. (2002). A critical period for right hemisphere recruitment in American Sign Language processing. *Nature Neuroscience, 5*(1), 76–80.

Newman, J. P., & Lorenz, A. R. (2003). Response modulation and emotion processing: Implications for psychopathy and other dysregulatory psychopathology. In R. J. Davidson, K. R. Scherer, & H. H. Goldsmith (Eds.), *Handbook of affective sciences* (pp. 904–929). New York: Oxford University Press.

Nichols, S. R., Svetlova, M., & Brownell, C. A. (2010). Toddlers' understanding of peers' emotions. *Journal of Genetic Psychology, 171*(1), 35–53.

Nicolosi, J. J. (2009). *Shame and attachment loss: The practical work of reparative therapy.* Downers Grove, IL: InterVarsity Press.

Nisbett, R. E., & Miyamoto, Y. (2005). The influence of culture: Holistic versus analytic perception. *Trends in Cognitive Sciences, 9*(10), 467–473.

Nobre, A. C., Correa, A., & Coull, J. T. (2007). The hazards of time. *Current Opinion in Neurobiology, 17*(4), 465–470.

Nobre, A. C., Coull, J. T., Frith, C. D., & Mesulam, M. M. (1999). Orbitofrontal cortex is activated during breaches of expectation in tasks of visual attention. *Nature Neuroscience, 2*, 11–12.

Noll, J., & Shenk, C. E. (2010). Introduction to the special issue: The physical health consequences of childhood maltreatment implications for public health. *Journal of Pediatric Psychology, 35*(5), 447–449.

Noll-Hussong, M., Otti, A., Laer, L., Wohlschlaeger, A., Zimmer, C., Lahman, C., et al. (2010). Aftermath of sexual abuse history on adult patients suffering from chronic functional pain syndromes: An fMRI pilot study. *Journal of Psychometric Research, 68*(5), 483–487.

Noriuchi, M., Kikuchi, Y., & Senoo, A. (2008). The functional neuroanatomy of maternal love: Mother's response to infant's attachment behaviors. *Biological Psychiatry, 63*(4), 415–423.

Norman, G. J., Cacioppo, J. T., & Berntson, G. G. (2009). Social neuroscience. *Wiley Interdisciplinary Reviews: Cognitive Science, 1*(1), 60–68.

Normann, C., Schmitz, D., Fürmaier, A., Döing, C., & Bach, M. (2007). Long-term plasticity of visually evoked potentials in humans is altered in major depression. *Biological Psychiatry, 62*(5), 373–380.

Northoff, G., & Bermpohl, F. (2004). Cortical midline structures and the self. *Trends in Cognitive Sciences, 8*(3), 102–107.

Oatley, K. (2007). Narrative modes of consciousness and selfhood. In P. D. Zelazo, M.

Moscovitch, & E. Thompson (Eds.), *The Cambridge handbook of consciousness* (pp. 375–402). Cambridge, UK: Cambridge University Press.

Obhi, S. S., Hogeveen, J., & Pascual-Leone, A. (2011). Resonating with others: The effects of self-construal type on motor cortical output. *Journal of Neuroscience, 31*(41), 14531–14535.

Ochsner, K., Ray, R., Hughes, B., McRae, K., Cooper, J., Weber, J., et al. (2009). Bottom-up and top-down processes in emotion generation: Common and distinct neural mechanisms. *Psychological Science, 20*(11), 1322–1331.

Ochsner, K. N., & Schacter, D. L. (2003). Remembering emotional events: A social cognitive neuroscience approach. In R. J. Davidson, K. R. Scherer, & H. H. Goldsmith (Eds.), *Handbook of affective sciences* (pp. 643–660). New York: Oxford University Press.

Oddo, S., Lux, S., Weiss, P., Schwab, A., Welzer, H., Markowitsch, H., et al. (2010). Specific role of medial prefrontal cortex in retrieving recent autobiographical memories: An fMRI study of young female subjects. *Cortex: A Journal Devoted to the Study of the Nervous System and Behavior, 46*(1), 29–39.

O'Doherty, J. P. (2007). Lights, Camembert, action!: The role of human orbitofrontal cortex in encoding stimuli, rewards, and choices. *Annals of the New York Academy of Sciences, 1121*, 254–272.

O'Donohue, J. (1997). *Anam cara: A book of Celtic wisdom.* New York: HarperCollins.

Ogawa, J. R., Sroufe, L. A., Weinfeld, N. S., Carlson, E. A., & Egeland, B. (1997). Development and the fragmented self: Longitudinal study of dissociative symptomatology in a nonclinical sample. *Development and Psychopathology, 9*, 855–880.

Ogren, M. P., & Lombroso, P. J. (2008). Epigenetics: Behavioral influences on gene function. Part I. Maternal behavior permanently affects adult behavior in offspring. *Journal of the American Academy of Child and Adolescent Psychiatry, 47*(3), 240–244.

Oliveira-Souza, J. M., Moll, J., & Grafman, J. (2011). Emotion and social cognition: Lessons from contemporary human neuroanatomy. *Emotion Review, 3*(3), 310–312.

Oliver, B. R., & Plomin, R. (2007). Twins' Early Development Study (TEDS): A multivariate, longitudinal genetic investigation of language, cognition and behavior problems from childhood through adolescence. *Twin Research and Human Genetics, 10*(1), 96–105.

O'Neill, J., Pleydell-Bouverie, B., Dupret, D., & Csicsvari, J. (2010). Play it again: Reactivation of waking experience and memory. *Trends in Neurosciences, 33*(5), 220–229.

Oppenheim, D., Goldsmith, D. F., & Koren-Karie, N. (2004). Maternal insightfulness and preschoolers' emotions and behavior problems: Reciprocal influences in a therapeutic preschool program. *Infant Mental Health Journal, 25*, 352–367.

Oppenheim, D., & Koren-Karie, N. (2002). Mothers' insightfulness regarding their children's internal worlds: The capacity underlying secure child–mother relationships. *Infant Mental Health Journal, 23*, 593–605.

Ornstein, R., Herron, J., Johnstone, J., & Swencionis, C. (1979). Differential right hemisphere involvement in two reading tasks. *Psychophysiology, 16*, 398–401.

Ortigue, S., King, D., Gazzaniga, M., Miller, M., & Grafton, S. (2009). Right hemisphere dominance for understanding the intentions of others: Evidence from a split-brain patient. *BMJ Case Reports. doi:10.1136/bcr.07.2008.0593*

Öztekin, I., Davachi, L., & McElree, B. (2010). Are representations in working memory distinct from representations in long-term memory? *Psychological Science, 21*(8), 1123–1133.

Packard, M. G., & Cahill, L. (2001). Affective modulation of multiple memory systems. *Current Opinion in Neurobiology, 11*(6), 752–756.

Palaszynski, K. M., & Nemeroff, C. B. (2009). The medical consequences of child abuse and neglect. *Psychiatric Annals, 39*(12), 1004–1012.

Paller, K. A., & Voss, J. (2004). Memory reactivation and consolidation during sleep. *Learning and Memory, 11*(6), 664–670.

Paller, K. A., Voss, J. L., & Westerberg, C. E. (2009). Investigating the awareness of remembering, *Perspectives on Psychological Sciences, 4*(2), 185–199.

Paller, K. A., & Wagner, A. D. (2002). Observing the transformation of experience into memory. *Trends in Cognitive Sciences, 6*(2), 93–102.

Palombo, J., Bendicsen, H. K., & Koch, B. J. (2009). *Guide to psychoanalytic developmental theories.* New York: Springer.

Panksepp, J. (1982). Toward a general psychobiological theory of emotions. *Behavioral and Brain Sciences, 5,* 407–467.

Panksepp, J. (1998). *Affective neuroscience: The foundations of human and animal emotions.* New York: Oxford University Press.

Panksepp, J. (2001). The long-term psychobiological consequences of infant emotions: Prescriptions for the twenty-first century. *Infant Mental Health Journal, 22*(1–2), 132–173.

Panksepp, J. (2009). Brain emotional systems and qualities of mental life: From animal models of affect to implications for psychotherapeutics. In D. Fosha, D. J. Siegel, & M. F. Solomon (Eds.), *The healing power of emotion: Affective neuroscience, development and clinical practice* (pp. 1–26). New York: Norton.

Panksepp, J. (2010). The basic affective circuits of mammalian brains: Implications for healthy human development and the cultural landscapes of ADHD. In C. M. Worthman, P. M. Plotsky, D. S. Schechter, & C. A. Cummings (Eds.), *Formative experiences: The interaction of caregiving, culture, and developmental psychobiology* (pp. 470–503). New York: Cambridge University Press.

Panksepp, J., & Biven, L. (2012). *The archaeology of mind: Neuroevolutionary origins of human emotions.* New York: Norton.

Pascual-Leone, A., Amedi, A., Fregni, F., & Merabet, L. B. (2005). The plastic human brain cortex. *Annual Review of Neuroscience, 28,* 377–401.

Pasupathi, M., Mansour, E., & Brubaker, J. R. (2007). Developing a life story: Constructing relations between self and experience in autobiographical narratives. *Human Development, 50,* 85–110.

Patrick, M., Hobson, R. P., Castle, D., Howard, R., & Maughan, B. (1994). Personality disorder and the mental representation of early social experience. *Development and Psychopathology, 6*(2), 375–388.

Paulson, S., Flanagan, O., Bloom, P., & Baumeister, R. (2011). Quid pro quo: The ecology of the self. *Annals of the New York Academy of Sciences, 1234*(1), 29–43.

Paz, R., Pelletier, J. G., Bauer, E. P., & Paré, D. (2006). Emotional enhancement of memory via amygdala-driven facilitation of rhinal interactions. *Nature Neuroscience, 9,* 1321–1329.

Pearson, J. L., Cohn, D. A., Cowan, P. A., & Cowan, C. P. (1994). Earned- and continuous-security in adult attachment: Relation to depressive symptomatology and parenting style. *Development and Psychopathology, 6*(2), 358–373.

Perani, D., Saccuman, M. C., Scifo, P., Spada, D., Andreolli, G., Rovelli, R., et al. (2010). Functional specializations for music processing in the human newborn brain. *Proceedings of the National Academy of Sciences USA, 107*(10), 4758–4763.

Perlman, S. B., & Pelphrey, K. A. (2010). Regulatory brain development: Balancing emotion and cognition. *Social Neuroscience, 5*(5–6), 1–10.

Perner, J., & Dienes, Z. (2003). Developmental aspects of consciousness: How much theory of mind do you need to be consciously aware? *Consciousness and Cognition,* 63–82.

Perry, B. D. (2002). Childhood experience and the expression of genetic potential: What childhood neglect tells us about nature and nurture. *Brain and Mind: A Transdisciplinary Journal of Neuroscience and Neurophilosophy, 3*(2), 79–100.

Perry, B. D., Pollard, R. A., Blakely, T. L. Baker, W. L., & Vigilante, D. (1995). Childhood trauma, the neurobiology of adaptation, and "use-dependent" development of the brain: How states become traits. *Infant Mental Health Journal, 16*, 271–291.

Pessoa, L. (2008). On the relationship between emotion and cognition. *Nature Reviews Neuroscience, 9*, 148–158.

Peters, J., Daum, I., Gizewski, E., Forsting, M., & Suchan, B. (2009). Associations evoked during memory encoding recruit the context-network. *Hippocampus, 19*(2), 141–151.

Peterson, C., McDermott Sales, J., Rees, M., & Fivush, R. (2006). Parent–child talk and children's memory for stressful events. *Developmental Psychology, 21*(8), 1057–1075.

Pettit, G. S., Laird, R. D., Dodge, K. A., Bates, J. E., & Criss, M. M. (2001). Antecedents and behavior-problem outcomes of parental monitoring and psychological control in early adolescence. *Child Development, 72*(2), 583–598.

Pfeifer, J. H., Masten, C. L., Borofsky, L. A., Dapretto, M., Fuligni, A. J., & Lieberman, M. D. (2009). Neural correlates of direct and reflected self-appraisals in adolescents and adults: When social perspective-taking informs self-perception. *Child Development, 80*(4), 1016–1038.

Phelps, E. A. (2004). Human emotion and memory: Interactions of the amygdala and hippocampal complex. *Current Opinion in Neurobiology, 14*(2), 198–202.

Phillips, M. L., Drevets, W. C., Rauch, S., & Lane, R. (2003). Neurobiology of emotion perception: II. Implications for major psychiatric disorders. *Biological Psychiatry, 52*, 525–528.

Phillips, M. L., Ladouceur, C. D., & Drevets, W. C. (2008). A neural model of voluntary and automatic emotion regulation: Implications for understanding the pathophysiology and neurodevelopment of bipolar disorder. *Molecular Psychiatry, 13*, 833–857.

Pillow, J. W., Shlens, J., Paninski, L., Sher, A., Litke, A. M., Chichilnisky, E. J., et al. (2008). Spatio-temporal correlations and visual signalling in a complete neuronal population. *Nature, 454*, 995–999.

Pinker, S. (1999). *How the mind works.* New York: Norton.

Pinker, S. (2005). So how 'does' the mind work? *Mind and Language, 20*(1), 1–24.

Piolino, P., Desgranges, B., & Eustache, F. (2009). Episodic autobiographical memories over the course of time: Cognitive, neuropsychological and neuroimaging findings. *Neuropsychologia, 47*(11), 2314–2329.

Piolino, P., Desgranges, B., Manning, I., North, P., Jokic, C., & Eustache, F. (2007). Autobiographical memory, the sense of recollection and executive functions after severe traumatic brain injury. *Cortex, 43*(2), 176–195.

Plaut, D., & McClelland, J. (2010). Locating object knowledge in the brain: Comment on Bowers's (2009) attempt to revive the grandmother cell hypothesis. *Psychological Review, 117*(1), 284–288.

Polan, H. J., & Hofer, M. A. (2008). Psychobiological origins of infant attachment and its role in development. In J. Cassidy & P. R. Shaver (Eds.), *Handbook of attachment: Theory, research, and clinical applications* (2nd ed., pp. 158–172). New York: Guilford Press.

Poldrack, R., Wagner, A. D., Phelps, E. A., & Sharot, T. (2008). How (and why) emotion enhances the subjective sense of recollection. *Current Directions in Psychological Science, 17*(2), 147–152.

Pollak, S. D. (2005). Early adversity and mechanisms of plasticity: Integrating affective neuroscience with developmental approaches to psychopathology. *Development and Psychopathology, 17*(3), 735–752.

Polyn, S., Norman, K., & Kahana, M. (2009). Task context and organization in free recall. *Neuropsychologia, 47*(11), 2158–2163.

Porges, S. W. (2009). Reciprocal influences between body and brain in the perception and expression of affect: A polyvagal perspective. In D. Fosha, D. J. Siegel, & M. F. Solomon (Eds.), *The healing power of emotion: Affective neuroscience, development and clinical practice* (pp. 27–54). New York: Norton.

Porges, S. W. (2011). *The polyvagal theory.* New York: Norton.

Posner, J., Russell, J. A., & Peterson, B. S. (2005). The circumplex model of affect: An integrative approach to affective neuroscience, cognitive development, and psychopathology. *Development and Psychopathology, 17*(3), 715–734.

Posner, M. I., & Rothbart, M. K. (1998). Attention, self-regulation and consciousness. *Philosophical Transactions of the Royal Society of London: Series B. Biological Sciences, 353*(1377), 1915–1927.

Post, R. M., Leverich, G. S., Xing, G., & Weiss, S. R. B. (2001). Developmental vulnerabilities to the onset and course of bipolar disorder. *Development and Psychopathology, 13*(3), 581–598.

Post, R. M., & Weiss, S. R. B. (1997). Emergent properties of neural systems: How focal molecular neurobiological alterations can affect behavior. *Development and Psychopathology, 9*, 907–930.

Post, R. M., Weiss, S. R. B., Li, H., Smith, M. A., Zhang, L. X., Xing, G., et al. (1998). Neural plasticity and emotional memory. *Development and Psychopathology, 10*, 829–856.

Princeton University. (2010). Sentience. *WordNet.* Retrieved from *wordnetweb.princeton.edu/perl/webwn?s=sentience&sub=Search+WordNet&o2=&o0=1&o8=1&o1=1&o7=&o5=&o9=&o6=&o3=&o4=&h=*.

Purvis, K. B., Cross, D. R., & Sunshine, W. L. (2007). *The connected child: Bring hope and healing to your adoptive family.* New York: McGraw-Hill.

Putnam, F. W., & Carlson, E. B. (1998). Hypnosis, dissociation, and trauma: Myths, metaphors, and mechanisms. In J. D. Bremner & C. R. Marmar (Eds.), *Trauma, memory, and dissociation* (pp. 27–56). Washington, DC: American Psychiatric Press.

Quoidbach, J., Hansenne, M., & Mottet, C. (2008). Personality and mental time travel: A differential approach to autonoetic consciousness. *Consciousness and Cognition, 17*(4), 1082–1092.

Race, E., Keane, M. M., & Verfaellie, M. (2011). Medial temporal lobe damage causes deficits in episodic memory and episodic future thinking not attributable to deficits in narrative construction. *Journal of Neuroscience, 31*(28), 10262–10269.

Raffone, A., & Pantani, M. (2010). A global workspace model for phenomenal and access consciousness. *Consciousness and Cognition, 19*(2), 580–596.

Raffone, A., & Van Leeuwen, C. (2001). Activation and coherence in memory processes: Revisiting the parallel distributed processing approach to retrieval. *Connection Science, 13*(4), 349–382.

Ragozzino, M. E. (2007). The contribution of the medial prefrontal cortex, orbitofrontal cortex, and dorsomedial striatum to behavioral flexibility. *Annals of the New York Academy of Sciences, 1121*, 355–375.

Raichle, M. E. (2010). Two views of brain function. *Trends in Cognitive Sciences, 14*(4), 180–190.

Raichle, M. E., & Snyder, A. Z. (2007). A default mode of brain function: A brief history of an evolving idea. *NeuroImage, 37*(4), 1083–1090.

Rakel, D. P., Hoeft, T. J., Barrett, B. P., Chewning, B. A., Craig, B. M., & Niu, M. (2009).

Practitioner empathy and the duration of the common cold. *Family Medicine, 41*(7), 494–501.

Rakison, D. H. (2007). Is consciousness in its infancy in infancy? *Journal of Consciousness Studies, 14* (9–10), 66–89.

Ramirez-Esparza, N., & Pennebaker, J. W. (2006). Do good stories produce good health?: Exploring words, language, and culture. *Narrative Inquiry, 16*(1), 211–219.

Ramus, S., Davis, J., Donahue, R., Discenza, C., & Wait, A. (2007). Interactions between the orbitofrontal cortex and the hippocampal memory system during the storage of long-term memory. *Annals of the New York Academy of Sciences, 1121,* 216–231.

Ranganath, C., Cohen, M., & Brozinsky, C. (2005). Working memory maintenance contributes to long-term memory formation: Neural and behavioral evidence. *Journal of Cognitive Neuroscience, 17*(7), 994–1010.

Raposo, A., Han, S., & Dobbins, I. (2009). Ventrolateral prefrontal cortex and self-initiated semantic elaboration during memory retrieval. *Neuropsychologia, 47*(11), 2261–2271.

Rauch, S. L., Shin, L. M., & Phelps, E. A. (2006). Neurocircuitry models of posttraumatic stress disorder and extinction: Human neuroimaging research—past, present, and future. *Biological Psychiatry, 60*(4), 376–382.

Raval, V. V., Martini, T. S., & Raval, P. H. (2007). 'Would others think it is okay to express my feelings?' Regulation of anger, sadness and physical pain in Gujarati children in India. *Social Development, 16*(1), 79–105.

Ravassard, P., Pachoud, B., Comte, J., Mejia-Perez, C., Scoté-Blachon, C., Gay, N., et al. (2009). Paradoxical (REM) sleep deprivation causes a large and reversible decrease in long-term potentiation, synaptic transmission, glutamate receptor protein levels, and ERK/MAPK activation in the dorsal hippocampus. *Sleep, 32*(2), 227–240.

Reck, C., Hunt, A., Fuchs, T., Weiss, R., Noon, A., Moehler, E., et al. (2004). Interactive regulation of affect in postpartum depressed mothers and their infants: An overview. *Psychopathology, 37*(6), 272.

Reed, E. S. (1994). Perception is to self as memory is to selves. In U. Neisser & R. Fivush (Eds.), *The remembering self: Construction and accuracy in the self-narrative* (pp. 278–292). Cambridge, UK: Cambridge University Press.

Rees, C.A. (2010). Understanding emotional abuse. *Archives of Disease in Childhood, 95*(1), 59–67.

Reese, E., & Newcombe, R. (2007). Training mothers in elaborative reminiscing enhances children's autobiographical memory and narrative. *Child Development, 78*(4), 1153–1170.

Reilly, J., & Seibert, L. (2003). Language and emotion. In R. J. Davidson, K. R. Scherer, & H. H. Goldsmith (Eds.), *Handbook of affective sciences* (pp. 535–559). New York: Oxford University Press.

Rempel-Clower, N. L. (2007). Role of orbitofrontal cortex connections in emotion. *Annals of the New York Academy of Sciences, 1121,* 72–86.

Renken, B., Egeland, B., Marvinney, D., Magelsdorf, S., & Sroufe, L. A. (1989). Early childhood antecedents of aggression and passive-withdrawal in early elementary school. *Journal of Personality, 57,* 257–281.

Rentesi, G., Antoniou, K., Marselos, M., Fotopoulos, A., Alboycharali, J., & Konstandi, M. (2010). Long-term consequences of early maternal deprivation in serotonergic activity and HPA function in adult rat. *Neuroscience Letters, 480*(1), 7–11.

Repacholi, B., & Meltzoff, A. (2007). Emotional eavesdropping: Infants selectively respond to indirect emotional signals. *Child Development, 78*(2), 503–521.

Ridley, M. (2003). *Nature via nurture: Genes, experience, and what makes us human.* New York: HarperCollins.

Ridout, N., Dritschel, B., Matthews, K., McVicar, M., Reid, I., & O'Carroll, R. (2009). Memory for emotional faces in major depression following judgement of physical facial characteristics at encoding. *Cognition and Emotion, 23*(4), 739–752.

Riegler, A. (2008). Natural or internal selection?: The case of canalization in complex evolutionary systems. *Artificial Life, 14*(3), 345–362.

Riessman, C. K. (2003). Analysis of personal narratives. In J. A. Holstein & J. F. Gubrium (Eds.), *Inside interviewing* (pp. 331–345). Thousand Oaks, CA: Sage.

Riggs, S. A., & Jacobvitz, D. (2002). Expectant parents' representations of early attachment relationships: Associations with mental health and family history. *Journal of Consulting and Clinical Psychology, 70*(1), 195–204.

Riggs, S. A., Paulson, A., Tunnell, E., Sahl, G., Atkinson, H., & Ross, C. A. (2007). Attachment, personality, and psychopathology among adult inpatients: Self-reported romantic attachment style versus Adult Attachment Interview states of mind. *Development and Psychopathology, 19*(1), 263–291.

Rimol, L. M., Panizzon, M. S., Fennema, C.-N., Eyler, L.T., Fischl, B., Franz, C. E., et al. (2010). Cortical thickness is influenced by regionally specific genetic factors. *Biological Psychiatry, 67*(5), 493–499.

Rippon, G., Brock, J., Brown, C., & Boucher, J. (2007). Disordered connectivity in the autistic brain: Challenges for the new psychophysiology. *International Journal of Psychophysiology, 63*(2), 164–172.

Risch, N., Herrell, R., Lehner, T., Liang, K. Y., Eaves, L., Hoh, J., et al. (2009). Interaction between the serotonin transporter gene (5-HTTLPR), stressful life events, and risk of depression. A meta-analysis. *Journal of the American Medical Association, 301*(23), 2462–2471.

Ritblatt, S. N. (2000). Children's level of participation in a false-belief task, age, and theory of mind. *Journal of Genetic Psychology, 161*(1), 53–64.

Ritter, M., Bucci, W., Beebe, B., Jaffe, J., & Maskit, B. (2007). Do mothers of secure infants speak differently than mothers of avoidant infants in natural conversation?: An interpersonal exploration of language differences. *Journal of the American Psychoanalytic Association, 55*(1), 269–275.

Rizzolatti, G., Fogassi, L., & Gallese, V. (2001). Neurophysiological mechanisms underlying the understanding and imitation of action. *Nature Reviews Neuroscience, 2,* 661–670.

Rizzolatti, G., Fogassi, L., & Gallese, V. (2006, November). Mirrors in the mind. *Scientific American,* pp. 54–61.

Roberson, D., Damjanovic, L., & Filling, M. (2007). Categorical perception of facial expressions: Evidence for a "category adjustment" model. *Memory and Cognition, 35*(7), 1814–1829.

Robertson, R., & Combs, A. (Eds.). (1995). *Chaos theory in psychology and the life sciences.* Mahwah, NJ: Erlbaum.

Rodrigues, S. M., LeDoux, J. E., & Sapolsky, R. M. (2009). The influence of stress hormones on fear circuitry. *Annual Review of Neuroscience, 32,* 289–313.

Rogers, L. J. (2000). Evolution of hemisphere specialization: Advantages and disadvantages. *Brain and Language, 73*(2), 236–253.

Rogers, T., & McClelland, J. (2008). Précis of semantic cognition: A parallel distributed processing approach. *Behavioral and Brain Sciences, 31*(6), 689–749.

Rogoff, B. (2003). *The cultural nature of human development.* New York: Oxford University Press.

Roisman, G. I., Clausell, E., Holland, A., Fortuna, K., & Elieff, C. (2008). Adult romantic relationships as contexts of human development: A multi-method comparison of same-sex couples with opposite-sex dating, engaged, and married dyads. *Developmental Psychology, 44*(1), 91–101.

Roisman, G. I., Fraley, R. C., & Belsky, J. (2007a). A taxometric study of the Adult Attachment Interview. *Developmental Psychology, 43*(3), 675–686.

Roisman, G. I., Holland, A., Fortuna, K., Fraley, R. C., Clausell, E., & Clarke, A. (2007b). The Adult Attachment Interview and self-reports of attachment style: An empirical rapprochement. *Journal of Personality and Social Psychology, 92*(4), 678–697.

Roisman, G. I., Padrón, E., Sroufe, L. A., & Egeland, B. (2002). Earned-secure attachment status in retrospect and prospect. *Child Development, 73*(4), 1204–1219.

Rolls, E. T. (2004). The functions of the orbitofrontal cortex. *Brain and Cognition, 55*(1), 11–29.

Rolls, E. T., & Grabenhorst, F. (2008). The orbitofrontal cortex and beyond: From affect to decision-making. *Progress in Neurobiology, 86*(3), 216–224.

Roozendaal, B., Barsegyan, A., & Lee, S. (2007). Adrenal stress hormones, amygdala activation, and memory for emotionally arousing experiences. *Progress in Brain Research, 167*, 79–97.

Roozendaal, B., McEwen, B. S., & Chattarji, S. (2009). Stress, memory and the amygdala. *Nature Reviews Neuroscience, 10*, 423–433.

Rosa, M. G. P., Palmer, S. M., Gamberini, M., Burman, K. J., Yu, H., Reser, D. H., et al. (2009). Connections of the dorsomedial visual area: Pathways for early integration of dorsal and ventral streams in extrastriate cortex. *Journal of Neuroscience, 29*(14), 4548–4563.

Rose, A. J., & Rudolph, K. D. (2006). A review of sex differences in peer relationship processes: Potential trade-offs for the emotional and behavioral development of girls and boys. *Psychological Bulletin, 132*(1), 98–131.

Rosenzweig, E., Barnes, C., & McNaughton, B. (2002). Making room for new memories. *Nature Neuroscience, 5*(1), 6–8.

Ross, E. D. (1996). Hemispheric specialization for emotions, affective aspects of language and communication and the cognitive display behaviors in humans. *Progress in Brain Research, 107*, 583–594.

Ross, E. D., Homan, R. W., & Buck, R. (1994). Differential hemispheric lateralization of primary and social emotions: Implications for developing a comprehensive neurology of emotions, repression, and the subconscious. *Neuropsychiatry, Neuropsychology, and Behavioral Neurology, 7*, 1–19.

Ross, E. D., Prodan, C. I., & Monnot, M. (2007). Human facial expressions are organized functionally across the upper-lower facial axis. *The Neuroscientist, 13*(5), 433–446.

Rotenber, V. S. (2004). The peculiarity of the right-hemisphere function in depression: Solving the paradoxes. *Progress in Neuro-Psychopharmacology and Biological Psychiatry, 28*(1), 1–13.

Rubin, D. C. (1986). *Autobiographical memory.* Cambridge, UK: Cambridge University Press.

Rubin, K. H., Coplan, R. J., & Bowker, J. C. (2009). Social withdrawal in childhood. *Annual Review of Psychology, 60*, 141–171.

Ruchkin, D., Grafman, J., Cameron, K., & Berndt, R. (2003). Working memory retention systems: A state of activated long-term memory. *Behavioral and Brain Sciences, 26*(6), 709–777.

Rueckert, L., & Naybar, N. (2008). Gender differences in empathy: The role of the right hemisphere. *Brain and Cognition, 67*(2), 162–167.

Rueda, M. R., Posner, M. I., & Rothbart, M. K. (2005). The development of executive attention: Contributions to the emergence of self-regulation. *Developmental Neuropsychology, 28*, 573–594.

Rutter, M. (2005). How the environment affects mental health. *British Journal of Psychiatry, 186*, 4–6.

Ryan, L., Cox, C., Hayes, S., & Nadel, L. (2008). Hippocampal activation during episodic and semantic memory retrieval: Comparing category production and category cued recall. *Neuropsychologia, 46*(8), 2109–2121.

Saarni, C. (2007). The development of emotional competence: Pathways for helping children become emotionally intelligent. In R. Bar-On, J. G. Maree, & M. J. Elias (Eds.), *Educating people to be emotionally intelligent* (pp. 15–36). Westport, CT: Praeger.

Sagi, A., van IJzendoorn, M. H., Scharf, M. H., Koren-Karie, N., Joels, T., & Mayseless, O. (1994). Stability and discriminant validity of the Adult Attachment Interview: A psychometric study in young Israeli adults. *Developmental Psychology, 30*, 771–777.

Sahin, N. T. T., Pinker, S., Cash, S. S., Schomer, D., & Halgren, E. (2009). Sequential processing of lexical, grammatical, and phonological information within Broca's area. *Science, 326*(5951), 445–449.

Salomons, T., Osterman, J., Gagliese, L., & Katz, J. (2004). Pain flashbacks in posttraumatic stress disorder. *Clinical Journal of Pain, 20*(2), 83–87.

Sander, L. W. (1964). Adaptive relationships in early mother–child interaction. *Journal of the American Academy of Child Psychiatry, 3*, 231–264.

Sanford, A. J., & Emmott, C. (2012). *Mind, brain and narrative.* Cambridge, UK: Cambridge University Press.

Sato, W., & Aoki, S. (2006). Right hemispheric dominance in processing of unconscious negative emotion. *Brain and Cognition, 62*(3), 261–266.

Saur, D., Kreher, B. W., Schnell, S., Kummerer, D., Kellmeyer, P., Vry, M., et al. (2008). Ventral and dorsal pathways for language. *Proceedings of the National Academy of Sciences USA, 105*(46), 18035–18040.

Sauter, D., Eisner, F., Ekman, P., & Scott, S. (2009). Universal vocal signals of emotion. In N. Taatgen & H. Van Rijn (Eds.), *Proceedings of the 31st Annual Meeting of the Cognitive Science Society* (pp. 2251–2255). Amsterdam: Cognitive Science Society.

Saxe, R. (2006). Uniquely human social cognition. *Current Opinion in Neurobiology, 16*(2), 235–239.

Saxena, S., Gorgis, E., O'Neill, J., Baker, S. K., Mandelkern, M. A., Maidment, K. M., et al. (2009). Rapid effects of brief intensive cognitive-behavioral therapy on brain glucose metabolism in obsessive–compulsive disorder: PET study of brief intensive CBT for OCD. *Molecular Psychiatry, 14*, 197–205.

Schacter, D. L. (1996). *Searching for memory: The brain, the mind, and the past.* New York: Basic Books.

Schacter, D. L., Addis, D., & Buckner, R. (2007). Remembering the past to imagine the future: The prospective brain. *Nature Reviews Neuroscience, 8*(9), 657–661.

Schafe, G., Doyère, V., & LeDoux, J. (2005). Tracking the fear engram: The lateral amygdala is an essential locus of fear memory storage. *Journal of Neuroscience, 25*(43), 10010–10015.

Scherf, K. S., Behrmann, M., Humphreys, K., & Luna, B. (2007). Visual category-selectivity for faces, places and objects emerges along different developmental trajectories. *Developmental Science, 10*(4), F15–F30.

Schick, B., De Villiers, P., De Villiers, J., & Hoffmeister, R. (2007). Language and theory of mind: A study of deaf children. *Child Development, 78*(2), 376–396.

Schmidt, L. A. A. (1999). Frontal brain electrical activity in shyness and sociability. *Psychological Science, 10*(4), 316–320.

Schmidt, S. R., & Saari, B. (2007). The emotional memory effect: Differential processing or item distinctiveness? *Memory and Cognition, 35*(8), 1905–1916.

Schmidt-Hellerau, C. (2002). Where models intersect: A metapsychological approach. *Psychoanalytic Quarterly, 71,* 503–544.

Schmitz, T. W., & Johnson, S. C. (2006). Self-appraisal decisions evoke dissociated dorsal–ventral aMPFC networks. *NeuroImage, 30*(3), 1050–1058.

Schnell, K., Dietrich, T., Schnitker, R., Daumann, J., & Herpertz, S. (2007). Processing of autobiographical memory retrieval cues in borderline personality disorder. *Journal of Affective Disorders,* 97(1–3), 253–259.

Schönenberg, M., Reichwald, U., Domes, G., Badke, A., & Hautzinger, M. (2008). Ketamine aggravates symptoms of acute stress disorder in a naturalistic sample of accident victims. *Journal of Psychopharmacology, 22*(5), 493–497.

Schore, A. N. (1994). *Affect regulation and the origin of the self: The neurobiology of emotional development.* Hillsdale, NJ: Erlbaum.

Schore, A. N. (1996). The experience-dependent maturation of a regulatory system in the orbital prefrontal cortex and the origin of developmental psychopathology. *Development and Psychopathology, 8*(1), 59–87.

Schore, A. N. (1997). Early organization of the nonlinear right brain and development of a predisposition to psychiatric disorders. *Development and Psychopathology, 9,* 595–631.

Schore, A. N. (1998). The experience-dependent maturation of an evaluative system in the cortex. In K. H. Pribram & J. King (Eds.), *Brain and values: Is a biological science of values possible?* (pp. 337–358). Mahwah, NJ: Erlbaum.

Schore, A. N. (2000). Attachment and the regulation of the right brain. *Attachment and Human Development, 2*(1), 23–47.

Schore, A. N. (2001). The effects of a secure attachment relationship on right brain development, affect regulation, and infant mental health. *Infant Mental Health Journal, 22*(1–2), 7–66.

Schore, A. N. (2002). Dysregulation of the right brain: A fundamental mechanism of traumatic attachment and the psychopathogenesis of posttraumatic stress disorder. *Australian and New Zealand Journal of Psychiatry, 36*(1), 9–30.

Schore, A. N. (2003a). *Affect dysregulation and disorders of the self.* New York: Norton.

Schore, A. N. (2003b). *Affect regulation and the repair of the self.* New York: Norton.

Schore, A. N. (2005). Back to basics: Attachment, affect regulation, and the developing right brain: Linking developmental neuroscience to pediatrics. *Pediatrics in Review, 26*(6), 204–217.

Schore, A. N. (2009a). Relational trauma and the developing right brain. *Annals of the New York Academy of Sciences, 1159,* 189–203.

Schore, A. N. (2009b). Right-brain affect regulation: An essential mechanism of development, trauma, dissociation, and psychotherapy. In D. Fosha, D. J. Siegel, & M. F. Solomon (Eds.), *The healing power of emotion: Affective neuroscience, development and clinical practice* (pp. 112–144). New York: Norton.

Schore, A. N. (2010). The right brain implicit self: A central mechanism of the psychotherapy change process. In J. Petrucelli (Ed.), *Knowing, not-knowing and sort-of-knowing: Psychoanalysis and the experience* (pp. 177–203). London: Karnac Books.

Schore, J. R., & Schore, A. N. (2008). Modern attachment theory: The central role of affect regulation in development and treatment. *Clinical Social Work Journal, 36*(1), 9–20.

Schultheiss, O. C., Riebel, K. J., & Jones, N. M. (2009). Activity inhibition: A predictor of lateralized brain function during stress? *Neuropsychology, 23*(3), 392–404.

Schwartz, C. E., Kunwar, P. S., Greve, D. N., Moran, L. R., Viner, J. C., Covino, J. M., et al. (2010). Structural differences in adult orbital and ventromedial prefrontal cortex predicted by infant temperament at 4 months of age. *Archives of General Psychiatry, 67*(1), 78–84.

Scott-Van Zeeland, A. A., Dapretto, M., Ghahremani, D. G., Poldrack, R. A., & Bookheimer, S. Y. (2010). Reward processing in autism. *Autism Research, 3*(2), 53–67.

Sergerie, K., Lepage, M., & Armony, J. L. (2006). A process-specific functional dissociation of the amygdala in emotional memory. *Journal of Cognitive Neuroscience, 18*(8), 1359–1367.

Seung, Y., Kyong, J.-S., Woo, S.-H., Lee, B.-T., & Lee, K.-M. (2005). Brain activation during music listening in individuals with or without prior music training. *Neuroscience Research, 52*(4), 323–329.

Shamay-Tsoory, S. G., Tomer, R., Berger, B. D., & Aharon-Peretz, J. (2003). Characterization of empathy deficits following prefrontal brain damage: The role of the right ventromedial prefrontal cortex. *Journal of Cognitive Neuroscience, 15*(3), 324–337.

Shanker, S., & Stieben, J. (2009). The roots of mindblindness. In I. Leudar & A. Costall (Eds.), *Against theory of mind* (pp. 126–144). New York: Palgrave Macmillan.

Shatz, C. J. (1990). Impulse activity and the patterning of connections during CNS development. *Neuron, 5*(6), 745–756.

Shatz, C. J. (1992). The developing brain. *Scientific American, 267*(3), 60–67.

Shatz, C. J. (1996). Emergence of order in visual system development. *Proceedings of the National Academy of Sciences USA, 93*(2), 602–608.

Sherwood, C., Subiaul, F., & Zawidzki, T. (2008). A natural history of the human mind: Tracing evolutionary changes in brain and cognition. *Journal of Anatomy, 212*(4), 426–454.

Shimada, S., & Hiraki, K. (2006). Infant's brain responses to live and televised action. *NeuroImage, 32*(2), 930–939.

Shin, L. M., Rauch, S., & Pitman, R. K. (2006). Amygdala, medial prefrontal cortex, and hippocampal function in PTSD. *Annals of the New York Academy of Sciences, 1071*, 67–79.

Shinbrot, T., Grebogi, C., Ott, E., & Yorke, J. A. (1993). Using small perturbations to control chaos. *Nature, 363*, 411–417.

Shmueli-Goetz, Y., Target, M., Fonagy, P., & Datta, A. (2008). The Child Attachment Interview: A psychometric study of reliability and discriminant validity. *Developmental Psychology, 44*(4), 939–956.

Showers, C. J., & Zeigler-Hill, V. (2007). Compartmentalization and integration: The evaluative organization of contextualized selves. *Journal of Personality, 75*(6), 1181–1204.

Shulman, G. L. L., Pope, D. L. W., Astafiev, S. V., McAvoy, M. P., Snyder, A. Z., & Corbetta, M. (2010). Right hemisphere dominance during spatial selective attention and target detection occurs outside the dorsal frontoparietal network. *Journal of Neuroscience, 30*(10), 3640–3651.

Shulman, R. G. (2001). Functional imaging studies: Linking mind and basic neuroscience. *American Journal of Psychiatry, 158*, 11–20.

Siegel, D. J. (1995a). Memory, trauma and psychotherapy: A cognitive science view. *Journal of Psychotherapy Practice and Research, 4*(2), 93–122.

Siegel, D. J. (1995b). Dissociation, psychotherapy, and the cognitive sciences. In J. Spira (Ed.), *Treating dissociative identity disorder* (pp. 39–79). San Francisco: Jossey-Bass.

Siegel, D. J. (1996a). Cognition, memory and dissociation. *Child and Adolescent Psychiatric Clinics of North America on Dissociative Disorders, 5*, 509–536.

Siegel, D. J. (1996b). Dissociation, psychotherapy and the cognitive sciences. In J. Spira (Ed.), *The treatment of dissociative identity disorder* (pp. 39–80). San Francisco: Jossey-Bass.

Siegel, D. J. (2001a). Toward an interpersonal neurobiology of the developing mind: Attachment relationships, mindsight, and neural integration. *Infant Mental Health Journal, 22*(1–2), 67–94.

Siegel, D. J. (2001b). Memory: An overview, with emphasis on developmental, interpersonal, and neurobiological aspects. *Journal of the American Academy of Child and Adolescent Psychiatry, 40*(9), 997–1011.

Siegel, D. J. (2004). Attachment and self-understanding: Parenting with the brain in mind. *Journal of Prenatal and Perinatal Psychology and Health, 18*(4), 273–285.

Siegel, D. J. (2006). An interpersonal neurobiology approach to psychotherapy: How awareness, mirror neurons and neural plasticity contribute to the development of well-being. *Psychiatric Annals, 36*(4), 248–258.

Siegel, D. J. (2007a). *The mindful brain: Reflection and attunement in the cultivation of well-being.* New York: Norton.

Siegel, D. J. (2007b). Mindfulness training and neural integration. *Social Cognitive and Affective Neuroscience, 2*(4), 259–263.

Siegel, D. J. (2009a). Emotion as Integration: A possible answer to the question, What is emotion? In D. Fosha, D. J. Siegel, & M. F. Solomon (Eds.), *The healing power of emotion: Affective neuroscience, development and clinical practice* (pp. 145–171). New York: Norton.

Siegel, D. J. (2009b). Mindful awareness, mindsight, and neural integration. *Journal of Humanistic Psychology, 37*(2), 137–158.

Siegel, D. J. (2010a). *Mindsight: The new science of personal transformation.* New York: Bantam/Random House.

Siegel, D. J. (2010b). *The mindful therapist: A clinician's guide to mindsight and neural integration.* New York: Norton.

Siegel, D. J. (2012). *Pocket guide to interpersonal neurobiology: An integrative handbook of the mind.* New York: Norton.

Siegel, D. J., & Bryson, T. P. (2011). *The whole-brain child: Twelve revolutionary strategies to nurture your child's developing mind.* New York: Random House.

Siegel, D. J., & Hartzell, M. (2003). *Parenting from the inside out: How a deeper self-understanding can help you raise children who thrive.* New York: Tarcher.

Siegel, D. J., & Pierce-McCall, D. (2009). Mindsight at work: An interpersonal neurobiology lens on leadership. *NeuroLeadership Journal*, No. 2, 23–34.

Siegel, J. M. (2001). The REM sleep–memory consolidation hypothesis. *Science, 294*(5544), 1058–1063.

Sigman, M., & Siegel, D. J. (1992). The interface between the psychobiological and cognitive models of attachment. *Behavioral and Brain Sciences, 15*, 523.

Sim, T.-C., & Martinez, C. (2005). Emotion words are remembered better in the left ear. *Laterality, 10*(2), 149–159.

Simeon, D., Knutelska, M., Yehuda, R., Putnam, F., Schmeidler, J., & Smith, L. M. (2006). Hypothalamic–pituitary–adrenal axis function in dissociative disorders, post-traumatic stress disorder, and healthy volunteers. *Biological Psychiatry, 61*(8), 966–973

Simon, D., Kaufmann, C., Müsch, K., Kischkel, E., & Kathmann, N. (2010). Fronto-striato-limbic hyperactivation in obsessive–compulsive disorder during individually tailored symptom provocation. *Psychophysiology, 47*(4), 728–738.

Simpson, J. A., & Belsky, J. (2008). Attachment theory within a modern evolutionary framework. In J. Cassidy & P. R. Shaver (Eds.), *Handbook of attachment: Theory, research, and clinical applications* (2nd ed., pp. 131–157). New York: Guilford Press.

Sinnet, S., Synder, J. J., & Kingstone, A. (2009). Role of the lateral prefrontal cortex in visual object-based selective attention. *Experimental Brain Research, 194*(2), 191–196.

Slade, A., Grienenberger, J., Bernbach, E., Levy, D., & Locker, A. (2005). Maternal reflective functioning, attachment, and the transmission gap: A preliminary study. *Attachment and Human Development, 7*(3), 283–298.

Slingerland, E., & Collard, M. (Eds.). (2011). *Consilience: Integrating the sciences and humanities.* New York: Oxford University Press.

Slotnick, S. D., & Moo, L. R. (2006). Prefrontal cortex hemispheric specialization for categorical and coordinate visual spatial memory. *Neuropsychologia, 44*(9), 1560–1568.

Smith, S. D., & Bulman-Fleming, M. B. (2004). A hemispheric asymmetry for the unconscious perception of emotion. *Brain and Cognition, 55*(3), 452–457.

Smith, S. D., & Bulman-Fleming, M. B. (2005). An examination of the right-hemisphere hypothesis of the lateralization of emotion. *Brain and Cognition, 57*(2), 210–213.

Smith, S. D., & Bulman-Fleming, M. B. (2006). Hemispheric asymmetries for the conscious and unconscious perception of emotional words. *Laterality: Asymmetries of Body, Brain and Cognition, 11*(4), 304–330.

Sodian, B., & Frith, U. (2008). Metacognition, theory of mind, and self-control: The relevance of high-level cognitive processes in development, neuroscience, and education. *Mind, Brain, and Education, 2*(3), 111–113.

Sohur, U. S., Emsley, J. G., Mitchell, B. D., & Macklis, J. D. (2006). Adult neurogenesis and cellular brain repair with neural progenitors, precursors and stem cells. *Philosophical Transactions of the Royal Society of London: Series B. Biological Sciences, 361*(1473), 1477–1497.

Solomon, J., & George, C. (2008). The measurement of attachment security and related constructs in infancy and early childhood. In J. Cassidy & P. R. Shaver (Eds.), *Handbook of attachment: Theory, research, and clinical applications* (2nd ed., pp. 383–418). New York: Guilford Press.

Solomon, M. F., & Siegel, D. J. (2003). *Healing trauma: Attachment, mind, body, and brain.* New York: Norton.

Someya, T., Uehara, T., Kadowaki, M., Tang, S. W., & Takahashi, S. (2000). Effects of gender difference and birth order on perceived parenting styles, measured by the EMBU scale, in Japanese two-sibling subjects. *Psychiatry and Clinical Neurosciences, 54*(1), 77–81.

Sommer, I. E. C. E., Aleman, A., Bouma, A., & Kahn, R. S. (2004). Do women really have more bilateral language representation than men?: A meta-analysis of functional imaging studies. *Brain, 127*(8), 1845–1852.

Soto, J. A., Levenson, R. W., & Ebling, R. (2005). Cultures of moderation and expression: Emotional experience, behavior, and physiology in Chinese Americans and Mexican Americans. *Emotion, 5*(2), 154–165.

Sowell, E. A. (2011, January 13). *Imaging the developing human brain.* Oral presentation at the UCLA Center for Culture, Brain, and Development Winter Seminar, UCLA.

Spaniola, J., Davidson, P. S., Kim, A. S., Han, H., Moscovitch, M., & Grady, C. L. (2009). Event-related fMRI studies of episodic encoding and retrieval: Meta-analyses using activation likelihood estimation. *Neuropsychologia, 47*(8–9), 1765–1779.

Spencer, P. E. E. (2004). Individual differences in language performance after cochlear implantation at one to three years of age: Child, family, and linguistic factors. *Journal of Deaf Studies and Deaf Education, 9*(4), 395–412.

Spere, K. A., Schmidt, L. A., Riniolo, T. C., & Fox, N. A. (2005). Is a lack of cerebral hemisphere dominance a risk factor for social "conflictedness"?: Mixed-handedness in shyness and sociability. *Personality and Individual Differences, 39*(2), 271–281.

Sporns, O. (2010). Brain networks and embodiment. In B. Mesquita, L. F. Barrett, & E. R. Smith (Eds.), *The mind in context* (pp. 42–64). New York: Guilford Press.

Sporns, O., Chialvo, D. R., Kaiser, M., & Hilgetag, C. C. (2004). Organization, development and function of complex brain networks. *Trends in Cognitive Sciences, 8*(9), 418–425.

Sporns, O., & Tononi, G. (2007). Structural determinants of functional brain dynamics. In V. K. Jirsa & A. R. McIntosh (Eds.), *Handbook of brain connectivity: Understanding complex systems* (pp. 117–148). New York: Springer.

Sporns, O., Tononi, G., & Edelman, G. M. (2000). Connectivity and complexity: The relationship between neuroanatomy and brain dynamics. *Neural Networks, 13*(8–9), 909–922.

Springer, S. P., & Deutsch, G. (1993). *Left brain, right brain* (4th ed.). New York: Freeman.

Squire, L. R. (2004): Memory systems of the brain: A brief history and current perspective. *Neurobiology of Learning and Memory, 82*(3), 171–177.

Squire, L. R., Rolls, E. T., Johnson, M. K., & Buckner, R. L. (2007). Memory systems. In H. Roediger, Y. Dudai, & S. Fitzpatrick (Eds.), *Science of memory* (pp. 337–365). New York: Oxford Scholarship Online Monographs.

Sroufe, A., & Siegel, D. J. (2011, March–April). The verdict is in: The case for attachment theory. *Psychotherapy Networker.* Retrieved from *www.psychotherapynetworker.org/magazine/recentissues/1271=the=verdict=is=in.*

Sroufe, L. A. (1996). *Emotional development: The organization of emotional life in the early years.* New York: Cambridge University Press.

Sroufe, L. A., Coffino, B., & Carlson, E. A. (2010). Conceptualizing the role of early experience: Lessons from the Minnesota longitudinal study. *Developmental Review, 30*(1), 36–51.

Sroufe, L. A., Egeland, B., Carlson, E., & Collins, A. (2005). *The development of the person: The Minnesota study of risk and adaptation from birth to adulthood.* New York: Guilford Press.

Stanislawa, L. (2000). Characteristics of attachment behavior in institution-reared children. In P. M. Crittenden & A. H. Claussen (Eds.), *The organization of attachment relationships: Maturation, culture, and context* (pp. 141–170). New York: Cambridge University Press.

Stark, D. E. E., Margulies, D. S., Shehzad, Z. E., Reiss, P., Kelly, A. M. C., Uddin, L. Q., et al. (2008). Regional variation in interhemispheric coordination of intrinsic hemodynamic fluctuations. *Journal of Neuroscience, 28*(51), 13754–13764.

Starmans, C., & Bloom, P. (2011). What do you think you are? *Annals of the New York Academy of Sciences, 1234*(1), 44–47.

Steele, H., & Steele, M. (Eds.). (2008). *Clinical applications of the Adult Attachment Interview.* New York: Guilford Press.

Steele, M., Hodges, J., Kanuk, J., Hillman, S., & Henderson, K. (2003). Attachment representations and adoption: Associations between maternal states of mind and emotional narratives in previously maltreated children. *Journal of Child Psychotherapy, 29*(2), 187–205.

Steele, M., Hodges, J., Kanuk, J., Steele, H., Hillman, S., & Asquith, K. (2008). Forecasting outcomes in previously maltreated children: The use of the AAI in a longitudinal adoption study. In H. Steele & M. Steele (Eds.), *Clinical applications of the Adult Attachment Interview* (pp. 426–451). New York: Guilford Press.

Steinvorth, S., Corkin, S., & Halgren, E. (2005). Ecphory of autobiographical memories: An fMRI study of recent and remote memory retrieval. *NeuroImage, 30*(1), 285–298.

Stemmler, G. (2003). Methodological considerations in the psychophysiological study of emotion. In R. J. Davidson, K. R. Scherer, & H. H. Goldsmith (Eds.), *Handbook of affective sciences* (pp. 225–255). New York: Oxford University Press.

Stephan, K. A., Marshall, J. C., Penny, W. D., Friston, K. J., & Fink, G. R. (2007).

Interhemispheric integration of visual processing during task-driven lateralization. *Journal of Neuroscience, 27*(13), 3512–3522.

Stern, D. N. (1985). *The interpersonal world of the infant: A view from psychoanalysis and developmental psychology.* New York: Basic Books.

Sterpenich, V., Albouy, G., Darsaud, A., Schmidt, C., Vandewalle, G., Vu, T. T. D., et al. (2009). Sleep promotes the neural reorganization of remote emotional memory. *Journal of Neuroscience, 29*(16), 5143–5152.

Stickgold, R., & Walker, M. P. (2007). Sleep-dependent memory consolidation and reconsolidation. *Sleep Medicine, 8*(4), 331–343.

Stoller, R. J. (1985). *Observing the erotic imagination.* New Haven, CT: Yale University Press.

Stoltenborgh, M., van IJzendoorn, M. H., Euser, E. M., & Bakermans-Kranenburg, M. J. (2011). A global perspective on child sexual abuse: Meta-analysis of prevalence around the world. *Child Maltreat, 16*(2), 79–101.

Storm, B., Bjork, E., & Bjork, R. (2005). Social metacognitive judgments: The role of retrieval-induced forgetting in person memory and impressions. *Journal of Memory and Language, 52*(4), 535–550.

Stovall-McClough, K. C., & Dozier, M. (2004). Forming attachments in foster care: Infant attachment behaviors during the first 2 months of placement. *Development and Psychopathology, 16*, 253–271.

Strathearn, L. (2011). Maternal neglect: Oxytocin, dopamine and the neurobiology of attachment. *Journal of Neuroendocrinology, 23*(11), 1054–1065.

Strayer, J., & Roberts, W. (2004). Children's anger, emotional expressiveness, and empathy: Relations with parents' empathy, emotional expressiveness, and parenting practices. *Social Development, 13*(2), 229–254.

Stroganova, T. A., Pushina, N. P., Orekhova, E. V., Posikera, I. N., & Tsetlin, M. M. (2004). Functional brain asymmetry and individual differences in hand preference in early ontogeny. *Human Physiology, 30*(1), 14–23.

Sulis, W. H., & Trofimova, I. N. (Eds.). (2001). *Nonlinear dynamics in the life and social sciences.* Burke, VA: IOS Press.

Surguladze, S., Young, A., Senior, C., Brébion, G., Travis, M., & Phillips, M. (2004). Recognition accuracy and response bias to happy and sad facial expressions in patients with major depression. *Neuropsychology, 18*(2), 212–218.

Sutton, J. (2006). Introduction: Memory, embodied cognition, and the extended mind. *Philosophical Psychology, 19*(3), 281–289.

Sutton, J. (2010). Observer perspective and acentred memory: Some puzzles about point of view in personal memory. *Philosophical Studies, 148*(1), 27–37.

Suveg, C., Jacob, M. L., & Payne, M. (2010). Parental interpersonal sensitivity and youth social problems: A mediational role for child emotion dysregulation. *Journal of Child and Family Studies, 19*(6), 677–686.

Svoboda, E., McKinnon, M., & Levine, B. (2006). The functional neuroanatomy of autobiographical memory: A meta-analysis. *Neuropsychologia, 44*(12), 2189–2208.

Swain, J. E., Lorberbaum, J. P., Kose, S., & Strathearn, L. (2007). Brain basis of early parent–infant interactions: Psychology, physiology, and *in vivo* functional neuroimaging studies. *Journal of Child Psychology and Psychiatry, 48*(3–4), 262–287.

Sweatt, J. D. (2004). Mitogen-activated protein kinases in synaptic plasticity and memory. *Current Opinion in Neurobiology, 14*(3), 311–317.

Sweatt, J. D. (2009). Experience-dependent epigenetic modifications in the central nervous system. *Biological Psychiatry, 65*(3), 191–197.

Szu-Han, W., & Morris, R. G. M. (2010). Hippocampal–neocortical interactions in memory formation, consolidation, and reconsolidation. *Annual Review of Psychology, 61*(1), 49–79.

Szyf, M., McGowan, P. O., Turecki, G., & Meaney, M. J. (2010).The social environment and the epigenome. In C. M. Worthman, P. M. Plotsky, D. S. Schechter, & C. A. Cummings (Eds.), *Formative experiences: The interaction of caregiving, culture, and developmental psychobiology* (pp. 53–81). New York: Cambridge University Press.

Talbot, N. L., Chapman, B., Yeates, C., McCollumn, K., Franus, N., Cotescu, S., et al. (2009). Childhood sexual abuse is associated with physical illness burden and functioning in psychiatric patients 50 years of age and older. *Psychosomatic Medicine, 71*(4), 417–422.

Tang, A. C. (2003). A hippocampal theory of cerebral lateralization. In K. Hugdahl & R. J. Davidson (Eds.), *The asymmetrical brain* (pp. 37–68). Cambridge, MA: MIT Press.

Tang, H., Li, H., & Yan, R. (2010). Memory dynamics in attractor networks with saliency weights. *Neural Computation, 22*(7), 1899–1926.

Tangney, J. P., & Dearing, R. L. (2002). *Shame and guilt.* New York: Guilford Press.

Tanji, J., & Hoshi, E. (2008). Role of the lateral prefrontal cortex in executive behavioral control. *Physiological Reviews, 88*(1), 37–57.

Tapiero, I., & Fillon, V. (2007). Hemispheric asymmetry in the processing of negative and positive emotional inferences. In F. Schmalhofer & C. A. Perfetti (Eds.), *Higher level language processes in the brain: Inference and comprehension processes* (pp. 355–377). Mahwah, NJ: Erlbaum.

Taylor, P. C. J., Nobre, A. C., & Rushworth, M. F. S. (2007). Subsecond changes in top–down control exerted by human medial frontal cortex during conflict and action selection: A combined transcranial magnetic stimulation–electroencephalography study. *Journal of Neuroscience, 27*(42), 11343–11353.

Taylor, S. E., Klein, L. C., Lewis, B. P., Gruenewald, T. L., Gurung, R. A. R., & Updegraff, J. A. (2000). Biobehavioral responses to stress in females: Tend-and-befriend, not fight-or-flight. *Psychological Review, 107*(3), 411–429.

Taylor, S. E., Klein, L. C., Lewis, B. P., Gruenewald, T. L., Gurung, R. A. R., & Updegraff, J. A. (2002). Sex differences in biobehavioral responses to threat: Reply to Geary and Flinn (2002). *Psychological Review, 109*(4), 751–753.

Tedeschi, R. G., & Calhoun, L. G. (2004). Posttraumatic growth: Conceptual foundations and empirical evidence. *Psychological Inquiry, 15*(1), 1–18.

Teicher, M. H. (2000). Wounds that time won't heal: The neurobiology of child abuse. *Cerebrum, 4*(2), 50–67.

Teicher, M. H. (2002, March). Scars that won't heal: The neurobiology of child abuse. *Scientific American*, pp. 54–61.

Teicher, M. H. (2007). Essay: The role of experience in brain development: Adverse effects of childhood maltreatment. In K. W. Fischer, J. H. Bernstein, & M. H. Immordino-Yang (Eds.), *Mind, brain, and education in reading disorders* (pp. 176–177). Cambridge, UK: Cambridge University Press.

Teicher, M. H. (2010). Commentary: Childhood abuse: New insights into its association with posttraumatic stress, suicidal ideation, and aggression. *Journal of Pediatric Psychology, 35*(5), 578–580.

Teicher, M. H., & Andersen, S. L. (2009). Delayed effects of early stress on hippocampal development. *Journal of Child and Adolescent Psychopharmacology, 13*(1), 41–51.

Teicher, M. H. Andersen, S. L., Polcari, A., Anderson, C. M., & Navalta, C. P. (2002). Developmental neurobiology of childhood stress and trauma. *Psychiatric Clinics of North America, 25*, 397–426.

Teicher, M. H. Andersen, S. L., Polcari, A., Anderson, C. M., Navalta, C. P., & Kim, D. M. (2003). The neurobiological consequences of early stress and childhood maltreatment. *Neuroscience and Biobehavioral Reviews, 27*(1–2), 33–44.

Teicher, M. H., Dumont, N. L., Ito, Y., Vaituzis, C., Giedd, J. N., & Andersen, S. L. (2004). Childhood neglect is associated with reduced corpus callosum area. *Biological Psychiatry, 56*(2), 80–85.

Teicher, M. H., Samson, J. A., Polcari, A., & Andersen, S. L. (2009). Length of time between onset of childhood sexual abuse and emergence of depression in a young adult sample: A retrospective clinical report. *Journal of Clinical Psychiatry, 70*(5), 684–691.

Teicher, M. H., Samson, J. A., Sheu, Y., Polcari, A., & McGreenery, C. E. (2010). Hurtful words: Association of exposure to peer verbal abuse with elevated psychiatric symptom scores and corpus callosum abnormalities. *American Journal of Psychiatry, 167,* 1464–1471.

Teicher, M. H., Tomoda, A., & Andersen, S. L. (2006). Neurobiological consequences of early stress and childhood maltreatment: Are results from human and animal studies comparable? *Annals of the New York Academy of Sciences, 1071,* 313–323.

Terr, L. C. (1991). Childhood traumas: An outline and review. *American Journal of Psychiatry, 148,* 10–20.

Thagard, P. (2002). *Coherence in thought and action.* Cambridge, MA: MIT Press.

Thatcher, R. W. (2007). Cycles and gradients in development of the cortex. In K. Fischer, J. H. Bernstein, & M. H. Immordino-Yang (Eds.), *Mind, brain, and education in reading disorders.* Cambridge, UK: Cambridge University Press.

Thatcher, R. W., Walker, R. A., & Guidice, S. (1987). Human cerebral hemispheres develop at different rates and ages. *Science, 236,* 1110–1113.

Thayer, J. F., Hansen, A. L. Saus-Rose, E., & Johnsen, B. H. (2009). Heart rate variability, prefrontal neural function, and cognitive performance: The neurovisceral integration perspective on self-regulation, adaptation, and health. *Annals of Behavioral Medicine, 37*(2), 141–153.

Thelen, E. (1989). Self-organization in developmental processes: Can systems approaches work?" In M. Gunnar & E. Thelen (Eds.), *Systems and Development: The Minnesota Symposium on Child Psychology* (Vol. 22, pp. 77–117). New York: Psychology Press.

Thelen, E., & Smith, L. B. (1994). *A dynamic systems approach to the development of cognition and action.* Cambridge, MA: MIT Press.

Thompson, K., Biddle, K. R., Robinson-Long, M., Poger, J., Wang, J., Yang, Q. X., et al. (2009). Cerebral plasticity and recovery of function after childhood prefrontal cortex damage. *Developmental Neurorehabilitation, 12*(5), 298–312.

Thompson, R. F., & Madigan, S. A. (2007). *Memory: The key to consciousness.* Princeton, NJ: Princeton University Press.

Thomsen, D. K., & Berntsen, D. (2008). The long-term impact of emotionally stressful events on memory characteristics and life story. *Applied Cognitive Psychology, 23*(4), 579–598.

Thomson, D., Milliken, B., & Smilek, D. (2010). Long-term conceptual implicit memory: A decade of evidence. *Memory and Cognition, 38*(1), 42–46.

Toga, A. W., & Thompson, P. M. (2003). Mapping brain asymmetry. *Nature Reviews Neuroscience, 4*(1), 37–48.

Tondowski, M., Kovacs, Z., Morin, C., & Turnbull, O. H. (2007). Hemispheric asymmetry and the diversity of emotional experience in anosognosia. *Neuropsychoanalysis, 9*(1), 67–81.

Toth, S. L., Rogosch, F. A., Struge-Apple, M., & Cicchetti, D. (2009). Building a secure base: Treatment of a child with disorganized attachment. *Child Development, 80*(1), 192–208.

Trachtenberg, J. T., Chen, B. E., Knott, G. W., Feng, G., Sanes, J. R., Welker, E., et al. (2002). Long-term *in vivo* imaging of experience-dependent synaptic plasticity in adult cortex. *Nature, 420*, 788–794.

Tranel, D., Damasio, H., Denburg, N., & Bechara, A. (2005). Does gender play a role in functional asymmetry of ventromedial prefrontal cortex? *Brain, 128*(12), 2872–2881.

Trevarthen, C. (1990a). Growth and education of the hemispheres. In C. Trevarthen (Ed.), *Brain circuits and functions of the mind: Essays in honour of Roger W. Sperry* (pp. 334–363). New York: Cambridge University Press.

Trevarthen, C. (1990b). Integrative functions of the cerebral commissures. In F. Boller & J. Grafman (Eds.), *Handbook of neurospsychology* (Vol. 4, pp. 49–83). Amsterdam: Elsevier.

Trevarthen, C. (1993). The self born in intersubjectivity: The psychology of infant communicating. In U. Neisser (Ed.), *The perceived self: Ecological and interpersonal sources of self-knowledge* (pp. 121–173). New York: Cambridge University Press.

Trevarthen, C. (1996). Lateral asymmetries in infancy: Implications for the development of the hemispheres. *Neuroscience and Biobehavioral Reviews, 20*, 571–586.

Trevarthen, C. (2001). Intrinsic motives for companionship in understanding: Their origin, development, and significance for infant mental health. *Infant Mental Health Journal, 22*(1–2), 95–131.

Trevarthen, C. (2005a). First things first: Infants make good use of the sympathetic rhythm of imitation, without reason or language. *Journal of Child Psychotherapy, 31*(1), 91–113.

Trevarthen, C. (2005b). Stepping away from the mirror: Pride and shame in adventures of companionship. Reflections on the nature and emotional needs of infant intersubjectivity. In C. S. Carter, L. Ahnert, K. E. Grossman, S. B. Hrdy, M. E. Lamb, S. W. Porges, et al. (Eds.), *Attachment and bonding: A new synthesis* (pp. 55–84). Cambridge, MA: MIT Press.

Trevarthen, C. (2005c). Action and emotion in development of the human self, its sociability and cultural intelligence: Why infants have feelings like ours. In J. Nadel & D. Muir (Eds.), *Emotional development* (pp. 61–91). Oxford, UK: Oxford University Press.

Trevarthen, C. (2007). Moving experiences: Perceiving as action with a sense of purpose. In G.-J. Pepping & M. A. Grealy (Eds.), *Closing the gap: The scientific writings of David N. Lee* (pp. 1–10). Mahwah, NJ: Erlbaum.

Trevarthen, C. (2009a). The functions of emotion in infancy: The regulation and communication of rhythm, sympathy, and meaning in human development. In D. Fosha, D. J. Siegel, & M. F. Solomon (Eds.), *The healing power of emotion: Affective neuroscience, development, and clinical practice* (pp. 112–144). New York: Norton.

Trevarthen, C. (2009b). Human biochronology: On the source and functions of 'musicality'. In R. Haas & V. Brandes (Eds.), *Music that works* (pp. 221–265). New York: Springer.

Trevarthen, C., & Aitken, K. J. (2001). Infant intersubjectivity: Research, theory, and clinical applications. *Journal of Child Psychology and Psychiatry, 42*(1), 3–48.

Trevarthen, C., & Aitken, K. J. (2003). Regulation of brain development and age related changes in infants' motives: The developmental function of regressive periods. In M. Heimann (Ed.), *Regression periods in human infancy* (pp. 107–184). Mahwah, NJ: Erlbaum.

Trevarthen, C., Aitken, K. J., Vandekerckhove, M., Delafield-Butt, J., & Nagy, E. (2006). Collaborative regulations of vitality in early childhood: Stress in intimate relationships and postnatal psychopathology. In D. Cicchetti & D. J. Cohen (Eds.), *Developmental psychopathology* (2nd ed., Vol. 1., pp. 66–114). Hoboken, NJ: Wiley.

Trevarthen, C., & Reddy, V. (2006). Consciousness in infants. In M. S. Velman (Ed.), *A companion to consciousness* (pp. 1–27). Oxford, UK: Blackwell.

Triandis, H. C., & Suh, E. M. (2002). Cultural influences on personality. *Annual Review of Psychology, 53*, 133–160.

Trickett, P. K., Noll, J. G., Susman, E. J., Shenk, C. E., & Putnam, F. W. (2010). Attenuation of cortisol across development for victims of sexual abuse. *Development and Psychopathology, 22*(1), 165–175.

Tronick, E. (2004). Why is connection with others so critical?: Dyadic meaning making, messiness and complexity governed selective processes which co-create and expand individuals' states of consciousness. In J. Nadel & D. Muir (Eds.), *Emotional development*(pp. 293–315). New York: Oxford University Press.

Tronick, E. (2007). *The neurobehavioral and social emotional development of infants and children.* New York: Norton.

Tronick, E. (2009). Multilevel meaning making and dyadic expansion of consciousness theory: The emotional and the polymorphic polysemic flow of meaning. In D. Fosha, D. J. Siegel, & M. F. Solomon (Eds.), *The healing power of emotion: Affective neuroscience, development, and clinical practice* (pp. 86–111). New York: Norton.

Tronick, E., & Reck, C. (2009). Infants of depressed mothers. *Harvard Review of Psychiatry, 17*(2), 147–156.

Trumbull, D. (2008). Humiliation: The trauma of disrespect. *Journal of the American Academy of Psychoanalysis and Dynamic Psychiatry, 36*(4), 643–660.

Tse, D., Langston, R. F., Kakeyama, M., Bethus, I., Spooner, P., Wood, E. R., et al. (2007). Schemas and memory consolidation. *Science, 316*(5821), 76–82.

Tsien, J. (2000). Linking Hebb's coincidence-detection to memory formation. *Current Opinion in Neurobiology, 10*(2), 266–273.

Tsukiura, T., & Cabeza, R. (2008). Orbitofrontal and hippocampal contributions to memory for face–name associations: The rewarding power of a smile. *Neuropsychologia, 46*(9), 2310–2319.

Tucker, D. M. (2002). Embodied meaning: An evolutionary-developmental analysis of adaptive semantics. In T. Givón & B. F. Malle (Eds.), *The evolution of language out of pre-language* (pp. 51–82). Amsterdam: Benjamins.

Tucker, D. M. (2007). *Mind from body: Experience from neural structure.* New York: Oxford University Press.

Tucker, D. M., Derryberry, D., & Luu, P. (2000). Anatomy and physiology of human emotion: Vertical integration of brainstem, limbic, and cortical systems. In J. Borod (Ed.), *Handbook of the neuropsychology of emotion* (pp. 56–79). New York: Oxford University Press.

Tucker, D. M., Frishkoff, G., & Luu, P. (2008). Microgenesis of language: Vertical integration of neurolinguistic mechanisms across the neuraxis. In B. Stemmer & H. A. Whitaker (Eds.), *Handbook of the neuroscience of language* (pp. 45–56). Boston: Elsevier/Academic Press.

Tucker, D. M., & Luu, P. (2006). Adaptive binding. In H. Zimmer, A. Mecklinger, & U. Lindenberger (Eds.), *Binding in human memory: A neurocognitive approach* (pp. 85–108). New York: Oxford University Press.

Tucker, D. M., Luu, P., & Pribram, K. H. (1995). Social and emotional self-regulation. *Annals of the New York Academy of Sciences, 769*, 213–239.

Tucker-Drob, E. M. (2009). Differentiation of cognitive abilities across the life span. *Developmental Psychology, 45*(4), 1097–1118.

Tulving, E. (2005). Episodic memory and autonoesis: Uniquely human?. In H. S. Terrace & J. Metcalfe (Eds.), *The missing link in cognition: Origins of self-reflective consciousness* (pp. 3–56). New York: Oxford University Press.

Tulving, E., Kapur, S., Craik, F. I. M., Moscovitch, M., & Houle, S. (1994). Hemispheric encoding/retrieval asymmetry in episodic memory: Positron emission tomography findings. *Proceedings of the National Academy of Sciences USA, 91,* 2016–2020.

Turk-Browne, N. B., Yi, D.-J., & Chun, M. M. (2006). Linking implicit and explicit memory: Common encoding factors and shared representations. *Neuron, 49*(6), 917–927.

Tyron, W. W., & McKay, D. (2009). Memory modification as an outcome variable in anxiety disorder treatment. *Journal of Anxiety Disorders, 23*(4), 546–556.

Uddin, L. Q., Davies, M. S., Scott, A. A., Zaidel, E., Bookheimer, S. Y., Iacoboni, M., et al. (2008). Neural basis of self and other representation in autism: An fMRI study of self-face recognition. *PLoS One, 3*(10), e3526.

Uddin, L. Q., Iacoboni, M., Lange, C., & Keenan, J. P. (2007). The self and social cognition: The role of cortical midline structures and mirror neurons. *Trends in Cognitive Sciences, 11*(4), 153–157.

Urry, H. L., Nitschke, J. B., Dolski, I., Jackson, D. C., Dalton, K. M., Mueller, C. J., et al. (2004). Making a life worth living: Neural correlates of well-being. *Psychological Science, 15*(6), 367–372.

Ursu, S., & Carter, C. (2009). An initial investigation of the orbitofrontal cortex hyperactivity in obsessive–compulsive disorder: Exaggerated representations of anticipated aversive events? *Neuropsychologia, 47*(10), 2145–2148.

Ustinova, K. I., Chernikova, L. A., Ioffe, M. E., & Sliva, S. S. (2001). Impairment of learning the voluntary control of posture in patients with cortical lesions of different locations: The cortical mechanisms of pose regulation. *Neuroscience and Behavioral Physiology, 31*(3), 259–267.

Vallacher, R., Read, S., & Nowak, A. (2002). The dynamical perspective in personality and social psychology. *Personality and Social Psychology Review, 6*(4), 264–273.

van Bakel, H. J., & Riksen-Walraven, J. M. (2008). Adrenocortical and behavioral attunement in parents with 1-year-old infants. *Developmental Psychobiology, 50*(2), 196–201.

van Dantzig, S., Pecher, D., Zeelenberg, R., & Barsalou, L. W. (2008). Perceptual processing affects conceptual processing. *Cognitive Science, 32*(3), 579–590.

Vandekerckhove, M. (2009). Memory, autonoetic consciousness and the self: Consciousness as a continuum of stages. *Self and Identity, 8*(1), 4–23.

Vandenberg, B. (1998). Hypnosis and human development: Interpersonal influence of intrapersonal processes. *Child Development, 69,* 262–267.

Vanderhasselt, M., De Raedt, R., Baeken, C., Leyman, L., Clerinx, P., & D'haenen, H. (2007). The influence of rTMS over the right dorsolateral prefrontal cortex on top-down attentional processes. *Brain Research, 1137,* 111–116.

van der Kolk, B. (2003). Posttraumatic stress disorder and the nature of trauma. In M. F. Solomon & D. J. Siegel (Eds.), *Healing trauma: Attachment, mind, body and brain* (pp. 168–195). New York: Norton.

van der Kolk, B., & Courtois, C. (2005). Editorial comments: Complex developmental trauma. *Journal of Traumatic Stress, 18*(5), 385–388.

van der Kolk, B., Roth, S., Pelcovitz, D., Sunday, S., & Spinazzola, J. (2005). Disorders of extreme stress: The empirical foundation of a complex adaptation to trauma. *Journal of Traumatic Stress, 18*(5), 389–399.

van der Velden, P. G., & Wittmann, L. (2008). The independent predictive value of peritraumatic dissociation for PTSD symptomatology after type I trauma: A systematic review of prospective studies. *Clinical Psychology Review, 28*(6), 1009–1020.

van Harmelin, A.-L., van Tol, M.-J., van der Wee, N. J. A., Veltman, D. J., Aleman, A., Spinhoven, P., et al. (2010). Reduced medial prefrontal cortex volume in adults reporting childhood emotional maltreatment. *Biological Psychiatry, 68*(9), 832–838.

van IJzendoorn, M. H., & Bakermans-Kranenburg, M. J. (2006). DRD4 7-repeat polymorphism moderates the association between maternal unresolved loss or trauma and infant disorganization. *Attachment and Human Development, 8*(4), 291–307.

van IJzendoorn, M. H., & Bakermans-Kranenburg, M.J. (2008). The distribution of adult attachment representations in clinical groups: A meta-analytic search for patterns of attachment in 105 AAI studies. In H. Steele & M. Steele (Eds.), *Clinical applications of the Adult Attachment Interview* (pp. 69–98). New York: Guilford Press.

van IJzendoorn, M. H., Bakermans-Kranenburg, M. J., & Mesman, J. (2008). Dopamine system genes associated with parenting in the context of daily hassles. *Genes, Brain and Behavior, 7*(4), 403–410.

van IJzendoorn, M. H., Bakermans-Kranenburg, M. J., & Sagi-Schwartz, A. (2006). Attachment across diverse sociocultural contexts: The limits of universality. In K. H. Rubin & O. Chung (Eds.), *Parenting beliefs, behaviors, and parent–child relations: A cross-cultural perspective* (pp. 107–142). New York: Psychology Press.

van IJzendoorn, M. H., Caspers, K., Bakermans-Kranenburg, M. J., Beach, S. R. H., & Philibert, R. (2010). Methylation matters: Interaction between methylation density and serotonin transporter genotype predicts unresolved loss or trauma. *Biological Psychiatry, 68*(5), 405–407.

Van Kleef, G. A., De Dreu, C. K. W., & Manstead, A. R. (2010). An interpersonal approach to emotion in social decision making: The Emotions as Social Information (EASI) model. In M. P. Zanna (Ed.), *Advances in experimental social psychology* (Vol. 42, pp. 45–96). San Diego, CA: Academic Press.

Van Lancker Sidtis, D., Pachana, N., Cummings, J. L., & Sidtis, J. J. (2006). Dysprosodic speech following basal ganglia insult: Toward a conceptual framework for the study of the cerebral representation of prosody. *Brain and Language, 97*(2), 135–153.

van Ooyen, A., & van Pelt, J. (1994). Activity-dependent neurite outgrowth and neural network development. *Progress in Brain Research, 102*, 245–259.

Van Opstal, F., de Lange, F. P., & Dehaene, S. (2011). Rapid parallel semantic processing of numbers without awareness. *Cognition, 120*(1), 136–147.

van Stegeren, A. H., Roozendaal, B., Kindt, M., Wolf, O. T., & Joels, M. (2010). Interacting noradrenergic and corticosteroid systems shift human brain activation patterns during encoding. *Neurobiology of Learning and Memory, 93*(1), 56–65.

Varela, F., Lachaux, J., Rodriguez, E., & Martinerie, J. (2001). The brainweb: Phase synchronization and large-scale integration. *Nature Reviews Neuroscience, 2*, 229–239.

Vaughn, B. E., Bost, K. K., & van IJzendoorn, M. H. (2008). Attachment and temperament: Additive and interactive influences on behavior, affect, and cognition during infancy and childhood. In J. Cassidy & P. R. Shaver (Eds.), *Handbook of attachment: Theory, research, and clinical applications* (2nd ed., pp. 192–216). New York: Guilford Press.

Velik, R. (2009). From single neuron-firing to consciousness: Towards the true solution of the binding problem. *Neuroscience and Biobehavorial Reviews, 34*(7), 993–1001.

Velmans, M. (2009). *Understanding consciousness* (2nd ed.). New York: Routledge.

Venn, H. R., Watson, S., Gallagher, P., & Young, A. H. (2006). Facial expression perception: An objective outcome measure for treatment studies in mood disorders? *International Journal of Neuropsychopharmacology, 9*(2), 229–245.

Vertes, R., & Eastman, K. (2003). The case against memory consolidation in REM sleep. In E. F. Pace-Schott (Ed.), *Sleep and dreaming: Scientific advances and reconsiderations* (pp. 75–84). New York: Cambridge University Press.

Vicentic, A., Francis, D., Moffett, M., Lakatos, A., Rogge, G., Hubert, G. W., et al. (2006). Maternal separation alters serotonergic transporter densities and serotonergic 1A receptors in rat brain. *Neuroscience, 140*(1), 355–365.

Voorhoeve, A., During, E., Jopling, D., Wilson, T., & Kamm, F. (2011). Who am I?:

Beyond "I think, therefore I am." *Annals of the New York Academy of Sciences, 1234*(1), 134–148.

Voss, J. L. L., Baym, C. L., & Paller, K. A. (2008). Accurate forced-choice recognition without awareness of memory retrieval. *Learning and Memory, 15*(6), 454–459.

Voss, J. L. L., & Paller, K. A. (2007). Neural correlates of conceptual implicit memory and their contamination of putative neural correlates of explicit memory. *Learning and Memory, 14,* 259–267.

Voss, J. L. L., & Paller, K. A. (2008). Brain substrates of implicit and explicit memory: The importance of concurrently acquired neural signals of both memory types. *Neuropsychologia, 46*(13), 3021–3029.

Voss, J. L. L., & Paller, K. A. (2009). An electrophysiological signature of unconscious recognition memory. *Nature Neuroscience, 12*(3), 349–355.

Vygotsky, L. S. (1986). *Thought and language* (A. Kozulin, Ed.). Cambridge, MA: MIT Press. (Original work published 1934)

Wade, T. D., & Kendler, K. S. (2000). The genetic epidemiology of parental discipline. *Psychological Medicine, 30*(6), 1303–1313.

Wager, T. D., Davidson, M. L., Hughes, B. L., Lindquist, M. A., & Ochsner, K. N. (2008). Prefrontal–subcortical pathways mediating successful emotion regulation. *Neuron, 59*(6), 1037–1050.

Walden, T. A. (1991). Infant social referencing. In J. Garber & K. A. Dodge (Eds.), *The development of emotion regulation and dysregulation* (pp. 69–88). Cambridge, UK: Cambridge University Press.

Walden, T. A., & Kim, G. (2005). Infants' social looking toward mothers and strangers. *International Journal of Behavioral Development, 29*(5), 356–360.

Walker, J. (2007). Unresolved loss and trauma in parents and the implications in terms of child protection. *Journal of Social Work Practice, 21*(1), 77–87.

Wallace, A. (2010). *Hidden dimensions: The unification of physics and consciousness.* New York: Columbia University Press.

Wallace, M. K., Krueger, J., & Royal, D. W. (2010). Neural development and plasticity of multisensory representations. In J. Kaiser & M. J. Naumer (Eds.), *Multisensory object perception in the primate brain* (pp. 329–349). New York: Springer.

Wallentin, M., Nielsen, A. H., Vuust, P., Dohn, A., Roepstorff, A., & Lund, T. E. (2011). Amygdala and heart rate variability responses from listening to emotionally intense parts of a story. *NeuroImage, 58*(3), 963–973.

Waller, E., & Scheidt, C. E. (2006). Somatoform disorders as disorders of affect regulation: A development perspective. *International Review of Psychiatry, 18*(1), 13–24.

Wallin, D. J. (2007). *Attachment in psychotherapy.* New York: Guilford Press.

Wallis, P., & Steele, H. (2001). Attachment representations in adolescence: Further evidence from psychiatric residential settings. *Attachment and Human Development, 3*(3), 259–268.

Walsh, W., Dawson, J., & Mattingly, M. (2010). How are we measuring resilience following childhood maltreatment? Is the research adequate and consistent? What is the impact on research, practice, and policy? *Trauma, Violence and Abuse, 11*(1), 27–41.

Wana, C. Y., Demaine, K., Zipse, L., Norton, A., & Schlaug, G. (2010). From music making to speaking: Engaging the mirror neuron system in autism. *Brain Research Bulletin, 82*(3–4), 161–168.

Wang, Q. (2001). Cultural effects on adults' earliest childhood recollection and self-description: Implications for the relation between memory and the self. *Journal of Personality and Social Psychology, 81*(2), 220–233.

Wang, Q. (2004). The emergence of cultural self-construct: Autobiographical memory and self-description in American and Chinese children. *Developmental Psychology, 40*(1), 3–15.

Wang, Q. (2006). Relations of maternal style and child self-concept to autobiographical memories in Chinese, Chinese immigrant, and European American 3-year-olds. *Child Development, 77*(6), 1794–1809.

Wang, Q. (2008a). Emotion knowledge and autobiographical memory across the preschool years: A cross-cultural longitudinal investigation. *Cognition, 108*(1), 117–135.

Wang, Q. (2008b). Being American, being Asian: The bicultural self and autobiographical memory in Asian Americans. *Cognition, 107*(2), 743–751.

Wang, Q., & Brockmeier, J. (2002). Autobiographical remembering as cultural practice: Understanding the interplay between memory, self and culture. *Culture and Psychology, 8*(1), 45–64.

Wang, Q., & Conway, M. A. (2004). The stories we keep: Autobiographical memory in American and Chinese middle-aged adults. *Journal of Personality, 72*(5), 911–938.

Wang, Q., Conway, M. A., & Hou, Y. (2007). Infantile amnesia: A cross cultural examination. In M.-K. Sun (Ed.), *New research in cognitive sciences* (pp. 95–105). New York: Nova Science.

Wang, Z., Neylan, T. C., Mueller, S. G., Lenoci, M., Truran, D., Marmar, C. R., et al. (2010). Magnetic resonance imaging of hippocampal subfields in posttraumatic stress disorder. *Archives of General Psychiatry, 67*(3), 296–303.

Ward, L. R. (2002). *Dynamical cognitive science.* Cambridge, MA: MIT Press.

Warren, S. L., Emde, R., & Sroufe, L. A. (2000). Predicting anxiety from children's play narratives, *Journal of the American Academy of Child and Adolescent Psychiatry, 39*, 100–107.

Wasserstein, J., & Stefanatos, G. A. (2000). The right hemisphere and psychopathology. *Journal of the American Academy of Psychoanalysis, 28*(2), 371–395.

Wataru, S., Sakiko, Y., Takanori, K., & Matsumura, M. (2004). The amygdala processes the emotional significance of facial expressions: An fMRI investigation using the interaction between expression and face direction. *NeuroImage, 22*(2), 1006–1013.

Waters, E., Merrick, S., Treboux, D., Crowell, J., & Albersheim, L. (2000). Attachment security in infancy and early adulthood: A twenty-year longitudinal study. *Child Development, 71*(3), 684–689.

Waugh, C. E., Hamilton, J. P., & Gotlib, I. H. (2010). The neural temporal dynamics of the intensity of emotional experience. *NeuroImage, 49*(2), 1699–1707.

*Webster's New World College Dictionary* (3rd ed.). (1997). New York: Simon & Schuster/Macmillan.

Weinberger, N. M. (2008). The nucleus basalis and memory codes: Auditory cortical plasticity and the induction of specific, associative behavioral memory. *Neurobiology of Learning and Memory, 80*, 268–284.

Weinfield, N. S., Sroufe, L. A., Egeland, B., & Carlson, E. (2008). Individual differences in infant–caregiver attachment: Conceptual and empirical aspects of security. In J. Cassidy & P. R. Shaver (Eds.), *Handbook of attachment: Theory, research, and clinical applications* (2nd ed., pp. 78–101). New York: Guilford Press.

Weinfield, N. S., Whaley, G. J., & Egeland, B. (2004). Continuity, discontinuity, and coherence in attachment from infancy to late adolescence: Sequelae of organization and disorganization. *Attachment and Human Development, 6*(1), 73–97.

Wendelken, C., Bunge, S., & Carter, C. (2008). Maintaining structured information: An investigation into functions of parietal and lateral prefrontal cortices. *Neuropsychologia, 46*(2), 665–678.

Wheeler, M. A. (2000). Episodic memory and autonoetic awareness. In E. Tulving &

F. I. M. Craik (Eds.), *The Oxford handbook of memory* (pp. 597–608). New York: Oxford University Press.

Wheeler, M. A., Stuss, D. T., & Tulving, E. (1997). Toward a theory of episodic memory: The frontal lobes and autonoetic consciousness. *Psychological Bulletin, 121,* 331–354.

Whittle, S., Yap, M. B. H., Yucel, M., Fornito, A., Simmons, J. G., Barrett, A., et al. (2009). Prefrontal and amygdala volumes are related to adolescents' affective behaviors during parent–adolescent interactions. *Proceedings of the National Academy of Sciences USA, 105*(9), 3653–3657.

Wiesel, T. N., & Hubel, D. H. (1963). Single cell responses in striate cortex of kittens deprived of vision in one eye. *Journal of Neurophysiology, 26,* 1003–1007.

Wig, G. S., Buckner, R. L., & Schacter, D. L. (2009). Repetition priming influences distinct brain systems: Evidence from task-evoked data and resting-state correlations. *Neurophysiology, 101*(5), 2631–2684.

Willis, M., Palermo, R., Burke, D., McGrillen, K., & Miller, L. (2010). Orbitofrontal cortex lesions result in abnormal social judgments to emotional faces. *Neuropsychologia, 48*(7), 2182–2187.

Wilson, E. O. (1998). *Consilience: The unity of knowledge.* New York: Vintage.

Wiltgen, B. J., Brown, R. A. M., Talton, L. E., & Silva, A. J. (2004). New circuits for old memories. *Neuron, 44*(1), 101–108.

Winsler, A. (2009). Still talking to ourselves after all these years: A review of current research on private speech. In A. Winsler, C. Fernyhough, & I. Montero (Eds.), *Private speech, executive functioning, and the development of verbal self-regulation* (pp. 3–41). New York: Cambridge University Press.

Winson, J. (1993). The biology and function of rapid eye movement sleep. *Current Opinion in Neurobiology, 3,* 243–248.

Wise, S. P., Murray, E. A., & Gerfen, C. R. (1996). The frontal cortex–basal ganglia system in primates. *Critical Reviews in Neurobiology, 10,* 317–356.

Witherington, D. (2007). The dynamic systems approach as metatheory for developmental psychology. *Human Development, 50*(2–3), 127–153.

Wittmann, L., Moergeli, H., & Schnyder, U. (2006). Low predictive power of peritraumatic dissociation for PTSD symptoms in accident survivors. *Journal of Traumatic Stress, 19*(5), 639–651.

Wolf, D. P. (1990). Being of several minds: Voices and versions of the self in early childhood. In D. Cicchetti & M. Beeghly (Eds.), *The self in transition: Infancy to childhood* (pp. 183–212). Chicago: University of Chicago Press.

Woltering, S., & Lewis, M. D. (2009). Developmental pathways of emotion regulation in childhood: A neuropsychological perspective. *Mind, Brain, and Education, 3,* 160–169.

Wooley, A. W., Charbris, C. F., Pentland, A., Hashmi, N., & Malone, T. W. (2010). Evidence for a collective intelligence factor in the performance of human groups. *Science, 330*(6004), 686–688.

Worthman, C. M., Plotsky, P. M., Schechter, D. S., & Cummings, C. A. (Eds.). (2010). *Formative experiences: The interaction of caregiving, culture, and developmental psychobiology.* New York: Cambridge University Press.

Yagmurlu, B., & Altan, O. (2009). Maternal socialization and child temperament as predictors of emotion regulation in Turkish preschoolers. *Infant and Child Development, 19*(3), 275–296.

Yehuda, R., & McFarlane, A. C. (1995). Conflict between current knowledge about posttraumatic stress disorder and its original conceptual basis. *American Journal of Psychiatry, 152,* 1705–1713.

Yoshida, T., Yoshino, A., Takahashi, Y., & Soichiro, N. (2007). Comparison of hemispheric asymmetry in global and local information processing and interference in divided and selective attention using spatial frequency filters. *Experimental Brain Research, 181*(3), 519–529.

Yu, C., & Ballard, D. H. (2004). A multimodal learning interface for grounding spoken language in sensory perceptions. *ACM Transactions on Applied Perception, 1*(1), 57–80.

Zahn-Waxler, C. (2010). Socialization of emotion: Who influences whom and how? *New Directions for Child and Adolescent Development, 2010*(128), 101–109.

Zajac, K., & Kobak, R. (2009). Caregiver unresolved loss and abuse and child behavior problems: Intergenerational effects in a high-risk sample. *Development and Psychopathology, 21*(1), 173–187.

Zelazo, P. D. (2004). The development of conscious control in childhood. *Trends in Cognitive Science, 8* (1), 12–17.

Zelazo, P. D., Carlson, S. M., & Kesek, A. (2008). The development of executive function in childhood. In C. Nelson & M. Luciana (Eds.), *Handbook of developmental cognitive neuroscience* (2nd ed., pp. 553–574). Cambridge, MA: MIT Press.

Zelazo, P. D., Hong Hao, H., & Todd, R. (2007). The development of consciousness. In P. D. Zelazo, M. Moscovitch, & E. Thompson (Eds.), *Cambridge handbook of consciousness* (pp. 405–434). New York: Cambridge University Press.

Zhang, D., & Raichle, M. E. (2010). Disease and the brain's dark energy. *Nature Reviews Neurology, 6*(1), 15–28.

Zhang, T., & Meaney, M. (2010). Epigenetics and the environmental regulation of the genome and its function. *Annual Review of Psychology, 61*, 439–466.

Zhong, J., Wang, A., Qian, M., Zhang, L., Gao, J., Yang, J., et al. (2008). Shame, personality, and social anxiety symptoms in Chinese and American nonclinical samples: A cross-cultural study. *Depress Anxiety, 25*(5), 449–460.

Zhou, C., Zemanova, L., Zamora, G., Hilgetag, C. C., & Kurths, J. (2006). Hierarchical organization unveiled by functional connectivity in complex brain network. *Physical Review Letters, 97*(23), 238103.

Zilberstein, K., & Messer, E. A. (2010). Building a secure base: Treatment of a child with disorganized attachment. *Clinical Social Work Journal, 38*(1), 85–97.

Zion-Golumbic, E., Kutas, M., & Bentin, S. (2010). Neural dynamics associated with semantic and episodic memory for faces: Evidence from multiple frequency bands. *Journal of Cognitive Neuroscience, 22*(2), 263–277.

Zuckerman, B., Zuckerman, P. M., & Siegel, D. J. (2005). Promoting self-understanding in parents—for the great good of your patients. *Contemporary Pediatrics, 22*(4), 77–90.

# Index

Note: f or t following a page number indicates a figure or table.